Dr. Keith E. Evans.

[Q.E.H.C.   Nov. 1968.]

PRACTICAL
PAEDIATRIC PROBLEMS

Practical
Paediatric Problems

JAMES H. HUTCHISON
O.B.E., M.D.(Glas.), F.R.S.E., F.R.C.P.(Lond.),
F.R.C.P.(Ed.), F.R.C.P.(Glas.)

*Professor of Child Health, University of Glasgow;
Visiting Physician, Royal Hospital for Sick Children
Glasgow; Consultant Paediatrician, The Queen
Mother's Hospital, Glasgow*

Second edition

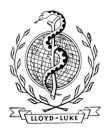

LLOYD-LUKE (MEDICAL BOOKS) LTD
49 NEWMAN STREET
LONDON
1967

FIRST EDITION . . . 1964

PRINTED AND BOUND IN ENGLAND BY
HAZELL WATSON AND VINEY LTD
AYLESBURY, BUCKS

This book is dedicated to
MY WIFE

PREFACE TO SECOND EDITION

WHEN a publisher informs an author that another edition of his text-book is required within three years of the first his initial reactions are a mixture of satisfaction that the first effort has been so well received, and of dismay at the work which lies ahead. In actual fact, the request reflects principally the continuing and remarkable progress in all fields of scientific medicine. The preparation of the Second Edition has involved a great deal of re-writing and many additions to nearly every chapter. The new additions include such subjects as dysmaturity and its characteristic complications which have been more clearly recognized during the last few years; the value of spectrophotometric analysis of the liquor amnii in haemolytic disease of the newborn and its practical implications; new inborn errors of metabolism such as homocystinuria, tyrosinosis and hereditary fructose intolerance; the problem of the undescended testis; and several others. An account of the parasitic infestations of the bowel has been added to Chapter XVI. A completely new chapter has been included on Accidental Poisoning in Childhood. The areas of re-writing are too numerous to detail. They vary from a complete revision of the agammaglobulinaemias to major changes in the discussions on malignant disease, on dehydration in gastro-enteritis, on the aetiology of nephritis, on endocrine disorders, and they include substantial changes in the chapter on diseases of the nervous system. The references at the end of each chapter have been brought up to date. All this has inevitably involved some increase in the size of the book but it is still of a convenient size for comfortable reading.

The contents have been maintained at a strictly practical level, and the problems considered could be encountered by any doctor in his daily routine. I have been encouraged to believe, by friends and col-leagues, that this type of book is a useful aid to study for both under-graduates and postgraduates, and many general practitioners have been kind enough to state that they have found it helpful in practice. I will be well content if readers find that the Second Edition brings the subject as up-to-date as any textbook can in this era of startling advance. I am again greatly indebted to my secretaries, Mrs. Margaret Stirling and Mrs. Dorothea Douglas, for their cheerful co-operation; and to Mr. J. Devlin for five additional illustrations.

JAMES H. HUTCHISON

Royal Hospital for Sick Children,
Oakbank,
Glasgow, C.4

February 1967

PREFACE TO FIRST EDITION

THE invitation to write a book on practical paediatric problems is an almost irresistible challenge to one who has spent most of his professional life, as I have, in paediatric practice in hospital and in the homes of sick children. The fact that I have recently been immured in the "ivory tower" of a University Chair, if anything, heightens the challenge. The latter circumstance is, however, unrelated to the unexpected difficulty, encountered as the book took shape, of recognizing a practical paediatric problem. The experimental approach of today is quite likely to become the routine practice of tomorrow. Diagnostic and therapeutic methods which are looked upon as research tools in some hospitals have become matters of everyday routine in the large centres which introduced them. The present book is intended to be an account of clinical paediatrics as it has been experienced by a paediatrician in a large medical school with responsibility for both undergraduate and postgraduate teaching. There has always seemed to me to be a need for a textbook which in content lies somewhere between the usual undergraduate text (often of little value to the qualified physician) and the large work of reference by many authors (usually consulted only by the specialist). In this book I have tried to deal with the problems of the paediatrician and the family doctor in a fairly detailed fashion. Treatment in particular has been accorded sufficient space to be of value to the practising physician. References to original work and to books of a specialized nature have been included in every chapter as a guide to those who would wish to go more deeply into the subject.

It is obviously unavoidable that a textbook by a single author on a subject as vast as paediatrics must to some extent be selective; for the author must write only of what he knows. I have omitted from consideration diseases of the eyes, ears and skin of which others can write more authoritatively. Most textbooks of medicine deal with the common infectious fevers and I have, therefore, left them out in order to have more space for present-day paediatrics. My object, in short, has been to provide a manageable account of clinical paediatrics for undergraduates, for postgraduates specializing in paediatrics, and for general practitioners who find that a large proportion of their daily routine is concerned with the care of sick children. It is inevitable, and not necessarily disadvantageous, that a personal approach should be evident. None the less, the considerable space devoted to the neonatal period reflects the fact that 70 per cent of the total infant mortality in the United Kingdom now falls within the first twenty-eight days of life. Moreover, the major paediatric advances of recent years have been made possible only by the evolution of new laboratory methods; for this reason the help to be obtained from the laboratory in many diseases has been discussed in some detail. The illustrations have been chosen with the sole object of amplifying the textual descriptions.

I count myself fortunate in having lived through a period of such rapid advances in medicine. I hope that in this book the reader will find a practical account of today's paediatrics, so different from that of thirty years ago when I qualified in medicine. It would be impossible for me to make suitable acknowledgements to the many colleagues, both senior and junior, who have helped to form the opinions and outlook of this book. I owe a special debt to Professor Stanley Graham and to the late Professor Noah Morris whose teaching and example set the feet of a young man upon the path of paediatrics. My colleague Dr. R. A. Shanks has read the manuscript of this book and I am grateful to him for many helpful suggestions. Mr. J. Devlin prepared the illustrations and gave me his expert advice. Finally, the work would have been impossible without the willing assistance of my secretaries Mrs. Margaret Stirling and Mrs. Dorothea Douglas.

I am indebted to the Editor of the *British Medical Journal* for permission to reproduce Fig. 68; to the Editor of the *Archives of Disease in Childhood* for permission to reproduce Fig. 65; and to the Editor of *Surgo* for permission to reproduce Fig. 60.

JAMES H. HUTCHISON

University Department of Child Health,
Royal Hospital for Sick Children,
Yorkhill,
Glasgow, C.3

June 1964

CONTENTS

CHAPTER I

ASPHYXIA NEONATORUM

The term "asphyxia neonatorum" has long been used by clinicians to indicate failure on the part of a newborn infant to establish spontaneous respiration immediately following complete delivery. This leads to a succession of serious consequences affecting various systems of the body, and unless adequate respiration can be quickly initiated the infant will die, or survive with permanent damage in the brain. The first consequence of failure to breathe is anoxia, rapidly followed by the excess accumulation in the blood of carbon dioxide, and by a fall in the blood pH. The clinician must have a sound understanding of the causes of asphyxia neonatorum and of its physiological effects if his management of this extreme emergency is to be rational. Indeed, an understanding of the aetiological factors will often enable him to foresee an emergency and so reach a better state of preparedness.

AETIOLOGY

(A) **Foetal anoxia.**—In the great majority of cases the causes of asphyxia neonatorum have been operating before the birth of the baby. Unfortunately, there is at the present time no reliable method of measuring foetal anoxia. Slowing and irregularity of the foetal heart, or the intra-uterine passage of meconium are indications of foetal distress but they can, nevertheless, be absent even when the foetus is in imminent danger of death *in utero*. The probability of foetal anoxia can often, however, be deduced from the state of the mother before or during labour.

1. *Anoxic anoxia* results from an inadequate supply of oxygen. This may arise from a diminution of the oxygen tension in the mother's circulation, as in congestive cardiac failure, pneumonia, bronchitis and emphysema or during an eclamptic fit. A particularly frequent cause of maternal anoxia is the use of inhalational anaesthesia. Donald (1957) has stressed the disastrous effects of mismanaged anaesthesia, often complicated by inhalation of vomit, during labour. There is also great danger to the foetus if the mother's blood pressure is allowed to fall abruptly during spinal anaesthesia. On the other hand, the oxygen supply from mother to foetus is entirely dependent upon the efficiency of the placenta. Maternal toxaemia and hypertension lead to reduced placental blood flow and this may exist for some time before the onset of labour (Morris *et al.*, 1955). Walker (1954) found evidence of a diminished transfer of oxygen due to placental insufficiency in post-

maturity. The foetal life-line may also be cut when the placenta separates prematurely, as in placenta praevia or accidental haemorrhage. Finally, the foetus is in danger during a long and severe labour because his oxygen supply is reduced during every uterine contraction.

2. *Anaemic anoxia* exists when the foetal blood is so anaemic that it cannot carry sufficient oxygen to meet the needs of the tissues. This may arise in rhesus incompatibility or from foetal haemorrhage.

3. *Stagnant anoxia* can arise from compression, prolapse or knotting of the umbilical cord. Accidents to the cord can rarely be foreseen.

4. *Histotoxic anoxia* arises when the foetal tissues, especially the nervous system, are so poisoned by drugs or damaged by haemorrhage that the cells can no longer utilize the oxygen delivered to them. Every drug which has so far been devised for the relief of pain during labour is capable of depressing the foetal respiratory centre if unskilfully used. This is true of pethidine, trichloroethylene, and even more so of morphine, hyoscine and related drugs. Their dangers are particularly great during premature labours.

(B) **Natal and postnatal anoxia.**—It is important that the clinician should appreciate that the causes of foetal anoxia often produce the very circumstances in which further anoxia becomes inevitable during or immediately after birth. For example, foetal anoxia occurs in abruptio placentae which is a common cause of premature birth, and the respiratory centre of the premature infant is immature and functionally inadequate. It may, indeed, have been further depressed by foetal anoxia, drugs administered to the mother, or by raised intracranial pressure due to haemorrhage or cerebral oedema. Barcroft (1946) showed that when rendered anoxic the foetus makes vigorous gasping movements *in utero* so that his lungs may be deeply filled with irritating meconium. The premature infant may suffer the further disadvantage of a soft unduly pliable thoracic cage surrounded by a weak musculature, so that he is unable to produce the negative intrathoracic pressure required to expand his immature lungs. Infrequently asphyxia appears for the first time after birth due to some congenital abnormality which does not cause trouble during foetal life, such as a laryngeal web or a diaphragmatic hernia.

PHYSIOLOGY

The physiological consequences of failure by the newborn infant to breathe have been described by Cross (1966). A fall in the arterial blood oxygen tension (Po_2) is associated with a rapid rise in carbon dioxide tension (Pco_2) and a fall in the blood pH. This rise in the hydrogen-ion concentration is due not only to CO_2 excess but to the anaerobic metabolism of glucose with lactic acid accumulation. It is characteristic of the newborn animal that the heart continues to beat for some time after the cessation of respiration, and the blood CO_2 and acid concentrations may reach much higher levels with a lower blood pH than are ever encountered in asphyxiated adults.

When a newborn animal is acutely asphyxiated as soon as the umbilical cord is severed, a characteristic sequence of events is observed (Dawes *et al.*, 1963). There is first an exaggerated respiratory activity and a change of skin colour from pink to blue or grey. This is succeeded by a period of "primary apnoea" which is ended by the appearance of spontaneous gasping. Finally "the last gasp" is followed by "secondary or terminal apnoea", although even at this stage resuscitation by cardiac massage and tracheal intubation with intermittent positive pressure ventilation is possible. In these circumstances it would be more correct to refer to "the last spontaneous gasp". At the onset of asphyxia the heart rate and blood pressure show a transient rise, soon to be followed by a precipitous fall. The fall in heart rate is directly related to the fall in the blood pH. Expansion of the lungs in the healthy newborn animal is accompanied by a great increase in pulmonary blood flow, a rise in left atrial pressure and a fall in pulmonary arterial pressure. The presence of hypoxia and failure of the lungs fully to expand result in pulmonary arteriolar constriction and a rise in pulmonary arterial pressure. Permanent damage to the brain occurs after 7–8 minutes total asphyxia in newly delivered monkeys and, if very severe, results in ataxia, tremors, athetosis and spastic paralysis. There is no reason to think that these consequences of asphyxia observed in various experimental animals differ materially in the human infant, although the actual duration of the different phases such as primary apnoea, spontaneous gasping and terminal apnoea are known to differ in rabbits, monkeys and lambs. They are also known to be prolonged by drugs and anaesthetics.

PATHOLOGY

Asphyxia produces congestive circulatory failure with over-filling of the chambers of the heart and pooling of the blood in the viscera (Morrison, 1961). The blood vessels are engorged. From the circulatory stasis and anoxic damage to the capillary walls petechial haemorrhages and oedema may result. If intra-uterine anoxia has been produced in the premature infant from retroplacental haemorrhage, which increases the pressure in the intervillous space and so drives blood from the placental channels into the foetal circulation, widespread petechial haemorrhages may be found in the brain and viscera. The severity of these various changes varies in different organs. The basic lesions in the lungs tend to be congestion, accumulation of oedema fluid in the air spaces and interstitial spaces, primary atelectasis and patchy haemorrhages. There appears to be a close relationship, not yet clearly understood, between perinatal anoxia and the subsequent development of hyaline membranes in the alveolar ducts. A big defect in our knowledge concerns the mechanism whereby overloading of the pulmonary circulation is prevented in the normal newborn, and how the capillary bed of the lung is protected by the pulmonary arteries and arterioles. The development of intraventricular and subarachnoid haemorrhages, especially in premature infants, is well known. It is much more difficult to assess the importance and significance of cerebral oedema and petechial haemorrhages in the brain substance, especially in regard to their possible relationship to neurological disorders in later life. In the other organs, haemorrhages are the most common evidence of anoxia. Adrenal haemorrhages are uncommon but they are probably rarely compatible with survival. Furthermore, anoxia increases the severity of bleeding from traumatic lesions, for example, in subdural haemorrhage or subscapsular haematoma of the liver.

Clinical Features

The traditional descriptions of "asphyxia livida" and "asphyxia pallida" are still useful provided it is appreciated that the latter is only a more severe degree of the former and in which peripheral circulatory failure has supervened. Donald (1957) prefers the term "foetal shock".

The nature of the stimulus to breathe in the normal newborn infant has long been a subject of interest. Cutaneous stimuli, especially those from the area supplied by the fifth cranial nerves, seem to play an important role, but probably much less so than the low blood level of oxygen and high carbon dioxide level at the time of birth.* In fact, every healthy newborn is asphyxiated by normal adult standards. Asphyxia of a degree requiring special measures should be diagnosed if the period of apnoea following complete delivery of an infant from the mother lasts longer than one minute. In asphyxia livida the infant is apnoeic or gasping and cyanosed, but muscle tone is normal or increased, the heart-rate is over 100 per minute and regular in rhythm, good pulsation is palpable in the umbilical cord, and there may be flexion movements or grimacing on cutaneous stimulation. Recovery is heralded by periodic ineffectual gasps proceeding to more effective inspiratory efforts. These result in a clearing of the cyanosis. Finally, there is a welcome cry. The deadly asphyxia pallida may be present from birth or develop subsequent to a deteriorating state of asphyxia livida. The infant has a deathly grey pallor and flaccidity of muscles, the heart-rate is below 100 per minute, and may be irregular, pulsation in the umbilical cord is barely perceptible, and there is no response to stimulation. Recovery is preceded by an acceleration in the heart-rate and occasional gasps, but it is often not sustained so that death supervenes.

* It may be that the most important stimulus for the initiation of respiration is the hydrogen ion concentration (pH) in the blood at the moment of birth (Reardon *et al.* 1960).

Assessment and Early Prognosis

In some hospitals special clinical methods of assessment of the degree of neonatal anoxia have been devised. Although these cannot accurately reflect blood chemical changes, their purpose is to give members of the staff some guide to those infants in whom continuing and possibly fatal respiratory difficulties may be expected. These infants can thereby be assured of more individual and careful supervision. Apgar *et al.* (1958) evolved a scoring system which evaluates five objective signs sixty seconds after complete delivery of the infant. These are skin colour, muscle tone, respiratory effort, heart-rate and response to stimulation. Each is given a score of 0–2. Thus, a good skin colour = 2, peripheral cyanosis = 1, and generalized cyanosis or pallor = 0; good muscle tone = 2, flexion movements of the limbs or trunk = 1, complete flaccidity = 0; rhythmic breathing or crying = 2, gasping = 1, apnoea = 0; heart rate over 100/min. = 2, under 100/min. = 1, absent = 0; brisk response to stimulation by suction applied to nostrils or by flicking the soles of the feet = 2, poor response = 1, no response = 0. A total score of 10 indicates an infant in optimum condition. A mortality rate of 15 per cent may be expected when the score is 2 or less. However, Apgar's method permits of considerable subjective variation between different observers, and Auld *et al.* (1961) have found it unreliable as a method of prediction in individual infants. Miller and Calkins (1961) graded newborn infants by measuring the time (in minutes and seconds) which elapsed between the birth of the infant and the onset of spontaneous respirations, and subsequently recording the respiratory rates at frequent intervals for 48 hours. Infants who cleared their cyanosis in a few minutes and whose respiratory rates did not increase were classified in Grade I; when the cyanosis disappeared in a few minutes but the respiratory rates were high for an hour with a subsequent decline, the infants were placed in Grade II; when there was failure to lose the cyanosis or when the respiratory rate was increased by more than 15 per minute after the first hour the infants were placed in Grade III. In a group of infants born by Caesarean section and in a series of premature births all the neonatal deaths had been classified in Grade III. It is clearly impracticable to assess every newborn infant by these methods which demand experienced observers. However, this type of evaluation of infants known to be at special risk, such as those born prematurely, by Caesarean section or to diabetic mothers, would at the least ensure the adequate and frequent observation which they demand.

TREATMENT

When the birth of an asphyxiated infant can be foreseen as a reasonable probability from the condition of the mother before or during labour, the delivery should, if possible, be conducted in hospital where adequate facilities exist. The first essential in the management of an apnoeic infant is to avoid chilling. Indeed, no doctor should agree to conduct a confinement at home unless he can be assured of a room temperature not below 65° F. After complete delivery from the mother and section of the umbilical cord the infant should be received into a sterile towel which lies over warm non-woollen blankets. He should be placed with head at a lower level than his feet, on the attendant's lap or preferably on a resuscitation trolley or in a suitable cot. Drainage of fluid from the mouth and pharynx by gravity should be assisted by suction. If a mucus extractor is used the end for the infant's mouth must be of soft rubber with a square-cut open end, and there should be a trap between the infant's mouth and that of the operator (Fig. 1). In

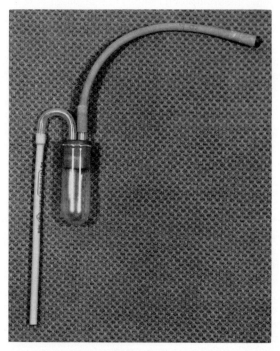

Fig. 1.—Mucus extractor with suitable trap and square-cut soft rubber end for infants.

hospital a mechanical or electric suction apparatus should be available. The nostrils should be sucked out as well as the pharynx. It is likely, in fact, that suction may do more good by stimulation than by removal of fluid from the respiratory tract. If the infant has not started to gasp within one minute pure oxygen must be given. This may be as a steady flow over the mouth and nose through a plastic filter funnel, or as intermittent short puffs from a small face-mask attached to the anaesthetic machine. The objectives thus far have been the avoidance of further shock by chilling, and the revival of the respiratory centre by getting oxygen to the brain after obtaining a patent airway.

It has been traditional practice to administer one of the analeptic group of drugs such as lobeline 3 mg., nikethamide 1 ml., or vanillic acid diethylamide 25 mg. They are, however, quite ineffective in severe asphyxia, and they can be dangerous by causing an abrupt fall in blood pressure, or convulsions, or even gangrene of the leg following accidental injection into an umbilical artery. Their use should be discontinued. On the other hand, in the baby who has been depressed by drugs such as morphine or pethidine administered to the mother shortly before delivery nalorphine is valuable. The dose 0·5 mg., is given into the umbilical vein which is then "milked" towards the infant. After spontaneous respiration has been established it is sound practice to raise the head above the level of the feet as respiration in the newborn is mainly diaphragmatic, and to aspirate the stomach contents with a sterile soft rubber catheter and 20 ml. syringe. This eliminates the danger of aspiration of vomitus into the lungs of an infant whose cough reflex is likely to be suppressed. Thereafter, if the infant's cyanosis is not completely cleared, he should be placed in an incubator or oxygen box of some type at an oxygen concentration of 35 to 40 per cent. Considerably higher concentrations may, in fact, be used safely for short periods in severely anoxic cases. On the other hand, mildly asphyxiated infants, who form the great majority, require no extra oxygen after respiration has become established.

The simple and conservative steps so far described will suffice to resuscitate the vast majority of apnoeic babies. There are, however, some severely asphyxiated infants who fail to breathe spontaneously in response to warmth, gentleness, pharyngeal suction, and the facial administration of oxygen. Many of these are premature. An understandable lack of complacency about this kind of tragic ending to pregnancy has led to the development of some ingenious techniques of assisted respiration. None the less, they have been accompanied by some difficult problems. Firstly, they can only be operated by trained personnel. Secondly, it is difficult to decide at what point of time the decision to use them should be made and impossible to know whether a successful outcome might not have taken place in any event had the physician but held his hand. Thirdly, the doubt arises whether they have not sometimes ensured the survival of a permanently brain-damaged child and whether this is sociologically justifiable is debatable. The fact must be faced that the number of severely asphyxiated infants who can survive undamaged only by the use of special resuscitative techniques is relatively small. However, it is impossible to withhold such methods in hospital where trained staff and suitable equipment are available. They should be used if an infant has not established adequate respiration within 3 minutes of complete delivery.

The most effective technique is probably the passage of an endotracheal tube, using a suitable infant-size laryngoscope. The plastic tube may be one which fits and occludes the larynx, or it may leave sufficient space within the trachea to allow of the escape of gas around it (Fig. 2). The bronchial contents are sucked out through the tube, and oxygen is then administered intermittently by the alternating squeezing and relaxing of a rubber bag filled with oxygen and connected also to a manometer, or by means of a water manometer. The positive pressure applied must not exceed 30 cm. H_2O because of the danger of rupturing lung tissue. There can be no doubt that this method can expand the infant's chest and improve oxygenation. Unfortunately, pressures of 30 cm. H_2O are sometimes insufficient to overcome the moist cohesion of the alveolar walls, and unless alveolar expansion takes place the infant will not long survive. Donald (1957) and others have shown that the newborn infant, even the premature, produces negative intrathoracic pressures of 40 cm. H_2O and more during the spontaneous onset of respiration. These pressures, which we dare not employ artificially, are probably safe because they are so briefly sustained during the initial respiratory efforts of the healthy baby (Day *et al.*, 1952). Intermittent positive pressure respiration may also be used with face-mask or intratracheal catheter by means of the electronically controlled "Pneumotron" devised by Donald (1957) and which is so triggered that its preset rhythm is altered automatically to augment any spontaneous inspiratory efforts which the infant may make.

For some years intragastric oxygen was popular, especially for the resuscitation of premature infants who sometimes withstand intubation poorly. However, Coxon (1960) failed to show any benefit from its use in hypoxic animals and its value in human infants is probably negligible. Furthermore, its use is likely to delay the institution of more effective techniques. Drinker or tank types of respirator which produce inspiratory movements by intermittent negative intrathoracic pressures have also been proved to be unable to bring about alveolar expansion. Donald and Lord (1953) devised a servo patient-cycled tank respirator which could improve oxygenation. Its value is limited by the difficulty of mounting a very ill infant within it and endotracheal intubation is much easier. Apparatus to apply Eve's rocking method has been devised but its value in the presence of airless lungs is open to question. Rhythmic faradic stimulation of the phrenic nerves has been reported to be capable of moving air or oxygen in and out of the chest with recovery from asphyxia pallida (Cross and Roberts, 1951).

At the present time tracheal intubation and intermittent positive

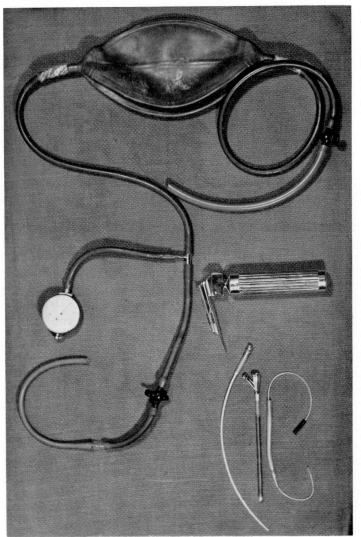

FIG. 2.—Apparatus for intratracheal intubation and intermittent positive pressure resuscitation. Note various types of intratracheal catheters in lower left corner.

pressure inflation, as described above, should be regarded as the standard technique of resuscitation in severe cases. In dire emergency outside hospital mouth-to-mouth breathing may be life-saving, but it carries a risk of introducing infection.

In Glasgow the author and his colleagues have used hyperbaric oxygen for the resuscitation of the apnoeic newborn infant (Hutchison *et al.*, 1963). The infant is placed in a perspex cylinder pressure chamber constructed by Vickers Ltd. (Fig. 3). This apparatus which uses pure oxygen has a maximum working pressure of 45 lb. per sq. in. (4 atmospheres absolute), and the rate of compression and decompression can be varied up to 8 lb. per sq. in. per min. There is a constant volume flow of oxygen through the chamber at 7 litres per min. which prevents any build-up of carbon dioxide. The indications which we employ for this form of treatment are an Apgar Score of 5 or less, and the failure of conservative methods of resuscitation such as pharyngeal and nasal suction, oxygen and nalorphine to initiate respiration within 3 minutes of birth. The average time spent by an infant in the chamber is about 15 minutes. The maximum permissible time is probably 30 minutes. The physiological basis for this form of treatment is that the hypoxic infant is totally immersed in pure oxygen at 2 to 4 atmospheres of pressure so that there will be a steep gradient of 1,500 to 3,000 mm./Hg between the environment and his plasma and tissue fluids. Under these circumstances oxygen diffuses into the circulating blood. In most severely asphyxiated infants a few feeble gasps occur after delivery and only a few alveoli need to open to allow oxygen to flood into the circulation under hyperbaric conditions. The relief of hypoxia permits the respiratory centre to function and spontaneous respiration is established with rapid full expansion of the lungs and elimination of the excess CO_2. This method of resuscitation has been criticized on the basis that it is less effective than tracheal intubation and intermittent positive pressure, particularly in experimental animals asphyxiated to beyond "the last spontaneous gasp" (Campbell *et al.*, 1966). On the other hand, controlled trials in human infants have failed to show that one method is superior to the other (Hutchison *et al.*, 1966). Certainly hyperbaric oxygen is an easier method for staff unskilled in the techniques of tracheal intubation, and free from risk with reasonable safeguards. Its efficacy must await confirmation by other workers before it can be regarded as an established technique of neonatal resuscitation.

Long-term Effects of Neonatal Anoxia

There is a large and conflicting literature on the long-term prognosis in the survivors from asphyxia neonatorum. Many of these studies have been retrospective with the well-known disadvantages of this method of investigation. The subject has been well discussed by Illingworth (1966). Even when the severely anoxic infant later shows signs of mental

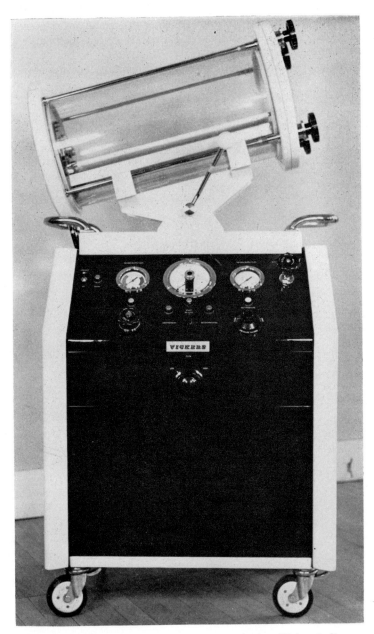

FIG. 3.—Infant pressure chamber for resuscitation (*Vickers Ltd.*)

retardation, cerebral palsy, epilepsy or behaviour disturbances, and some do, it is impossible to know whether the infant was damaged by the anoxia or whether the anoxia might not have been due to an underlying abnormality of the brain. There is, however, no doubt that the great majority of infants who survive neonatal anoxia develop normally.

REFERENCES

APGAR, V., HOLADAY, D. A., JAMES, L. S., WEISBROT, I. M., and BERRIEN, C. (1958). *J. Amer. med. Ass.*, **168**, 1985.

AULD, P. A. M., RUDOLPH, A. J., AVERY, M. E., CHERRY, R. B., DRORBAUGH, J. E., KAY, J. L., and SMITH, C. A., (1961). *Amer. J. Dis. Child.*, **101**, 713.

BARCROFT, J. (1946). *Researches on Prenatal Life.* Oxford: Blackwell Scientific Publications.

CAMPBELL, A. G. M., CROSS, K. W., DAWES, G. S., and HYMAN, A. I. (1966). *J. Pediat.*, **68**, 153

COXON, R. V. (1960). *Lancet*, **1**, 1315.

CROSS, K. W. (1966). *Brit. med. Bull.*, **22**, 73.

CROSS, K. W., and ROBERTS, P. W. (1951). *Brit. med. J.*, **1**, 1043.

DAWES, G. S., JACOBSON, H. N., MOTT, J. C., SHELLEY, H. J., and STAFFORD, A. (1963). *J. Physiol. (Lond.)*, **169**, 167.

DAY, R., GOODFELLOW, A. M., APGAR, V., and BECK, G. I. (1952). *Pediatrics*, **10**, 593.

DONALD, I. (1957). *Brit. J. Anaesth.*, **29**, 553.

DONALD, I., and LORD, J. (1953), *Lancet*, **1**, 9.

HUTCHISON, J. H., KERR, M. M., INALL, J. A., and SHANKS, R. A. (1966). *Lancet*, **1**, 935.

HUTCHISON, J. H., KERR, M. M., WILLIAMS, K. G., and HOPKINSON, W. I. (1963). *Lancet*, **2**, 1019.

ILLINGWORTH, R. S. (1966). *The Development of the Infant and Young Child*, 3rd edit. Edinburgh: E. & S. Livingstone.

MILLER, H. C., and CALKINS, L. A. (1961). *Amer. J. Dis. Child.*, **101**, 3.

MORRIS, N., OSBORN, S. B. and PAYLING WRIGHT, H. (1955). *Lancet*, **1**, 323.

MORRISON, J. E. (1961). *Cerebr. Palsy Bull.*, **3**, 559.

REARDON, H. S., BAUMANN, M. L., and HADDAD, E. J. (1960). *J. Pediat.*, **57**, 151.

WALKER, J. (1954). *J. Obstet. Gynaec. Brit. Emp.*, **61**, 162.

CHAPTER II

LOW BIRTH WEIGHT

In the United Kingdom today about 70 per cent of the neonatal deaths and more than half the stillbirths are associated with low birth weights. While many of these infants are small because they are born before their time others have an abnormally low birth weight for their gestational age. While both types of low birth weight infant require special care in the neonatal period it has been increasingly recognized that they are clinically distinguishable and that they present different problems. These facts have been recognized in this chapter by allocating separate sections to the consideration of "prematurity" and "dysmaturity".

PREMATURITY

The international definition of a *premature (or immature) infant is a live-born infant with a birth weight of* $5\frac{1}{2}$ *lb.* (*2·5 Kg.*) *or less*, or specified as immature. In most countries the diagnosis is based on the birth weight.

There is no entirely satisfactory definition of prematurity. For example, a low birth weight may be associated with post-maturity and placental insufficiency as described below. In some underdeveloped countries a weight limit of $5\frac{1}{2}$ lb. may be too high because there is a low average birth weight for all babies. Infants born to diabetic mothers are usually premature (Chapter XVIII) but they frequently have high birth weights. Small women tend to have small babies and some of these will be recorded as premature although they behave like full-term infants. Calculation of the period of gestation is notoriously inaccurate. None the less, the longer the period of gestation up to ten lunar months the better the infant's chances of survival, other things being equal. It is probable that the most reliable method of estimating maturity is the measurement of length. After 28 weeks of intra-uterine life an approximate figure for the maturity of a foetus in weeks may be arrived at by multiplying by two its length in inches, e.g. 28 weeks for a 14-in. foetus, 32 weeks for a 16-in. foetus and so forth (Crosse, 1961). The upper limit for premature infants has been given as $18\frac{1}{2}$ inches (Corner, 1960). Unfortunately, it is not easy in ordinary clinical practice to obtain reliable measurements of length, whereas a sufficiently precise weight can usually be obtained.

INCIDENCE

The incidence of premature births in the United Kingdom, although not accurately known, probably lies between 6 and 7 per cent of all births.

CAUSAL FACTORS

Not enough is known about the causes of prematurity to allow us to plan new measures to reduce its incidence. None the less, some factors are well known to predispose to premature labour, and our present increasingly effective antenatal and social services should be able to reduce their importance.

(1) *Maternal diseases* which may be directly related to pregnancy, such as toxaemia and antepartum haemorrhage, or coincidental, such as diabetes mellitus, chronic nephritis, acute infections or surgical operations are frequently the causes of premature delivery. In the U.K. this is seldom due to tuberculosis or syphilis. The actual percentage of premature births in which maternal diseases are responsible varies widely in different countries and in different social classes. However, in over 50 per cent no cause is discoverable in the mother.

(2) *Maternal age* is an obvious factor. The lowest incidence of prematurity is in the age period 26–35 years. Abnormally high rates have been found in primigravidae less than 20 years of age and in multigravidae with too closely spaced pregnancies. It should be noted, however, that these facts do not apply to the most prosperous 9 per cent of the community (Douglas, 1950).

(3) *Social and economic status* play an important part in the incidence of prematurity, as indeed they do in most medico-social problems. The incidence of premature birth is considerably higher among lower income groups than among professional and salaried classes (Baird, 1945; Douglas, 1950). This may be partly due to poor nutrition (Cameron and Graham, 1944), and the incidence can be diminished by supplementing the diet during pregnancy (Ebbs *et al.*, 1941; Peoples' League of Health, 1942). None the less, there is evidence that in the U.K. other social and economic factors concerned with a low standard of living play a more important part. Some of these are inadequate antenatal care, employment in industry in the later months of pregnancy, over-crowding and poor housing. The same factors have to do with the high rates of prematurity in illegitimate births.

(4) *Foetal abnormalities and disease* account for about 5 per cent of all premature births. Hydramnios is, of course, a well-known cause of premature labour.

(5) *Multiple pregnancies* frequently terminate prematurely, and twins or triplets are usually of low birth weight.

(6) *Sex of the infant* plays a minor role in that the average birth weight is lower for girls, with an apparent rather than real increase in the incidence of prematurity.

THE DISADVANTAGES OF PREMATURE BIRTH

The behaviour of the small premature infant and the elaborate measures required to keep him alive will be better appreciated if the disadvantages under which he labours are understood. It must be stated, however, that too little is yet known about the physiology of the premature infant for us to be confident about the optimum environment in which to nurse him. It is probable that time and increasing knowledge will make what seems reasonable today appear even ridiculous tomorrow.

The premature infant's immaturity and frailty make him very vulnerable to anoxia and intracranial haemorrhage. The well recognized instability of body temperature is due to several factors such as a relatively large surface area, lack of subcutaneous fat, muscular inactivity, an inadequate sweating mechanism and an immature heat regulating centre. Respiratory insufficiency is brought about by his underdeveloped and often incompletely expanded lungs, by his poor musculature and soft pliable thoracic cage and by the immaturity of the respiratory centre. Aspiration of gastric contents into the lungs is favoured also by a summation of several deficiencies. The cough, sucking and swallowing reflexes are often absent. The cardio-oesophageal sphincteric action is inefficient so that regurgitation of stomach contents into the oesophagus is common. Fat is poorly tolerated and abdominal distention not infrequent. Hepatic immaturity shows in the low levels of serum proteins and in the tendency to hyperbilirubinaemia. Tyrosine metabolism is also defective if strained by a high protein diet in the absence of vitamin C (Levine *et al.*, 1943). The kidneys show both anatomical and functional immaturity. Urinary output is small, urea clearance values are low, and there is a diminished ability to get rid of excess water and electrolytes. Acid-base balance is precarious and largely dependent on pulmonary function. The frequent occurrence of oedema is not fully understood but is partly related to hypoproteinaemia, partly to poor renal function. Several of the clotting factors, such as prothrombin, factor VII and Christmas factor are diminished so that the already fragile blood vessels bleed readily when torn. Iron stores at birth are low so that iron-deficiency anaemia is frequent after the fourth month of life. His rapid rate of growth renders him highly susceptible to rickets unless he is supplied with a high intake of vitamin D. Last but not least is his extreme susceptibility to infection. This may be partly due to the low serum levels of gamma globulin encountered in very small premature infants.

CLINICAL FEATURES

The appearance and behaviour of the premature baby is, of course, dependent on his degree of immaturity. The small ($3-3\frac{1}{2}$ lb.) infant has a disproportionately large head and abdomen. Lack of subcutaneous fat is reflected in his thin, lined face, loose skin over the limbs, and in the frequent appearance of intestinal peristalsis which is visible through the abdominal wall. He sleeps more or less continuously and his cry is infrequent and feeble. Respiration may be rhythmic but is often jerky and irregular, and periodic spells of apnoea are not uncommon. Hypotonicity produces the characteristic posture in which he lies with thighs widely abducted, knees and ankles flexed, head lolling to one side. The tonic neck reflex is little in evidence but the Moro reflex is usually brisk. Muscular movements are much less frequent and vigorous than in the full-term infant. The ability to suck is absent or feeble, especially during the first 48 to 96 hours of life. Hunger is indicated by crying, restlessness and threshing movements of the arms. If signs of hunger do not appear within 96 hours this should arouse suspicion of infection or intracranial haemorrhage. It is to be noted, however, that response to cutaneous stimuli is usually brisk soon after birth. Slight oedema is often present at birth and may become more marked during the next 24–48 hours. The skin appears shiny and smooth, pitting may be demonstrable, and the oedema may shift with changes of posture. Severe oedema is an unfavourable omen. It is most frequently associated with antepartum haemorrhage, toxaemia and maternal diabetes mellitus. The heart rate in premature infants averages 140 per min. and irregularities are not usually of great significance. The respiratory rate varies quite widely. In healthy infants rates of 40 to 50 per min. are usual in the first 12 to 24 hours, thereafter falling to 35 to 45. A continued rapid rate should arouse suspicion of the pulmonary syndrome or pneumonia. Contrary to popular belief the premature infant's nails are well formed and not particularly short.

MANAGEMENT

There are four major problems in the care of small feeble infants, (1) maintenance of body temperature, (2) feeding, (3) protection against infection, (4) prevention of vitamin and iron deficiencies.

These will be considered individually but as the problems differ according to whether the infant is to be supervised in hospital or at home, it is necessary first to discuss the difficult problem which faces the physician when an infant is prematurely born at home. It is, of course, obvious that every effort should be made to avoid this, because in every premature labour the full resources of a hospital are desirable. None the less, the premature infant will at times have to be delivered in a private house. The decision to keep him there will depend upon the availability of reasonable and adequately heated accommodation, and of trained nurses and reliable domestic help. In many areas nurses specially trained in the home-care of premature babies are available from the Local Health Authority. The condition of the infant at birth will also weigh heavily. Strong indications for immediate transfer to hospital are respiratory distress, signs of cerebral involvement, and a birth weight of under 4 lb. Transfer to hospital should be in a specially heated cot or portable incubator. Many large maternity units will send out such apparatus in the charge of a trained nurse for the collection from a private house of a premature or sick infant.

(1) **Maintenance of body temperature** is much easier in hospital. It is probably wise to maintain the premature infant's rectal temperature 1 to 2° F. below the level of 97° F. which is accepted as normal for a mature infant. The nursery temperature should be 80 to 85° F. and it is an advantage when humidity can also be controlled. A relative humidity of 50 to 55 per cent is acceptable by the staff who must work in the nursery for long periods. Small feeble infants are best nursed in incubators controlled at a temperature range of 90 to 95° F. and humidity over 65 per cent. Larger and more vigorous infants are more conveniently nursed in cots. All infants are best nursed naked, except for the napkin. This has several advantages. Any change in condition, respiration or colour can be quickly noted. Movements are in no way restricted. Handling is reduced to a minimum. Cyanosis must be prevented by oxygen which can be given in the incubator or by covering the cot with a plastic lid. The concentration of oxygen, in the incubator or cot should not exceed 40 per cent, and it should be checked periodically by means of a pyrogallic acid or an electromagnetic analyser (see p. 25). = Beckman.

When the premature infant is nursed at home the room temperature must never fall below 65° F. This can only be achieved by gas or electric fires in the absence of central heating. Coal fires are dangerous as the room temperature may fall abruptly during the night. Reasonable humidity can be obtained by placing a bowl of water before the fire or a damp blanket over a central heating radiator. The cot temperature must be kept at 85 to 90° F. by means of hot water bottles, suitably covered, or with a small electric pad. Strict precautions to avoid burning the infant are essential. In the home it is necessary to dress the infant in loose, non-restrictive, and heat-retaining clothing. Suitable clothes and equipment for the domiciliary care of feeble infants are provided by many Local Health Authorities.

(2) **Feeding** is always a difficult problem in premature infants who require a high protein intake (over 5 gm./Kg./day) and a high intake of carbohydrate (as cane sugar or lactose) if they are to gain weight adequately after the initial loss during the first week of life. On the other hand, they tolerate fat poorly.

It has been common practice to withhold oral feeds from premature infants for 36 to 48 hours, or even longer, after birth to minimize the risks of regurgitation and aspiration pneumonia. In the past few years it has been appreciated that this regime may well increase the risks of hyperbilirubinaemia, symptomatic hypoglycaemia and possibly even of later cerebral diplegia. Many now advise that the first feed be given between 12 and 24 hours after birth, by nasogastric polyvinyl tube if the infant is unable to suck. We are not yet convinced of the wisdom or advantages of giving the first tube feed within 2 hours of birth as recommended by Smallpeice and Davies (1964). Most premature babies can suck from a bottle within 48 to 72 hours provided a soft teat with a large enough hole is used. The experienced nurse can assist the infant's rather feeble efforts by applying gentle upward pressure on the infant's chin with her forefinger. The infant should be propped with head raised during and for 15 minutes after each feed to lessen the risk of regurgitation, and to help him to bring up wind. Infants over 4½ lb. birth weight can usually feed from the breast, but until the fourth day fluid intake may have to be supplemented with 5 per cent glucose in water after each feed. Infants under 3½ lb. may be unable to suck. They should be tube fed, either by passing a No. 4 or 5 Jacques rubber catheter by mouth for each feed, or by a plastic (polyvinyl) tube passed into the stomach through the nose and left *in situ* for 5 days. The use of polyvinyl disposable tubes, sterilized by gamma radiation, is a great advantage for the smallest infants. Feeding by means of pipette, Belcroy feeder or spoon carries great risk of inhalation and in our view is best eschewed. Indeed the danger of aspiration of feeds and stomach contents into the lungs is considerable in feeble infants and the necessity for expert nursing care in its prevention constitutes a major reason why small premature infants should rarely be nursed at home.

Human milk is the food of choice and most large maternity hospitals run breast milk banks for their own requirements. A few are willing to supply breast milk to other hospitals. Breast milk, undiluted, is particularly valuable during the first few days of life and in the smallest babies. Excellent results can also be obtained with Half-cream National Dried Milk or Cow and Gate Special Half-Cream. Humanized dried milks such as Trufood and Glaxo's Ostermilk No. 1 may also be used. Evaporated milks such as Regal or Carnation are popular in some centres, but sweetened condensed milk is not recommended because of its low protein content in the reconstituted state. Whichever formula is used should contain about 20 Cals. per fl. oz. A suitable formula for half-cream dried milk is 3 measures of milk powder made up 3 fl. oz. (90 ml.) with water plus a rounded-off teaspoonful of sugar (21 Cals. per fl. oz.). This formula can be given from the start of feeding. We have not encountered increased feeding difficulties from this practice, nor can we see great advantage in the common custom of diluting either breast milk or the dried milk formula during the first two weeks of life. Specially modified milks, such as Frailac and S.M.A., have not been proved to have material advantages over those already mentioned.

During the first week or two of life small feeds must be given frequently to lessen the risks of regurgitation. Most premature infants can tolerate feeds of 2 fl. drachms (8 ml.) of milk formula every three hours from the first or second day of life. The volume is increased gradually so as to avoid abdominal distention or vomiting, and the physician will do well to proceed cautiously during the first two weeks. Thereafter, a fluid intake of 2½ to 3 fl. oz. per lb. body weight per day (150–180 ml./ Kg./day) should be achieved. Caloric requirements vary considerably from one infant to another. The aim after the second week is as rapid weight gain as possible. At least 60 Cals. per lb. body weight per day (3×20) (120 Cals./Kg./day) are required. The intervals between feeds should be altered from 3 hours to 4 when a weight of 5 lb. (2·5 Kg.) has been reached. These quantities and times should be regarded as a guide, but those experienced in the care of premature infants will frequently modify their normal routine to meet the needs of individual infants.

(3) **Protection against infection** can probably never be complete and maximum protection can only be obtained in maternity hospitals with specially designed nurseries for premature and sick infants. Even more important is an adequate nursing staff fully trained in the techniques of barrier-nursing. There must be separate nurseries for infants born within the hospital and those transferred from outside. A small isolation unit is essential for infected infants or those born to infected mothers. The modern nursery consists of cubicles for 2 to 6 cots, with a few single cot cubicles for very feeble or ill babies. The intervening partitions are of glass to permit full visibility. Each cubicle contains a wash-hand basin with elbow operated taps. The cots should be of metal or plastic to allow of efficient cleaning with soap and water or antiseptic solution, and each should include a suitable cupboard for the infant's personal requisites such as thermometer, containers for clean and used swabs, cleansing materials, etc. Incubators must also be cleaned or fumigated with formaldehyde vapour after use. The floors should be cleaned by vacuum apparatus daily and washed with soap and water at least once a week. The walls are washed monthly. Linen and equipment must be protected from dust in cupboards and covered containers. Dirty linen is received into a covered bin or bag. Disposable napkins are advised. They should be incinerated within the premature unit itself. If blankets are used at all they must be of Terylene or cotton weave to withstand sterilization. Procedures such as exchange transfusion, subdural taps and lumbar puncture should be carried out in a separate surgical room within the premature unit.

The preparation and storage of feeds require the strictly aseptic conditions of a properly designed milk kitchen which should supply the needs of all infants in the hospital. Breast milk after expression must be sterilized by boiling or in an autoclave. It can then be stored in a refrigerator at 4° C. for 48 hours. The milk kitchen normally consists of two rooms. In one the used bottles and teats are washed. In the other, nurses who wear gowns, masks and caps prepare the feeds. Sterilization of bottles may be carried out in a double-ended autoclave which communicates with both rooms, or in a 1 in 80 solution of sodium hypochlorite (Milton) which is made up once every 24 hours. In some hospitals terminal sterilization of the prepared feeds in the bottles is carried out in the autoclave.

Precise details of nursing technique will vary in different hospitals but the basic principles are always the same. All staff wear adequate masks, preferably of the paper disposable type. When the nurses change into special sterile cotton dresses in the premature unit we have abandoned the use of gowns. The custom of putting on a gown before handling each infant is very wasteful of nurses' time and it has not, in our experience, reduced the incidence of cross-infection. Hand washing technique is of vital importance. The hands must be washed on entering a cubicle and before and after handling each infant. They should be dried on disposable towels. Hexachlorophene soaps considerably reduce skin bacteria. The methods used for cleansing the premature babies' very delicate skin vary from soap and water to inactivity. Our own preference is for whole body cleansing every second day by gentle lathering with hexachlorophene skin cleanser (pHisoHex). This is also applied to the buttocks when napkins are soiled. All nursing measures, including administration of feeds or drugs, must be carried out within the cot or incubator. Changing tables are a highly dangerous source of cross-infection. Practice varies greatly in regard to the umbilical cord. We re-ligature the cord and cut it off 1 in. from the umbilicus on admission to the premature nursery. Some prefer to cover it with a sterile dressing or collodion. The infant's eyes, nose and mouth must be inspected daily, but routine cleansing is inadvisable. Temperatures are taken rectally twice daily, or more frequently if they are elevated or subnormal. Weighing routines vary from daily to twice weekly. The nurse's hands must be washed before the infant is placed on tissue paper previously put on the scales at the cot-side.

(4) **Prevention of vitamin and iron deficiency** should be a routine procedure. Supplements of vitamins A, D, and C are started gradually about the fourteenth day. Suitable preparations are adexolin (Glaxo) 10 drops twice daily (vitamin D 800 units; vitamin A 8,000 units), and ascorbic acid 5 mg. tablets in each feed. Iron can be given from the sixth week of life as:

$$\begin{array}{ll} \text{Ferrous sulphate} & \tfrac{1}{2} \text{ gr. (30 mg.)} \\ \text{Dilute hypophosphorous acid} & \tfrac{1}{2} \, \mathrm{\eta}. \text{ (0·03 ml.)} \\ \text{Dextrose} & 15 \text{ gr. (1 gm.)} \end{array}$$

Chloroform water to 60η. (4 ml.), thrice daily.

It should be continued during the first year.

COMPLICATIONS OF PREMATURITY

(1) **The idiopathic respiratory distress syndrome (RDS).**—This condition is characterized by pulmonary resorption atelectasis associated with intense congestion, the presence of an eosinophilic hyaline membrane within dilated alveolar ducts, and sometimes intrapulmonary

See P. 57, in Synopsis (Kindle-Short)

haemorrhage of widely variable extent. The term *hyaline membrane disease* is less suitable because membrane formation is not invariably present and, indeed, may be the result rather than the cause of the condition. Another name for the disease is *the pulmonary syndrome of the newborn*. The hyaline membrane material appears to be composed largely of fibrin although it does not give the usual histochemical reactions of this substance (Gitlin and Craig, 1956). It is seen only in infants who have lived at least one hour. This condition is the commonest cause of death in premature infants, but it is relatively rare in mature infants. Predisposing factors are antepartum haemorrhage, caesarean section and maternal diabetes mellitus. The aetiology is still elusive although it seems certain that it starts before birth and is in some way related to intrapartum hypoxia. An important finding has been the demonstration by Pattle (1965) that the normally complete lung-lining film or surface active material, identifiable histochemically as a phospholipid and which greatly reduces the surface tension in the alveoli, is absent or defective in the lungs of these infants. (*i.e. Surfactant ?= lecithin dipalmitate*)

Clinical Features

Some affected infants appear to breathe normally for a short period, but the majority are in poor condition with grunting respiration from birth. Within a few hours there is inspiratory retraction of the subcostal margin, sternum and intercostal spaces. Expiratory grunting is associated with violent inspiratory efforts, but breath sounds are greatly diminished. The respiratory rate rises to 75 per minute and remains high. Muscle flaccidity causes the infant to lie with thighs widely abducted and knees flexed, while the arms are flexed at the elbows, and the hands are held in supination alongside the head. Greyish cyanosis is present. Oedema often becomes severe during the first 12 hours. Spells of apnoea occur with increasing frequency in deteriorating babies. Radiographs show a characteristic granular mottling. As this becomes more confluent the bronchial tree stands out clearly as an "air bronchogram" (Donald and Steiner, 1953) (Fig. 4).

Severe biochemical disturbances have been stressed by Usher (1961*a*, *b*) and ourselves (Hutchison *et al*., 1962). Respiratory acidosis (high Pco_2) is associated with metabolic acidosis. The arterial Po_2 is reduced. The serum potassium level rises between 12 and 60 hours of age and this is associated with electro-cardiographic changes such as widening of P–R and QRS, prolongation of Q–T and left ventricular preponderance. The kidneys seem unable to conserve base, probably because of an inability to excrete phosphate to act as a buffer, so that the bicarbonate level falls in the plasma. The presence of an increased catabolic rate releases excess potassium, nitrogen and phosphorus from the cells. As the kidneys cannot increase their excretion of solutes these substances reach high levels in the serum. Other chemical disorders are

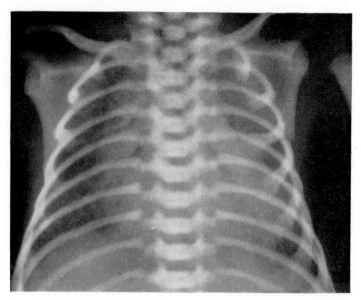

FIG. 4.—Appearances in hyaline membrane disease. Note granular mottling in lung fields with bronchi showing clearly outlined by air.

hypoproteinaemia and an excessive urinary output of 17-hydrocorti-costeroids.

Treatment

The present routine care amounts to placing the infant in an incubator at a relative humidity of 80 to 100 per cent and administering oxygen so that the concentration is between 35 and 40 per cent. The stomach contents should be aspirated every 12 hours and feeds are withheld until recovery starts. Antibiotics such as cloxacillin (50 mg. per Kg. per day) combined with ampicillin (50 mg. per Kg. per day), or cephalori-dine (30 mg. per Kg. per day) should be given intramuscularly to prevent bacterial infection. It is often necessary to increase the oxygen saturation in the incubator considerably above 40 per cent to abolish cyanosis, but the level should be reduced as soon as possible. In some centres oxygen therapy is monitored by periodic measurements of the arterial Po_2 by means of cannulation of an umbilical artery with a poly-vinyl catheter. The object should be to achieve a Po_2 above 70 mm. Hg and concentrations of oxygen as high as 90 per cent may be needed to achieve this.

The results of these well-intentioned therapeutic measures are disappointing. Mild cases do well, but severe cases in which there is cyanosis even in 90 per cent oxygen with severe sternal recession show a mortality rate in the region of 45 per cent. Some have advocated digitalization but this has produced little benefit in our experience. Usher (1961b) has reported a greatly reduced mortality from the administration of 10 to 15 per cent glucose solutions containing 5 to 25 mEq. of sodium bicarbonate per 100 ml. by continuous intravenous infusion (65 ml./Kg./day) according to the blood pH levels. If hyperkalaemia develops he gives insulin (1 unit per 3 gm. glucose) in the fluid. This is an arduous routine possible only in large hospitals, and scalp vein infusions in small premature infants involve considerable handling and exposure.

The author and his colleagues (Hutchison et al., 1962) have reported a substantial fall in their mortality rates when a more rapid correction of metabolic acidosis was obtained with much larger doses of sodium bicarbonate. This became a safe and practicable procedure with the development of the Astrup micro-method whereby on small volumes (100 μl.) of capillary blood it is possible within a few minutes to determine the blood pH, Pco_2, and plasma standard bicarbonate (Andersen et al., 1960; Astrup et al., 1960). These estimations can be repeated at hourly intervals, thus permitting accurate control of the pH and standard bicarbonate which are raised to normal in these acidotic infants by hourly intravenous doses of 8·4 per cent sodium bicarbonate (1 ml. contains 1 mEq. of $NaHCO_3$). We have given the intravenous fluids through a polyvinyl catheter which has been passed into the umbilical vein. In addition to frequent doses of sodium bicarbonate we bring the total daily fluid intake up to 60 ml./Kg. with 20 per cent fructose solution which is non-irritant to veins, and from which the infant's seriously depleted glycogen stores can be replenished. It has been our experience that the mortality rate in severe cases of the pulmonary syndrome (respiratory distress syndrome) has been reduced to about 11·5 per cent with this therapeutic regime (Hutchison et al., 1964). This too requires a fairly large medical team and our methods do not correct severe respiratory acidosis which, if persistent, signifies a poor prognosis. We have also shown that hyperbaric oxygen in a pressure chamber is ineffective in combating respiratory acidosis and a high blood Pco_2 (Hutchison et al., 1962).

Bound and his co-workers (1962) have suggested that delay in ligation of the umbilical cord, and encouragement of the transfusion of placental blood into the infant by gravity decreases the incidence of the pulmonary syndrome. Bonham Carter et al. (1956) had earlier suggested that a raised venous pressure is beneficial to infants with respiratory difficulty, and Wallgren et al. (1960) have shown that placental transfusion can compensate for the increased vascular capacity of the lungs after they have expanded. Delayed ligation would seem to be a rational measure when this is practicable.

Another therapeutic approach has been to assist respiration in these very distressed infants by means of mechanical ventilation, either through a tracheostomy (Delivoria-Papadopoulos *et al.*, 1965) or an in-dwelling plastic intratracheal tube (Thomas *et al.*, 1965; Reid, 1966). It is obvious that this regime is only possible in large centres and its value has yet to be established. Another ingenious approach is the attempt to reduce the severe pulmonary arteriolar constriction, with high pulmonary arterial pressure, by the injection of acetylcholine through a catheter the tip of which has been placed as near the pulmonary artery as possible (Chu *et al.*, 1965).

(2) **Intraventricular haemorrhage.**—Spontaneous bleeding into one or both lateral ventricles arises from anoxia and is peculiar in site to the premature infant. It is usually associated with hyaline membrane formation in the lungs. Indeed, it is probably secondary to the anoxia which occurs in this syndrome. Unfortunately, it is often impossible to differentiate those infants whose respiratory distress and apnoeic spells are associated with intraventricular haemorrhage, and this condition is frequently found at autopsy when death has followed many hours of skilled nursing and medical care.

(3) **The retinopathy of prematurity.**—This name is preferred to *retrolental fibroplasia* because it takes account of the important fact that some cases are arrested early before advancing to complete blindness. The disease first appeared in the U.S.A. in 1942 and in the U.K. in 1946. These dates coincide with the widespread use of modern incubators in the two countries and this fact aroused early suspicion that oxygen therapy might have aetiological importance. Experimental proof of the role of oxygen came from a series of observations on newborn kittens by Ashton and his colleagues in London (1953). The kitten was chosen because its retinal vessels at birth are about the same stage of development as in the 7-month human foetus. While the kittens are exposed to high concentration of oxygen the retinal vessels undergo intense vasoconstriction. On subsequent transfer to air these vessels show gross vasodilatation followed by the proliferation of new vessels in a completely disordered fashion. In the human infant the same sequence of events is directly related to the degree of immaturity, the concentration of oxygen and the duration of exposure.

Clinical Features

This disorder is seen only in infants under $4\frac{1}{2}$ lb., who have received oxygen. The acute stage is first seen with the ophthalmoscope between the ages of 3 and 6 weeks in the form of dilatation of the retinal veins and arteries. This is followed by the growth, in a disorderly pattern, of new capillaries at the growing ends of the veins. Clusters of new capillaries may simulate haemorrhages. Subsequently, some of the new vessels begin to grow forwards into the vitreous towards the lens. Retinal oedema occurs and is followed by peripheral retinal detachment when the condition becomes irreversible. In the cicatricial stage there may be complete retinal detachment, leaving only a stalk of rolled-up retina connected posteriorly around the optic disc (Fig. 5). Finally, there is a retrolental mass of fibrous tissue visible behind a clear lens with the naked eye. In severe cases the condition is bilateral with microphthalmos, a narrow anterior chamber, irregular small pupil and gross loss of vision. Squint is common, and glaucoma frequently occurs. There is also an increased incidence of mental retardation and cerebral palsy in these children (Williams, 1958; McDonald, 1962).

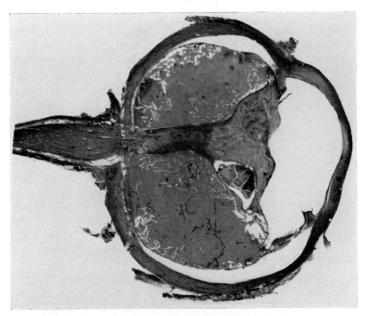

FIG. 5.—Fully established retrolental fibroplasia showing complete retinal detachment and retrolental retinal chaos.

Management

There is some evidence that the process may be arrested in the early stages with ACTH or corticosteroids. It is obviously much better to prevent this tragic sequel to premature birth by attention to the following rules:

    (a) Oxygen concentrations in incubators must not be allowed to rise above 40 per cent save in grave emergency.

    (b) Oxygen should never be given in the absence of respiratory distress or cyanosis.

    (c) The administration of oxygen should not be continued longer than is necessary.

    (4) **The early anaemia of prematurity.**—This condition must be

clearly distinguished from the hypochromic anaemia of iron-deficiency to which the premature infant is unduly susceptible after the age of 4 months (Chapter XIX). The latter condition may be thought of as "the late anaemia of prematurity". Unlike the early anaemia of prematurity it can be prevented or cured with iron.

The haemoglobin level at birth in the venous blood of both mature and premature infants is high by adult standards (19–21 gm. per 100 ml.). In all infants there is a fairly rapid fall during the early weeks of life. This is because the oxygen saturation of the blood rises at birth from the foetal level of 65 per cent to the normal adult value of 95 per cent when the lungs take over this function from the placenta. There is, in consequence, a drop in the need for circulating haemoglobin and the bone marrow goes into a resting phase with relative erythropoietic inactivity. Gairdner et al. (1952) have shown that the total circulating haemoglobin falls at a rate of 1 per cent per day. However, the rate of fall of haemoglobin concentration depends also upon the infant's rate of growth. As this is more rapid in premature infants there is an exaggerated rate of fall in haemoglobin concentration. A level of 8 gm. per 100 ml. is not uncommon at the age of 6 to 8 weeks. This early anaemia of prematurity is normochromic (Gairdner et al., 1955). Recovery from this anaemia tends to take place as the bone marrow responds to the low level of oxygenation of the tissues. However, as rapid growth also continues this spontaneous rise in the haemoglobin concentration is slow. It will also be ill-sustained if adequate supplies of iron are not made available from the age of 6–8 weeks.

Treatment

When the early anaemia of prematurity is aggravated by infection or haemorrhage of any kind blood transfusion is indicated. Cobalt has been used successfully to stimulate erythropoiesis, but as it is also goitrogenic its use cannot be recommended.

(5) **Jaundice of prematurity (hyperbilirubinaemia).**—The incidence of non-obstructive jaundice in small premature infants is considerable, particularly in those who survive hyaline membrane disease. The danger of kernicterus (nuclear jaundice) arises when the serum "indirect" bilirubin level rises above 20 to 24 mg. per 100 ml. The incidence of kernicterus is increased by the administration of vitamin K analogues, sulphafurazole and novobiocin. Vitamin K should never be given in a dose exceeding 2 mg. Sulphafurazole and novobiocin should not be prescribed at all during the neonatal period. The pathogenesis of jaundice and its management are discussed in Chapter IV.

DYSMATURITY

This section deals with those infants whose low birth weight in relation to their gestational age is the result of intra-uterine deprivation.

Various names have been used for the condition including dysmaturity, postmaturity syndrome, pseudoprematurity, placental insufficiency, intra-uterine growth retardation and foetal malnutrition. Excellent reviews of the problem have been supplied by Warkany *et al.* (1961) and Wigglesworth (1966).

AETIOLOGY

Little definite is yet known of the factors leading to depression of foetal growth. Gruenwald (1963) attributed the condition to placental insufficiency and it seems certain that there is interference with the supplies of essential nutrients and oxygen to the foetus in late pregnancy. The placenta, which is normally about a sixth of the weight of the infant at term, is abnormally small in most cases of dysmaturity and the villous surface-area is much reduced (Aherne and Dunhill, 1966). In some instances genetic factors may be involved. Ounsted (1965) made a prospective study of 225 pregnant women alongside a study of 90 women who gave birth to infants whose birth weights were more than two standard deviations below the mean for gestational age. There were no significant differences between the two groups in duration of pregnancy, maternal age or height, reproductive history, duration of gestation of previous liveborn siblings, or the incidence of antepartum haemorrhage or hypertension. There was, however, a highly significant difference in the birth weights of the liveborn siblings in the two groups. In the prospective series these birth weights were distributed around a median of 3,345 gm. whereas in the growth-retarded series the median for siblings was 2,608 gm. A third series of short-gestation prematures was then studied and here the birth weight of the siblings approximated closely to that of the prospective or control group.

Whatever may be the precise aetiology the dysmature infant shows the signs of a low income and high capital expenditure. The total carbohydrate and glycogen stores of the liver, heart and skeletal muscle are reduced, while the growth of the brain and mature lungs contrast with the shrunken liver. A not uncommon post-mortem finding is massive pulmonary haemorrhage.

CLINICAL FEATURES

The external appearance of the dysmature infant varies somewhat with the duration of pregnancy and placental insufficiency. He is thin and underweight for his length, although the latter is usually less than that to be expected at the gestational age. By contrast, head circumference is much less affected so that it may appear disproportionately large. The skin looks dry, loose, and wrinkled and it frequently shows transverse cracks as well as desquamation. Foetal distress during labour is a common incident in cases of dysmaturity often resulting in meconium staining of the skin, nails and umbilical cord. However, it is unlikely that the term "dysmaturity" comprises a homogeneous group of infants sharing a common environmental or genetic aetiology. Indeed, even the external appearances vary, a few infants appearing normally proportioned while most look long and skinny; in some the appearances suggest recent marked loss of weight, others merely appear miniature. A somewhat striking feature of the dysmature low birth weight infant is the lively wide-awake expression which is not seen in the truly premature baby.

MANAGEMENT

The dysmature infant is usually eager to feed and oral feeds should be started between 4 and 12 hours after birth to reduce the danger of hypoglycaemia. The blood glucose levels should be checked every few hours by the Dextrostix (Ames & Co.) method, and a true blood glucose estimation should be performed if the reading is below 40 mg. per 100 ml. on the Dextrostix. A careful watch should be kept on the respiratory rate as continued tachypnoea one to two hours after birth may well indicate the presence of meconium aspiration.

COMPLICATIONS OF DYSMATURITY

Meconium Aspiration Syndrome

Whereas we associate the idiopathic respiratory distress syndrome with the premature baby the usual cause of respiratory distress in the dysmature infant is the aspiration of meconium which is intensely irritating to the bronchiolar epithelium. In this situation the oxygen supply to the foetus has been interrupted with the result that the distressed foetus has made vigorous gasps *in utero* while at the same time passing meconium into the liquor amnii. The clinical picture closely simulates that of RDS but the infant, although of low birth weight, shows the clinical signs of dysmaturity. The radiographic appearances of the lung fields are, however, quite different, amounting to a more coarse streaking with varying degrees of aeration and emphysema (Fig. 6). The treatment should be along the lines laid down for RDS.

Transient Symptomatic Hypoglycaemia of the Newborn

It is now clear that this dangerous condition occurs predominantly in the male infant who is of low birth weight for his period of gestation. If it is not promptly recognized and vigorously treated permanent brain damage is a common sequel. The only complication of pregnancy known to increase the risk of spontaneous hypoglycaemia in the infant is pre-eclamptic toxaemia, present in about half the cases. The pathogenesis is not yet clear although the extremely poor glycogen stores of the dysmature infant is likely to be an important factor. There may be an insufficiency of glucose available for the relatively large glucose-dependent brain and the metabolically active mature body. Excellent accounts of this disorder can be found in the papers by Shelley and Neligan (1966) and Chance and Bower (1966), and in the textbook by Cornblath and Schwartz (1966).

Clinical Features

The infant usually appears well for a period which may vary from six hours to seven days after birth. Then various symptoms manifest

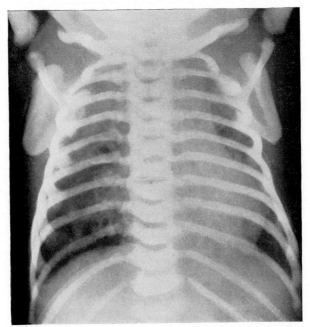

FIG. 6.—Meconium aspiration syndrome. Radiograph shows generalized streaky shadows and areas of emphysema.

themselves such as jitteriness or twitchings, attacks of apnoea and cyanosis, pallor, reluctance to feed, limpness, apathy or generalized convulsions. When these manifestations occur in an infant showing the signs of dysmaturity the diagnosis should be suspected and a true blood glucose estimation be arranged without delay. The diagnosis can be regarded as confirmed if the blood glucose level is below 20 mg. per 100 ml.

Treatment

An intravenous injection of 50 per cent glucose in water, 2 ml. per kg. body weight, should be given immediately upon receipt of the blood glucose result. Thereafter a continuous infusion of 10 per cent glucose in water, 60 to 75 ml. per Kg. per day, should be set up in a scalp vein. In some cases there is a prompt recovery, when oral feeds should be resumed. In others, the symptoms persist for several days. If the intravenous 10 per cent glucose has to be given for longer than 24 hours it should then be dissolved in quarter-strength physiological saline to prevent hyponatraemia. If this treatment fails to maintain the blood glucose level above 30 mg. per 100 ml. corticosteroids (such as oral hydrocortisone 5 mg. per Kg. per day) or ACTH (4 units per Kg. per day) should be added. In a few cases the serum calcium level is also low (below 8 mg. per 100 ml.) when oral calcium chloride 5 gr. (0·3 gm.) should be given four-hourly for three days. After discharge from hospital the infant should be followed up until the presence or absence of brain damage can be ascertained.

REFERENCES

PREMATURITY

ANDERSEN, O. S., ENGEL, K., JØRGENSEN, K., and ASTRUP, P. (1960). *Scand. J. clin. Lab. Invest.*, **12**, 172.
ASHTON, N., WARD, B., and SERPELL, G. (1953). *Brit. J. Ophthal.*, **37**, 513.
ASTRUP, P., JØRGENSEN, K., ANDERSEN, O. S., and ENGEL, K. (1960). *Lancet*, **1**, 1035.
BAIRD, D. (1945). *J. Obstet. Gynaec. Brit. Emp.*, **52**, 217, 339.
BONHAM CARTER, R. E., BOUND, J. P., and SMELLIE, J. M. (1956). *Lancet*, **2**, 1320.
BOUND, J. P., HARVEY, P. W., and BAGSHAW, H. B. (1962). *Lancet*, **1**, 1200.
CAMERON, C. S., and GRAHAM, S. (1944). *Glasg. med. J.*, **142**, 1.
CHU, J., CLEMENTS, J. A., COTTON, E., KLAUS, M. H., SWEET, A. Y., THOMAS, M. A., and TOOLEY, W. H. (1965). *Pediatrics*, **35**, 733.
CORNER, B. (1960). *Prematurity*. London: Cassell & Co.
CROSSE, V. M. (1961). *The Premature Baby*, 5th edit. London: J. & A. Churchill.
DELIVORIA-PAPADOPOULOS, M., LEVINSON, H., and SWYER, P. (1965). *Arch. Dis. Childh.*, **40**, 474.
DONALD, I., and STEINER, R. E. (1953). *Lancet*, **2**, 846.
DOUGLAS, J. W. B. (1950). *J. Obstet. Gynaec. Brit. Emp.*, **57**, 143.
EBBS, J. H., TISDALL, F. F., and SCOTT, W. A. (1941). *J. Nutr.*, **22**, 515.
GAIRDNER, D., MARKS, J., and ROSCOE, J. D. (1952). *Arch. Dis. Childh.*, **27**, 214.
GAIRDNER, D., MARKS, J., and ROSCOE, J. D. (1955). *Arch. Dis. Childh.*, **30**, 203.
GITLIN, D., and CRAIG, J. M. (1956). *Pediatrics*, **17**, 64.
HUTCHISON, J. H., KERR, M. M., McPHAIL, M. F. M., DOUGLAS, T. A., SMITH, G., NORMAN, J. N., and BATES, E. H. (1962). *Lancet*, **2**, 465.
HUTCHISON, J. H., KERR, M. M., DOUGLAS, T. A., INALL, J. A., and CROSBIE, J. C. (1964). *Pediatrics*, **33**, 956.
LEVINE, S. Z., DANN, M., and MARPLES, E. (1943). *J. clin. Invest.*, **22**, 551.
McDONALD, A. D. (1962). *Brit. med. J.*, **1**, 895.
PATTLE, R. E. (1965). *Physiol. Rev.*, **45**, 48.
PEOPLES' LEAGUE OF HEALTH. (1942). *Lancet*, **2**, 10.
REID, D. H. S. (1966). *Lancet*, **1**, 784.
SMALLPEICE, V., and DAVIES, P. A. (1964). *Lancet*, **2**, 1349.
THOMAS, D. V., FLETCHER, G., SUNSHINE, P., SCHAFFER, I. A., and KLAUS, M. H. (1965). *J. Amer. med. Ass.*, **193**, 183.
USHER, R. H. (1961a). *N.Y. St. J. Med.*, **61**, 1677.
USHER, R. H. (1961b). *Pediat. Clin. N. Amer.*, **8**, 525.

WALLGREN, G., KARLBERG, P., and LIND, J. (1960). *Acta paediat.* (*Uppsala*), **49**, 843.
WILLIAMS, C. E. (1958). *Brit. J. Ophthal.*, **42**, 549.

DYSMATURITY

AHERNE, W., and DUNHILL, M. S. (1966). *Brit. med. Bull.*, **22**, 5.
CHANCE, G. W., and BOWER, B. D. (1966). *Arch. Dis. Childh.*, **41**, 279.
CORNBLATH, M., and SCHWARTZ, R. (1966). *Disorders of Carbohydrate Metabolism in Infancy*, Chap. 5. Philadelphia: W. B. Saunders Co.
GRUENWALD, P. (1963). *Biologia Neonat.* (*Basel*), **5**, 215.
OUNSTED, M. (1965). *Develop. Med. child. Neurol.*, **7**, 479.
SHELLEY, H. J., and NELIGAN, G. A. (1966). *Brit. med. Bull.*, **22**, 34.
WARKANY, J., MONROE, B. B., and SUTHERLAND, B. S. (1961). *Amer. J. Dis. Child.*, **102**, 249.
WIGGLESWORTH, J. S. (1966). *Brit. med. Bull.*, **22**, 13.

CHAPTER III

NEONATAL INJURIES

In this chapter we shall discuss only the common neonatal injuries of the present day. Gross injuries of the liver, spine and lungs caused by now discarded obstetric procedures and misguided methods of resuscitation are rarely seen. It should be stressed at the outset that it is frequently impossible to separate the effects of anoxia from those due to injury during delivery. Indeed, the one often aggravates the other and both commonly coexist. For example, a difficult labour may well place insupportable stresses on the membranous septa within the skull so that a tear develops in the tentorium cerebelli or the falx cerebri. It is likely also to result in foetal anoxia which will cause venous distension. If a blood vessel has been involved in the septal tear this distension may encourage profuse haemorrhage. In fact, venous distension from anoxia can itself cause rupture of one of the thin-walled poorly supported blood vessels of various organs such as the brain or adrenal glands. This is especially true of the premature infant.

SUPERFICIAL INJURIES

Abrasions, ecchymoses and patches of erythema are not infrequently caused by forceps blades. They are a possible site of entry for infection and must be treated with respect. Subconjunctival haemorrhages and petechiae over the head, neck and upper chest may arise during a long labour. They require no treatment. *Subcutaneous fat necrosis* due to localized pressure during labour is revealed by a well-circumscribed area of subcutaneous thickening. It may soften in the process of resolution and be mistaken for an abscess. There is no constitutional upset. This condition is not seen on those parts of the body such as the abdomen, axillae or inner aspects of the thighs which are protected from direct intra-uterine pressure.

CEPHALHAEMATOMA

This condition is a subperiosteal haemorrhage, most often overlying the parietal bone, rarely the frontal or occipital. It becomes obvious during the second or third days of life as the caput succedaneum subsides. It takes the form of a soft fluctuant swelling, sometimes bilateral (Fig. 7), and always limited by the periosteal attachments at the suture lines. After a week or two when the blood begins to organize and calcify there may be a hard edge with a depressed soft centre. This stage may be mistaken for a depressed fracture until it is remembered that a

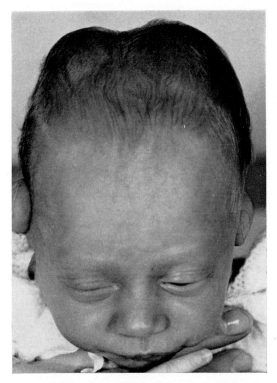

Fig. 7.—Bilateral cephalhaematoma showing distinct separation along line of the sagittal suture.

cephalhaematoma must be limited to one bone, whereas a fracture has less regard for anatomy. The condition is itself benign provided there is no intracranial lesion. Aspiration of blood from the cephalhaematoma carries the risk of introducing sepsis. It will subside spontaneously in some weeks or months if left alone.

INTRACRANIAL HAEMORRHAGE

This is the most dreaded of birth injuries, not only as one of the common causes of neonatal mortality, but also as a cause of permanent physical and mental handicap.

Aetiology

There are three important and frequently inter-related causal factors, (1) prematurity, (2) anoxia, (3) trauma. It is unlikely that hypopro-thrombinaemia plays a part, unless the intracranial bleeding is but an incident in haemorrhagic disease of the newborn (Chapter V). Prematurity is a factor in over 50 per cent of deaths from intracranial haemorrhage (Craig, 1938). Anoxia is, of course, particularly common in premature infants, either at birth or later due to hyaline membrane disease. It is especially likely to cause rupture of the fragile venae terminales in the subependymal areas surrounding the lateral ventricles. Trauma is an important cause of intracranial haemorrhage in mature infants. Manipulations, the use of forceps, breech delivery, contracted pelvis, precipitate labour and the injudicious use of oxytocic drugs all increase the risk, but the incidence has fallen with improved antenatal care and obstetric techniques.

Pathology

This has been well described by Claireaux (1959, 1960). Anoxic intracranial haemorrhage is commonest in premature infants in whom subependymal haemorrhage from the venae terminales in the walls of the lateral ventricles may disrupt the primitive glia and finally rupture into one or both ventricles. In other premature infants massive subarachnoid haemorrhage is encountered. In mature infants anoxia may cause less severe subarachnoid bleeding due to oozing from congested meningeal veins, or damage to the intracerebral capillaries may result in multiple perivascular petechiae. Traumatic haemorrhage, on the other hand, is always subdural. The bleeding arises from one of the venous sinuses which have been involved in a tear of the tentorium or falx, or from the great cerebral vein of Galen before it enters the straight sinus. Less frequently a superficial cerebral vein is torn near to its point of entry into the superior longitudinal sinus. When a subdural haemorrhage tracks beneath the tentorium it may endanger the vital centres of the medulla. Sometimes it spreads upwards over the cerebral hemispheres on one or both sides.

Clinical Features

Signs of cerebral disturbance or irritation are a common occurrence in infants who have survived a period of apnoea and anoxia in the labour room. It is, as a rule, impossible to determine whether the signs are due to temporary cerebral oedema and congestion, or whether there has been actual intracranial bleeding. The precise diagnosis is in any case academic as the treatment is the same. Such infants are born asphyxiated and shocked. Subsequently, they remain unduly lethargic, unable to suck, with irregular jerky respirations and with absence of the Moro reflex. Alternatively, they may be hyperirritable, unduly sensitive to stimuli such as noise, bright light and touch, and convulsive twitchings may occur. Some infants develop a constant wailing, or whimpering cry but the classical high-pitched "cerebral cry" is not of great diagnostic significance. The anterior fontanelle may be tense and bulging, but this may arise from cerebral oedema alone, and it need not be present in cases of intracranial haemorrhage. In premature infants the position may be complicated by the pulmonary syndrome of the newborn (RDS) (Chapter II). In fact, intracranial haemorrhage may not produce any neurological signs in these patients.

Traumatic subdural haemorrhage in the mature infant following a difficult birth can often be diagnosed with more assurance. This is especially true of the cases in which the infant appears to be in good condition at birth and who suddenly develops cerebral signs some hours or days later. When the haemorrhage is below the tentorium the infant becomes lethargic or comatose, has disordered respiration or frequent spells of apnoea, and may exhibit neck rigidity or head retraction. When the haemorrhage spreads upwards over one or other cerebral hemisphere a somewhat characteristic clinical picture is produced. There is an acute onset of irritability and convulsive movements which are often unilateral. On the side of the subdural haemorrhage the pupil is dilated and sluggish, and ptosis may be present. The anterior fontanelle is bulging and feels tense or "boggy". Diagnosis is easily confirmed by tapping the subdural space by inserting a needle through the coronal suture about ½ inch from the lateral angle of the fontanelle when dark fluid blood will drip from the needle.

Treatment

The great majority of newborn infants who exhibit signs of cerebral disturbance should be treated along conservative lines. This amounts to a minimum of gentle handling, warmth under incubator control, sufficient oxygen to abolish cyanosis, and aspiration of excess mucus from pharynx and stomach. Hyperirritability, convulsions or constant whimpering should be treated with chloral hydrate 2 gr. (120 mg.) or phenobarbitone ⅛ gr. (8 mg.) four-hourly. An intramuscular 1 mg. dose of vitamin K analogue is at least harmless. Tube-feeding is likely to be required until recovery begins. There is considerable doubt as to the value of lumbar puncture, either as a diagnostic or a therapeutic measure. Furthermore, the procedure involves handling and exposure of a gravely ill infant. There is no doubt as to the value of repeated subdural taps in relieving increased intracranial pressure in clear-cut cases of supratentorial subdural haemorrhage. Nelson (1960) has advocated turning down a bone-flap with evacuation of subdural clot in such cases. We have usually found it possible to achieve success by subdural tapping alone.

Prognosis

The frequency with which intracranial haemorrhage at birth is followed by permanent brain damage is open to doubt. One difficulty is to separate the effects of anoxia from those of actual bleeding. Massive haemorrhage is probable always fatal. There can be no doubt that less severe bleeding accounts for some cases of mental deficiency, cerebral palsy and epilepsy. It is probable, however, that most infants who survive a period of cerebral involvement in the neonatal period do not, subsequently, suffer from mental or physical handicap (Craig, 1950; 1960).

CHRONIC SUBDURAL HAEMATOMA OR HYGROMA

This condition needs to be clearly distinguished from the acute sub-dural haematoma discussed above. The aetiology of the chronic sub-dural collection of fluid is not yet satisfactorily explained. No doubt some are related to trauma occurring at birth or subsequently (Ingraham and Matson, 1944), but in the majority of cases no convincing history is obtainable and considerable doubt exists as to their traumatic origin (Baar, 1957). It may be, in fact, that the original name of *pachymeningitis haemorrhagica interna* better describes the condition.

Pathology

The condition consists of an accumulation of proteinous fluid within a membranous envelope, the outer and thicker layer of which is fused with the dura while the inner layer, fused with the arachnoid, is thinner. In early cases the fluid looks like brown altered blood, but it gradually changes to a protein-rich xanthochromic fluid which looks rather like serum but has a lower concentration of protein. This "hygroma" usually overlies the frontoparietal area and is, not infrequently, bilateral. In untreated cases irreversible cortical atrophy results from compression of the brain and permanent mental and physical disability become inevitable.

Clinical Features

Examples of this disease are rare before the age of six weeks. Most cases are not diagnosed until four months or more after birth. The affected infant becomes irritable, suffers from vomiting and fails to thrive. Intercurrent infections, fever and anaemia are commonly found. In some cases scurvy has complicated the issue. In about one half of the cases attention is drawn to the nervous system by the occurrence of convulsions. The fontanelle is often tense and bulging, a sufficiently unusual finding in the presence of marasmus to be of great diagnostic significance. Enlargement of the head may simulate hydrocephalus, but the frequent finding of retinal haemorrhages on ophthalmoscopy points towards the true diagnosis. Focal neurological signs such as hemiparesis are late in appearing and of unwelcome prognostic significance. The diagnosis must be confirmed by subdural taps which should always be performed on both sides. The extent of the fluid-containing space may be outlined by radiographs taken after replacement of some fluid by an equal volume of air.

Treatment

The head should be decompressed by frequent subdural taps. Not more than 10–15 ml. of fluid should be removed from each side at one time because of the dangers associated with too sudden a relief of intracranial pressure. In early cases this routine itself may result in complete resolution. In more chronic cases proteinous fluid which is always xanthochromic continues to accumulate. In such cases some surgeons wash out the space through burr holes, others prefer to turn down a flap and remove as much of the enveloping membrane as possible. Surgery must, however, be preceded by the measures necessary to improve the infant's general condition. These include blood transfusion for anaemia, eradication of any intercurrent infection and the correction of vitamin deficiency. Late cases are frequently associated with permanent sequelae such as hemiparesis, mental handicap and epilepsy.

FRACTURES

Fractures during the process of delivery have become infrequent in modern obstetric practice. None the less, their early diagnosis is necessary if only to save the physician the embarrassment of explaining to parents the nature of the large lump which a characteristic exuberant formation of callus subsequently produces in the newborn. Recovery is usually excellent.

Skull.—Common types are the linear or furrow-shaped groove, and the spoon-shaped or pond fracture. Surgical intervention is rarely necessary, although some recommend elevation of the pond fracture through a burr hole if it has shown no evidence of flattening out within a month. Fracture of the occipital-bone with separation of the squamous and basal portions due to traction on the head during breech delivery is, fortunately, now rare. It is usually associated with rupture of the underlying venous sinuses and fatal haemorrhage.

Clavicle.—The Moro reflex is absent in the arm of the affected side. The supraclavicular fossa may be filled in by swelling and crepitus can be elicited. The brachial plexus may also have been damaged. No specific treatment need be applied to the clavicle.

Humerus.—There may be a pseudo-paresis of the affected arm and it will not react in the Moro reflex. Crepitus can be elicited. The arm should be strapped to the chest wall for 10–14 days.

Femur.—This bone may be heard to crack during delivery. The affected leg tends to be held immobile, the Moro reflex is absent and crepitus can be felt. Treatment is to extend the limb by suspending the infant by both ankles so that the buttocks are just off the mattress. (ä· gallows traction)

NERVE INJURIES

Facial palsy.—Contusion of the extracranial portion of the facial nerve is commonly due to the pressure of a forceps blade, although it can occur in spontaneous deliveries. Diagnosis is easy. The unaffected side of the face is drawn over when the infant cries. The eye on the affected side cannot be completely closed. Recovery is usually complete within a few weeks. Absence of any recovery should suggest the possibility of the rare congenital absence of the seventh cranial nucleus. The intracranial portion of the nerve is occasionally damaged by intracranial haemorrhage or infection.

Brachial plexus palsies.—The common *Erb's palsy* is due to traction damage to the fifth and sixth cervical spinal roots. The paralyzed muscles are the supraspinatus, infraspinatus, teres minor, deltoid, brachialis anticus and supinator longus. The arm lies limp at the infant's side with the hand pronated. It does not respond in the Moro reflex. First-aid treatment is to pin the sleeve to the pillow alongside the infant's head with the hand in the position of supination. Subsequently a splint is fitted to hold the arm abducted, elbow flexed and hand supinated in front of the chest. Most patients recover in a few weeks. A few are left with permanent weakness. In the uncommon *Klumpke's palsy* the eighth cervical and first dorsal roots are damaged. This causes paralysis of the flexors and of all the intrinsic muscles of the hand. There may also be homolateral meiosis and ptosis if the cervical sympathetic fibres in the first dorsal root are involved. Treatment is to put the hand and forearm in a cock-up splint.

Phrenic nerve palsy.—As the phrenic nerve derives from the third, fourth and fifth cervical spinal segments it is sometimes associated with an Erb's type of paralysis. It should be suspected if an infant so damaged shows also dyspnoea and if the breath sounds are diminished on the affected side. Fluoroscopy reveals elevation and paradoxical movement of the paralyzed side of the diaphragm. Oxygen may be required to relieve cyanosis but the prognosis is good.

Radial nerve palsy.—Strong uterine contractions during labour sometimes damage the radial nerve as it passes round the outer side of the arm. There is often a circumscribed area of subcutaneous fat necrosis at the site of compression. The muscles affected by paralysis are the supinators and also the extensors of the hand and fingers so that there is a drop-wrist. The shoulder muscles are unaffected. The appropriate treatment is a cock-up splint.

STERNOMASTOID TUMOUR

This condition is not noticed until the third or fourth day of life when a visible swelling, palpable as a firm painless lump about 1 inch in diameter, makes its appearance in the middle or lower third of the sternomastoid muscle. It is no longer believed to be a haematoma. Some have reported it as an area of ischaemic necrosis, others regard it as a developmental dysplasia. Torticollis is not a common sequel and the condition is probably best left alone. ℞. Physiotherapy.

VISCERAL INJURIES

A relatively common injury is *subcapsular haematoma of the liver*. It is usually associated with severe anoxia especially in breech deliveries, and may develop in haemorrhagic disease of the newborn (Chapter V). The signs are pallor, shock, restlessness and a palpable mass in the right hypochondrium. Blood transfusion should be followed by laparotomy for evacuation of clot and arrest of haemorrhage. *Adrenal haemorrhage* is also more common in breech cases and is also probably an anoxic phenomenon. It is most often fatal and the infant becomes rapidly shocked and cyanosed. Less severe cases are compatible with recovery, and bilateral adrenal calcification has occasionally been found in radiographs of older children (Stevenson *et al.*, 1961). *Renal vein thrombosis* is usually related to postnatal infections or severe dehydration, but it may also occur in severe neonatal anoxia. The presenting signs are albuminuria and haematuria. The resulting haemorrhagic infarction of the kidney may cause such enlargement as to produce a palpable mass in the loin. Bilateral cases end in death from uraemia. When a unilateral mass is found nephrectomy should be undertaken. In a review of cases of renal vein thrombosis from a variety of causes McFarland (1965) reached the conclusion that nephrectomy is best delayed until the acute episode has subsided, the only exception to this rule being when it is not possible to differentiate between renal infarction and tumour.

COLD INJURY OF THE NEWBORN

This injury differs from the others discussed in this chapter in that it happens after the second stage of labour has been completed. The cause is almost always chilling of the body surface at or after delivery in a cold room. It may occur without undue exposure to cold in premature infants and in the presence of intracranial haemorrhage or severe infection. None the less, infants die needlessly every winter because the danger of leaving the newborn in a cold room is insufficiently appreciated by doctors as well as parents. The ritual of the daily bath is particularly dangerous in a poorly warmed room. The condition is by no means confined to poorer homes and many a British middle-class house is uncomfortably cold in winter. Good accounts have been given of cold injury by Mann and Elliott (1957), Bower *et al.* (1960), and Arneil and Kerr (1963).

Clinical Features

The affected infant after a good start to life becomes lethargic, cries only infrequently and feebly, and becomes disinclined for feeds. Pitting oedema often develops over the limbs, and the eyelids may appear puffy. The body skin feels cold to the touch, and the face, hands and feet often have a striking red colour which we have seen to be misinterpreted as a sign of wellbeing. A rubbery hardening of the skin and subcutaneous tissues (sclerema) may be found, especially over the cheeks, buttocks and thighs. The heart rate is at first elevated but this gives way to bradycardia when the rectal temperature falls below 90° F. Haemorrhage from stomach or bowel may occur, but most common is massive intrapulmonary haemorrhage which may result in the appearance of blood-stained frothy mucus in the nose and throat. Hypoglycaemia is a common finding and there may be raised levels of urea, potassium and phosphate.

Prevention

It cannot be stressed too strongly that the newborn infant must not be delivered or nursed in a room temperature below 65° F. The coal fire is an inadequate source of heat as it is apt to go out during the hours of sleep. Daily bathing should be forbidden unless an adequately heated room is assured. The infant must be warmly but not tightly clothed, and the cot temperature maintained above 85° F. with hot-water bottles or an electric pad. Rectal temperature should be recorded by the doctor or nurse at each visit, using a low-reading thermometer (85–110° F.). A rectal temperature below 95° F. is a clear danger signal. If a newborn infant requires to be transferred to hospital a portable incubator should be used.

Treatment

The hypothermic infant should not be warmed up quickly as this warms up the superficial tissues while the deep vital organs remain hypothermic and unable to cope with increased demands upon them. The infant is best placed in an incubator at a temperature of 80–85° F. and slowly warmed to 95° F. over the next 36 hours. The hypoglycaemia can be corrected with an intragastric drip of 20 per cent glucose solution, but the dangers of regurgitation and aspiration are thought by some to outweigh the advantages. Protection against bacterial infection must be obtained by the intramuscular administration of a broad spectrum antibiotic. A rectal temperature below 90° F. is associated with a mortality rate of at least 25 per cent.

REFERENCES

ARNEIL, G. C., and KERR, M. M. (1963). *Lancet*, **2**, 765.
BAAR, H. S. (1957). *Lancet*, **1**, 1349.

BOWER, B. D., JONES, L. F., and WEEKS, M. M. (1960). *Brit. med. J.*, **1**, 303.

CLAIREAUX, A. E. (1959). *Guy's Hosp. Rep.*, **108**, 2.

CLAIREAUX, A. E. (1960). *J. Obstet. Gynaec. Brit. Emp.*, **67**, 763.

CRAIG, W. S. (1938). *Arch. Dis. Childh.*, **13**. 89

CRAIG, W. S. (1950). *Arch. Dis. Childh.*, **25**, 325.

CRAIG, W. S. (1960). *Arch. Dis. Childh.*, **35**, 336.

INGRAHAM, F. D., and MATSON, D. D. (1944). *J. Pediat.*, **24**, 1.

MCFARLAND, J. B. (1965). *Quart. J. Med.*, **34**, 269.

MANN, T. P., and ELLIOTT, R. I. K. (1957). *Lancet*, **1**, 229.

NELSON, T. Y. (1960). *Clin. Rep. Adelaide Child. Hosp.*, **3**, 215.

STEVENSON, J., MACGREGOR, A. M., and CONNELLY, P. (1961). *Arch. Dis. Childh.*, **36**, 316.

CHAPTER IV

NEONATAL JAUNDICE

Jaundice developing during the neonatal period has always interested physicians. Its causes, until recent years, were poorly understood and it was frequently followed by permanent neurological sequelae of a type not seen in jaundiced adults. Recent advances in our knowledge of the physiology of bilirubin excretion (Billing and Lathe, 1958; Schmid, 1958; Sherlock, 1962) have made possible a much clearer understanding of the pathogenesis and effects of neonatal jaundice.

PHYSIOLOGY OF BILIRUBIN EXCRETION

The chemical steps by which haemoglobin is converted into bilirubin are not fully understood but the process is a function of the reticulo-endothelial system. The bilirubin so formed gives an indirect reaction with the Van den Bergh reagents and is often called "indirect" or free bilirubin. It is carried in the plasma bound to albumin. In the liver it is mostly conjugated to glucuronic acid to form bilirubin diglucuronide which is then excreted into the intercellular bile canaliculi. Conjugated bilirubin is not normally present in the blood in significant amounts, but reflux into the circulation occurs if there is an obstruction in the biliary system or severe damage to the liver parenchymal cells. It will then give a direct Van den Bergh reaction and it is often called "direct" bilirubin.

The conjugation of free or "indirect" bilirubin to glucuronic acid to form conjugated or "direct" bilirubin takes place in the liver parenchyma by a series of enzyme reactions (Fig. 8). The final step is dependent on a microsomal enzyme, glucuronyl transferase, which brings about the transfer of glucuronic acid from uridine diphosphoglucuronic acid (UDPGA) to bilirubin, thus forming bilirubin diglucuronide. UDPGA is the only form in which glucuronic acid is available for conjugation. It should be stated that several other substances, including steroids, salicylates, menthol, aniline and chloramphenicol are excreted along the same pathway. It should also be noted that the various steps in bilirubin conjugation involve both nucleotide and carbohydrate metabolism (Fig. 8). The availability of glucose is, therefore, of importance in bilirubin excretion. Another pigment, identified as bilirubin monoglucuronide has also been demonstrated in human serum (Cole and Lathe, 1953; Billing, 1955). It seems to be formed outside the liver but its function, if any, in the newborn is unknown. It also gives a direct Van den Bergh reaction. There is, furthermore, evidence that other pathways of bilirubin excretion exist besides glucuronation (Isselbacher and McCarthy, 1958). One of these is by conjugation to sulphate, but the newborn is apparently unable to use this pathway to compensate for defective glucuronation.

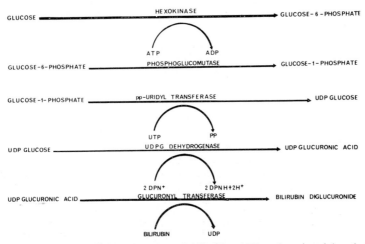

FIG. 8.—Enzyme steps in conjugation of bilirubin. ATP=adenosinetriphosphate; ADP=adenosinediphosphate; UTP=uridinetriphosphate; PP=pyrophosphate; DPN=oxidised diphosphopyridine nucleotide; DPNH=reduced diphosphopyridine nucleotide; UDP=uridine diphosphate.

From the point of view of the newborn infant the importance of the conjugation of bilirubin to glucuronic acid lies in the change in the solubility of bilirubin which this process brings about. Free or "indirect" bilirubin is insoluble in water so that it cannot be excreted by the kidneys or in the bile. Because it is fat-soluble, however, it can enter the brain or the subcutaneous adipose tissues, especially if high serum levels exist. As the premature infant lacks subcutaneous fat there may be greater danger of "indirect" bilirubin entering the nervous system where it is highly toxic (kernicterus—p. 53). Conjugated or "direct" bilirubin is, on the other hand, soluble in water and so readily excreted in the urine or bile, and as it is not soluble in fat it is not toxic to the nervous system.

An abnormally high level of "indirect" bilirubin may develop in the blood of the newborn under two conditions. Firstly, a deficiency in the liver of the activity of glucuronyl transferase will result in a high serum "indirect" bilirubin, derived from the normal rate of red cell breakdown. Such a deficiency or immaturity of this enzyme system is common, especially in the premature infant (Brown and Zuelzer, 1958). The situation in the premature infant may be further complicated by a lack of available glucose for the formation of UDPGA (Zuelzer and Brown, 1961). Secondly, a raised serum "indirect" bilirubin level can arise from increased production due to haemolytic anaemia. In some cases both factors are operative. For example, dangerous levels of "indirect" bilirubin are rare in the adult with haemolytic anaemia because the liver has an enormous reserve capacity for glucuronation, whereas a similar degree of haemolysis in the newborn is quite beyond the capacity of the enzyme system concerned. The danger of a high serum "indirect" bilirubin level is, of course, that this fat-soluble pigment may gain entry to the cells of the central nervous system (Claireaux *et al.*, 1953). On the other hand, an abnormally high level of "direct" or conjugated bilirubin may develop in the blood if there is biliary obstruction or severe hepatocellular damage. There is, however, no danger of the water soluble "direct" bilirubin entering the nervous system.

The type of jaundice due to a high level of "indirect" bilirubin is called *non-obstructive*, whereas that involving reflux into the blood from the liver of "direct" bilirubin is *obstructive*. It is, of course, possible for both types to co-exist.

NON-OBSTRUCTIVE JAUNDICE

"PHYSIOLOGICAL" JAUNDICE

The serum "indirect" bilirubin level rises above the adult level (0·8 mg. per 100 ml.) in most newborn infants. Some develop icterus on the second or third day of life. These infants are not ill and they show no evidence of excess haemolysis. The icterus fades in 7–10 days. This has long been known as "physiological jaundice" although it is better regarded as a functional immaturity of the glucuronyl transferase enzyme system. No treatment is required.

JAUNDICE OF PREMATURITY

(see also Chapter II)

In premature infants jaundice is commonly due to an even more immature enzyme system. The postnatal rise in serum "indirect" bilirubin occurs somewhat later than in mature infants, but dangerously high levels (above 24 mg. per 100 ml.) may develop between the sixth and eighth days of life—*hyperbilirubinaemia*. In premature infants recovering from hyaline membrane disease the hyperbilirubinaemia may be further aggravated by a diminished supply of available glucose for the formation of UDPGA. The occurrence of brain damage from high serum levels of "indirect" bilirubin (kernicterus) in prematurity is well established. There is, however, wide variation in the reported incidence of this complication of the hyperbilirubinaemia of prematurity. No doubt several factors can explain these differences. Three are the variable use and dosage of water soluble vitamin K analogues (e.g. Synkavit), of sulphafurazole (Gantrisin), and of novobiocin.

Vitamin K analogues.—There can be no doubt that Synkavit and other diphosphate derivatives of menaphthone raise the serum bilirubin levels in premature infants when given intramuscularly in doses of 10 mg. or more (Bound and Telfer, 1956; Meyer and Angus, 1956). Their action is probably haemolytic. As it is known that a dose of 1 mg. is as effective in preventing hypoprothrombinaemia as are larger doses, it is important that the maximum permissible dosage be limited to 2 mg. Vitamin K_1 (phytomenadione B.P.) does not raise the serum bilirubin level and is now available for intramuscular injection (see p. 63).

Sulphafurazole.—This sulphonamide is widely used because of its solubility. However, it increases the risk of kernicterus in premature infants (Silverman *et al.*, 1956), even when the serum bilirubin levels are below the 24 mg. per 100 ml. "danger" level. It seems that sulphafurazole has a greater affinity for circulating serum albumin than bilirubin which is, thereby, displaced to enter the tissues of the brain. This drug should, obviously, never be prescribed in the neonatal period.

Novobiocin.—More recently evidence has accrued to show that this antibiotic can interfere with the enzyme glucuronyl transferase, and that it increases the risk of kernicterus in the newborn (Sutherland and Keller, 1961; Hargreaves and Holton, 1962). It is probably never essential to prescribe this drug during the first month of life.

Several other factors are also concerned in influencing the susceptibility of the jaundiced premature infant to kernicterus. Thus, salicylates or heparin administered to the pregnant woman may cross the placenta and displace bilirubin from its binding sites on the infant's serum albumin. Hypoalbuminaemia is not uncommon in small prematures and the reduced amount of albumin available for binding bilirubin may well be crucial. Situations which result in asphyxia, a lowered blood pH or hypoglycaemia predispose to kernicterus, probably by damaging the nerve cells and rendering them more permeable to bilirubin.

Treatment

There is only one method of proven efficiency in lowering the bilirubin levels of the serum and tissues and that is replacement transfusion. The value of this technique in haemolytic disease of the newborn is beyond doubt. The indications are less clear in the hyperbilirubinaemia of prematurity. The risks in feeble premature infants are not inconsiderable. It is often impossible to determine in which infants dangerous levels of bilirubin may develop. Furthermore, the incidence of kernicterus seems to vary widely from one centre to another, probably being affected by iatrogenic factors like the use of vitamin K, and the incidence in different regions of such maternal influences as toxaemia and antepartum haemorrhage. It is our practice to administer vitamin K in 1–2 mg. doses only in overt haemorrhagic disease, and the incidence of kernicterus in premature infants has been almost nil. We only advocate replacement transfusion in the jaundice of prematurity if the serum bilirubin level remains over 24 mg. per 100 ml. for several successive days. We have found this to be rare.

OTHER NON-HAEMOLYTIC CAUSES OF HYPERBILIRUBINAEMIA

In rare circumstances abnormally high levels of "indirect" bilirubin may develop in the serum of the mature infant in the absence of excess haemolysis. One of these is *congenital familial non-haemolytic jaundice* (Crigler and Najjar, 1952) in which several infants in a family, often of a consanguineous mating, develop severe jaundice in the neonatal period. Some of these patients have died of kernicterus. This disease is an inborn error of metabolism in which there is an absence or deficiency of glucuronyl transferase enzyme activity. In *cretinism* there is sometimes a prolonged postnatal jaundice (Åkerrén, 1954), probably due to delayed maturation of the enzyme system in the presence of hypothyroidism. We have also seen prolonged jaundice in a few infants with *pyloric stenosis.* It has been suggested that this could be due to a disturbed carbohydrate metabolism leading to an insufficient production of UDPGA (Zuelzer and Brown, 1961). The jaundice in cretinism and pyloric stenosis disappears when the primary disease is treated.

HAEMOLYTIC DISEASE IN THE NEWBORN

Excessive haemolysis in the newborn infant most often results from incompatibility of the maternal and foetal blood groups. The Rhesus groups are the most important but other systems such as ABO, Kell, Lewis, Duffy and Kidd may also result in haemolytic disease. In certain parts of the world a genetically determined deficiency of the erythrocytic enzyme glucose-6-phosphate dehydrogenase is a common and important cause.

RHESUS INCOMPATIBILITY

Aetiology

About 83 per cent of Europeans carry the Rhesus antigen in their red cells (Rh positive). The remaining 17 per cent do not possess this antigen and are referred to as Rh negative. Haemolytic disease of the newborn occurs when the mother (usually Rh negative) and the foetus (usually Rh positive) are of different groups. When foetal red cells enter the maternal circulation the mother may become sensitized to the Rh antigen and form Rh antibodies (isoimmunization). Later in pregnancy these maternal Rh antibodies cross the placenta in the opposite direction to act upon the foetal red cells. It is exceedingly rare for the first infant to be affected but this can occur if a mother has been previously sensitized to the Rh antigen by a transfusion of Rh incompatible blood or the miscarriage of a Rh positive foetus. It is most important, therefore, to avoid transfusing a female patient with Rh incompatible blood. Although some 14 per cent of marriages are between Rh negative women and Rh positive men the incidence of haemolytic disease is only about 6 per 1000 births (Walker, 1959).

Since Landsteiner and Wiener first described the Rhesus factor in 1940 it has been shown that it includes, in fact, six antigens in the red cells, C,c, D,d, E,e, which are determined by three allelomorphic pairs of genes, similarly labelled. A mother may, therefore, be sensitized by any of these antigens which she herself does not possess. The most important is D antigen, those who possess it being called Rh (D) positive, whereas those who do not are Rh (D) negative. The three genes C or c, D or d, and E or e are carried close together on the same chromosome. There are eight possible combinations of genes on one chromosome, in descending order of frequency, CDe, cde, cDE, cDe, cdE, Cde, CDE and CdE. In the somatic cells there are, of course, two such chromosomes. The commonest genotypes in the U.K. are CDe/cde, CDe/CDE, cde/cde, CDe/cDE, and cDE/cde (Mollison *et al.*, 1948). The genotype of the husband of a Rh negative woman is important. If he is homozygous (D/D) with two D genes all his children must receive a D gene, so that once haemolytic disease has made its appearance all subsequent children of the marriage will be similarly affected. When, however, the father is heterozygous Rh positive (D/d) half his children will inherit d. As they will also have inherited d from their Rh negative (d/d) mother they will be Rh (D) negative and so unaffected by the disease. The great majority of cases of Rh sensitization involve D antigen but in a few cases other antigens (e.g. c) are at fault. These explain the cases of haemolytic disease which occur in the offspring of Rh (D) positive women.

Pathology

The liver and spleen are greatly enlarged and they are the seat of extensive extramedullary erythropoiesis. The liver parenchyma cells and Kupffer cells contain haemosiderin and the Prussian blue reaction is positive (Claireaux, 1960).

Clinical Features

(A) **Foetus affected.**—The disease develops severely during foetal life in a minority of cases. It may then result in a stillbirth, intra-uterine death with the subsequent delivery of a macerated foetus, or in the birth of a live infant with *hydrops foetalis*. The last is rarely compatible with life beyond a few hours. The infant is born grossly oedematous and with hepatosplenomegaly. The placenta is large, pale and oedematous, and the liquor amnii has a golden yellow colour. The presence of hydrops foetalis may frequently be recognized antenally by radiography. The oedematous scalp may be visualized as a "halo" around the foetal skull. The greatly distended foetal abdomen may cause a loss of flexion of the vertebral column and flaring outwards of the subcostal angle. The overall risk of stillbirth is 15 per cent. If no previous infant has been affected it is about 8 per cent. A previous severely affected infant increases the incidence to 50 per cent. A previous stillbirth increases it still further to 70 per cent (Walker, 1959).

(B) **Infant affected.**—In the great majority of cases the infant is born apparently normal but subsequently develops signs of the disease. In the most common form, *icterus gravis*, jaundice appears within minutes or hours of birth. It may become intense and has a characteristic golden yellow colour. In severe untreated cases purpura and other haemorrhages may develop. The spleen and liver are greatly enlarged. The peripheral blood shows anaemia, reticulocytosis, many erythroblasts and normoblasts, and immature white cells of the granular series. The serum "indirect" bilirubin reaches high levels in untreated cases. There is also some increase in the "direct" bilirubin with bile in the urine. Indeed, before the days of exchange transfusion some infants showed a subsequent prolonged elevation of serum "direct" bilirubin with pale acholic stools. This is called the *inspissated bile syndrome*, and it recovered spontaneously but slowly. The danger of kernicterus (p. 53) in untreated cases of icterus gravis is great. Less frequently the disease takes the form of a *haemolytic anaemia* which develops shortly after birth and in which jaundice is absent or quite minimal. The presenting sign is pallor of a rapidly progressive degree in association with splenomegaly, erythroblastaemia and reticulocytosis. Bile is absent from the urine although there is an excess of urobilinogen.

Diagnosis

It is, in most instances, possible to predict the appearance of haemolytic disease during pregnancy, and by timely treatment to prevent most of the serious manifestations described above. The rhesus and ABO blood groups of every pregnant woman should be determined early in pregnancy. In the case of Rh (D) negative women the serum should be tested for Rh antibodies then and periodically throughout the pregnancy. The finding of antibody is a strong indication that the infant may be affected and the mother should be delivered in hospital where replacement transfusion can be carried out. In the case of women who have had previously affected infants the husband's Rh genotype must also be determined to help in more accurate prediction. The history of the previous pregnancies is often some indication of the probable severity of the disease. In some families the disease pattern tends to be similar in each pregnancy; in others succeeding infants show a worsening severity (Allen and Diamond, 1958).

Antenatal Management

Following the publication of Liley (1961) we have increasingly used the technique of spectrophotometric examination of amniotic fluid obtained by amniocentesis from about the 28th week of pregnancy, or even earlier in a few cases, to predict the probable severity of the disease. This method gives an accuracy of prediction above 95 per cent, so permitting infants seriously at risk to be delivered *before* they are hydropic or moribund and considerably reducing the over-all mortality rate (Bowman and Pollock, 1965).

When fresh normal liquor is examined by spectrophotometry, the optical density being plotted on a logarithmic scale against wave length, virtually a straight line is obtained from 365 mμ to 600 mμ. In the presence of haemolytic disease of the newborn a peak is found, centred on 450 mμ. This rise in optical density at 450 mμ, due to at least seven bilirubinoid protein-bound pigments, is the figure of prognostic value. The actual figure is obtained by drawing a tangent to the absorption curve connecting 550 mμ with 365 mμ and measuring from the point at which this line intersects 450 mμ to the actual optical density reading at 450 mμ. This figure of the optical density line is then plotted using optical density as the logarithmic vertical co-ordinate and the gestation in weeks as the horizontal linear co-ordinate. Liley (1961) divided this graph into three zones. Liquor falling into the upper zone (Zone III) indicates severe foetal disease and impending intra-uterine death. Liquor falling into the middle zone (Zone II) indicates moderately severe disease. Liquor falling into the lowest zone (Zone I) indicates a mildly affected or unaffected foetus. The pigment peak measured as outlined above shows a close correlation with simultaneous cord haemoglobin level (Liley, 1961). Even more accurate prediction is achieved by repeating the amniocentesis and spectrophotometric examination every few weeks, because a pigment peak which is not remarkable at 28 weeks gestation may become sinister by 35 or 36 weeks.

The indications for amniocentesis must be determined in relation to the risks, which are sufficient to negative its use in all iso-immunized women. The maternal risk is very small provided it is never performed after 36 weeks gestation. There is, however, a risk to the foetus if the placenta is damaged so that leakage of foetal erythrocytes takes place into the maternal circulation with an increase in the severity of the iso-immunization. Improved methods of placentography as by ultra-sonography, may in future reduce this hazard. Our present indications for amniocentesis are, (i) in all sensitized pregnant women with a history of a preceding stillbirth or of an infant severely enough affected to require exchange transfusion; (ii) in all first sensitized pregnancies in which the indirect Coombs' antibody titre exceeds 1:8 by 32 weeks gestation.

By means of such serial amniocenteses it is possible to follow the progression of the haemolytic disease and the graphs can be used to arrange the optimal management. Thus, cases falling into Zone I may safely be allowed to go to full term. On the other hand, in Zone II are the babies with significant anaemia; while premature delivery is necessary a reasonable maturity, not less than 34 weeks, can still be obtained. It is in this group of patients that amniocentesis produces the greatest improvement in mortality because it obviates stillbirth or the birth of a moribund infant, while still permitting the best possible maturity in the individual case. The small number of cases falling in Zone III, and which show very large pigment peaks, will end in foetal death or hydrops before 34 weeks gestation. Premature induction has little to offer in this group because the combination of extreme prematurity and severe haemolytic disease constitutes a desperate situation. It is for these babies that the technique of *intra-uterine transfusion* has been developed and seems likely to be a considerable advance (Liley, 1965). Our own experience with this treatment has been encouraging although the actual technique is, of course, a matter for the obstetrician after consultation with the haematologist and the paediatrician. It must be stressed that intra-uterine transfusion is only indicated in a small minority of cases, probably under 10 per cent of sensitized pregnancies. Technical details have been given by Liley (1965). The first transfusion is usually indicated, on the results of amniocentesis, between 28 and 32 weeks. Second and third transfusions at intervals of $1\frac{1}{2}$ to 3 weeks may be required to delay delivery of the baby until 34 weeks or later. Thereafter the management of the infant, who will certainly require one or more replacement transfusions, becomes the responsibility of the paediatrician.

Postnatal Management

The correct use of replacement transfusion is the only means whereby death from heart failure or kernicterus can be prevented in severe cases. Prompt treatment can ensure the survival of more than 95 per cent of all affected infants who are born alive. At birth a specimen of blood should be collected from the maternal end of the umbilical cord. The diagnosis is then confirmed by Coombs' direct anti-human-globulin test (Mollison *et al.*, 1948) which detects the presence of antibody bound to the infant's red cells. The same specimen of cord blood is tested for haemoglobin and bilirubin levels. The indications for replacement transfusion are:

1. A birth weight of $5\frac{1}{2}$ lb. or less.
2. A history of a previous severely affected infant or stillbirth.

In the absence of 1 and 2 the indications are:

3. A cord Hb. level below 15 mg. per 100 ml.
4. A cord bilirubin level above 5 mg. per 100 ml.
5. The development of more than mild jaundice in the first 24 hours of life.

The purposes of the early exchange transfusion are to correct anaemia, to remove damaged and antibody-coated red cells from the circulation, and to remove unfixed antibodies. The donor blood should be Rh negative, preferably of the same ABO group as the infant's, and it should also be compatible with the mother's serum by the indirect antiglobulin technique. It should not be more than 5 days old. As ill infants usually have a metabolic acidosis which can readily be aggravated by donor blood with a low pH (Barrie, 1965) it has become our practice to inject 1 ml. (1 mEq.) of 8·4 per cent sodium bicarbonate after each 100 ml. of acid-citrate-dextrose blood during the first exchange transfusion. As the citrate is metabolized there is a later tendency towards metabolic alkalosis and sodium bicarbonate should not be given during subsequent exchanges. We also inject 1 ml. of 10 per cent calcium gluconate with each 100 ml. of blood. The total volume of blood usually removed amounts to 80 ml. per lb. (175 ml. per Kg.) with the replacement of about 40 ml. less over the complete transfusion. When possible the supernatant plasma should be removed so that concentrated red cells are given to the infant.

Subsequent exchange transfusions will be required if the serum "indirect" bilirubin level rises above 20 mg. per 100 ml. during the first 5 days. The aim here is simply to remove the toxic "indirect" bilirubin from the serum and tissues of the infant, and so to obviate the danger of kernicterus. It is important that the exchange transfusion be performed slowly because this has been shown to result in the removal of larger quantities of bilirubin from the tissues.

After the immediate emergency has passed the infant should be kept under careful supervision as an out-patient for some weeks. It is not uncommon for red cell production to be low for some weeks and a small "boost" transfusion (10 ml. per lb. body weight; 20 ml./Kg.) is indicated if the Hb. level falls below 9 gm. per 100 ml. This may also be necessary in those infants who develop haemolytic anaemia as the sole manifestation of the disease.

The sophisticated techniques which have been described above to rescue the most severely affected foetuses may in the future be rendered rarely necessary by the development of methods which will prevent the production of anti-rhesus antibodies in Rhesus negative mothers (Combined Study, 1966). This protection is obtained by giving to mothers, in whose blood foetal cells are discovered after the delivery of a Rhesus positive baby, an injection of a suitable gamma globulin containing a very high titre of incomplete anti-D rhesus antibody. This technique is not yet a practical proposition because of the difficulty of obtaining large quantities of suitable gamma globulin, but when this difficulty is overcome haemolytic disease due to Rhesus incompatibility is likely to become rare.

ABO INCOMPATIBILITY

Cases of ABO incompatibility are probably not uncommon but tend to be mild, so that some are mistaken for "physiological" jaundice. However, jaundice which develops within 24 hours of birth is never to be regarded as benign. An unusually severe degree of jaundice (about 18 mg. per 100 ml.) in a mature infant should also indicate the need for full haematological investigation. The blood groups of both infant and mother should be determined if they are not already known. If they are potentially incompatible (e.g. mother O, infant A or B) the mother's serum must be examined for immune type antibodies specific for A or B antigens. In ABO incompatibility the direct Coombs' test in the infant is usually negative. This type of haemolytic disease is rarely predictable antenatally. Fortunately, there is no emergency in this situation. Replacement transfusion is only required if the serum "indirect" bilirubin rises above 20 mg. per 100 ml. Group O blood of homologous Rhesus group should be used.

GLUCOSE-6-PHOSPHATE DEHYDROGENASE (G.-6-P.D.) DEFICIENCY

A variety of substances which include primaquine, nitrofurantoin, naphthalene and fava beans can produce an acute haemolysis in certain apparently healthy people. It has been shown that this is due to the defective activity of an enzyme, G.-6-P.D., which has the function of maintaining glutathione in a reduced state in the erythrocytes (Carson *et al.*, 1956). This inborn deficiency is transmitted as a sex-linked recessive characteristic. It is common in certain races and areas of the world, e.g. in negroes, and in Greece, Sardinia, Spain, Singapore and Israel.

In the neonatal period G.-6-P.D. deficiency can cause a degree of haemolysis sufficient to raise the serum "indirect" bilirubin to dangerous levels in the absence of an exogenous factor such as primaquine etc. There have been several reports from Greece (Doxiadis *et al.*, 1961), Singapore (Smith and Vella, 1960) and Hong Kong (Yue and Strickland, 1965) that neonatal jaundice requiring exchange transfusion to prevent kernicterus was often due to G.-6-P.D. deficiency. Blood group incompatibility and prematurity were excluded in these cases although no doubt transient immaturity of the glucuronyl transferase enzyme system would often coexist. In these neonatal cases the jaundice has not been confined to male infants so that the sex-linked gene cannot be completely recessive (Doxiadis and Valaes, 1964). This is not a common cause of neonatal jaundice in the United Kingdom but it is clearly of great importance to the clinician practising amongst certain racial groups.

ACHOLURIC JAUNDICE (CONGENITAL SPHEROCYTOSIS)

It is uncommon for this hereditary disease which is transmitted as a Mendelian dominant trait (Chapter XIX) to manifest itself during the neonatal period. On occasion it may do so, and we have had to submit three infants in one family to splenectomy during early infancy because of persistent jaundice and anaemia. Whenever possible, however, splenectomy should be avoided during the first year of life because of the subsequent increased susceptibility to bacterial infection. Rarely, exchange transfusion is necessary in the neonatal period to prevent kernicterus. The spleen is enlarged. The blood shows anaemia with a reticulocytosis, some erythroblastaemia, increased fragility of the red cells and microspherocytosis. The "indirect" serum bilirubin is raised and there is urobilinogenuria.

KERNICTERUS

Kernicterus or nuclear jaundice may arise from any cause which raises the serum "indirect" bilirubin level above 20 mg. per 100 ml. The most common are prematurity when it appears between 6–8 days, and haemolytic disease of newborn when it develops in the first 4 days. It may be caused by congenital familial non-haemolytic jaundice, cytomegalic inclusion disease, neonatal hepatitis and congenital spherocytosis. Its relationship to vitamin K, sulphafurazole, novobiocin and other factors has already been discussed (p. 45).

Pathology

It is believed that bilirubin damages the neurones by interfering with certain enzyme actions, particularly oxidative phosphorylation (Zetterström and Ernster, 1956). Its conjugation with glucuronic acid renders it non-toxic because it loses its fat-solubility. The brain is stained yellow but certain structures, the corpus striatum, thalamus, sub-thalamic nuclei, hippocampus, nucleus of the third nerve, mammillary bodies, red nucleus and nuclei on the floor of the fourth ventricle, are intensely coloured. In older infants who have survived the acute stage there is a marked loss of nerve cells and replacement gliosis (Claireaux, 1960).

Clinical Features

In the acute stage various obvious neurological disturbances are seen. These include rolling of the eyes, marked lethargy, convulsions, refusal to suck, increased muscle tone, head retraction or opisthotonus. The

Moro reflex is absent or diminished. If the infant survives the period of intense jaundice, later in the first year he develops spasms of muscular rigidity, opisthotonus and sometimes convulsive seizures. After the age of 2 years he shows the typical picture of athetosis with muscle tension. There may be pyramidal signs but extrapyramidal rigidity is more common. High-tone deafness is present and this leads to interference with the acquisition of speech. This in turn tends to make the mental retardation which is always present seem more severe than is really the case. In addition to producing nuclear jaundice, hyperbilirubinaemia affects the growing tooth buds so that the first dentition may show an unwelcome green staining, sometimes a visible line of hypoplasia of the enamel and dentine between the antenatal and postnatal parts.

Prevention

Once established kernicterus is irreversible. The only means of prevention of proved effectiveness is replacement transfusion. This not only removes bilirubin from the plasma but also from the tissue cells themselves (Lathe, 1955). The indications for replacement transfusion have already been discussed (p. 51).

OBSTRUCTIVE JAUNDICE

While the differential diagnosis between the different causes of non-obstructive jaundice is rarely difficult, it is often extremely hard to establish the correct diagnosis in cases of obstructive jaundice characterized by a high serum "direct" bilirubin, pale acholic stools and the presence of bile in the urine.

Congenital Biliary Atresia

This is the most common form of neonatal biliary obstruction with an incidence of 1 in 20,000 births. There may be other congenital anomalies especially of the renal tract.

Pathology

There are two types, extrahepatic and intrahepatic (Claireaux, 1960). The former is more common. Many variants occur but in most cases the whole extrahepatic biliary apparatus is missing. Biliary cirrhosis develops with perilobular fibrosis and proliferation of the small bile ducts. Bile plugs are numerous in the intercellular canaliculi. The intrahepatic variety is rare and compatible with life for several years. The gall-bladder and common bile duct may be normal but there is periportal fibrosis and intrahepatic bile ducts are scanty or absent. Bile thrombi are present in the intercellular canaliculi.

Clinical Features

The presenting sign is jaundice. This may appear soon after birth, more often during the second or third weeks. It may fluctuate in intensity but is of a deep green colour. The liver becomes enormously enlarged with a hard smooth edge. The veins over the abdominal wall are often dilated. Ascites is common. The stools are acholic and putty-coloured, although in some cases a little pigment reaches the stools from desquamation of intensely bile-stained intestinal epithelium. Bile is present in the urine but urobilinogen is absent. Liver function tests are usually normal and unhelpful in diagnosis. Intrahepatic cases are less severe and the jaundice may never become deep. The serum cholesterol level is often high and xanthomatous plaques frequently develop in the skin.

Management

It is frequently impossible to differentiate between biliary atresia and neonatal hepatitis without liver biopsy. Our practice is to observe such cases for several weeks in the hope that spontaneous recovery may begin. If the serum level of conjugated bilirubin remains constant or increases progressively, laparotomy is advised. This permits of an adequate biopsy and direct cholangiography with radio-opaque medium on which evidence a firm diagnosis and prognosis can be based. It is, unfortunately, quite rare for the surgeon to be able to construct a channel between the liver and the intestine and most infants with extrahepatic biliary atresia die within a year. Intrahepatic cases, on the other hand, have been known to survive into adolescence.

Other Causes of Obstruction of the Bile Ducts

It is well always to keep in mind the possibility of such rare causes of jaundice in the infant as intrahepatic tumours like primary hepatoma, haemangioma, and malignant reticulosis (Letterer-Siwe disease). We have also seen congenital myelogenous leukaemia present with deep jaundice and spontaneous haemorrhages. Very rarely a choledochal cyst may present in the young infant with jaundice and an abdominal mass.

Neonatal Hepatitis

Aetiology

This relatively common disease has often been assumed to be a viral infection. This is based on the observation by Stokes *et al.* (1951) that serum from an affected infant and his mother produced hepatitis in volunteers. It is, however, quite exceptional for the mother of an infant with hepatitis to give any history of recent illness and there is no direct evidence that a virus is, in fact, the cause of this disease. An alternative explanation has been that the condition is not infective at all but represents a maldevelopment of the intercellular bile canaliculi (Smetana and Johnson, 1955). Hsia *et al.* (1958) conducted a statistical analysis which suggested that the "hepatitis" might be determined by an autosomal recessive gene. Danks and Bodian (1963) have reached a similar conclusion.

Pathology

The characteristic histological features are a complete loss of the normal pattern of hepatic lobules, and the presence of many multinucleated giant cells, showing degenerative changes and the intracellular deposition of bile pigment and haemosiderin (Claireaux, 1960; Zuelzer and Brown, 1961). There is an increase of fibrous tissue around the necrotic liver cells and in the portal tracts. Bile thrombi may be numerous. The extrahepatic bile ducts are normally formed.

Clinical Features

The onset is insidious. It is frequently difficult to determine the date of onset because "physiological" jaundice may be immediately followed by the obstructive jaundice of this disease. Weight gain slows down or stops and vomiting is common. The jaundice is usually but not invariably intense in degree. The stools are pale but not always completely acholic. The urine is heavily bile stained, but urobilinogen may or may not be detectable. The liver is grossly enlarged with a hard smooth edge. Splenomegaly is almost invariable. Liver function tests are only sometimes abnormal but this finding would make biliary atresia less likely as a diagnosis. Significant in this respect would be abnormal thymol or zinc sulphate turbidity tests or a raised serum level of glutamic oxalacetic transaminase. Frequently the differential diagnosis is only made after a liver biopsy, which we prefer to accomplish by laparotomy.

Management

The mortality rate in neonatal hepatitis is at least 25 per cent. It is doubtful if any form of treatment influences the outcome and we have been unimpressed by the results of steroid therapy. Recovery takes from 2–3 months.

OTHER TYPES OF VIRAL HEPATITIS

Cytomegalic inclusion disease is acquired in utero from mothers with inapparent infection. Indeed, the virus seems to be widespread in the community but only rarely causes clinical disease after the neonatal period (Stern and Elek, 1965). The clinical features have been described by Stern and Tucker (1965). In some neonates the illness is mild with hepatosplenomegaly and some lowering of the platelet count. Recovery is usual although these patients may continue to excrete the virus into the urine and respiratory tract for as long as eighteen months. In many cases there is a grave illness with deep obstructive jaundice, gross hepatosplenomegaly, purpura, erythroblastaemia, thrombocytopenia, pulmonary signs with respiratory distress, and encephalitic signs with subsequent permanent brain damage. Intracranial calcification, micro-cephaly and choroidoretinitis may be found. The prognosis is poor. On post-mortem examination inclusion bodies are found in enlarged cells in the salivary glands, liver, lungs, kidneys, pancreas and thyroid (Claireaux, 1960). The diagnosis can be established during life by (i) a search for "owl's eye" inclusion bodies in renal tubular cells in the urine, (ii) successful culture of the virus from urine or throat swabs, or (iii) demonstrating a rising titre in the serum of complement-fixing antibodies. There is no specific treatment but corticosteroids may be used in severe cases.

Herpes simplex hepatitis is part of a generalized infection involving liver, lungs, adrenals and brain. It is not transplacentally acquired but from the mother during passage through the birth canal or subsequently. The mother may or may not have obvious herpetic lesions of the vulva or around the mouth. The infant is ill with hepatosplenomegaly, jaundice, dyspnoea, purpura and thrombocytopenia. Convulsions may reflect brain damage which is likely to be permanent. In some cases herpetic vesicles may be found on the skin. Choroidoretinitis has been reported. Post-mortem examination shows characteristic white or pale yellow nodules in the affected tissues. The diagnosis may be confirmed by antibody tests.

NON-VIRAL TYPES OF HEPATITIS

Jaundice with a rise in both "indirect" and "direct" forms of bili-rubin may appear in *severe bacterial infections* such as pyelonephritis, gastroenteritis and meningitis due to *E. coli*. Indeed, septicaemia due to Gram-negative bacilli is a common cause of jaundice in the neonatal period. It may also develop as the consequence of direct spread of staphylococcal sepsis from the umbilical stump to the liver. The urine contains bile and the stools may be pale. Recovery accompanies success-ful treatment of the primary bacterial infection. *Congenital toxo-plasmosis* may cause severe jaundice, hepatosplenomegaly, purpura, erythroblastaemia, thrombocytopenia and myocarditis in the newborn (Chapter X). Appropriate serological tests on both the patient's and the mother's blood will confirm the diagnosis. Promising results have been obtained by treatment with pyrimethamine (Daraprim) and sulpha-diazine. *Congenital syphilis* has often been recorded as a cause of neonatal jaundice. While the spirochaete can cause pericellular hepatic cirrhosis we have never seen jaundice due to congenital syphilis.

REFERENCES

ÅKERRÉN, Y. (1954). *Acta paediat.* (*Uppsala*), **43**, 411.
ALLEN, F. H., and DIAMOND, L. K. (1958). *Erythroblastosis Fetalis, including Exchange Transfusion Technic.* Boston, Mass.: Little Brown & Co.
BARRIE, H. (1965). *Lancet*, **2**, 712.
BILLING, B. H. (1955). *J. clin. Path.*, **8**, 130.
BILLING, B. H., and LATHE, G. H. (1958). *Amer. J. Med.*, **24**, 11.
BOUND, J. P., and TELFER, T. P. (1956). *Lancet*, **1**, 720.
BOWMAN, J. M., and POLLOCK, J. M. (1965). *Pediatrics*, **35**, 815.
BROWN, A. K., and ZUELZER, W. W. (1958). *J. clin. Invest.*, **37**, 332.
CARSON, P. E., FLANAGAN, C. L., ICKES, C. E., and ALVING, A. S. (1956). *Science*, **124**, 484.
CLAIREAUX, A. E. (1960). *Brit. med. J.*, **1**, 1528.
CLAIREAUX, A. E., COLE, P. G., and LATHE, G. H. (1953). *Lancet*, **2**, 1226.
COLE, P. G., and LATHE, G. H. (1953). *J. clin. Path.*, **6**, 99.
COMBINED STUDY FROM CENTRES IN ENGLAND AND BALTIMORE (1966). *Brit. med. J.*, **2**, 907.
CRIGLER, J. F., and NAJJAR, V. A. (1952). *Pediatrics*, **10**, 169.
DANKS, D., and BODIAN, M. (1963). *Arch. Dis. Childh.*, **38**, 378.
DOXIADIS, S. A., FESSAS, Ph., and VALAES, T. (1961). *Lancet*, **1**, 297.
DOXIADIS, S. A., and VALAES, T. (1964). *Arch. Dis. Childh.*, **39**, 545.
HARGREAVES, T., and HOLTON, J. B. (1962). *Lancet*, **1**, 839.
HSIA, D. Y. Y., BOGGS, J. D., DRISCOLL, S. G., and GELLIS, S. S. (1958). *Amer. J. Dis. Child.*, **95**, 485.
ISSELBACHER, K. J., and MCCARTHY, E. A. (1958). *Biochim biophys. Acta* (*Amst.*), **29**, 658.
LATHE, G. H. (1955). *Brit. med. J.*, **1**, 192.
LILEY, A. W. (1961). *Amer. J. Obstet. Gynec.*, **82**, 1359.
LILEY, A. W. (1965). *Pediatrics*, **35**, 836.
MEYER, T. C., and ANGUS, J. (1956). *Arch. Dis. Childh.*, **31**, 212.
MOLLISON, P. L., MOURANT, A. E., and RACE, R. R. (1948). *Memor. med. Res. Coun.* (*Lond.*) No. 19.
SCHMID, R. (1958). *Arch. intern. Med.*, 101, 669.
SHERLOCK, S. (1962). *Brit. med. J.*, **1**, 1359.
SILVERMAN, W. A., ANDERSON, D. H., BLANC, W. A., and CROZIER, D. N. (1956). *Pediatrics*, **18**, 614.
SMETANA, H. F., and JOHNSON, F. B. (1955). *Amer. J. Path.*, **31**, 747.
SMITH, G., and VELLA, F. (1960). *Lancet*, **1**, 1133.
STERN, H., and ELEK, S. D. (1965). *J. Hyg.* (*Lond.*), **63**, 79.
STERN, H., and TUCKER, S. M. (1965). *Lancet*, **2**, 1269.
STOKES, J., WOLMAN, I. J., BLANCHARD, M. C., and FARQUHAR, J. D. (1951). *Amer. J. Dis. Child.*, **82**, 213.
SUTHERLAND, J. M., and KELLER, W. H. (1961). *Amer. J. Dis. Child.*, **101**, 447.
WALKER, W. (1959). *Brit. med. Bull.*, **15**, 123.
YUE, P. C. K., and STRICKLAND, M. (1965). *Lancet*, **1**, 350.
ZETTERSTRÖM, R., and ERNSTER, L. (1956). *Nature* (*Lond.*), **178**, 1335.
ZUELZER, W. W., and BROWN, A. K. (1961). *Amer. J. Dis. Child.*, **101**, 87.

CHAPTER V

NEONATAL HAEMORRHAGE

The newborn infant is peculiarly liable to bleed under a variety of circumstances. These include anoxia, birth trauma, hypothermia, haemolytic disease, infections of bacterial, viral or protozoal origin, and inadequacies of the complicated blood clotting mechanism. In this chapter we shall confine our attention to those conditions in which haemorrhage is itself the main danger to life.

FOETAL HAEMORRHAGE

Whereas haemorrhage in the newborn infant is most often visible and, when severe, accompanied by the usual signs of shock, haemorrhage in the foetus is often invisible and its effects are hidden from view. None the less, an awareness of the circumstances under which foetal bleeding may occur will frequently enable the physician to act promptly enough after the birth to save the life of an exsanguinated baby.

Aetiology

Bleeding from the foetus may occur if the placenta is accidentally incised during lower segment Caesarean section for anterior placenta praevia. Experienced obstetricians are aware of this risk and take steps to avoid it (Neligan and Russell, 1954; Butler and Martin, 1954). The foetus may also suffer severe blood loss if there is rupture of a velamentous vessel overlying the cervix (Potter, 1959) or of a blood vessel on the foetal aspect of the placenta (Wickster and Christian, 1954), or from haemorrhage into the placenta itself (Chown, 1955). Damage to the placenta and foetal blood vessels has been reported as a result of artificial rupture of the membranes (Russell *et al.*, 1956). It should be suspected whenever blood is obtained at this procedure.

Haemorrhage is invisible when the foetus bleeds across the placenta into the mother's circulation. This syndrome is called *foetomaternal transfusion.* It was first suggested as a cause of anaemia in the infant at birth by Wiener (1948), and subsequently proved by differential agglutination techniques by Chown (1954). This type of foetal haemorrhage has now been quite frequently reported (Chown, 1957; Gunson, 1959). The factors which cause transplacental bleeding are not clear. Damage to the placenta from high rupture of the membranes with a catheter has been reported (Apley *et al.*, 1961), and one case was associated with a choriocarcinoma (Benson *et al.*, 1962), but in most instances no abnormality of the placenta is obvious.

A rare but intriguing situation arises when one monovular twin bleeds into the other (Kerr, 1959; Potter, 1959) so that one is anaemic and the other is polycythaemic, while one portion of the monochorionic placenta is pale and bloodless and the other is purple and engorged.

Clinical Features

Foetal haemorrhage during labour should be suspected if there is a sudden flow of bright red blood from the mother's vagina. The same applies to the appearance of blood during the operation of artificial rupture of the membranes. The foetal origin of the blood can be quickly confirmed by testing it for foetal haemoglobin which is alkali-resistant (Singer *et al.*, 1951; Beaven *et al.*, 1956). In this situation early delivery and ligation of the umbilical cord are imperative to stop haemorrhage from the foetal surface of the placenta. The infant will be delivered from the mother in a state of oligaemic shock with severe pallor, but there will rarely be the apnoeic state of asphyxia pallida and the heart rate will be rapid in contrast to the bradycardia which is usual in severe asphyxia. When the bleeding has been less severe or has been taking place for some time before birth, as in cases of foetomaternal transfusion, the presenting sign is pallor alone. Indeed, this may not become manifest for some hours after birth. Examination of the infant's blood will show a hypochromic anaemia with reticulocytosis and increased numbers of circulating erythroblasts and normoblasts. When the mother in a case of foetomaternal transfusion receives a large volume of foetal blood she may have back pain or a rigor during pregnancy or labour. This is especially likely if she is Rhesus (D) negative and has been previously sensitized by Rhesus (D) positive pregnancies (Goodall *et al.*, 1958).

Diagnosis

The presence of foetomaternal transfusion may be confirmed by various methods of examination of the mother's blood, but these depend for their success on an early clinical suspicion leading to collection of maternal blood in a suitable anticoagulant soon after delivery. Direct serological proof may be obtained by differential agglutination provided there is a major blood group difference between mother and her infant (Chown, 1954; Gunson, 1959). Goodall *et al.* (1958) found Coombs' positive red cells in the mother's blood in a case which was also complicated by Rhesus immunization. Direct chemical evidence of transplacental haemorrhage may be forthcoming if there has been sufficient foetal bleeding to raise the level of foetal haemoglobin in the mother's blood substantially above the normal adult level of 2 per cent (Singer *et al.*, 1951). Examination of the buffy coat in the mother's blood may reveal many small foetal erythroblasts. In one mother, previously Rhesus sensitized, evidence of foetomaternal transfusion was found by the demonstration of phagocytosis of nucleated red cells in the buffy coat (Goodall *et al.*, 1958). A quick method of diagnosis when there has been a fairly severe foetomaternal transfusion is to treat methanol-fixed blood films of the maternal blood with an acid buffer at pH 3·4. Foetal erythrocytes resist lysis by the buffer solution so that they react subsequently with ordinary haemoglobin stains, whereas the adult maternal red cells appear as "ghosts" (Kleihauer *et al.*, 1957; Apley *et al.*, 1961). In all cases of suspected foetal haemorrhage the placenta itself should be inspected by an experienced pathologist for evidence of damage.

Treatment

The only treatment is blood transfusion, but this is life-saving. When the haemorrhage has taken place shortly before birth the haemoglobin level may not be much reduced, but as restoration of the blood volume takes place over the next few hours serial determinations will reveal a fall. A haemoglobin level below 13 gm. per 100 ml. is an indication for transfusion. In some rare instances the foetal haemorrhage during labour is so severe that the state of exsanguination of the infant at birth precludes the normal blood grouping procedures. In such an eventuality Group O Rhesus negative blood should be given.

HAEMORRHAGIC DISEASE OF THE NEWBORN

It must first be stressed that haemorrhagic disease in spite of the similarity in name to haemolytic disease of the newborn (Chapter IV) is quite unrelated thereto and has nothing to do with blood group incompatibility. In fact, the term haemorrhagic disease of the newborn (or *melaena neonatorum*) has been used in the past somewhat indiscriminately to include a wide variety of blood coagulation defects. Many of these have now been precisely defined by modern investigative techniques and should no longer be included within this diagnosis. The term should be confined to those cases in which a temporary coagulation defect is associated with spontaneous haemorrhage between the second and fifth days of life and which disappears within a few days thereafter (Van Creveld, 1959).

Aetiology

There is a deficiency in the blood of affected infants of Factor VII (proconvertin) required in the second phase of coagulation to convert prothrombin to thrombin, of plasma thromboplastin component (PTC; Christmas factor) which is required in the first phase of coagulation for the formation of circulating thromboplastin; and of Stuart-Prower factor (Schulz and Van Creveld, 1958) which is necessary for both the first and second phases. It has often been accepted that hypoprothrombinaemia is a basis for this disease, but there is good evidence that the apparent decrease in prothrombin is, in fact, largely due to Factor VII deficiency. There is at present no agreement as to the level of prothrombin in the blood of newborn infants. Haemorrhagic disease of the newborn is, therefore, due to multiple but temporary deficiencies of factors required for blood clotting. Similar deficiencies are demonstrable in many newborn infants who do not bleed, so that the complete explanation has not yet been reached. No doubt an important element producing these deficiencies is hepatic immaturity and they tend to be more marked in the premature. Furthermore, the newborn infant's bowel during the first week is lacking the bacterial flora which can synthesize vitamin K.

Clinical Features

The presenting sign is bleeding although it varies greatly in severity. The most common form is melaena. In severe cases frank blood is passed per rectum and the infant then looks shocked and pale. Haematemesis, haematuria, vaginal bleeding, and haemorrhage from the umbilicus or into the skin may also occur. Visceral haemorrhages are uncommon but we have occasionally seen retroperitoneal haemorrhage, subcapsular haematoma of the liver and intracranial bleeding. The laboratory findings vary somewhat. The prothrombin time is always prolonged. The thromboplastin generation test (Medical Research Council, 1955) is abnormal with the patient's serum due to deficiency of Stuart-Prower factor and sometimes of PTC. More detailed laboratory procedures (Schulman and Smith, 1957) are only infrequently required.

Differential Diagnosis

Various permanent inherited abnormalities in the clotting mechanism (Chapter XIX) may rarely present in the neonatal period and simulate haemorrhagic disease. They are difficult to define at this time because of the multiple temporary deficiencies already mentioned. None the less, they should be suspected if bleeding continues or recurs in spite of treatment.

The *swallowed blood syndrome* is a term often used to apply to the swallowing of maternal blood either during labour or from cracked nipples, This can, of course, lead to haematemesis or melaena. The diagnosis should be confirmed by testing the vomitus or stool for foetal haemoglobin. The result will be negative when the source of the blood is maternal. Mild vaginal bleeding is not uncommon about the third day of life in an otherwise healthy infant. It is not associated with bleeding elsewhere and is probably an oestrogen withdrawal effect. Peptic ulcer is a rare cause of haematemesis and melaena during the neonatal period. The haemorrhage is often copious and it leads to sudden collapse, frequently with respiratory difficulty and cyanosis if there is co-incidental perforation. The ulcer can often be demonstrated by fluoroscopy after the instillation of lipiodol by stomach tube (Barger, 1958).

Treatment

In the first instance haemorrhage in the newborn is an indication for the intramuscular administration of vitamin K analogue (Synkavit; Kapilon) in a 1 mg. dose which can be repeated within the next 12 hours or of vitamin K_1 (phytomenadione) in a single 5 mg. dose. The dangers of larger doses, which are unnecessary in any case, have already been discussed (Chapters II and IV). The value of vitamin K in treatment, or given to the mother during labour as a prophylactic measure, has been questioned (Craig, 1961), and assessment is difficult because the disease does in the event recover spontaneously. In cases where blood loss is severe and sudden, transfusion of fresh blood (20–30 ml. per Kg. body weight; 10–15 ml./lb.) is life-saving.

UMBILICAL HAEMORRHAGE

Bleeding from the umbilicus may develop from several causes and routine periodic examination of the cord should be part of newborn nursery routine. In haemorrhagic disease of the newborn umbilical bleeding is rarely if ever the sole source of haemorrhage and so it seldom passes unobserved. Umbilical bleeding by itself may, however, be due to a wrongly applied ligature (too loose or too tight), to injudicious attempts to accelerate separation of the cord or to sepsis. In these circumstances it is possible for a dangerous degree of bleeding to pass unobserved for some hours. It is our practice to insist upon re-ligaturing of the cord proximal to the ligature applied in the labour room when the infant is admitted to the newborn nursery or lying-in ward with the mother.

REFERENCES

APLEY, J., COLLEY, P. A. N., and FRASER, I. D. (1961). *Lancet*, **1**, 1375.
BARGER, A. J. (1958). *Amer. J. Roentgenol.*, **80**, 426.
BEAVEN, G. H., ELLIS, M., and WHITE, J. C. (1956). *Nature (Lond.)*, **178**, 857.
BENSON, P. F., GOLDSMITH, K. L. G., and RANKIN, G. L. S. (1962). *Brit. med. J.*, **1**, 841.
BUTLER, N. R., and MARTIN, J. D. (1954). *Brit. med. J.*, **2**, 1455.
CHOWN, B. (1954). *Lancet*, **1**, 1213.
CHOWN, B. (1955). *Amer. J. Obstet. Gynec.*, **70**, 1298.
CHOWN, B. (1957). *Pediat. Clin. N. Amer.*, 371.
CRAIG, W. S. (1961). *Arch. Dis. Childh.*, **36**, 575.
GOODALL, H. B., GRAHAM, F. S., MILLER, M. C., and CAMERON, C. (1958). *J. clin. Path.*, **11**, 251.

GUNSON, H. H. (1959). *J. Pediat.*, **54**, 602.

KERR, M. M. (1959). *Brit. med. J.*, **1**, 902.

KLEIHAUER, E., BRAUN, H., and BETKE, K. (1957). *Klin. Wschr.*, **35**, 637.

MEDICAL RESEARCH COUNCIL (1955). *The Diagnosis and Treatment of Haemophilia and its Related Conditions* (Memorandum No. 32). London: H.M. Staty. Office.

NELIGAN, G. A., and RUSSELL, J. K. (1954). *J. Obstet. Gynaec. Brit. Emp.*, **61**, 206.

POTTER, E. L. (1959). *J. Pediat.*, **54**, 552.

RUSSELL, J. K., SMITH, D. F., and YULE, R. (1956). *Brit. med. J.*, **2**, 1414.

SCHULMAN, I., and SMITH, C. H. (1957). *Advanc. Pediat.*, **9**, 231.

SCHULZ, J., and VAN CREVELD, S. (1958). *Neo-Natal Studies*, **7**, 133.

SINGER, K., CHERNOFF, A. I., and SINGER, L. (1951). *Blood*, **6**, 413.

VAN CREVELD, S. (1959). *J. Pediat.*, **54**, 633.

WICKSTER, G. Z., and CHRISTIAN, J. R. (1954). *Pediat. Clin. N. Amer.*, 555.

WIENER, A. S. (1948). *Amer. J. Obstet. Gynec.*, **56**, 717.

CHAPTER VI

NEONATAL INFECTIONS

The problem of infection in the newborn has for several reasons received much attention during the past 20 years. It is more common in infants born in hospital than in those born in private homes, and there has been a steady trend during this period towards more frequent hospital confinement. Antibiotic resistance has assumed major proportions within our hospitals although it is not yet a serious problem in the general community. Furthermore the high incidence of infections among infants born in hospitals constitutes a great source of anxiety to their staffs. Deaths from infection acquired during the neonatal period are particularly tragic, and largely preventable with the knowledge already available to us. Indeed, they are a constant reminder of Florence Nightingale's famous dictum that "the first requirement of a hospital is that it should do the sick no harm".

Sources of Infections

The sources and routes of spread of infections which affect the newborn may be conveniently discussed according to their time of onset.

(1) **Antenatal.**—During pregnancy the infecting organism passes from the maternal circulation to the intervillous spaces of the placenta from whence it penetrates into the foetal circulation (Blanc, 1961). A variety of viruses are known to cross the placenta including rubella, poliomyelitis, Coxsackie, variola, vaccinia and cytomegalic inclusion disease. Some of these, such as the rubella virus, produce early damage to the developing embryo, others such as cytomegalic inclusion disease or Coxsackie produce late effects such as hepatitis or myocarditis in the newborn infant. The spirochaete of syphilis has become a rare cause of neonatal infection in the U.K. but is a common problem in some parts of the world. A protozoon, toxoplasma gondii, not uncommonly causes severe damage to the foetus. Bacteria rarely cross the placenta although *Escherichia coli* and *Listeria monocytogenes* can do so. Congenital tuberculosis can arise from transplacental infection. In other instances a tuberculous focus in the placenta ruptures into the liquor amnii so that the foetus inhales the bacteria.

(2) **Intranatal.**—Infection during the process of birth is a much more frequent occurrence. In most cases it is due to the ascent of vaginal organisms into the uterine cavity after rupture of the membranes. Premature rupture of the membranes before or during labour, and a long interval before delivery, are important predisposing factors to the

development of a placentitis and infection of the liquor amnii. Infection may also occur even while the membranes are intact if labour is prolonged, and especially if there has been excessive manipulation or if hands or instruments are contaminated. Most commonly the foetus inhales the infected liquor so that congenital pneumonia is the result. Indeed, this condition has been considered to be responsible for about 10 per cent of the perinatal mortality (Cook *et al.*, 1960). Alternatively, the infection may spread from the septic placenta to the foetal circulation with resulting septicaemia, although this is probably uncommon. Infection of the eyes by the gonococcus during passage of the foetal head through the birth canal was once greatly feared as the commonest cause of blindness in childhood. It has become so rare in the U.K., and so easily treated, that most centres have given up the use of prophylactic eye drops at the time of birth. Thrush may also occur at this time if the mother's vagina is infected with *Candida albicans*.

(3) **Postnatal.**—While intrapartum infection is an important cause of perinatal mortality most fatal infections occur after birth. Whereas the other principal causes of neonatal mortality—asphyxia, intracranial haemorrhage, hyaline membrane disease—destroy life during the first 72 hours, most of the infective deaths occur between the end of the first week and the first month of life (Department of Health for Scotland, 1947). The problem is largely one of hospital nurseries, and while hospital confinement may well increase the safety of the mother it undoubtedly exposes the baby to greater risk of infection. Thus, Ravenholt and his colleagues (1957) revealed that the incidence of skin sepsis alone in infants born in 15 Seattle hospitals was 18 per cent, while 4 per cent of their mothers developed mastitis.

In British hospitals the total incidence of neonatal infections has been estimated to be from 20–25 per cent. On the other hand, although the incidence of infections has probably not fallen much in recent years, the mortality rate has greatly diminished. For example, in the period 1939–1943 the incidence of infection in 618 neonatal deaths in Glasgow Royal Maternity Hospital was 36·4 per cent, whereas in the period 1953–1957 evidence of infection was found in only 10 per cent of 451 neonatal deaths. Among the infants who died of infection in 1953–1957, 76 per cent were premature. There has also been a marked change in the incidence of the different types of infection. In the Simpson Memorial Maternity Pavilion, Edinburgh, in the period 1939–1943, of 182 neonatal infective deaths 24·7 per cent were due to gastro-enteritis. In the Glasgow 1953–1957 series there were no deaths from this cause. Although the *Esch. coli*, *Strept. pyogenes*, Pneumococcus and *H. influenzae* trouble us from time to time the big problem has become the ubiquitous coagulase-positive *Staphylococcus aureus* which is notoriously able to develop resistance to antibiotics. The staphylococcal menace may present in three forms:

(a) The sudden outbreak within a newborn nursery of severe sepsis with a considerable mortality (Timbury *et al.*, 1958). This type of epidemic has usually been caused by certain particular strains of staphylococci, such as phage types 80/81, which are always penicillin-resistant and frequently resistant to several of the other commonly used antibiotics, e.g. streptomycin and the tetracyclines. In recent years the staphylococcus has tended to cause pneumonia, osteitis and other pyaemic lesions, while pemphigus neonatorum which was so often lethal in the past seems largely to have disappeared from our hospitals.

(b) Apart from the occasional epidemics of severe sepsis, there is the ever-present problem of minor lesions in newborn nurseries—septic spots, paronychiae, conjunctivitis and umbilical sepsis—which come and go from time to time. While the staphylococci concerned show a wide scatter of phage types, and while they seem to be less virulent than the epidemic strains, they also show an increasing tendency to develop antibiotic resistance. It is an inescapable fact that where antibiotics have been widely used in hospitals the staphylococcal population develops a high incidence of antibiotic resistance, while outside the hospitals they remain mostly penicillin-sensitive.

(c) The third problem is the symptomless colonization of infants and their mothers by pathogenic staphylococci. Hurst (1957) found that 99 per cent of 106 infants born in hospital carried pathogenic staphylococci when they left hospital, and 33 of 34 babies carried at least one penicillin-resistant strain. At least one half of the infants continued to carry hospital staphylococci at the end of their first year of life. On the other hand, of 36 infants born at home 72 per cent acquired staphylococci during the first two weeks of life, although only 18 per cent were penicillin-resistant. The figures for infant carriage of staphylococci have varied widely, e.g. 75 per cent (Barber *et al.*, 1953), 60 per cent (Forfar *et al.*, 1953), and 40·1 per cent (Edmunds *et al.*, 1955). The incidence of penicillin resistance in these series was 90 per cent; 64·4 per cent and 64·7 per cent respectively. All investigators have confirmed that a much higher incidence of penicillin-resistant staphylococci are found in infants born in hospital than among those born at home. A similar situation has been revealed in the mothers. Hutchison and Bowman (1957) found that on admission to hospital the staphylococci isolated from the mothers were 86 per cent penicillin-sensitive, but that on their discharge the same mothers yielded staphylococci 60 per cent of which were penicillin-resistant. These figures are by no means of mere academic interest. It is now well recognized that many newborn infants who show no evidence of disease during their sojourn in the maternity unit develop serious lesions, particularly staphylococcal pneumonia, weeks or months after their return home. Furthermore, they are frequently a source of infection (e.g. boils, whitlows, otitis media, breast abscess) in their mothers and other members of their families (Nelson, 1960).

The routes whereby infection may travel are not yet fully understood. The severe epidemic of staphylococcal sepsis due to phage type 80 is probably initiated by a member of the staff who is harbouring a staphylococcal lesion on his or her person (Colbeck, 1949). This is almost certainly not the source of the more common minor sepsis or of the symptomless colonization of the infant's nose, umbilical stump or perineum. It is true that there is often a high nasal carrier-rate (from 50–68 per cent) of coagulase-positive staphylococci among nurses in maternity units (Barber *et al.*, 1949; Rowntree and Thomson, 1952; Edmunds *et al.*, 1955), and understandable that it should have been suggested that they might be an important source of infection both by droplet spray and handling (Allison and Hobbs, 1947). However, the phage types and antibiotic sensitivities of the staphylococci isolated from the nurses and from the infants have sometimes been the same (Forfar *et al.*, 1955), sometimes different (Forfar *et al.*, 1953), even within the same hospital at different times. This would suggest that nurses are not a major source of infection. It would, in fact, be surprising if nurses and infants living in the same environment did not at times pick up the same organisms (Forfar and Maccabe, 1958). It is also rare for infection to be transferred from mother to baby although the opposite is quite common (Edmunds *et al.*, 1955; Hutchison and Bowman, 1957). It is much more probable that staphylococcal neonatal sepsis spreads from infant to infant via the attendants' hands, on blankets, or in the dust which arises from personal clothing, bedding, towels, etc. Rigorous methods of self discipline, including hand washing, have had a fair measure of success in recent years. Woollen blankets should no longer be used in hospitals.

BACTERIOLOGY

The infant in the first month of life reacts poorly to bacterial infection so that the patterns of disease differ from those with which we are familiar in older persons. Thus, *E. coli* while it may produce urinary infections also causes pneumonia, pyogenic meningitis and gastroenteritis. The staphylococcus may produce not only infections of areolar tissue but also pneumonia, osteitis, parotitis, meningitis and brain abscess. The poor local resistance of the newborn tissues favour the development of generalized septicaemia or pyaemia, and the paucity of local signs explains the well-known difficulties of diagnosis in the neonatal period. Infection by *Candida albicans* is also common. It is usually relatively benign but may cause death in feeble or premature infants. Virus infections have already been mentioned, but comparatively little is yet known of their frequency in the newborn. On the other hand, the young infant is normally given a passive but temporary immunity to diphtheria, measles and mumps by the transplacental passage of maternal antibodies. This does not apply to chickenpox or pertussis.

DIAGNOSIS

The diagnosis of infection during the neonatal period can be very difficult. Localizing signs are frequently absent and the primary portal of entry is often not obvious. In fact the infection may so quickly become a generalized septicaemia or pyaemia that a "local diagnosis" has little relevance. On the other hand, although a precise diagnosis in anatomical terms is often impossible, an *early diagnosis* is usually possible if the physician is aware enough of the fact that apparently small abnormalities of behaviour in a newborn infant can herald the onset of a fulminating infection. He should bear in mind always that if the infant survives the first 72 hours of life without obvious distress, and if he is free from severe congenital abnormalities, any subsequent deterioration in his condition is almost certainly due to infection. None the less, the features of a severe infection in the newborn are usually fairly typical to the experienced observer (Moncrieff, 1953).

The first indications are a sudden reluctance to finish feeds, vomiting, undue drowsiness sometimes alternating with excessive irritability, or a rise in the respiratory rate. A sudden loss of weight in an infant who has been progressing satisfactorily is very significant. There is usually a rather characteristic greyish pallor and anxious facies. Diarrhoea is not uncommon. Oedema, jaundice, purpura and other haemorrhages, and convulsive twitchings indicate severe sepsis. Hepatosplenomegaly is common in septicaemic infections. Fever may or may not be present. In premature infants, indeed, hypothermia and sclerema are frequent concomitants of an infective process. The appearance of any of these manifestations should indicate the need for a careful physical examination of the whole infant followed by relevant laboratory investigations. These may include urine analysis, blood culture, white cell count, lumbar puncture and radiography. They should precede treatment and they brook no delay whatever the hour. The diagnosis of infection is always urgent not only in the interests of the patient but, in a newborn nursery, the immediate isolation of such a source of infection is of vital importance.

CLASSIFICATION OF INFECTIONS

For descriptive purposes it is convenient to subdivide the common neonatal infections into *major* and *minor*. In this context a major infection is one which endangers life. This may be a septicaemia or a severe infection confined to one system of the body. A minor infection is one which does not endanger the patient's life. The description must not be taken to imply that the physician may regard a minor infection lightly, because the causal organism may spread within the nursery and produce major sepsis in other infants. Furthermore, a minor infection such as a septic spot can occasionally lead to the development of a severe metastatic lesion elsewhere in the body, e.g. osteitis, brain abscess, etc.

MAJOR INFECTIONS

(1)   PNEUMONIA IN THE NEWBORN

The most commonly fatal infection during the neonatal period is pneumonia. It can be most usefully described under several distinct aetiological types.

(*a*) **Congenital (intra-uterine) pneumonia** is often mistaken for asphyxia neonatorum, hyaline membrane disease or intracranial haemorrhage. Indeed, accurate diagnosis may be impossible because the affected infant is often apnoeic at birth, and later shows the same type of grunting respiration with subcostal and sternal recession, and cyanosis which is seen in hyaline membrane disease (Chapter II). Pneumonia, however, is equally common in mature and premature infants. It should always be suspected when more than 24 hours have elapsed between rupture of the membranes and delivery, and particularly if the mother is febrile (Anderson *et al.*, 1962). The chest radiograph shows softer and more confluent opacities than in hyaline membrane disease (Fig. 9). Clinical signs over the lungs are usually few and unhelpful. The air entry may be poor and crepitations may be heard.

Treatment

Treatment amounts to incubator care in 40 per cent oxygen, humidity above 75 per cent, and broad spectrum antibiotics given intramuscularly. A useful combination is cloxacillin (50 mg./Kg. body weight/day) and ampicillin (50 mg./Kg. body weight/day), each given in four equal doses. An alternative and single antibiotic which promises to be valuable in this type of situation where bacteriological studies are usually impracticable is cephaloridine (30 mg./Kg. body weight/day) given in two equal doses. Chloramphenicol is also effective in a dose of 25 mg./Kg. body weight/day. Larger doses must not be prescribed during the neonatal period because chloramphenicol is detoxicated by glucuronation in the liver and this enzyme system is immature in the newborn (Chapter IV). There is, therefore, a danger of poisoning from excessively high blood levels. These result in peripheral circulatory collapse, abdominal distension, diarrhoea and vomiting—"the grey baby syndrome" (Lischner *et al.*, 1961). It is now rarely necessary to use chloramphenicol during the first month of life.

(*b*) **Aspiration pneumonia** used to be a common cause of death in premature infants who had been fed before the swallowing and cough

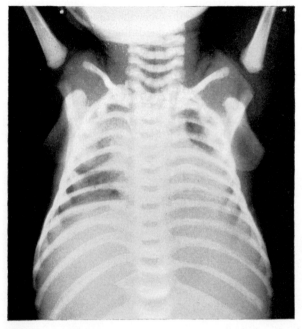

FIG.9.—Intra-uterine pneumonia producing soft confluent shadows in right upper and left lower zones.

reflexes were established. It is uncommon when feeds are given by skilled nurses. The introduction of polyvinyl chloride catheters which can be passed intranasally and left *in situ* for several days has also made tube-feeding a much safer process in very feeble infants. Aspiration pneumonia should be suspected if a premature infant becomes lethargic and anorexic, if weight gain suddenly ceases and if there have been apnoeic or cyanotic attacks during feeds. There may be crepitations over the lung bases and the diagnosis may be established by radiography. The treatment is the same as that outlined for congenital pneumonia.

(*c*) **Staphylococcal pneumonia** is particularly common in the newborn who has been born in hospital. It is especially likely to appear when there have been minor staphylococcal lesions in other infants in the nursery. The staphylococcus produces massive consolidation in many infants, and this may proceed to abscess formation, empyema or pyopneumothorax. The onset is sudden with listlessness, dyspnoea, reluctance to feed and sometimes cyanosis. Cough is not usually severe, but when it is spasmodic and distressing the possibility of fibrocystic disease of the pancreas (Chapter XVI) should be borne in mind.

Physical signs are often marked with dullness to percussion, diminished or bronchial breath sounds and numerous crepitations over the affected areas. Empyema produces marked dullness and displacement of the heart to the opposite side. Tension pneumothorax is associated with severe respiratory distress and collapse which will rapidly prove fatal unless emergency measures are taken. The X-ray at first shows a homogeneous opacity which may be extensive. Subsequently emphysematous bullae (pneumatoceles) can be visualized, an appearance which is almost diagnostic of staphylococcal pneumonia (Fig. 10). Metastatic abscesses may develop elsewhere and we have seen them in the brain, kidneys, liver and bones.

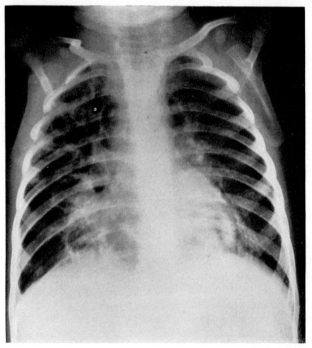

Fig. 10.—Staphylococcal pneumonia with emphysematous bullae in right lung.

Treatment

In addition to oxygen the urgent need is for an effective antibiotic. The organism is always penicillin-resistant, and the antibiotic sensitivities should be determined from throat swabs, laryngeal swabs or pleural fluid when present. The drug of first choice is cloxacillin (50 mg./Kg./day), but a change may prove necessary to erythromycin, cephaloridine or fucidin. Intramuscular administration is indicated in very ill infants. An empyema may frequently be successfully treated by repeated aspiration of pus and intrapleural replacement with a suitable antibiotic such as streptomycin, the intravenous preparation of tetracycline, or methicillin. Alternatively an in-dwelling intrapleural catheter may be connected with under-water drainage and suction.

(*d*) **Air-borne bronchopneumonia** does not differ essentially from the broncho-pneumonia of older infants (Chapter XIII). It is derived from the upper respiratory tracts of adult contacts and is probably initially a virus infection. It is not more common in babies born in hospital. The bacterial invaders may be pneumococci, haemolytic streptococci or *H. influenzae* as in older infants, but in the newborn organisms not usually associated with pneumonia may infect lung tissue, e.g. *E. coli*; enterococci; proteus and pseudomonas. The onset of the pneumonia is often preceded by an upper respiratory infection with rhinitis and nasal discharge which interferes with sucking. The infant then develops the signs of severe infection with dyspnoea and inspiratory dilation of the alae nasi. Cough is often slight. Local signs over the lungs vary from a few crepitations to dullness, diminished breath sounds and numerous crepitations. The radiographic appearances are those of patchy to confluent opacities, but in premature infants they may be singularly unrevealing. Treatment is along the lines indicated above. If nasal obstruction interferes with feeding 1 per cent ephedrine in normal saline nasal drops may be instilled before feeds.

(2) EPIDEMIC DIARRHOEA OF THE NEWBORN

This name for infantile gastro-enteritis stresses the fact that in newborn nurseries the disease tends to occur in explosive epidemics with a considerable mortality. Such outbreaks have been reported much less often within recent years, no doubt reflecting improved standards of care in newborn nurseries. Most cases are due to one of a number of serotypes of specific agglutinable *E. coli* which are classified by their somatic (O) antigens (Kauffmann, 1947). The most common are *E. coli* O·111; O·55; O·26; O·119; and O·128. Some outbreaks have been due to organisms of the Salmonella group (Graham, 1939), and in some a virus may have been causal (Light and Hodes, 1949).

Clinical Features

The illness may vary from a mild upset with lethargy, anorexia, slight loss of weight and a few loose stools to a fulminating outburst of severe diarrhoea and vomiting. The stools are large, fluid, green or orange coloured, and losses of body water and electrolytes may be very heavy with resultant diminution in plasma volume. A severe metabolic acidosis may arise from the considerable losses of sodium and potassium, with renal failure due to the diminished blood flow through the kidneys.

Within a few hours of the onset the infant may have developed the classical picture of severe dehydration with sunken eyes, depressed fontanelle, over-riding sutures, scaphoid abdomen, glazed corneae and semi-coma. The extremities, lips and ears may be cold and cyanosed due to peripheral circulatory failure (Hutchison, 1961).

Treatment

Oral feeds should be discontinued and replaced with quarter strength physiological saline (180 ml./Kg./day; 90 ml./lb.) given in small quantities every hour. If dehydration or vomiting is severe, fluid and electrolytes must be given by continuous intravenous infusion for 24–72 hours. A suitable fluid is 5 per cent glucose in quarter strength saline (120–150 ml./Kg./day; 60–75 ml./lb.). When there are signs of peripheral circulatory collapse citrate plasma diluted with equal parts of 10 per cent glucose in water, can be given rapidly by syringe initially (30–40 ml./Kg.; 15–20 ml./lb.). Severe acidosis is best corrected with 1/6 molar sodium lactate solution (30 ml./Kg.; 15 ml./lb.) repeated in four hours if necessary or by intravenous doses of 8·4 per cent sodium bicarbonate if the Astrup micro-method is available. After 24–48 hours small milk feeds are started and gradually increased, the intravenous fluids being correspondingly reduced. Oral antibiotic therapy should be based on bacterial sensitivity tests. A useful drug is neomycin, 50 mg./Kg./day in four divided doses. If a potassium deficit is revealed by hypokalaemia *after dehydration has been corrected*, oral potassium chloride 1 gm. twice daily should be prescribed. Full details of the complicated measures required to correct severe dehydration in infancy can be obtained in M.R.C. Memorandum No. 26 (1952).

(3) Pyogenic Meningitis

This very grave infection of the newborn is most commonly due to *E. coli.* Other organisms have been salmonella, pneumococci, haemolytic streptococci and staphylococci.

Clinical Features

The onset is insidious with loss of weight, drowsiness, reluctance to feed and vomiting. Convulsive twitchings are frequently seen. Significant signs are a bulging anterior fontanelle and head retraction. Nuchal rigidity and Kernig's sign do not occur in the newborn. The most important aid to diagnosis is a marked degree of suspicion when a newborn infant develops the general signs of severe infection and becomes excessively drowsy. The diagnosis must be confirmed by lumbar puncture. The cerebrospinal fluid is turbid due to large numbers of pus cells. Gram-negative bacilli are usually found in smears. Culture is required to determine the antibiotic sensitivities.

Treatment

The mortality rate is high and many of the survivors suffer permanent brain damage. Early diagnosis is, therefore, paramount. We have found the most effective treatment to be intramuscular chloramphenicol 25 mg./Kg./day, and sulphadiazine 0·25 gm. six-hourly, plus prednisolone 5 mg. six-hourly. The steroid dosage should be halved after one week and withdrawn in two weeks. The antibacterial drugs should be continued until the cerebrospinal fluid has returned to normal. Supportive measures such as intravenous fluids may also be necessary.

(4) PYELONEPHRITIS

There seems to have been a tendency for Gram-negative infections to become more common in recent years as the problem of staphylococcal sepsis has to some extent been controlled. Pyelonephritis is among the most common.

Clinical Features

The infant becomes ill with fever, and there is reluctance to feed, vomiting, greyish pallor and loss of weight. The diagnosis will, however, be missed unless the urine is obtained and subjected to microscopy and culture. In the newborn a urinary white cell count is significant if it exceeds 15 per c.mm. Pyuria may also be part of the clinical picture in a jaundiced baby suffering from a dangerous Gram-negative septicaemia (Chapter IV). In this event the pyelonephritis arises from the blood stream and sometimes there is also present a pyogenic meningitis. In such cases blood culture, and sometimes lumbar puncture, should be performed in addition to urine culture.

Treatment

When the infant is not severely ill the choice of antibacterial drug (e.g. sulphadimidine 200 mg./Kg./day, or nitrofurantoin 8 mg./Kg.day) can await the results of bacterial sensitivities. In septicaemic cases a combination of chloramphenicol and sulphadiazine is likely to be effective and must not be delayed. Intramuscular colistin methosulphate, 150,000 units/Kg./day, may also be added in dire emergency.

(5) ACUTE OSTEITIS (Osteomyelitis)

Osteitis in the newborn is a metastatic lesion which is almost invariably due to a penicillin-resistant *Staph. aureus*. The organism is also frequently resistant to streptomycin and the tetracyclines.

Clinical Features

In most cases the infant is seriously ill although fever is inconstant. Localizing signs are sometimes slow to appear and should be diligently sought in every ill infant. These are local swelling with or without discoloration; extreme irritability on handling the affected part or limb; or immobility of the affected limb (pseudoparesis) (Dennison, 1955; Boyes *et al.*, 1957). In the newborn osteitis is not infrequently multiple, and sites of predilection are the superior maxilla and the pelvis. When the maxilla is involved retro-orbital cellulitis causes proptosis as a presenting sign. If diagnosis is delayed extensive bone destruction and disorganization of the neighbouring joint (Fig. 11) may lead to permanent crippling. In some infants general systemic illness is remarkably slight, when the dangers of late diagnosis are even greater.

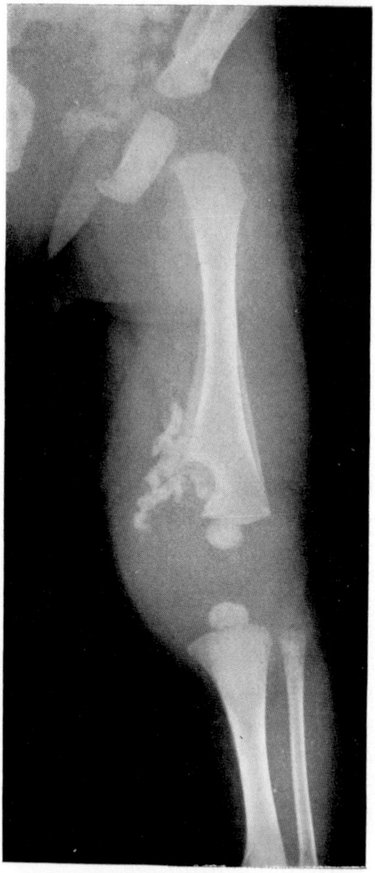

FIG. 11.—Osteitis in femur of young infant showing extensive destruction of bone and periostitis.

Treatment

An attempt should be made to isolate the causal organism and determine its antibiotic sensitivities by marrow puncture over the affected bone. Aspiration of pus through a wide-bore needle is preferable in most cases to open operation. A suitable antibiotic should be instilled locally and this may have to be repeated on several occasions. However, the life-saving measure is the systemic administration of an effective antibiotic or combination of antibiotics for a period of at least three weeks. We have recently obtained good results with intramuscular cloxacillin 50 mg./Kg./day in four divided doses.

(6) TETANUS NEONATORUM

Although now almost unknown in the U.K. neonatal tetanus is still an important cause of death in many tropical and subtropical countries, where the umbilical cord may be cut with a dirty knife, spear or piece of broken glass, may be tied with a makeshift ligature, or dressed with animal dung (Trowell and Jelliffe, 1958).

Clinical Features

The onset is between the third and tenth day of life, with difficulty in sucking due to masseteric spasm followed by tetanic spasms which result in risus sardonicus and opisthotonus. Between the spasms there is continuous muscle rigidity with clenched jaw, risus sardonicus and stiff back, neck, abdominal wall and limbs. Death can result from arrest of breathing during a spasm or from intercurrent pneumonia.

Treatment

The mortality is high and most infants die within a few days. Tetanus antitoxin should be given intramuscularly (50,000–75,000 units) and also locally around the umbilicus (15–25,000 units). A broad spectrum antibiotic should also be given intramuscularly. Sedation should be achieved by the regular administration of phenobarbitone soluble 15 mg., paraldehyde 0·5–1·0 ml., or chlorpromazine hydrochloride 5 mg. Feeds should be given through an intranasal polyvinyl chloride catheter. The value of muscle relaxants is doubtful in the newborn and their use requires the constant availability of a skilled anaesthetist. Smythe (1963) has reported good results from their use in association with carefully controlled intermittent positive pressure respiration.

MINOR INFECTIONS

(1) Infections of Skin and Areolar Tissues

Minor staphylococcal septic spots and pustules are probably the commonest types of infection seen in nurseries for the newborn. While trivial in themselves they are an important source of infection which may assume a virulent form in other infants. A much more severe form of skin sepsis is *pemphigus neonatorum* or bullous impetigo. The initial lesion is a clear blister, soon becoming purulent, surrounded by an area of erythema. There may be multiple bullae and severe constitutional upset. Occasionally the epidermis peels off which results in a highly dangerous exfoliative dermatitis (*Ritter's disease*). Pemphigus neonatorum used to be a common epidemic disease in maternity units and it carried a high mortality. In recent years outbreaks of staphylococcal sepsis have rarely taken this form, and the accurate choice of an antibiotic should make death a rarity. Another common minor staphylococcal lesion is paronychia, often involving fingers which the infant has enjoyed sucking. There is redness and oedema round the nail and sometimes the exudation of a little pus. Breast abscess may complicate the physiological mastitis neonatorum, especially if injudicious and unnecessary manipulation or binding has been practised. There are the usual signs of swelling, redness, oedema, shiny skin and fluctuation.

Treatment

Minor septic lesions can be quite safely treated with methylated spirit and powder, or with an antibiotic ointment containing neomycin and bacitracin. Systemic antibiotic therapy should be strictly reserved for infants who show obvious constitutional upset, to lessen the risk of the emergence of resistant organisms. Antibiotics should only be used in superficial sepsis after arrangements have been made to determine the bacterial sensitivities. An abscess in the breast, or elsewhere, should be incised and drained.

(2) CONJUNCTIVITIS (OPHTHALMIA NEONATORUM)

In the past gonococcal ophthalmia, acquired during passage of the foetal head through the birth canal, was the most common cause of blindness in children in the U.K. Today the disease has become so rare that in most maternity hospitals the use of prophylactic eye drops at birth has been abandoned. Indeed drops such as argyrol or silver nitrate, although effective prophylactics, can themselves cause an un-pleasant chemical conjunctivitis. The vast majority of cases of con-junctivitis now encountered in the newborn are staphylococcal. The organisms are acquired after birth from other infants, being carried on the attendants' hands or on blankets. In these cases the palpebral con-junctiva is hyperaemic and oedematous and the eyelids tend to get stuck together by pus ("sticky eye"). The disease may be unilateral or it may spread to both eyes. In marked contrast to the mild staphylococcal cases, gonococcal conjunctivitis is a severe infection with a profuse creamy discharge and grave risk of corneal ulceration and permanent scarring.

Treatment

It is essential that swabs be taken before any applications are pre-scribed. Cultures should be set up and a smear should be stained by Gram's method. Gonococcal cases can be diagnosed within a few minutes by the demonstration of the typical Gram-negative intracellular diplococci. Staphylococcal cases are almost always penicillin resistant. We have found the local application of an ointment containing neo-mycin and bacitracin (Neobacrin) every 6 hours to be an effective measure of treatment. Gonococcal cases must be immediately trans-ferred outwith the maternity unit. Treatment is highly effective but it requires intensive medical and nursing attention. Penicillin drops (2,500 units per ml.) should be instilled into both conjunctival sacs every 5 minutes until all discharge has ceased. Thereafter the drops are instilled every $\frac{1}{2}$ hour for 12 hours, hourly for another 12 hours, and finally every 2 hours for a further 24 hours. Alternative preparations for both types of conjunctivitis are 30 per cent sulphacetamide or 0·5 per cent chloramphenicol solutions.

(3) UMBILICAL SEPSIS

Infection of the umbilical stump is most often due to *Staph. aureus*. It is usually mild and presents as a scanty purulent discharge. In more severe cases the surrounding skin may be red and oedematous. In rare instances the infection may spread along the falciform ligament to the liver where multiple abscesses may form and produce jaundice and severe systemic upset. Direct spread into the peritoneal cavity is excessively uncommon. Much less infrequently pyaemic lesions may develop in bones or other organs. In chronic or neglected cases a granuloma may develop in the umbilicus itself.

Treatment

Umbilical sepsis is largely preventable by adequate care of the umbilical cord and efficient nursing techniques (Chapter II). It can be treated simply with a neomycin-bacitracin powder and an occlusive dressing. A granuloma may have to be touched up with solid silver nitrate or copper sulphate. Systemic antibiotic therapy is only indicated in the rare cases where the infant is ill.

(4) THRUSH (MONILIASIS)

This infection is due to the fungus *Candida albicans* and may be acquired during birth from the mother's vagina. The organism is not infrequently present in the mouths of healthy adults and the infant's feeding utensils can be contaminated when the attendants' personal hygiene is defective. The lesions are usually found in the mouth, but often spread to involve the oesophagus and cardiac end of the stomach. Sometimes the perianal skin is involved. Rarely the disease becomes blood-borne with lesions in brain and kidneys. Pulmonary moniliasis, which is not uncommon in adults treated with broad spectrum antibiotics, is rare in the newborn.

The lesions in the mouth are small greyish white patches on the gums, palate, buccal mucosa and tongue. They are to be distinguished from milk curd by the fact that they do not rub off easily on a swab and when they are detached a raw surface remains. A swab from the mouth smeared on a slide, fixed, and stained with methylene blue will reveal the typical mycelium and spores. Thrush is usually mild but occasionally causes death in premature or debilitated infants.

Treatment

A cheap and efficient method of treatment is to place 1 ml. of 0·5 per cent *freshly prepared* aqueous solution of gentian violet into the infant's mouth thrice daily for 3 days. A more expensive but less messy form of treatment is nystatin in liquid form, 100,000 units 4-hourly for 7–10 days.

PREVENTION OF NEONATAL SEPSIS

The general prophylactic measures required in nurseries for the new-born have been described in Chapter II. It is probably impossible to abolish minor sepsis completely from our hospitals. Indeed, the problem of staphylococcal sepsis is much more frequently recognized in the best hospitals with adequate laboratory services than in others where it tends to be missed until a severe epidemic occurs.

There are, however, several additional points which should be stressed:

(1) In every maternity unit there must be separate cubicle accommodation for the immediate isolation of an infant or mother who contracts an infection. The most important source of infection in the newborn nursery is the infant himself. Even the most trivial infection is potentially dangerous and an indication for isolation.

(2) It has frequently been shown that outbreaks of severe sepsis are preceded by a period of serious over-crowding and over-loading of the staff. We believe that clinicians who are responsible for the safety of their patients must resist administrative pressure to admit patients beyond the safe level which their medical and nursing staffs can handle efficiently.

(3) Antibiotics must be used intelligently. The emergence of resistant strains of organisms are, at least in part, due to the indiscriminate use of antibiotics, often to combat minor lesions which would recover without them, sometimes because the medical staff were too busy to undertake sufficiently frequent clinical observations of patients at risk. They should never be used without adequate laboratory control. They have also been used in some hospitals as a substitute for an efficient aseptic routine. Combinations of antibiotics have frequently been used in a blunderbuss fashion to combat infections which adequate laboratory investigation would have shown to be resistant from the outset.

(4) There is evidence that some outbreaks due to virulent strains of staphylococci (e.g. phage type 80/81) have originated from a member of the staff with a minor septic lesion like a boil. It is essential that members of the medical and nursing staffs do *not* go on duty when they are suffering from infections, however trivial they may seem.

(5) The value of treating staphylococcal nasal carriers among the staff with antiseptic creams is open to doubt. Some people are perineal carriers who are likely to remain undetected. There is little evidence to suggest that infants are infected from healthy carriers among the staff. On the other hand, there is no doubt that the incidence of staphylococcal colonization of the nose and umbilicus among the infants can be reduced with hexachlorophene powder or cream to the skin, and with chlorhexidine

(Hibitane) cream to the nose. Such measures are often used as a routine, but should certainly be instituted in any nursery in which minor sepsis is prevalent.

(6) The importance of thorough hand washing before *and* after handling any infant cannot be over-emphasized. The use of a hexachlorophene-impregnated soap serves further to reduce the staphylococcal population on the skin. Disposable paper towels must be used for drying the hands. It should be regarded as unthinkable in any neonatal unit that any doctor or nurse will depart from this essential self discipline.

REFERENCES

ALLISON, V. D., and HOBBS, B. C. (1947). *Brit. med. J.*, **2**, 1.

ANDERSON, G. S., GREEN, C. A., NELIGAN, G. A., NEWELL, D. J., and RUSSELL, J. K. (1962). *Lancet*, **2**, 585.

BARBER, M., HAYHOE, F. G. J., and WHITEHEAD, J. E. M. (1949). *Lancet*, **2**, 1120.

BARBER, M., WILSON, B. D. R., RIPPON, J. E., and WILLIAMS, R. E. O. (1953). *J. Obstet. Gynaec. Brit. Emp.*, **60**, 476.

BLANC, W. A. (1961). *J. Pediat.*, **59**, 473.

BOYES, J., BREMNER, A. E., and NELIGAN, G. A. (1957). *Lancet*, **1**, 544.

COLBECK, J. C. (1949). *Canad. med. Ass. J.*, **61**, 557.

COOK, C. D., BARRIE, H., and AVERY, M. E. (1960). *Advanc. Pediat.*, **11**, 11.

DENNISON, W. (1955). *Lancet*, **2**, 474.

DEPT. OF HEALTH FOR SCOTLAND (1947). *Neonatal Deaths due to Infection.* Edinburgh: H.M. Staty. Office.

EDMUNDS, P. N., ELIAS-JONES, T. F., FORFAR, J. O., and BALF, C. L. (1955). *Brit. med. J.*, **1**, 990.

FORFAR, J. O., BALF, C. L., ELIAS-JONES, T. F., and EDMUNDS, P. N. (1953). *Brit. med. J.*, **2**, 170.

FORFAR, J. O., and MACCABE, A. F. (1958). *Brit. med. J.*, **1**, 76.

FORFAR, J. O., MACCABE, A. F., BALF, C. L., WRIGHT, A. A., and GOULD, J. C. (1955). *Lancet*, **1**, 584.

GRAHAM, S. (1939). *Arch. Dis. Childh.*, **14**, 277.

HURST, V. (1957). *J. Hyg. (Lond.)*, **55**, 299 and 313.

HUTCHISON, J. G. P., and BOWMAN, W. D. (1957). *Acta Paediat. (Uppsala)*, **46**, 125.

HUTCHISON, J. H., (1961). *Practitioner*, **186**, 179.

KAUFFMANN, F. (1947). *J. Immunol.*, **57**, 71.

LIGHT, J. S., and HODES, H. L. (1949). *J. exp. Med.*, **90**, 113.

LISCHNER, H., SELIGMAN, S. J., KRAMMER, A., and PARMELEE, A. H. (1961). *J. Pediat.* **59**, 21.

MEDICAL RESEARCH COUNCIL (1952). *The Treatment of Acute Dehydration in Infants* (Memorandum No. 26). London: H.M. Staty. Office.

MONCRIEFF, A. (1953). *Brit. med. J.*, **1**, 1.

NELSON, W. E. (1960). *J. Pediat.*, **56**, 274.

RAVENHOLT, R. T., WRIGHT, P., and MULHERN, M. (1957). *New Engl. J. Med.*, **257**, 789.

ROWNTREE, P. M., and THOMSON, E. F. (1952). *Lancet*, **2**, 262.

SMYTHE, P. M. (1963). *Brit. med. J.*, **1**, 565.

TIMBURY, M. C., WILSON, T. S., HUTCHISON, J. G. P., and GOVAN, A. D. T. (1958). *Lancet*, **2**, 1081.

TROWELL, H. C., and JELLIFFE, D. B. (1958). *Diseases of Children in the Subtropics and Tropics.* London: Edward Arnold.

CHAPTER VII

INFANT FEEDING

The past twenty-five years have seen a vast change in our approach to the problems of infant feeding. In the earlier years of this century paediatricians enforced rigid time-tables on infants, and presented their mothers with authoritarian prescriptions of milk formulae in which the relative proportions of protein, fat and carbohydrate were carefully detailed. These have now been replaced by a more realistic and sympathetic understanding of the needs of both infant and mother (Smellie, 1952). It has been appreciated that the food requirements of different infants at the same age and weight may vary enormously. The rigidity and dogmatism of earlier paediatricians must, however, be viewed against the social background of their times in which an appalling infant mortality, much of it due to the diarrhoeal diseases, was coexistent with a poor understanding of intestinal pathogens. At that time failure to thrive and diarrhoea were often ascribed to faulty milk formulae instead of underfeeding and infection which we now recognize to be their principal causes. Furthermore, the introduction of the dried and evaporated preparations of cow's milk has greatly reduced the risks of enteral infection. The use of liquid cow's milk, often supplied by unhygienic producers to equally unhygienic consumers, has been largely abandoned.

A much less satisfactory change in custom has been the great reduction in the incidence of breast feeding in the more highly developed countries. At first sight it seems paradoxical that material prosperity and improved standards of education should be associated with a falling incidence of the physiological nutrition of infants. The causal factors are probably quite complex. An important one is the increasing tendency for mothers to continue in gainful employment after marriage and childbirth, some because they find in homekeeping insufficient intellectual satisfaction, but most because by augmenting the family income a higher material standard of living can be assured. Indeed, the materialism of the twentieth century may be the basic causal factor. Another important influence lies in custom itself, and the human is an animal with a well-developed herd instinct. The increased safety and simplicity of artificial feeding also must aggravate the trend away from natural feeding. The much greater infant mortality rates which were previously reported in artificially-fed infants (Grulee *et al.*, 1934) are no longer in evidence, although there is still a considerably higher incidence of morbidity among bottle-fed, as against breast-fed infants. A reflection of this can be seen in our children's hospitals where it is exceptional to find among infants suffering from infections one who is entirely breast-fed. A factor which must not be ignored is the comparative lack of enthusiasm and interest among doctors and midwives in the matter of breast feeding. It is, of course, easier to give a mother with lactation difficulties some stilboestrol tablets with one hand and a tin of dried milk with the other than to spend time and mental effort in trying to understand and resolve her problems. The best time to ensure troublefree breast feeding is during the pregnancy, as part of the routine antenatal care. This opportunity is too often allowed to go by default. Exhortations about the advantages of breast feeding *after* the baby is born are apt to sound unconvincing and insincere. It is, in fact, very doubtful if at that stage a doctor is wise to press a mother to breast feed against her inclination, and it is certainly not often successful.

In this chapter the management of infant feeding is approached in a relatively brief manner and personal preferences have not been eliminated. More detailed accounts can be obtained in books written by Graham and Shanks (1954), Evans and MacKeith (1954), and Ellis (1966).

BREAST FEEDING

ANTENATAL PREPARATION

The great value of preparing the expectant mother for lactation during her pregnancy was stressed by Waller (1946) in his admirable studies of the problems of breast feeding.

1. **Psychological.**—The doctor can do much to convince the young expectant mother of the value and advantages of breast feeding, and to neutralize the bad advice she so often gets from her own mother, other relatives and friends. He can, by using his position of trust, inculcate a positive attitude of conviction in the young mother who has probably never previously been educated in these aspects of female physiology. Among the advantages of breast feeding over artificial feeding are:

(a) Breast-milk is the natural food for the human infant. Its composition is very different from that of cow's milk (Table I) which was obviously never intended by nature as a source of infant nutrition.

(b) Breast-milk goes direct from "producer" to "consumer"; it is free from pathogenic bacteria while still in the mother's breasts, and there is little opportunity for it to become contaminated.

(c) Both baby, who enjoys the comfort of contact with a soft breast in contrast to a hard bottle, and mother, who derives great satisfaction from doing "what comes naturally", should obtain a feeling of well-being from the act of breast-feeding. The baby makes his first emotional contact with the person who feeds him. It is well that this should be his mother and that the contact should be as intimate as possible, because an infant learns to love through the pleasure and comfort connected with the satisfaction of his hunger instincts.

TABLE I

RELATIVE COMPOSITION OF HUMAN MILK AND COW'S MILK

Constituents	Human Milk	Cow's Milk
Protein	1·25 per cent	3·50 per cent
Lactalbumin	0·75 ,, ,,	0·50 ,, ,,
Caseinogen	0·50 ,, ,,	3·00 ,, ,,
Carbohydrate (lactose)	7·50 ,, ,,	4·50 ,, ,,
Fat	3·50 ,, ,,	4·00 ,, ,,
Calories per ounce	20	18–20

Calcium content of cow's milk is 4 times that of human milk.
Iron content of human milk is 2–3 times that of cow's milk.

2. **Diet.**—A mother who is to feed her baby should obviously have a good diet herself during pregnancy and lactation. Many women in the U.K. still fail to eat a properly balanced diet.

Important constituents to be advised are:

(*a*) First-class protein, e.g. milk, butter, eggs, cheese, fish, meat.

(*b*) Calcium and vitamin D, e.g. milk as the source of calcium, tab. calciferol conc. B.P., 1 daily (or substitute) as the source of vitamin D.

(*c*) Iron, e.g. vegetables, oatmeal, eggs. If the expectant mother is anaemic she should be given medicinal iron in a suitable preparation and dosage, e.g. ferrous sulphate 3 grains (0·2 gm.) t.d.s.

(*d*) Vitamin C, e.g. fruit, vegetables, salads.

3. **Preparation of the breasts.**—The breasts should be bathed every day during pregnancy. They should be massaged with the mother's two hands from the chest wall towards the nipple a dozen times each day. The nipples should then be rolled gently between the thumb and forefinger to clear the nipple ducts of the cheesy material which often blocks them, especially in primigravida. When this is done it will frequently be observed that colostrum can be freely expressed in the last week or two before term. When the nipples are retracted they can be drawn forwards during pregnancy by Waller's nipple shields (Maw and Sons, Watford), which should be worn under a well-fitting brassière.

TECHNIQUE OF BREAST FEEDING

Breast feeding is more likely to be successfully established in hospital-born babies when their cots are kept alongside their mothers' beds.

This custom, which is much to be preferred to isolating healthy infants in nurseries, also allows the mother to fondle and acquire confidence in handling her infant. The healthy infant should be put to the breast 12 hours after birth. To begin with 1 to 3 minutes at each breast will suffice at each feeding time, but after a week or so he should be allowed to suck for 10 minutes at each breast per feed. During the first 3 days of the puerperium the breasts secrete small volumes of colostrum. About the 4th day the milk comes in and the best stimulation to lactation is a healthy infant emptying the breasts at frequent intervals. In the early weeks of life the "feeding on demand" system is advocated. It is a pity that more maternity units do not encourage it, because this is obviously the natural behaviour which is likely to put the least stress on both mother and baby. It avoids the mother having to worry about her baby crying until the next feeding time falls due and in the baby it develops the sense of security which comes from knowing that he will be fed when he is hungry. In practice it will be found that most infants demand to be fed about every 3 hours 7–8 times in each 24 hours for the first 4 to 6 weeks, after which they settle down spontaneously to a fairly regular 4-hourly schedule. If the mother has too many other duties it is usually very easy *after* the first few weeks to change from self-demand feeding to a 4-hourly time-table which suits her convenience. Indeed, the introduction of breast feeding requires only reasonable commonsense. There is certainly none in laying down arbitrary rules about feeding times. These should be restful periods, and the mother should be comfortably seated in a low chair with a foot-stool on which to place her foot. In this way she can support her baby in the bend of her elbow with his head and shoulders raised to prevent regurgitation of gastric contents. Most modern mothers prefer to be alone while feeding their infants.

It is important, also, that the mother should be instructed in allowing her infant to gulp into his mouth as much of the breast as possible. This allows him to get his gums on the skin behind the areola where he can squeeze the milk out of the lacteal sinuses into the lactiferous ducts. It also ensures that the nipple is up against the infant's soft palate and so protected from the forces of suction or trauma from his gums. Sucking on the nipple alone is not only useless but may cause its delicate covering to crack with the risk of a breast abscess. The breast must not, however, be allowed to obstruct the infant's nostrils.

When lactation is well established, and this phase of adaptation takes 3–4 weeks, the "draught reflex" may be experienced by the mother (Waller, 1943; 1947). Many women experience bodily pleasure during the draught of milk into the breasts. This is especially likely if an explanation of the sensation has been given to her during pregnancy, so that she is not then troubled by it. This is analogous to the process known in the cow as the "let-down reflex". It is a nervous reaction which stimulates the secretion of oxytocin by the posterior pituitary, so that milk from the secreting areas of the breast is brought rapidly and under pressure into the lacteal sinuses below the areola. The mother experiences a feeling of tingling and tension in the breasts when about to feed her baby. In some, milk is actually ejected from the nipples. The draught reflex is a reliable sign that lactation is well established.

After the feed the infant should be propped over the mother's shoulder or into a sitting position on her lap to help him to "burp" up air which has been swallowed during the feed. Rubbing or patting his back is of further assistance.

The nipples should be cleaned with boiled water before and after each feed, and they should be protected from friction by the brassière with cotton wool. Mothers should be advised regarding the need for good personal hygiene. In particular, they should always wash their hands before feeding the baby. If the nipples should get sore some lanolin can be rubbed in gently every evening.

WEANING

In the Western countries weaning is usually recommended about the age of six months. In primitive communities breast feeding is often continued well into the second year of life. By then, however, milk alone is not an adequate diet and there is an especial liability to iron-deficiency anaemia in these circumstances. Weaning is easier if the infant has already been started on cereals or vegetables about the age of four months (see below). At six months one of the five breast feeds, to suit the mother's convenience, is replaced by a cow's milk preparation—from bottle or cup according to the infant's preference. On each subsequent week another breast feed is dropped so that by nine months of age the infant is off the breast entirely. It is unnecessary to replace all of the breast feeds by cow's milk. Indeed, some infants do not like cow's milk, and it is then more reasonable to use other sources of first-class protein, e.g. cereals, vegetables, egg-yolk, potato, minced meat and fish. If the mother's breasts are uncomfortable, and this is rarely a problem when weaning is gradual, she may be given stilboestrol 5 mg. t.d.s. for a few days.

CONTRA-INDICATIONS TO BREAST FEEDING

In the vast majority of instances breast feeding is replaced by bottle feeding for reasons which have no sound medical basis. In some cases breast feeding is impracticable because the infant is premature and too feeble to suck, or has some deformity such as cleft lip and palate, or micrognathia. Every effort should be made, however, to maintain lactation by regular expression of milk from the mother's breasts, either manually or by means of a breast-pump. The milk so obtained can be boiled and fed to the infant by bottle or tube until he is strong enough to feed for himself. It must also be stressed that although the breast-milk may be inadequate in quantity in some mothers, it is never inadequate in quality. It is, therefore, always wrong to abandon breast feeding because the infant is having digestive symptoms. The only exceptions to this rule are the rare conditions of galactosaemia and phenylketonuria (Chapter IX).

None the less, there are a few clear contra-indications, temporary or permanent, to breast feeding:

1. **Tuberculosis in the mother.**—In fact, the tuberculous mother should not look after her infant at all until he has been immunized with B.C.G. and isolated from her for at least six weeks. It is obvious that the mother should also receive appropriate drug treatment to render her non-infectious.

2. **Heart disease.**—In most cases breast feeding would over-burden the mother's already diminished reserve. Exceptions can, however, be made in the case of well-compensated valvular lesions.

3. **Thyrotoxicosis.**—This is an obvious contra-indication. It should be pointed out, further, that antithyroid drugs such as the thiouracils and carbimazole are excreted in breast-milk and would, if ingested by the infant, cause goitre and possible hypothyroidism.

4. **Puerperal insanity.**

5. **Chronic renal disease.**

6. **Diabetes mellitus.**—Mothers whose diabetes is well stabilized on diet and insulin may, however, be allowed to breast feed their infants.

7. **Acute infections.**—In practice, severe infections, such as pneumonia, usually result in discontinuance of breast feeding. They need not always do so because modern antibiotics can so quickly cure some conditions that the infant could be put back to the breast after some days.

8. **Other chronic diseases,** e.g. cancer, disseminated sclerosis.

9. **Acute engorgement of the breasts.**—This is only an indication for the *temporary* cessation of breast feeding. It develops about the third or fourth day of the puerperium and should be treated as a medical emergency. The breasts should be emptied by manual expression, both hands working from the chest wall towards the areola, followed by rhythmic expression of the breast just behind the areola between thumb and forefinger. The milk so expressed should be collected in a sterile container every four hours. Some experienced nurses become exceedingly expert at this technique. However, if the engorged breasts are very tense and tender with distended veins, shininess of the skin and hard palpable nodules behind the areola, manual expression may be intolerable. The condition may then be relieved with stilboestrol 5–10 mg. every four hours for six doses (24 hours) only. This causes a temporary inhibition of lactation and the breasts soon become soft and comfortable. The infant should then be put back to them and the stimulus of sucking will re-establish lactation at an adequate level.

Provided engorgement is treated promptly it should only be necessary to stop breast feeding for a few days.

ARTIFICIAL FEEDING

Reference to Table I will show that cow's milk cannot be an entirely satisfactory substitute for human milk. None the less, if its tough casein curd is attenuated—by boiling, drying or evaporating—cow's milk can promote an entirely acceptable rate of growth in human infants. The many mothers who decline to breast feed their babies can, of course, observe this for themselves in almost every street in the land. Although cow's milk differs widely from human milk, not only in protein, fat and carbohydrate, but also in aminoacid composition and mineral content, artificial feeding need not be a complicated or difficult business. All the common infant milk preparations, dried or evaporated, are equally satisfactory, although it is advisable to reduce the fat content to about 2 per cent of the reconstituted liquid form during the first 6–8 weeks of life (Table II). The common claim that a particular infant thrived on

TABLE II

APPROXIMATE PROTEIN, FAT, CARBOHYDRATE AND CALORIC VALUES OF SOME COMMON INFANT FOODS ON THE BRITISH MARKET. ALL ARE FORTIFIED TO SOME DEGREE WITH VITAMIN D, NOT EXCEEDING 100 I.U. PER DRIED OUNCE.

Preparation	Strength or Dilution	Protein	Fat	CHO	Calories per fl. oz.
Half Cream National Dried	1:8	3·4	2·0	4·8	15
Full Cream National Dried	1:8	3·4	3·4	4·8	18
Half Cream Cow and Gate	1:8	2·4	1·9	7·1	16
Full Cream Cow and Gate	1:8	3·3	3·4	4·8	18
Half Cream Cow and Gate (Special)	1:8	3·8	2·0	5·5	16
Ostermilk No. 1 (Glaxo)	1:8	2·3	2·4	7·0	18
Ostermilk No. 2 (Glaxo)	1:8	2·9	3·3	5·3	18
Trufood (Humanized)	1:8	1·8	3·4	6·3	18
S.M.A.	1:8	1·5	3·5	6·8	20
Half Cream Regal (Evaporated)	1:1·3	3·8	2·0	5·0	18
Regal (Evaporated)	1:2	3·8	3·0	4·8	18
Carnation (Evaporated)	1:2	3·0	3·0	4·8	18

one proprietary food and not on another can safely be assumed to be a misinterpretation of the true situation. It is, however, preferable that artificial feeding should be carried out with any one of the available proprietary preparations than with liquid cow's milk which is too easily contaminated in the unhygienic home.

Successful artificial feeding of the healthy infant demands only that *four* simple requirements be satisfied:

1. An adequate intake of calories in the form of modified cow's milk.
2. Absence of pathogenic bacteria from feeds.
3. Reasonable regularity in feeding times and methods.
4. Vitamin supplementation to replace those lacking in modified cow's milk.

1. **An adequate intake.**—The fact has already been stressed that the food requirements of individual infants may vary widely. It follows, therefore, that the various formulae used for the calculation of infant feeds at different ages must be regarded as no more than guidance to those inexperienced in the matter of infant feeding. The only real danger lies in underfeeding (see below). Overfeeding of gross degree may cause excessive gain in weight and some regurgitation of excess milk, but it is not a serious or common problem. Indeed, the fear of overfeeding has not infrequently been the cause of a dangerous degree of underfeeding (Vining, 1952; Wickes, 1952). However, some basic principles in the calculation of feeds must be stated. They are based largely on the work of the late G. B. Fleming in Glasgow (Graham and Shanks, 1954), and they must be regarded as indicating the *minimum* food requirements of healthy infants. It is not claimed that this method is superior to any other, because none can indicate the *optimum* food requirements of individual infants. Some may criticize the weights given below for healthy infants as being too low. While this is probably true of our prosperous community, they could also be criticized as being too high in many parts of the world. It can be stated, however, that the feeds as set out below will ensure that no infant suffers materially from malnutrition and that infants so fed will grow at an acceptable rate.

An infant requires 50 calories per lb. (110 calories per Kg.) of his *expected* body weight per day. If he is fed according to his actual weight the underweight infant will be underfed, whereas the obese infant will be overfed. A normal full-term infant weighs about 7 lb. (3·2 Kg.). He should gain $1\frac{1}{3}$ lb. (0·6 Kg.) per month for the first six months, and $1\frac{1}{4}$ lb. (0·5 Kg.) per month for the second six months. For example, an infant aged three months should weigh $7 + (1\frac{1}{3} \times 3)$ lb. $= 11$ lb. His caloric requirements are $11 \times 50 = 550$ per day. A reconstituted liquid ounce (1 measure made up to 1 fl. oz. with water) of full cream dried milk contains 18 calories (Table II). Therefore, the infant would require $550/18 = 30$ fl. oz. of milk per day, or five four-hourly feeds of

6 fl. oz. But as full cream milk contains only 4·8 per cent of carbohydrate, 1 fl. oz. of milk from each feed (18 calories) should be replaced
by 1 rounded off teaspoonful of sugar (20 calories). The suitable feeding
regime for a three month infant would thus be 5 fl. oz. of reconstituted
full cream dried milk (5 measures of milk powder made up to 5 fl. oz.
with water) plus 1 teaspoonful (rounded off) of sugar every four hours
five times daily. The same type of calculation can, of course, apply to
half-cream dried and evaporated milks. There is no advantage is using
a more expensive sugar than sucrose for artificial feeds. In some preparations the carbohydrate content has already been sufficiently raised
by the manufacturers, e.g. Half Cream Cow and Gate, Ostermilk No. 1,
Trufood Humanized and S.M.A. After mixed feeding has become a
substantial fraction of the infant's diet the daily intake of milk will become less than that which the above calculations would indicate. A
healthy infant does not need larger single milk feeds than 7 fl. oz. It is
preferable during the first 6–8 weeks of life that a milk preparation containing approximately 2 per cent of fat be used, because a few young
infants find a higher fat intake indigestible. Subsequently, a gradual
change over (e.g. 1 fl. oz. per feed per day) to a full cream milk should be
advocated. The nearest chemical approach to human milk is at present
found in S.M.A. There is, however, no substantial evidence that the
greater cost is justified by any increased well-being or safety in
its use.

2. **Absence of pathogens.**—An advantage of the dried milks is that
bacteria do not readily grow in them, and as the milk should be reconstituted with boiled water immediately before use the risks of contamination are slight. Evaporated milk is safer when the household
possess a refrigerator, but in its absence the tin should be covered with a
saucer after it has been opened.

The feeding bottles, preferably of the single-ended Soxhlet type, must
be thoroughly cleaned after use in cold water which will not coagulate
the milk protein. A bottle brush is used to detach milk from the inner
surface of the bottle. Thereafter, hot water should be used to remove the
fat. The bottles can be sterilized by leaving them in boiling water for ten
minutes. Alternatively they should be immersed for at least four hours
in a 1:80 solution of sodium hypochlorite (Milton Pharmaceuticals
Ltd.). It is convenient to use six bottles and to sterilize them all together.
They can be left in the water in which they were sterilized or in Milton
solution until each is required. The spoon and half-pint measure which
are used for mixing the feeds should, of course, be similarly sterilized.
The teats can also be boiled or put into Milton, or they can be rendered
safe by pouring *boiling* water over them just before use. They should be
protected from dust between feeds by covering them with a cup or small
medicine glass. Some infants prefer plain, others bulb-ended teats. Wide-
necked bottles, which are easier to clean, require suitably designed teats.

The hole in a teat can be enlarged if necessary by a quick insertion of a fine red-hot needle.

Many poorly educated mothers are ignorant about the dangers of contamination and the methods of sterilization. They must be given detailed instructions in simple language, preferably in writing. It is also important to stress the necessity of hand-washing before the bottles are handled or feeds are prepared. This type of instruction in mothercraft is the responsibility of the family doctor, the child welfare medical officer, the health visitor or the mothercraft sister of a children's hospital.

3. **Regular feeding times.**—Most full-term infants are fed at four-hourly intervals, e.g. 6 a.m., 10 a.m., 2 p.m., 6 p.m. and 10 p.m. It is unnecessary to insist on absolute time-keeping. In particular, latitude should be permitted for the early morning and evening feeds. Very young infants frequently cry for food in the early hours of the morning and a sixth feed should be prepared in case of need before the parents retire at night. The infant should be held with his head and shoulders raised during feeds. The hole in the teat should be big enough to let him finish his feed within 20 minutes but not so large that too free a flow of milk chokes him. Too small a hole results in swallowing excessive amounts of air with resultant colic and crying. In any case, the infant should be propped up after each feed to let him break wind. The milk should be at about body temperature when it is offered to the infant.

4. **Vitamin supplements.**—The normal full-term baby requires about 2,500 units of vitamin A, 400 units of vitamin D, and 15–25 mg. of vitamin C (ascorbic acid) per day. These amounts are not available in cow's milk. However, all the dried and evaporated milks contain sufficient vitamin D to prevent rickets in normal infants. The Government issue of Cod-liver Oil Compound contains 2,500 units of vitamin A and 400 units of vitamin D_2 (calciferol) in a teaspoonful, which is recommended as a suitable daily dose. An adequate intake of vitamin C can be assured by two teaspoonfuls (diluted with water and sweetened with sugar) of the Government issues of Concentrated Orange Juice or Rose-hip Syrup. Alternatively vitamins A and D may be given in the form of one of the official B.P. or proprietary concentrates, and vitamin C as ascorbic acid tablets. Premature infants require larger doses (Chapter II).

INTRODUCTION OF MIXED FEEDING

Mixed feeding should be introduced before the 10 a.m. and 6 p.m. feeds by the age of four months. It is particularly important to ensure an adequate intake of iron after this age because both human milk and cow's milk are lacking in this mineral. A start may be made with two teaspoonfuls of one of the pre-cooked cereals suitable for infants, e.g. Cow and Gate Infant Cereal, Farex, Scott's Twinpack, Robrex etc.

These are mixed with some of the milk feed subsequently to be given. When the infant has learned to enjoy these foods (which are also fortified with calciferol) and to take about a tablespoonful at each feed he can be offered further variety before the 2 p.m. feed, e.g. potatoes and gravy, soft boiled egg yolk, mince, homogenized vegetables, meats and fruits, pulped banana, stewed apple etc. After the age of six months the average infant can hold in his hand and chew a rusk or crust. Finally, by the age of one year he should be on three main meals per day— breakfast, dinner and tea—plus fruit juice on awakening and a drink of pasteurized cow's milk at bedtime.

FEEDING DISORDERS

Feeding disorders in infancy are most often due to incorrect feeding (Hutchison, 1958). Their satisfactory treatment requires accurate diagnosis as to cause, and this rests largely upon careful history-taking. It is obviously necessary to separate digestive upsets which are caused by improper feeding from those due to some primary organic disease, but it is only occasionally necessary to have resort to special radiographic and biochemical investigations.

UNDERFEEDING

This is by far the commonest cause of digestive upset in both breast-fed and bottle-fed babies. Diagnosis depends upon eliciting the fact that the intake of milk amounts to less than 50 calories per lb. of expected body weight per day. This is done in breast-fed infants by test weighing before and after every feed for 24 hours, and by a careful feeding history in the case of bottle-fed babies. The underfed infant fails to gain weight satisfactorily and finally develops a state of marasmus (Chapter VIII). He is irritable and sleepless and he cries long before his feeds are due. He feeds eagerly and often swallows air so that colic aggravates his misery and restlessness. Constipation is an early sign. Later he passes only small dark green stains of mucus, "starvation stools". These must not be mistaken for the large, watery grass-green stools of gastro-enteritis. The underfed infant obviously requires more food and not the starvation regime employed in gastro-enteritis.

Treatment

The correction of underfeeding by gradually increasing the milk intake over a period of a few days results in a dramatic improvement in the infant's temperament, to be followed by gain in weight. In the case of the breast-fed infant complementary feeds of dried or evaporated milk should be given after every breast-feed. When the breast-milk supply from the mother amounts to less than half the value of 50 calories per lb. of expected weight per day the infant is best weaned and put entirely on to artificial feeding.

VOMITING

Possetting or the vomiting of mouthfuls of milk is fairly common, especially in breast-fed infants. It does not interfere with satisfactory weight gains and the food intake should not be reduced unless the infant is being grossly overfed. This is rare. The most common cause of vomiting is air swallowing. This may be due to underfeeding or to too small a hole in the teat. The treatment in each case is obvious and diagnosis is facilitated by watching the infant while he is feeding. Nasal obstruction from rhinitis can make feeding difficult and lead to vomiting. It can be relieved by the instillation of nose drops (1 per cent ephedrine in physiological saline) before each feed. Vomiting from organic causes such as pyloric stenosis when it is projectile and forcible, or intestinal obstruction when the vomitus is bile-stained, or infections whether enteral or parenteral, can usually be diagnosed on simple clinical examination. Hiatus hernia should be suspected and confirmed by barium-swallow when the vomitus contains excess mucus or altered blood. Cretinism frequently presents as a case of feeding difficulty with some vomiting and constipation, and this diagnosis is too often unnecessarily long in being reached. There is a small group of infants who suffer from "habitual vomiting" for which no cause can be found. They usually thrive quite well and the mothers rather than the infants are distressed. In fact, the parents of these babies are often tense over-anxious people, difficult to reassure. It is, of course, essential that incorrect feeding and organic abnormalities are safely excluded before a diagnosis of "habitual vomiting" is accepted. Sedation with chloral hydrate 1–3 grains before each feed is often helpful.

Finally, mention must be made of rumination. This habit allows the infant to obtain oral gratification by voluntarily bringing back into his mouth some of his feed which he partly vomits and partly chews. He can frequently be seen to curl his tongue into a funnel and to encourage the regurgitation of milk along it by rhythmic back and forward movements of his mandible. The treatment of this psychoneurosis of infancy is often difficult. The feeds should be thickened with cereal, and the infant should be propped up after feeds. His attention should be diverted, as far as practicable, when he indulges in his habit. Spontaneous recovery takes place when he learns to stand unsupported. Vomiting due to true *milk allergy* is very uncommon and virtually unknown in breast-fed infants. It demands gradual desensitization with carefully graduated milk dilutions, while a trial is made with soya flour or goat's milk. Alternatively, corticosteroids may be used, starting with large doses which are gradually reduced. The risks of this form of therapy must be carefully weighed against the advantages. The author has only once had to resort to it.

Constipation

It is common for mothers to complain that their infants are "constipated", by which they usually mean infrequent stools. In fact, in most cases the stools are of normal consistency and these mothers have failed to appreciate that the stool frequency varies widely from one infant to another, especially in breast-fed babies. In true constipation the stools are small and hard as well as infrequent, and apart from underfeeding and over-heating it is uncommon in infancy. The physician should only accept a diagnosis of constipation when he has himself confirmed that the stools are small and hard, or when he can palpate numerous hard masses of faeces in the abdomen. Other causes of constipation are infections, hypothyroidism, anal stenosis, Hirschsprung's disease and metabolic disorders such as idiopathic hypercalcaemia or the de Toni-Fanconi syndrome. It should be noted that in none of these conditions would laxatives achieve any benefit and they are rarely, if ever, indicated in young infants. Underfeeding and over-heating are readily correctable. The other causes require much more complicated treatment.

Diarrhoea

Diarrhoea in infancy is most often due to enteral infections by specific *E. coli* or other pathogens. Some cases are secondary to parenteral infections, e.g. pyelonephritis, osteitis and otitis media. It is most improbable that diarrhoea is ever due to relative excesses of fat, protein or carbohydrate in the diet, although this has often been claimed in the past. It is worth mention that some perfectly healthy breast-fed infants pass frequent loose mustard-coloured stools. The obvious well-being of these babies should be sufficient indication that they do not have diarrhoea.

Colic

In most cases loud crying associated with flexion of the thighs on to the abdominal wall does not indicate pain but hunger, discomfort from chilling or over-heating, a wet napkin, or anxiety due to a worried inexperienced mother. When there is severe abdominal pain, as in intussusception, the attacks of colic produce blanching and faintness. Air-swallowing as a cause of colic has already been mentioned as due to underfeeding, nasal obstruction or too small a hole in the teat. Illingworth (1954) has given a good description of the somewhat mysterious "three months' colic". This is encountered in infants between the hours of 6 and 10 p.m. The infant goes red in the face, draws up his legs, and screams loudly for 2–10 minutes. He is not quietened by an extra feed or by fondling. One line of treatment is sedation with choral hydrate 3–5 grains (0·2–0·3 gm.) or elixir methylpentynol 15–30 minims (1–2 ml.). Another is with dicyclomine hydrochloride 5–10 mg. (Merbentyl syrup 30–60 minims) before feeds. The condition is benign and disappears spontaneously.

REFERENCES

ELLIS, R. W. B. (1966). *Child Health and Development*, 4th edit. London: J. & A. Churchill.

EVANS, P., and MACKEITH, R. (1954). *Infant Feeding*, 2nd edit. London: J. & A. Churchill.

GRAHAM, S., and SHANKS, R. A. (1954). *Notes on Infant Feeding*, 4th edit. Edinburgh: E. & S. Livingstone.

GRULEE, C. G., SANFORD, H. N., and HERRON, P. H. (1934). *J. Amer. med. Ass.*, **103**, 735.

HUTCHISON, J. H. (1958). *Practitioner*, **180**, 401.

ILLINGWORTH, R. S. (1954). *Arch. Dis. Childh.*, **29**, 165.

SMELLIE, J. M. (1952). *Brit. J. Nutr.*, **6**, 220.

VINING, C. W. (1952). *Lancet*, **2**, 99.

WALLER, H. (1943). *Lancet*, **1**, 69.

WALLER, H. (1946). *Arch. Dis. Childh.*, **21**, 1.

WALLER, H. (1947). *Mth. Bull. Minist. Hlth. Lab. Serv.*, **6**, 73.

WICKES, I. G. (1952). *Brit. med. J.*, **2**, 1178.

CHAPTER VIII

FAILURE TO THRIVE IN INFANCY

An infant's failure to thrive and to gain weight at a satisfactory rate is one of the most common reasons for young parents to consult their family physician. Persistent failure to gain weight, or actual loss of weight, will lead to the clinical state of marasmus (infantile atrophy; wasting; athrepsia). This exists when an infant is below 75 per cent of the expected weight for his age. The state of marasmus can by itself endanger life, whatever the primary cause, and even if that cause is eliminated, when the infant's weight falls below 65 per cent of the expected weight for his age. Furthermore, if admission to hospital cannot be avoided, the marasmic infant is highly susceptible to cross infection which only too often proves fatal. It is, therefore, the physician's urgent responsibility when consulted about an infant who is not making satisfactory progress, to ascertain the primary cause. This can frequently be corrected at an early stage without recourse to the hospital.

It must be emphasized that the word "marasmus" implies only a clinical state, in the same way as words such as "acidosis", "ketosis" and "uraemia". It is not to be accepted as a satisfactory diagnosis because by itself it gives no clue to aetiology or to rational treatment. It should also be stressed that, with the exception of a few uncommon metabolic disorders (e.g. galactosaemia, hypercalcaemia), attempts to treat the marasmic infant by advising a change from one variety or preparation of infant food to another are misdirected. All too often this type of uninspired guesswork only delays the search for the true diagnosis and the start of correct treatment. The ability to arrive at a correct diagnosis requires firstly that the physician is familiar with the possible causes of marasmus. When this knowledge is associated with the information to be obtained from a thoughtful case-history followed by a careful clinical examination, the cause of an infant's failure to thrive is usually evident. It is only infrequently that admission to hospital for laboratory tests proves necessary. The contrast between the sound physician and the empiricist is never more obvious than when he is faced with a marasmic and unhappy infant. The practical problem of the management of the state of marasmus can conveniently be approached by a description of the clinical appearances, by an account of the possible causes and, finally, by a discussion of the differentiation between these causes as the clinical history and examination of the patient unfold and reveal significant clues.

Clinical Features of Marasmus

The most striking appearances (Fig. 12) are due to loss of the sub-cutaneous fat. This often gives the infant's face a lined and somewhat aged appearance. Over the limbs, and especially on the inner aspects of the thighs and arms and on the buttocks, the skin hangs in loose folds. The ribs are unduly prominent and the abdominal wall is hypotonic and loosely covered by skin. The appearances are quite similar to those

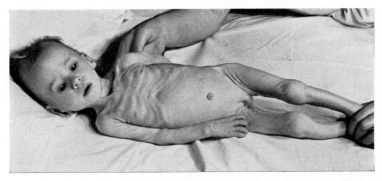

Fig. 12.—Marasmic infant aged 10 months. Note loss of subcutaneous fat, most marked over limbs and chest. Facial expression is unhappy and apathetic.

of old age, and for the same reason, there is a paucity of subcutaneous fat. In a few infants the subcutaneous fat over the face is less depleted than elsewhere on the body and the true extent of the body wasting may not be appreciated unless the infant is fully undressed. In others the face becomes so wasted that the so-called "sucking pads" of fat over the masseter muscles project visibly from each side of the face. The temperament of the marasmic infant is characterized by unhappiness, an anxious expression, and a disconsolate wailing irritability. Finally, this may be replaced by an ominous apathy. When his weight falls below 65 per cent of the expected body weight for his age it is common to find a low rectal temperature because the insulating and heat-conserving layer of subcutaneous fat has gone. Furthermore, there is a lack of spare tissue which may be used for endogenous heat production. The depletion of glycogen stores may be reflected in a low blood sugar, and a glucose tolerance test may reveal a diabetic type of curve. In the ter-minal stages the presence of hypoproteinaemia is frequently revealed by peripheral oedema ("starvation oedema"), and purpura may appear. Intercurrent infections, especially subcutaneous abscesses over pressure areas such as the occiput, scapulae and buttocks, suppurative otitis media, or bronchopneumonia due to aspiration of vomitus and gastric contents, are common. In fact, they commonly aggravate the marasmus so that a vicious circle is set up, marasmus—intercurrent infection—marasmus.

Causes of Marasmus

(1) **Underfeeding.**—While simple starvation is a common cause of wasting in some parts of the world, marasmus due to an insufficient intake of calories in Britain always results from an improper feeding regime by ignorant or negligent parents. The incidence of marasmus due to incorrect feeding has been greatly reduced by the widespread use of dried or evaporated milk preparations in preference to liquid cow's milk. Enteral infection has become much less frequent and an adequate caloric intake is usually assured when the mother follows the manufacturers' instructions on the labels. Notwithstanding, it is still not uncommon in paediatric practice among the less intelligent sections of our community to encounter infants whose failure to thrive is solely accountable to mismanagement (Chapter VII).

(2) **Infections.**—Any infection of enough severity and duration can lead to marasmus. It may be enteral (e.g. infantile gastro-enteritis) or parenteral (e.g. bronchopneumonia, osteitis, pyelonephritis, subcutaneous abscesses), and while not often the primary cause of marasmus nowadays is still commonly superimposed on the infant who has been already rendered marasmic by other factors.

(3) **Congenital abnormalities of structure.**—Any severe anatomical anomaly which is compatible with prolongation of life beyond a few weeks is likely to interfere with the infant's ability to thrive. There are many such congenital defects amongst which some of the commonest are cardiac anomalies (cyanotic and acyanotic), hydrocephalus, cerebral agenesis, renal anomalies (e.g. bladder neck obstruction, bilateral hydronephrosis, renal hypoplasia), hiatus hernia, pyloric stenosis, atresia of the bile ducts, Hirschsprung's disease, and deformities of the palate and jaws which interfere with feeding (e.g. severe cleft palate, micrognathia).

(4) **Fibrocystic disease of the pancreas.**—This disease may interfere with nutrition by deficient intestinal absorption, and also from the effects of the invariable staphylococcal lung sepsis which accompanies its course.

(5) **Metabolic disorders.**—A wide variety of metabolic disturbances, some inborn and others acquired, but each relatively rare in themselves, may cause failure to thrive in infancy. Their relative importance continues to increase as underfeeding and the infections have become less common in our prosperous economy, and as surgical treatment of the more serious congenital abnormalities becomes ever more successful. Among the more serious metabolic diseases are dysfunction of the renal tubules as in hyperchloraemic renal acidosis, the de Toni-Fanconi syndrome and nephrogenic diabetes insipidus; idiopathic hyper-

calcaemia; galactosaemia; and congenital diabetes mellitus. These conditions are fully discussed in the relevant sections of this book.

(6) **Hypothalamic tumour.**—Russell (1951) has described an exceedingly rare type of fatal emaciation which develops in a peculiarly euphoric over-active infant under the name of the "diencephalic syndrome of infancy". The tumour is usually an astrocytoma.

A common cause of tissue-wasting in young children is coeliac disease. This condition frequently has its onset during the last three months of the first year of life, but it rarely leads to a state of wasting until after the first birthday. It is, therefore, not properly included amongst the causes of marasmus as the term is customarily confined to the period of infancy (birth—one year).

Differential Diagnosis

The investigation of a marasmic infant is an intellectual exercise in which adherence to the basic principles of clinical medicine is essential. The unfortunate infant who falls into the hands of the practitioner who approaches the problem with a new proprietary infant food or tablets of sodium citrate, based on the nonsensical concept that the infant's digestion may be "weak", is in a sorry plight, nor will he be extricated from it by a battery of laboratory tests carried out in a haphazard manner and in the hope that "something will turn up". Unfortunately, we have seen these methods too often used with disastrous and avoidable results.

The first requirement of the physician is that he should take a thoughtful history, starting with the mother's health before and during pregnancy. A history of maternal rubella during the first trimester could indicate congenital heart disease. A detailed feeding history, although it may have to be elicited with difficulty from an unintelligent mother, is the only means whereby underfeeding can be diagnosed. It can certainly not be revealed by physical examination or by any laboratory investigation. A history of projectile vomiting would obviously suggest pyloric stenosis, whereas when the vomitus contains much mucus and/or altered blood hiatus hernia must be considered. When vomiting is accompanied by the frequent passage of loose grass-green stools the diagnosis is likely to be gastro-enteritis. The small dark green mucoid stains on the napkins which are often passed by grossly underfed infants ("starvation stools") must, of course, be distinguished from the large watery green stools of infection. On the other hand, when the stools are described as greasy and very foul-smelling, and especially if there is a history of a spasmodic cough, fibrocystic disease of the pancreas becomes a distinct possibility. Congestive cardiac failure in the young infant results in undue breathlessness on exertion, just as it does in the adult. However, the infant's most common form of exertion is in feeding and the mother may reveal the breathlessness at these times by saying that the baby "gets tired" halfway through his feeds, or that he takes over an hour to finish them.

A careful history will more often than not direct the physician to the probable cause of the marasmus. He may, in fact, have already reached a diagnosis, such as incorrect feeding or gastro-enteritis. Physical examination will then reveal most of the diseases which can cause marasmus. For example, there may be signs of respiratory infection, or there may be cardiac enlargement with audible murmurs and possibly cyanosis, hepatomegaly or oedema. In Hirschsprung's disease there will be a grossly distended abdomen and severe constipation, but the rectum is found empty by the examining little finger. Even in the early weeks of life the staphylococcal bronchiolitis and complicating obstructive emphysema of fibrocystic disease of the pancreas may be reflected in the chest, which is held permanently in an inspiratory position with taut sternomastoid muscles, prominent sternum and horizontal ribs. Each inspiration causes subcostal and intercostal recession. There may be crepitations over the lungs. Distressing spasms of coughing are typically seen. Pyloric stenosis must be confirmed by a test-feed as described in Chapter XVI. A bladder neck obstruction produces a large hypertrophied bladder, which is both visible and palpable in the hypogastrium. The kidneys and greatly dilated ureters may also be visible or palpable. Enquiry will elicit the fact that the infant never passes a normal stream of urine but only dribbles small volumes intermittently. Other congenital anomalies of the urinary tract usually present with pyuria. It is particularly important that a specimen of urine should be obtained, and examined chemically and microscopically, from any marasmic infant in whom the diagnosis is not already obvious. Not only may this simple procedure reveal pyuria, it may also lead to a diagnosis of galactosuria or congenital diabetes mellitus. At this stage well directed special investigations may be necessary to complete or confirm the diagnosis, e.g. barium swallow for hiatus hernia, X-rays of the abdomen for Hirschsprung's disease, X-rays and electrocardiographs for congenital heart disease, or chemical analysis of the duodenal juice for fibrocystic disease of the pancreas. These investigations are described in the appropriate sections, but it should be stressed that in most cases of marasmus a diagnosis upon which rational therapy can be based may be reached without them and without recourse to the hospital.

However, in a few instances the cause of the marasmus remains uncertain even after a careful history and examination of the patient. In these cases the suspicion of one of the somewhat rare metabolic diseases should be aroused, e.g. de Toni-Fanconi syndrome, hyperchloraemic renal acidosis, idiopathic hypercalcaemia or nephrogenic diabetes insipidus. All of these very different metabolic disturbances tend to share the same symptoms, such as failure to thrive, vomiting, marked constipation, and thirst with polyuria. Dehydration frequently accompanies the marasmus. Their differentiation requires detailed biochemical studies which are described elsewhere. It is in this type of case that the facilities of a hospital are essential.

Treatment

Enough has already been said in this short chapter to indicate the necessity that the physician, charged with the responsibility of caring for the infant who is not thriving, shall obey one of the golden rules of clinical medicine, namely, that diagnosis must always precede treatment. While this rule is admittedly sometimes difficult to keep, in the case of marasmus it cannot be overstressed that a careful history and diligent physical examination will, with rare exceptions, reveal the diagnosis and point to the logical line of treatment. Only in a minority of cases is it necessary to admit the infant to hospital with its attendant risks of cross-infection. When it is unavoidable, the debilitated infant should always be placed in a cubicle and full barrier nursing techniques be enforced.

The precise details of treatment will be found under the appropriate diseases which cause failure to thrive in infancy. The commonest, underfeeding, is most easily corrected by progressively, but not too suddenly increasing the infant's caloric intake (see Chapter VII). The most difficult problem arises in the infant who is already under 65 per cent of the expected body weight for his age, and in whom two causes coexist, e.g. underfeeding and infection. In these cases a considerable mortality is inevitable and the only reasonable course is prevention. This is, fortunately, practised by large numbers of family doctors and in our Child Welfare Clinics. Only too often, however, the admission of a severely wasted infant to a paediatric unit reflects a most regrettable neglect of the first principles of good doctoring on the part of some practitioner who has been previously consulted. It is in an attempt to avoid these incidents that the subject of failure to thrive has been accorded a separate chapter in this book.

REFERENCE

RUSSELL, A. (1951). *Arch. Dis. Childh.*, **26**, 274.

CHAPTER IX

INBORN ERRORS OF METABOLISM

There has been a remarkable increase in our knowledge of the inborn metabolic errors in recent years, largely brought about by the introduction of new biochemical techniques. The term "inborn errors of metabolism" was first used by Garrod in 1908 when he described albinism, alkaptonuria, cystinuria and pentosuria. Garrod, noting the frequency of consanguineous matings in the pedigrees of his patients, correctly inferred the genetic origin of these disorders. He went further and suggested that they arose through the medium of defective enzyme activities. At the present time over 80 inborn errors of metabolism have been defined and our concepts of their nature have considerably broadened since 1908. In this book it would clearly be impracticable to consider the whole subject which is, indeed, now far beyond the competence of any one individual. An attempt has been made to portray a broad outline of the subject, and some of the more common or important diseases in the group receive more detailed consideration. Others are considered in other chapters under the various systems of the body. Fairly extensive references to the literature are included for those wishing to pursue the subject in more detail. Textbooks entirely devoted to the metabolic errors have been prepared by Hsia (1959) and Stanbury *et al.* (1965). A symposium on the subject was published in the *American Journal of Medicine*, Vol. 22, 1957.

GENERAL AETIOLOGICAL CONSIDERATIONS

It is now certain that genes act through the control of complex intracellular biochemical reactions. In 1957, Dent wrote, "By an inborn metabolic error is meant a permanent inherited condition due to a primary enzyme abnormality. As a result one or more chemical compounds may follow an altered metabolic pathway and may be found in some body fluids in greatly increased or decreased quantities." The modern concept of "one gene—one enzyme" is now firmly established. It follows, therefore, that an abnormal or defective enzyme activity must be related to an abnormal or mutant gene.

Our understanding of the nature of gene activity was greatly furthered by the work of Watson and Crick (1952) when they described the structure of the deoxyribonucleic acid (DNA) molecule. A gene is composed of DNA combined in some way to protein, and it is believed that the structure of the DNA molecule determines the specific function of the gene. This structure consists of two helical chains of phosphate-sugar each coiled round the same axis. The chains are held together by purine and pyrimidine bases which are at right angles to the axis of the molecule. There are four such bases in the DNA molecule—adenine (a purine), thymine (a pyrimidine), guanine (a purine) and cytosine (a pyrimidine). The genetic function is coded, as it were, by the particular sequence of these alternating pairs of purine and pyrimidine bases along the length of the DNA molecule. It would appear that the activity of the DNA molecules on the chromosomes transmits information to the molecules of ribonucleic acid (RNA) within the cell nucleus. There are also four nitrogen bases in the RNA molecule—adenine, guanine, cytosine and uracil (instead of thymine as in DNA). The RNA or "messenger" molecules then diffuse out into the cytoplasm and pick up individual aminoacids which come together to form polypeptide chains and proteins. The sequence of bases along the RNA molecule is the code which determines the order of incorporation of aminoacids into the particular polypeptide chains. A mutation, therefore, consists of a single alteration in the sequence of bases in the DNA molecule and consequently in the RNA molecule. This results then in the substitution of one aminoacid for another in the polypeptide chain. For example, the haemoglobin in sickle cell anaemia (Hb.S) differs from normal haemoglobin (Hb.A) only in that valine occupies the position in the haemoglobin peptide sequence normally occupied by glutamic acid (Ingram, 1956 and 1957).

In the case of defective enzyme reactions it seems likely that the absence of activity is due to the formation of an enzyme protein which is only slightly abnormal in structure, possibly only involving one aminoacid, but because of this, lacking normal functional activity. The protein macromolecules built up along the RNA "messenger" molecules are often but not always in the form of enzymes. However, they are essential to the metabolism of the cells, and many workers now include among the inborn errors of metabolism all specific molecular abnormalities which are genetically determined whether they involve enzymes or not. Pauling has suggested the term "the molecular diseases". They can be divided into four types (Hsia, 1959):

1. *Disturbances in structure of protein molecules*, e.g. the haemoglobinopathies.
2. *Disturbances in synthesis of protein molecules*, e.g. haemophilia, Christmas disease, congenital afibrinogenaemia, congenital hypogammaglobulinaemia, and Wilson's disease where caeruloplasmin is deficient.
3. *Disturbances in function of protein molecules*, e.g. enzyme deficiencies like phenylketonuria, galactosaemia and many others.
4. *Disturbances in renal transport mechanisms*, e.g.

nephrogenic diabetes insipidus, renal glycosuria, de Toni-Fanconi syndrome, vitamin D-resistant rickets.

In 1961 a striking advance was made in the attempt to "break the code" which the base-pair sequences on the DNA and RNA molecules represent (Nirenberg and Matthaei, 1961; Crick *et al.*, 1961), and our understanding of the nature of gene mutation has proportionately increased. It would seem that the basic unit of the code which codes any individual aminoacid is a sequence of three of the four possible nitrogen bases on the RNA molecule. Mutation is thought to involve the addition or deletion of a base. The addition of one or two bases destroys the function of the gene, but the addition of a third largely restores the function. For example, if the normal base sequence is taken to be ABC, ABC, . . . , the effect of adding one base would be MAB, CAB, CAB, . . . , of adding two bases MMA, BCA, BCA, . . . , but of adding three bases MMM, ABC, ABC, ... It can be seen that the addition of three bases has largely restored the original sequence of bases. As a practical example it is known that a sequence of three uracil bases in the RNA molecule is the code for phenylalanine. As a code of three bases out of the four gives 64 different possibilities it is obvious that any one particular aminoacid must be able to be coded by several triplets of genes. This type of code is described as "degenerate". It is probable that when the code is fully worked out it will be the same for all living organisms from viruses to man. The day will come when the mutations which result in anatomical anomalies can be interpreted in biochemical terms. This will mean that these anatomical abnormalities and the physiological abnormalities which we call "inborn metabolic errors" will be inseparable.

It is hoped that this short introduction to a complicated subject will assist the reader to comprehend more fully the common factor in a group of diseases which in superficial symptomatology would seem to be totally unrelated one to another.

PHENYLKETONURIA

Aetiology

This condition is transmitted as an autosomal recessive trait, so that in any family in which the disease has appeared the chances of future children being affected will be 1 in 4. The incidence of phenylketonuria is at least 1 in 20,000 births.

Pathogenesis

In normal individuals phenylalanine, which is an essential aminoacid, is converted in the liver to tyrosine by the activity of phenylalanine hydroxylase. In persons homozygous for the gene there is an absence or gross deficiency of this enzyme. In consequence, phenylalanine rises to high levels in the blood and urine. It is also converted by oxidative deamination and transamination to phenylpyruvic acid, the easy detection of which is the basis for a simple diagnostic test in this disease. Other degradation products such as phenyllactic acid, phenylacetic acid and phenylacetylglutamine are also found in the urine in large amounts. Other abnormal urinary constituents are indole products—indolyllactic, indolylacetic and indolylpyruvic acids—derived from tryptophane. There may also be traces of tyrosine products—p-hydroxyphenyl-pyruvic-lactic, and -acetic acids. The precise mechanism of the brain damage in phenylketonuria is unknown but the fair hair and blue eyes are presumed to be due to deficient availability of tyrosine.

Clinical Features

Most phenylketonurics are low-grade mental defectives. A very few are only slightly retarded. They are frequently blue-eyed, fair-haired and with fair skins. Eczema is often troublesome. Some have convulsions, athetosis and electroencephalographic changes. Many show psychotic features such as abnormal posturings with hands and fingers, repetitive movements such as head-banging or rocking to-and-fro, and complete lack of interest in people as distinct from inanimate objects. The tendon reflexes are often accentuated.

It should be noted that infants born homozygous for the phenyl-ketonuric trait are not brain-damaged at birth. They only become so after they start to ingest phenylalanine in their milk.

Diagnosis

The presence of phenylpyruvic acid in the urine can be quickly detected by adding a few drops of 5 or 10 per cent aqueous solution of ferric chloride to 5 ml. of acidified urine, when a green colour will develop within 2–3 minutes. Alternatively, a moist napkin can be tested with Phenistix (Ames & Co.) which is pressed between two layers of the napkin to be followed by a similar green colour. A false positive result yielding a less stable green colour can be due to p-hydroxyphenyl-pyruvic acid in the urine. This occurs in the inborn error of meta-bolism called tyrosinosis (Medes, 1932) in which the enzyme p-hydroxy-phenylpyruvic oxidase is deficient, and also in some premature infants who are on high protein diets (Levine et al., 1943). A positive ferric chloride or Phenistix reaction must, therefore, be followed by the demonstration of a high serum phenylalanine level before the diagnosis of phenylketonuria can be accepted (La Du and Michael, 1960). A screening test designed to reveal high serum levels of phenylalanine has now been developed—the bacterial inhibition assay method of Guthrie. It is being widely used to detect cases of phenylketonuria in very early infancy, and it becomes positive by the seventh day of life. A positive Guthrie test should also be taken to indicate the need for chemical estimation of the serum phenylalanine level to confirm the diagnosis.

The heterozygous carriers of the phenylketonuric gene can be detected on the basis of abnormal phenylalanine tolerance tests (Hsia *et al.*, 1956).

Treatment

But not established *—may well be* *waste of effort* There is reason to believe that the early introduction of a low-phenylalanine diet can prevent brain damage in affected infants (Knox and Hsia, 1957; Woolf *et al.*, 1958). When the diagnosis is delayed for over a year there is an irreversible component in the brain damage and treatment can then only improve, but not abolish, the mental retardation and other neurological abnormalities. In many areas of Britain it is now routine practice to test the urine of every infant for phenylpyruvic acid between the ages of four and six weeks. In some districts the Guthrie test on blood is replacing urine testing in the belief that the results are more reliable. As a result an increasing number of patients are being placed on this complicated and extremely expensive diet. The full implications of this treatment have yet to be faced. It is not only very costly, but its satisfactory employment demands a greater level of intelligence and responsibility than some parents possess, and there is at present no long-term residential accommodation for phenyl-

TABLE III

Preparation	Phenylalanine mg. per 100 gm.	Protein per 100 gm. powder	Additions
Minafen (Trufood) *Reconstitute 1 : 8 (infants)*	20 mg.	17·5 gm.	Aminoacids Carbohydrate Fat Minerals Vitamins
Cymogran (Allen & Hanbury)	10 mg.	28 gm.	Aminoacids Carbohydrate Fat Minerals
Lofenalac (Mead Johnson)	60–100 mg.	15 gm.	Aminoacids Carbohydrate Fat Minerals Vitamins

Foods almost free of phenylalanine. Minafen is reconstituted with water as a 1 in 8 parts preparation for infants. Cymogran and Lofenalac are prepared either as soups (flavoured with vegetables, tomato juice etc.) or as puddings (flavoured with fruit essences).

ketonurics who cannot be adequately treated at home and who are of normal or near-normal intelligence.

The aim of treatment is to reduce the serum level of phenylalanine to normal (2–3 mg. per 100 ml.) (Hutchison, 1962). It is not satisfactory merely to keep the urine clear of phenylpyruvic acid because negative urine tests frequently coexist with serum phenylalanine levels over 8 mg. per 100 ml. Treatment is started with a phenylalanine-free preparation (Table III). This is a casein hydrolysate which is almost completely free of phenylalanine and to which has been added certain aminoacids, fats and minerals. When the serum phenylalanine level has come down to normal or less, some phenylalanine-containing foods are carefully added to the diet in measured quantities, e.g. milk, cornflour, vegetables, fruit, potato, gluten-free bread, butter and jam. Tables showing the phenylalanine content of many articles of diet have been published by Brimblecombe *et al.* (1961), from which a reasonably balanced diet can be constructed for the older child. The daily intake of phenylalanine which is compatible with normal serum levels varies from patient to patient. It may be as high as 50 mg./Kg. body weight/day in infants, but is rarely above 20 mg./Kg./day in older children. Vitamin supplements must be adequate for the patient's needs. Anaemia may necessitate the use of ferrous sulphate. During infancy the most useful preparation low in phenylalanine is Minafen. In older children (over 1 year) Cymogran or Lofenalac can be used. These diets are very restricted and require careful supervision in the older child who is at school. A detailed account of the treatment has been published by the Medical Research Council (1963).

OTHER DISTURBANCES OF AMINOACID METABOLISM

Tyrosinosis has already been mentioned as a rare inborn error of metabolism (Medes, 1932). It is due to a defect in the enzyme p-hydroxyphenylpyruvate oxidase so that p-hydoxyphenylpyruvic acid, derived from tyrosine, is not converted to homogentisic acid. The presence of p-hydroxyphenylpyruvic acid in the urine results in a positive ferric chloride test (as in phenylketonuria) and a positive Benedict's reaction. It is now recognized that tyrosinosis causes severe symptoms and may cause the death of several members of a family (Halvorsen *et al.*, 1966). In some infants the disease runs an acute course with vomiting and diarrhoea, marasmus, abdominal distension due to hepatosplenomegaly, ascites and paralytic ileus, and there may be haematemesis, melaena or haematuria. In other cases a more chronic course is seen with cirrhosis of the liver, steatorrhoea and multiple renal tubular defects which result in vitamin D-resistant rickets. A moderate thrombocytopenia is a frequent finding, and various deficiencies of the coagulation mechanism have been described. The diagnosis is based upon finding high levels of tyrosine and methionine in the serum, and excess p-hydroxyphenyl-lactic, -pyruvic, and -acetic acids in the urine. Carbohydrate metabolism is also disturbed and there may be hypoglycaemia or galactosuria and fructosuria. It seems likely that treatment with a diet low in both phenylalanine and tyrosine will be successful.

Alkaptonuria was one of the metabolic defects described by Garrod (1908). It is due to deficiency of homogentisic oxidase so that homogentisic acid, instead of being converted to maleylacetoacetate, accumulates in the tissues and is excreted in the urine. The urine is noted to turn dark on standing, or it can be made to do so immediately by the addition of ammonia or sodium hydroxide. It will also reduce Benedict's solution, but homogentisic acid does not ferment yeast nor rotate a beam of polarized light. The alkaptonuric is symptomless in childhood but in adult life develops ochronosis. This causes an ochre-like pigmentation of sclerae, ears, nasal cartilages and tendon sheaths, also kyphosis and osteoarthritis of the large joints (Galdston *et al.*, 1952). The disease is usually inherited as an autosomal recessive. A few families have shown dominant inheritance. There is no specific treatment.

Another disturbance which also arises from defective metabolism of the aromatic aminoacids is *total albinism.* Consanguineous mating has been especially frequently recorded in this autosomal recessive trait. One of the various pathways of tyrosine metabolism is its conversion to 3,4-dihydroxyphenylalanine (DOPA). This is then converted to DOPA quinone. These steps depend upon the availability of tyrosinase after which DOPA quinone is converted to melanin (Lerner and Fitzpatrick, 1950). In albinism tyrosinase is lacking. The patients are exceedingly fair-skinned and fair-haired with red pupils and a pink or bluish iris. Astigmatism and nystagmus are common. Some are mentally backward. The only available treatment is to protect the eyes and skin from bright sunshine and to correct any refractive errors. In recent years neurological defects have been associated with several other aminoacid disturbances. In *maple syrup urine disease,* so called because the urine from affected infants has an odour of maple syrup or burnt sugar, neurological disturbances appear soon after birth, e.g. difficulties with feeding, absence of the Moro reflex, irregular respirations, spasticity and opisthotonus (Menkes *et al.*, 1954). Death occurs within a few months. The ferric chloride test on the urine gives a colour reaction which could be mistaken for phenylpyruvic acid. However, urine chromatography will reveal abnormally high concentrations of the aliphatic aminoacids valine, leucine and isoleucine, and of their corresponding keto- and hydroxy-acids. Some interference with tryptophane metabolism is also shown by the presence of indolylacetic and indolyllactic acids. The abnormal presence in the urine of the hydroxyacids, which are responsible for the characteristic smell, suggests that the keto-acids are reduced by an abnormal pathway, possibly due to a carboxylase deficiency (Mackenzie and Woolf, 1959). The possibility of treatment by a diet low in the three branched chain aminoacids requires to be investigated.

Hartnup disease, first described by Baron *et al.* (1956), was so called after the family in which it was first detected. The presenting sign is a rash over the exposed areas of the face, hands and legs which is indistinguishable from pellagra. However, the neurological signs are different, e.g. cerebellar ataxia, mild pyramidal signs such as exaggerated deep reflexes, nystagmus, tremor, and involuntary movements of the tongue and hands. Mental deterioration progresses slowly, but the course of the disease is one of remissions and relapses. Chromatography shows gross aminoaciduria involving all aminoacids except proline; also large amounts of indican, indolylacetic acid, indolylacetyl glutamine, tryptophane and an unidentified indolic substance. The cause may be an enzyme block along the intermediary pathway from tryptophane to nicotinic acid or a specific defect in the transport of aminoacid in the cells of the gut and proximal renal tubules (Asatoor *et al.*, 1963). Doubtful improvement has been reported from large doses of nicotinamide.

Another metabolic error has been called the *oast-house syndrome* (Moncrieff, 1960). This was described in a young infant who had an unusual and unpleasant smell due to the presence of α-hydroxybutyric acid in her urine. She was severely mentally defective with unresponsiveness to stimuli and muscular flaccidity, and she had repeated attacks of generalized oedema. In addition to α-hydroxybutyric acid, her urine contained phenylpyruvic acid, which led initially to an erroneous diagnosis of phenylketonuria; also methionine, phenylalanine and tyrosine in excess (Smith and Strang, 1958). Further studies were described by Jepson *et al.* (1958). Leucine was also found in excess in the urine but many aminoacids normally found in small amounts were absent. A high concentration of indolyllactic acid contrasted with a normal amount of indolylacetic acid (in contrast to phenylketonuria). In spite of some resemblances this is obviously a different enzyme block from phenylketonuria. Jepson *et al.* (1958) suggest a general failure in the utilization of keto-acids.

In 1958, Allan and his colleagues, described a family in which two of four children suffered from mental deficiency, convulsions followed by ataxia, friable hair and cardiac murmurs. The urine contained large amounts of an abnormal peptide. This was associated with a low level in the plasma but a high level in the cerebrospinal fluid, suggesting the brain as its site of formation. This substance has since been identified (Dent, 1959) and the disease called *argininosuccinic aciduria.* Yet another metabolic error, recently defined, has been called *histidinaemia* (Auerbach *et al.*, 1962; Ghadimi *et al.*, 1961; Davies and Robinson, 1963). In this condition the salient biochemical features are an excess of histidine in the blood and urine. The urine also contains considerable quantities of imidazolepyruvic, imidazoleacetic and imidazolelactic acids, and the first of these gives positive results with ferric chloride and Phenistix. The cause of histidinaemia is thought to be a deficiency of histidine-alpha-deaminase, so that the principal metabolic pathway of histidine to urocanic acid and ultimately glutamic acid is blocked. As a result histidine takes the less efficient pathway of transamination to imidazole pyruvic acid. The clinical features have not been accurately defined but retardation of speech development may be the most important.

Homocystinuria is one of the most recently discovered metabolic errors (Carson et al., 1965). It is characterized by mental deficiency, congenital bilateral dislocation of the lens, bright pink patches of colour on each cheek, and erythematous blotches over the body skin. There may be a progressive spastic paraplegia, and also genu valgum or pes cavus. There may also be extensive fatty change in the liver. Elevated levels of homocystine are found on urine chromatography. As the child grows, other clinical features may become apparent such as arachnodactyly, kyphosis or scoliosis, and thrombo-embolic phenomena such as pulmonary embolism, renal artery thrombosis and hypertension and swelling of the legs. A clue to the pathogenesis is found in the fact that there are raised levels of homocystine and methionine in the plasma and cerebrospinal fluid whereas there is an almost complete absence of cystathionine in the brain tissue. This is due to deficiency of the enzyme cystathionine synthetase. The results of treatment with a diet low in methionine but supplemented with cystine are at present being evaluated (Brenton et al., 1966).

GALACTOSAEMIA

Aetiology

This disease, also called hereditary galactose intolerance, is another example of autosomal recessive inheritance and it results from the combination in one individual of two recessive genes (Holzel and Komrower, 1955; Schwarz et al., 1961).

Pathogenesis

The basic defect is an inability to convert galactose to glucose. Galactose is ingested as lactose in milk which undergoes splitting in the intestine into its component monosaccharides glucose and galactose. Galactose is then converted to glucose or energy in a series of four enzyme steps (Fig. 13). Although the liver is the main site of this conversion, the demonstration of a similar series of enzyme reactions in red cells and the excess accumulation of galactose-1-phosphate in the erythroeytes from galactosaemic patients (Schwarz et al., 1956) made it likely that the defect lay in the activity of galactose-1-phosphate uridyl transferase and in the inability to convert galactose-1-phosphate to glucose-1-phosphate (step 2 in Fig. 13). The accumulation in the erythrocytes of galactose-1-phosphate, believed to be the toxic substance in galactosaemia (Komrower *et al.*, 1956), is evidence that hexokinase activity is normal. In fact, galactosaemic red cells have been confirmed to be defective in G-1-P uridyl transferase (Isselbacher *et al.*, 1956), and a similar deficiency has now been demonstrated in liver tissue from affected patients (Anderson *et al.*, 1957).

Clinical Features

Two main clinical types occur. The more severe develops its symptoms within two weeks of birth, after milk feeding has been started, with vomiting, disinclination to feed, diarrhoea, loss of weight and dehydration. The liver is enlarged with a firm smooth edge and there may be jaundice. Splenomegaly is common. Cataracts may be seen with the slit-lamp. Finally, the infant becomes severely marasmic with hepatic cirrhosis, ascites, hypoprothrombinaemia. Obvious symptoms are later to appear in the less severe type although a history suggesting some early intolerance of milk may be obtained. The child is brought to the physician with mental retardation, bilateral cataracts and cirrhosis of the liver. The explanation for the less severe cases may be the existence of an alternative pathway for galactose metabolism in the liver (Issel-

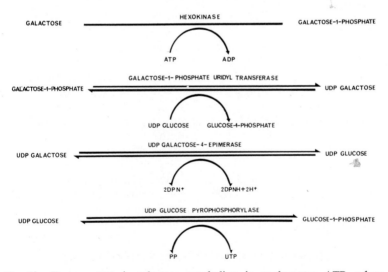

FIG. 13.—Enzyme steps in galactose metabolism in erythrocytes. ATP=adenosinetriphosphate;   ADP=adenosinediphosphate;   UDP=uridinediphosphate; UTP=uridinetriphosphate;   DPN$^+$=oxidised   diphosphopyridine   nucleotide; DPNH=reduced diphosphopyridine nucleotide; PP=pyrophosphate.

bacher, 1957). All the abnormalities in this disease may regress completely on a galactose-free diet save the mental deficiency. It is, therefore, of prime importance that diagnosis be made before irreversible brain-damage has occurred.

Diagnosis

The first clue to the disease is usually the finding of a reducing substance in the urine. Proteinuria is also present. However, although Benedict's test is positive, tests based on the enzyme glucose oxidase (Clinistix: Tes-tape) will be negative. Chromatography will then confirm that the reducing substance is galactose. There is, also, marked aminoaciduria due to renal tubular damage (Komrower, 1953). A valuable method of diagnosis, which can be used for umbilical cord blood in the infant born into a known galactosaemic family and before milk feeds have been started, is the demonstration of the absence of galactose-1-phosphate uridyl transferase activity in the red cells (Anderson et al., 1957). An alternative test for use in the newborn is based on the excess accumulation of galactose-1-phosphate in the erythrocytes in this disease (Schwarz et al., 1958). The galactose tolerance test is always abnormal in galactosaemia, but as it is not free from risk the indications for its use are few. It can be used to reveal heterozygous carriers of the gene but this can be better done by quantitative estimation of G-1-P uridyl transferase activity in lysed erythrocytes (Schwarz et al., 1961).

Treatment

The infant should be placed on a lactose-free diet as soon as the diagnosis has been established. When previously affected siblings are known to exist the diagnosis can and should be confirmed before the infant receives his first milk feed. Two suitable milk substitutes which are almost quite free from lactose are Low-Lactose Food (Cow and Gate) and Nutramigen (Mead Johnson). As the child gets older and on to a more varied diet the use of these expensive artificial feeds becomes less essential. Furthermore, as the child gets older he is often able to tolerate some galactose in his diet, presumably by utilizing the alternative metabolic pathway in the liver. The prognosis as regards both physical and mental growth is good provided diagnosis is made early and treatment is diligently controlled by periodic biochemical tests of urine and blood.

HEREDITARY FRUCTOSE INTOLERANCE

(FRUCTOSAEMIA)

Aetiology

This disease causes severe metabolic disturbances and it is inherited as an autosomal recessive trait, although in some families there may have been a dominant mode of inheritance (Cornblath and Schwartz, 1966). It must be clearly distinguished from *benign fructosuria* which is due to a deficiency of fructokinase and which produces no clinical disease.

Pathogenesis

The metabolic pathways of fructose are complicated and the reader is referred to the excellent account by Cornblath and Schwartz (1966). It is sufficient to state here that the primary enzymatic defect is in fructose-1-phosphate aldolase which in the liver and intestine splits fructose-1-phosphate into the two trioses, glyceraldehyde and dihydroxy-acetone phosphate. This defect results in the accumulation of fructose-1-phosphate which inhibits fructokinase and leads to high blood levels of fructose after its ingestion in the diet. The mechanisms of the gastro-intestinal symptoms and of the hypoglucosaemia in affected infants are not yet fully understood.

Clinical Features

Symptoms only appear when fructose is introduced into the diet as sucrose in milk feeds, or as fruit juices. They vary in severity, partly according to the amounts of fructose ingested, and the wholly breast-fed infant remains symptomless. Common features are failure to thrive and severe marasmus, anorexia and vomiting, diarrhoea and hepatomegaly. Hypoglucosaemia may cause convulsions or losses of consciousness. The liver damage may result in jaundice, and liver function tests give abnormal results. Albuminuria, fructosuria and excess aminoaciduria may be present. Hyperfructosaemia and hypoglucosaemia develop following upon the ingestion of fructose or sucrose (glucose + fructose). Death ensues in undiagnosed infants. In milder cases in older children gastro-intestinal symptoms predominate and in some a profound distaste for anything sweet develops spontaneously as a protective mechanism.

Diagnosis

An intravenous fructose tolerance test (0·25 gm. per Kg.) or an oral fructose tolerance test (1·75 gm. per Kg.) results in a marked and prolonged fall in the true blood glucose level, and also a fall in the inorganic phosphorus. There will also be raised blood levels of fructose, free fatty acids and lactic acid. Fructosuria may be detected.

Treatment

Early diagnosis is important. The treatment consists simply in the complete removal of all fructose-containing foods from the diet and of sucrose from the milk feeds. Vitamin C supplements must not be given in the form of fruit juices or rose-hip syrup.

THE GLYCOGEN STORAGE DISEASES

Glycogen is a complex polysaccharide of high molecular weight and composed of numerous glucosyl units linked together in the form of many branches. The glucosyl units are mainly linked together through carbon atoms 1 and 4, but at the branch points the bonds are between C1 and 6. Multiple enzymes are involved in the synthesis (glycogenesis) and breakdown (glycogenolysis) of glycogen. There are still several gaps and uncertainties which make classification of the metabolic errors in glycogen metabolism difficult. In practical paediatric practice, however, a somewhat over-simplified concept of these physiological steps will prove sufficient for the clinician's purpose. Those who seek detailed descriptions are referred to Cori (1952–53) and Stanbury *et al.* (1965). In health, human liver glycogen content varies from 0–5 per cent, while muscle glycogen is rarely as high as 1 per cent.

Glycogenesis.—Glucose reacts with ATP under the catalytic activity of hexokinase to form glucose-6-phosphate and ADP. Glucose-6-phosphate is then converted to glucose-1-phosphate by phosphoglucomutase. The next step is the conversion of glucose-1-phosphate to glucosyl units in 1,4 linkage. While this can be achieved *in vitro* by phosphorylase, it is possible that *in vivo* it proceeds independently of phosphorlyase and by means of two other steps involving UDP-glucose pyrophosphorlyase and UDPG glycogen-transglucosylase (Stanbury *et al.*, 1965). This could explain the observation of several workers that the activation of phosphorylase *in vivo* always lead to glycogen breakdown and never to glycogen synthesis. When a chain of the growing glycogen molecule reaches a critical level a branch point is established by transfer of the 1,4 linkage to a 1,6 linkage, this being mediated by amylo-(1,4-1,6)-transglucosidase (brancher enzyme).

Glycogenolysis.—Glycogen can be converted back to glucose-1-phosphate by the enzymes phosphorylase, which breaks the 1,4 linkage, and amylo-1,6-glucosidase (debrancher enzyme) which breaks the 1,6 linkage. Glucose-1-phosphate is then converted to glucose-6-phosphate, a reversible reaction, by phosphoglucomutase. Finally glucose-6-phosphate can be converted to free available glucose by glucose-6-phosphatase. This enzyme is found only in the liver and kidneys. Glycogen in the muscles cannot be converted to free glucose but only to pyruvate and lactate via the Embden-Meyerhof glycolytic pathway.

At least six types of glycogenosis can now be delineated, and this number is likely to increase as further enzyme deficiencies are detected by modern biochemical techniques (Illingworth and Cori, 1952; Cori and Cori, 1952; Illingworth *et al.*, 1956; Schmid and Mahler, 1959; Hers, 1959). The investigation of such cases nowadays can only be considered complete when the chemical structure of the deposited glycogen has been determined and when the various enzymes mentioned above have been assayed. Some types have so far only been described in adults, and we shall describe here only four types of glycogen storage disease which, not very infrequently, can provide diagnostic difficulties for the paediatrician.

GLYCOGEN STORAGE DISEASE OF LIVER AND KIDNEYS
(VON GIERKE'S DISEASE: GLUCOSE-6-PHOSPHATASE DEFICIENCY)

Aetiology

This was the first of the glycogenoses to be recognized. It is an autosomal recessive characteristic in which consanguinity is a common feature. The heterozygous, and apparently healthy, carriers of the gene can be detected by the elevated glucose-6-phosphate and fructose-6-phosphate levels in their erythrocytes (Hsia and Kot, 1959).

Pathogenesis

The absence of glucose-6-phosphatase activity has been proved in this form of the disease. This enzyme normally liberates free glucose from glucose-6-phosphate in the liver.

Clinical Features

Gross enlargement of the liver is the most constant feature and it is often recognized in early infancy. Growth is stunted, and the protuberant abdomen is often associated with an exaggerated lumbar lordosis. Genu valgum is common. There may be an excess deposition of fat, and xanthomatous deposits are commonly found on the knees, elbows and buttocks.

Biochemical Findings

Acetonuria is common in the fasting state. Hypoglycaemia may be so severe as to precipitate convulsions and even lead to mental impairment. Hyperlipaemia and hypercholesterolaemia are marked and may even interfere with accurate measurement of electrolytes and plasma CO_2. Episodes of severe metabolic acidosis develop in some cases. The serum pyruvate and lactate levels are raised. The serum phosphate may be low. Renal damage from glycogenosis can cause glycosuria and aminoaciduria.

Diagnosis

Strong presumptive evidence of Von Gierke's disease may be obtained from a variety of tests:

1. The glucose tolerance test (after 1·5 gm. glucose/Kg.) shows an abnormally high rise of blood sugar and a delayed fall.

2. There is a marked resistance to the hyperglycaemic actions of

adrenalin (0·2 ml. subcutaneously) or glucagon (1 mg. intravenously). In normal subjects these agents cause glycogen breakdown to glucose-1-phosphate, its subsequent conversion to glucose-6-phosphate, and liberation of free glucose therefrom by the action of glucose-6-phosphatase. The last step is, of course, deficient in this disease. The adrenalin or glucagon is given after an 8-hour fast and immediately after removal of a specimen of blood for estimation of the true glucose level. Thereafter the blood glucose levels are measured every 10 minutes for 1 hour. In healthy individuals the level rises 40–60 per cent above the fasting level. In Von Gierke's disease a "flat" curve is obtained.

3. Another indirect measurement of glucose-6-phosphatase activity can be obtained after an intravenous dose of galactose 1 gm./Kg., or fructose 0·5 gm./Kg. (Schwartz et al., 1957). Blood glucose levels at 10-minute intervals are compared with the pre-injection level. In healthy persons galactose and fructose are converted via glucose-6-phosphate to free glucose, but this metabolic pathway is blocked in Von Gierke's disease.

Conclusive proof of the diagnosis, however, can only be obtained from a specimen of liver removed at laparotomy. The findings in this type of glycogenosis will be:

(a) A liver glycogen content over 5 per cent of wet weight.

(b) Glycogen of normal chemical structure.

(c) Absent or very low glucose-6-phosphatase activity.

Treatment

Although the enzyme failure cannot be corrected, considerable benefit can accrue from a diet in which a high intake of protein and carbohydrate is given in frequent feeds throughout the 24 hours. Lowe et al. (1959) concluded from their experiments that glucagon inhibits postprandial glycogen deposition in this disease, and they reported good effects from a long-term therapeutic regime based on repeated injections of glucagon immediately after feeds. Episodes of severe metabolic acidosis, often precipitated by intercurrent infections, can endanger life. They must be promptly treated with intravenous glucose and sodium bicarbonate under careful biochemical control. If these children can be tided over the dangerous early years their health often improves greatly during adolescence.

GLYCOGEN STORAGE DISEASE OF LIVER AND MUSCLE

(LIMIT DEXTRINOSIS: DEBRANCHER ENZYME DEFICIENCY)

Aetiology

It is probable that this form of glycogen storage disease is also inherited as an autosomal recessive. It has only recently been possible to distinguish it from Von Gierke's disease and may not be uncommon.

Pathogenesis

The debrancher enzyme (amylo-1,6-glucosidase) is absent from liver, skeletal and cardiac muscle. Glycogen deposition in the heart and skeletal muscles does not, of course, occur in Von Gierke's disease.

Clinical Features

Hepatomegaly is marked but hypoglycaemic problems are less troublesome and there is less interference with growth. In some cases, the involvement of skeletal muscles gives rise to weakness and hypotonia.

Diagnosis

Acetonuria may appear during fasting, and there is a diminished hyperglycaemic response to adrenalin or glucagon. However, de-esterification of glucose-6-phosphate to glucose can proceed normally and there is, therefore, a normal hyperglycaemic response to intravenous galactose or fructose. The liver glycogen content is raised and it is abnormal in structure with short external chains and an increased number of 1,6 branch points. The activity of amylo-1,6-glucosidase is not detectable.

Treatment

The same dietary principles apply as in Von Gierke's disease but the disease runs a milder course. Cardiac involvement is rarely clinically demonstrable but strenuous exercise should probably be avoided.

FAMILIAL CIRRHOSIS OF THE LIVER WITH ABNORMAL GLYCOGEN

(AMYLOPECTINOSIS: BRANCHER ENZYME DEFICIENCY)

This appears to be an excessively rare disease in which amylo-(1,4-1,6)-transglucosidase deficiency results in deposition of an abnormal glycogen with a molecular structure resembling the amylopectins of plants. This substance is toxic so that the patient presents with cirrhosis of the liver, splenomegaly and jaundice. The liver function tests yield grossly abnormal results, and death is preceded by the development of ascites and deep jaundice. This diagnosis should be considered in all cases of familial hepatic cirrhosis.

GLYCOGEN STORAGE DISEASE OF THE HEART

(CARDIOMEGALIA GLYCOGENICA: IDIOPATHIC GENERALIZED

GLYCOGENOSIS; POMPE'S DISEASE)

Aetiology

Once again autosomal recessive inheritance is involved and consanguinity has been reported.

Pathogenesis

The disease may involve the central nervous system and skeletal muscles as well as the myocardium. It has recently been shown that the primary defect is of the lysosomal enzyme α-acid glucosidase (acid maltase) (Hers, 1963), although it is not yet quite clear how this defect permits the accumulation of glycogen granules which replace the normal cytoplasm of the cells. In biopsy specimens spontaneous glycogenolysis is rapid and the glycogen does not show the abnormal stability which is a characteristic finding in the other types of glycogenosis.

Clinical Features

The infant becomes ill in the early weeks of life with anorexia, vomiting, dyspnoea and failure to thrive. The heart is enlarged, tachycardia is present, and a systolic murmur is commonly heard. Oedema may also develop. The E.C.G. shows left axis deviation, inverted T waves and depression of the ST segments. When the skeletal muscles are severely involved the degree of hypotonia may simulate Werdnig-Hoffmann's disease. In some infants macroglossia has been so marked as to arouse the suspicion of cretinism. On the other hand, hepatomegaly is not prominent until cardiac failure is advanced. Glucose tolerance, adrenalin and glucagon responses are all normal. The diagnosis can be established by muscle biopsy (di Sant'Agnese, 1959).

Treatment

Death is inevitable, usually during the first year. Digoxin, and antibiotics when respiratory infection supervenes, can only have a temporary effect.

HYPOPHOSPHATASIA

Aetiology

This disease, first described by Rathbun (1948), is transmitted as an autosomal recessive characteristic in which the heterozygous carrier state can usually be detected (Rathbun et al., 1961).

Pathogenesis

In most inborn errors of metabolism the absence of an enzyme activity is deduced indirectly from the demonstration that a metabolic pathway has gone wrong. In hypophosphatasia the enzyme which is defective can be directly measured—alkaline phosphatase. Further evidence of the nature of hypophosphatasia was the demonstration by chromatography of an abnormal metabolite—phosphoethanolamine—in the plasma and urine of affected patients (Fraser et al., 1955; McCance et al., 1955). In fact, phosphoethanolamine seems to be a naturally occurring physiological substrate of alkaline phosphatase.

The consequence of this enzyme deficiency is a failure of mineralization of the skeleton, both membranous and cartilaginous. The long bones at the metaphyses show a wide irregular zone of proliferative cartilage with disorganized maturation of the cells and no evidence of calcification of the intercellular matrix. Osteoid tissue is deposited on the cartilaginous intercellular substance and on the outside of the shafts, and as it is almost completely uncalcified, fractures readily occur. There is, however, no shortage of osteoblasts which are the normal source of alkaline phosphatase in bone (MacDonald and Shanks, 1957).

Clinical Features

In severe cases the disease becomes obvious within a few weeks of birth. In one case, where a previous sibling had been affected, the diagnosis was established radiologically before birth (McCance et al., 1956). Many of the signs resemble those seen in rickets, e.g. enlarged epiphyses, "beading" of the ribs, kyphoscoliosis, and bowing of the long bones which sometimes show spontaneous fractures. However, as the membranous bones are also affected the skull may be so poorly mineralized (Fig. 14) that it feels like a balloon filled with water. The anterior fontanelle and sutures may be wide and tense, but subsequently there may be premature fusion with microcephaly (Schlesinger et al., 1955). In less

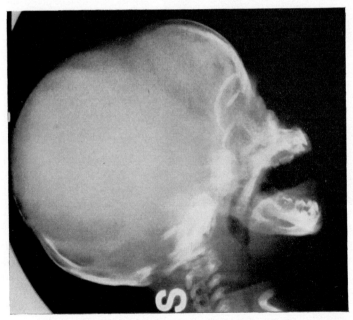

FIG. 14.—Radiograph of skull from infant with hypophosphatasia showing gross deficiency of mineralization of bones of vault.

severe cases the presenting sign may be premature loss of the deciduous and permanent teeth (Illingworth and Gardiner, 1955). Radiographs show an abnormal patchy calcification at the metaphyses producing an ill-defined margin distal to which there is a zone of poorly calcified osteoid (Fig. 15). The epiphyseal lines are irregularly widened. There may also be periosteal elevation due to deposition of osteoid.

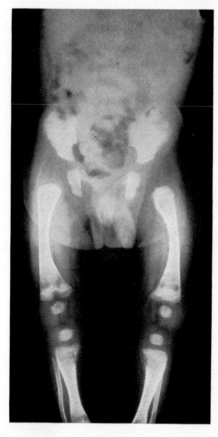

Fig. 15.—Radiograph of legs of infant with hypophosphatasia showing abnormal calcification at metaphyses, and zone of poorly calcified osteoid tissue. Note also widening of ephiphyseal lines.

Diagnosis

The diagnosis should be based on a very low level of serum alkaline phosphatase. Biopsy of tissues normally rich in alkaline phosphatase, such as bone, will also show a greatly reduced enzyme content (Sobel *et al.*, 1953; Schlesinger *et al.*, 1955; MacDonald and Shanks, 1957). An inconstant but serious finding is hypercalcaemia. It may lead to renal failure. Phosphoethanolamine may be demonstrated in the urine of patients and their heterozygous parents (Fraser, 1957).

Treatment

Cases which are diagnosed in early infancy do not long survive. In older patients massive doses of calciferol (vitamin D_2) encourage calcification, but toxic effects such as hypercalcaemia may limit their use for long periods.

HYPOGAMMAGLOBULINAEMIA

The first congenital form of hypogammaglobulinaemia was described in 1952 by Bruton. Since then the immunoglobulins have been divided into several types, and several types of immunological paralysis have been defined, of which that described by Bruton remains the commonest. The nomenclature of the immunoglobulins has been somewhat confused but the World Health Organization (1964) has made firm recommendations as follows:

WHO Terms	Old Terms
IgG or γG	7Sγ
IgA or γA	B_2A
IgM or γM	B_2M; 19Sγ; gamma macroglobulin
IgD or γD	

We propose to discuss separately those types of hypogammaglubulinaemia which have been reasonably well defined.

(1) CONGENITAL HYPOGAMMAGLOBULINAEMIA *IgG.↓*

Aetiology

This form of the disease is inherited as a sex-linked recessive and is confined to males (Peterson et al., 1965).

Pathogenesis

In this form of hypogammaglobulinaemia the deficiency is of IgG (7S) globulin. This is formed by the plasma cells of the normal child from about the age of 3 months. In the hypogammaglobulinaemic child the lymph nodes and other tissues are characteristically lacking in germinal centres and plasma cells. On the other hand, although their lymphoid structures and thymus may be somewhat smaller than normal the tissues of such patients contain relatively normal numbers of lymphocytes (Gitlin, 1964).

Clinical Features

Most commonly the disease presents in a young male child with repeated severe bacterial infections, e.g. pneumonia, otitis media, sinusitis, furunculosis and pyogenic meningitis. Gram-negative infections tend to be less common with the exception of pyelonephritis.

Virus infections are not particularly common in these children but they have a peculiar susceptibility to infection of the lungs by the protozoon *Pneumocystis carinii* (Hutchison, 1955; Bird and Thomson, 1957). This should be suspected when a child known to be hypogamma-globulinaemic develops progressive dyspnoea with few signs over the lungs. Radiographs show a characteristic symmetrical ground-glass opacity spreading outwards from the hilar regions. The parasites may be found in material obtained by lung puncture and stained by special methods (Gajdusek, 1957). Contrary to earlier suggestions, tuber-culosis seems to be commoner in patients with hypogammaglobulin-aemia than in normal people although response to anti-tuberculous drugs is good. In some children the mode of presentation has been with chronic bronchiectasis which extends inexorably in spite of treatment, medical or surgical. Another common symptom is chronic diarrhoea. In a few a rheumatoid type of arthritis has developed (Good *et al.*, 1957).

Diagnosis

More cases of this disease are being picked up by physicians aware of the possibilities of death in infancy from severe bacterial infections. Relatively simple tests may first be employed. Thus, the complete absence of any turbidity in Kunkel's zinc sulphate turbidity test, or extremely low titres of isoagglutinins against heterologous blood group substances would be strongly suggestive evidence of hypogamma-globulinaemia. Thereafter, the diagnosis should be fully confirmed by measurements of the various immunoglobulins, using techniques such as immuno-electrophoretic analysis. The Medical Research Council Working Party on Hypogammaglobulinaemia has laid down a gamma globulin level of under 200 mg. per 100 ml. as the criterion of diagnosis. Children with this disease also show a greatly reduced capacity to manu-facture antibodies against a wide variety of antigens, e.g. pertussis, T.A.B. and poliomyelitis vaccines, tetanus and diphtheria toxoids, and vaccination against smallpox.

Treatment

Infections should be treated with appropriate antibacterial drugs. Infection by *Pneumocystis carinii* has been successfully treated with pentamidine (Marshall *et al.*, 1964). The long-term management should be with weekly intramuscular injections of pooled gamma globulin, 0·05 gm. per Kg. body weight. These are capable of greatly reducing the incidence of severe infections. Although smallpox vaccination usually results in a normal response deaths have occurred from generalized vaccinia and it is best avoided. It is wise also to avoid BCG inoculation. There are no practical objections to the other common immunizations although their effectiveness in affected children is likely to be slight.

(2) FAMILIAL ("SWISS FORM") LYMPHOPENIA WITH AGAMMAGLOBULINAEMIA

G ↓
A ↓
M ↓

Aetiology

This form of immunoparalysis is inherited as an autosomal recessive and it affects infants of both sexes (Hitzig et al., 1965).

Pathogenesis

There is absence or gross deficiency in all three immunoglobulins (IgG., IgA and IgM). There is severe hypoplasia of the complete lymphreticular system. The thymus is rudimentary, virtually devoid of lymphocytes and without Hassall's corpuscles—*thymic alymphoplasia*. Indeed, not only is there an absence of plasma cells which normally produce IgG globulin but also of lymphocytes which appear at least to produce IgM globulin.

Clinical Features

This is a very severe form of immunoparalysis and affected infants have usually died of severe infection during the first few years of life. They show a characteristic and severe lymphopenia ($< 1,000$ per c.mm.). Malabsorption with foul-smelling stools has been present in some. Full thickness skin grafts are accepted without signs of rejection by these children, and delayed (tuberculin type) hypersensitivity reactions do not occur.

Treatment

Injections of gamma globulin have proved to be ineffective in reducing the incidence of severe infections. Transplants of foetal thymus have not so far been successful.

(3) DYSGAMMAGLOBULINAEMIA

Several reports have concerned patients with antibody deficiency syndromes who have shown different and selective deficiency of one or more of the immunoglobulins. In Type I there is a decrease in the levels of IgG and IgA with an increase in IgM. In Type II there is a decrease in IgG and IgM with a normal concentration of IgA. In such cases the total gamma globulin level of the serum is above 200 mg. per 100 ml. Treatment is being tried with injections of pooled gamma globulin.

CONGENITAL METHAEMOGLOBINAEMIA

Aetiology

(1) The most common form of congenital methaemoglobinaemia is inherited as an autosomal recessive trait and it is due to the absence of a normal intra-erythrocytic enzyme activity. A rare type, inherited as an

(2)

autosomal dominant, has a quite different aetiology in that it is due to the formation of an abnormal haemoglobin (haemoglobin M) with a defective globulin component.

Pathogenesis

In normal haemoglobin the iron of the four haem groups is in the reduced or ferrous state. In methaemoglobin the iron is in the oxidized or ferric state and it is incapable of combining with oxygen. In normal erythrocytes methaemoglobin is constantly being formed and in normal blood a small amount is always present. It is, however, continuously being reduced back to haemoglobin by a complex series of enzyme steps. In congenital methaemoglobinaemia there is an intra-erythrocytic defect in one of these enzyme reactions (Gibson, 1948; Breakey *et al.*, 1951). The other form of congenital methaemoglobinaemia belongs to the haemoglobinopathies (Chapter XIX), and haemoglobin M can be separated from normal haemoglobin by suitable electrophoretic techniques (Gerald, 1958).

Clinical Picture

The primary sign is a slaty-grey type of cyanosis which is present from birth. It is usually remarkably free from symptoms and clubbing of the fingers and toes does not develop. Some patients develop compensatory polycythaemia, and some have been severely retarded mentally.

Diagnosis

The presence of excess methaemoglobin in the blood should be demonstrated by spectrophotometry (Evelyn and Malloy, 1938).

It is important to distinguish the congenital and permanent form of methaemoglobinaemia from the temporary but dangerous acquired form, which may follow the entry into the body of certain poisons such as aniline dyes, nitrites, acetanilid, and potassium chlorate. Outbreaks of acquired methaemoglobinaemia have occurred in newborn nurseries when new napkins marked by aniline dyes have been used before laundering (personal observation), and cases have occurred in children drinking well-water containing nitrites.

It is also important to remember that cyanotic children without heart murmurs may have methaemoglobinaemia. We have seen the mistaken diagnosis of congenital heart disease made in two such cases and, in fact, one child was unnecessarily submitted to cardiac catheterization.

Treatment

Methaemoglobin may be reduced to haemoglobin with marked diminution or disappearance of the cyanosis by ascorbic acid 200–500 mg./day or methylene blue 5 mg./Kg./day, given orally or intravenously. These drugs do not, however, have any beneficial effect in haemoglobin M disease.

REFERENCES

General

CRICK, F. H. C., BARNETT, L., BRENNER, S., and WATTS-TOBIN, R. J. (1961). *Nature (Lond.)*, **192**, 1227.
DENT, C. E. (1957). *Amer. J. Med.*, **22**, 671.
GARROD, A. E. (1908). *Lancet*, **2**, 1, 73, 142, and 214.
HSIA, D. Y. Y. (1959). *Inborn Errors of Metabolism.* Chicago: Year Book Publishers.
INGRAM, V. M. (1956). *Nature (Lond.)*, **178**, 792.
INGRAM, V. M. (1957). *Nature (Lond.)*, **180**, 326.
NIRENBERG, M. W., and MATTHAEI, J. H. (1961). *Proc. nat. Acad. Sci. (Wash.)*, **47**, 1588.
STANBURY, J. B., WYNGAARDEN, J. B., and FREDRICKSON, D. S. (1965). *The Metabolic Basis of Inherited Disease*, 2nd edit. New York: McGraw-Hill Book Co.
WATSON, J. D., and CRICK, F. H. C. (1952). *Nature (Lond.)*, **171**, 737.

Aminoacid Disturbances

ALLAN, J. D., CUSWORTH, D. C., DENT, C. E., and WILSON, V. K. (1958). *Lancet*, **1**, 182.
ASATOOR, A. M., CRASKE, J., LONDON, D. R., and MILNE, M. D. (1963). *Lancet*, **1**, 126.
AUERBACH, V. H., DiGEORGE, A. M., BALDRIDGE, R. C., TOURTELLOTTE, C. D., and BRIGHAM, M. P. (1962). *J. Pediat.*, **60**, 487.
BARON, D. N,, DENT, C. E., HARRIS, H., HART, E. W., and JEPSON, J. B. (1956). *Lancet*, **2**, 421.
BRENTON, D. P., CUSWORTH, D. C., DENT, C. E., and JONES, E. E. (1966). *Quart. J. Med.*, **35**, 325.
BRIMBLECOMBE, F. S. W., BLAINEY, J. D., STONEMAN, M. E. R., and WOOD, B. S. B. (1961). *Brit. med. J.*, **2**, 793.
CARSON, N. A. J., DENT, C. E., FIELD, M. B., and GAULL, G. E. (1965). *J. Pediat.*, **66**, 565.
DAVIES, H. E., and ROBINSON, M. J. (1963). *Arch. Dis. Childh.*, **38**, 80.
DENT, C. E. (1959). *Proc. roy. Soc. Med.*, **52**, 885.
GALDSTON, M., STEELE, J. M., and DOBRINER, K. (1952). *Amer. J. Med.*, **13**, 432.
GHADIMI, H., PARTINGTON, M. W., and HUNTER, A. (1961). *New Engl. J. Med.*, **265**, 221.
HALVORSEN, S., PANDE, H., LØKEN, A. C., and GJESSING, L. R. (1966). *Arch. Dis. Childh.*, **41**, 238.
HSIA, D. Y. Y., DRISCOLL, K. W., TROLL, W., and KNOX, W. E. (1956). *Nature (Lond.)*, **178**, 1239.
HUTCHISON, J. H. (1962). *Practitioner*, **189**, 436.
JEPSON, J. B., SMITH, A. J., and STRANG, L. B. (1958). *Lancet*, **2**, 1334.
KNOX, W. E., and HSIA, D. Y. Y. (1957). *Amer. J. Med.*, **22**, 687.
LA DU, B. N., and MICHAEL, P. J. (1960). *J. Lab. clin. Med.*, **55**, 491.
LERNER, A. B., and FITZPATRICK, T. B. (1950). *Physiol. Rev.*, **30**, 91.
LEVINE, S. Z., DANN, M., and MARPLES, E. (1943). *J. clin. Invest.*, **22**, 551.
MACKENZIE, D. Y., and WOOLF, L. I. (1959). *Brit. med. J.*, **1**, 90.
MEDES, G. (1932). *Biochem. J.*, **26**, 917.
MEDICAL RESEARCH COUNCIL (1963). *Brit. med. J.*, **1**, 1691.
MENKES, J. H., HURST, P. L., and CRAIG, J. M. (1954). *Pediatrics*, **14**, 462.
MONCRIEFF, A. (1960). *Lancet*, **2**, 273.
SMITH, A. J., and STRANG, L. B. (1958). *Arch. Dis. Childh.*, **33**, 109.
WOOLF, L. I., GRIFFITHS, R., MONCRIEFF, A., COATES, S., and DILLISTONE, F. (1958). *Arch. Dis. Childh.*, **33**, 31.

Galactosaemia and Fructose Intolerance

ANDERSON, E. P., KALCKAR, H. M., and ISSELBACHER, K. J. (1957). *Science*, **125**, 113.
ANDERSON, E. P., KALCKAR, H. M., KURAHASHI, K., and ISSELBACHER, K. J. (1957). *J. Lab. clin. Med.*, **50**, 569.
CORNBLATH, M., and SCHWARTZ, R. (1966). *Disorders of Carbohydrate Metabolism in Infancy*, Chap. 9. Philadelphia: W. B. Saunders Co.
HOLZEL, A., and KOMROWER, G. M. (1955). *Arch. Dis. Childh.*, **30**, 155.
ISSELBACHER, K. J. (1957). *Science*, **126**, 652.
ISSELBACHER, K. J., ANDERSON, E. P., KURAHASHI, K., and KALCKAR, H. M. (1956). *Science*, **123**, 635.
KOMROWER, G. M. (1953). Arch. franç. Pédiat., **10**, 185.
KOMROWER, G. M., SCHWARZ, V., HOLZEL, A., and GOLDBERG, L. (1956). *Arch. Dis. Childh.*, **31**, 254.
SCHWARZ, V., GOLDBERG, L., KOMROWER, G. M., and HOLZEL, A. (1956). *Biochem. J.*, **62**, 34.
SCHWARZ, V., HOLZEL, A., and KOMROWER, G. M. (1958). *Lancet*, **1**, 24.
SCHWARZ, V., WELLS, A. R., HOLZEL, A., and KOMROWER, G. M. (1961). *Ann. hum. Genet.*, **25**, 179.

Glycogen Storage Diseases

CORI, G. T. (1952-53). *Harvey Lect.*, **48**, 145.
CORI, G. T., and CORI, C. F. (1952). *J. biol. Chem.*, **199**, 661.
DI SANT'AGNESE, P. A. (1959). *Ann. N.Y. Acad. Sci.*, **72**, 439.
HERS, H. G. (1959). *Rev. int. Hépat.*, **9**, 35.
HERS, H. G. (1963). *Biochem. J.*, **86**, 11.
HSIA, D. Y. Y., and KOT, E. G. (1959). *Nature (Lond.)*, **183**, 1331.
ILLINGWORTH, B., and CORI, G. T. (1952). *J. biol. Chem.*, **199**, 653.
ILLINGWORTH, B., CORI, G. T., and CORI, C. F. (1956). *J. biol. Chem.*, **218**, 123.
LOWE, C. U., SOKAL, J. E., DORAY, B. H., and SARCIONE, E. J. (1959). *J. clin. Invest.*, **38**, 1021.
SCHMID, R., and MAHLER, R. (1959). *J. clin. Invest.*, **38**, 1040.
SCHWARTZ, R., ASHMORE, J., and RENOLD, A. E. (1957). *Pediatrics*, **19**, 585.

Hypophosphatasia

FRASER, D. (1957). *Amer. J. Med.*, **22**, 730.
FRASER, D., YENDT, E. R., and CHRISTIE, F. H. E. (1955). *Lancet*, **1**, 286.
ILLINGWORTH, R. S., and GARDINER, J. H. (1955). *Arch. Dis. Childh.*, **30**, 449.
MCCANCE, R. A., FAIRWEATHER, D. V. I., BARRETT, A. M., and MORRISON, A. B. (1956). *Quart. J. Med.*, **25**, 523.
MCCANCE, R. A., MORRISON, A. B., and DENT, C. E. (1955). *Lancet*, **1**, 131.
MACDONALD, A. M., and SHANKS, R. A. (1957). *Arch. Dis. Childh.*, **32**, 304.
RATHBUN, J. C. (1948). *Amer. J. Dis. Child.*, **75**, 822.
RATHBUN, J. C., MACDONALD, J. W., ROBINSON, H. M. C., and WANKLIN, J. M. (1961). *Arch. Dis. Childh.*, **36**, 540.
SCHLESINGER, B., LUDER, J., and BODIAN, M. (1955). *Arch. Dis. Childh.*, **30**, 265.
SOBEL, E. H., CLARK, L. C. jnr., FOX, R. P., and ROBINSON, M. (1963). *Pediatrics*, **11**, 309.

Congenital Hypogammaglobulinaemia

BIRD, T., and THOMSON, J. (1957). *Lancet*, **1**, 59.
BRUTON, O. C. (1952). *Pediatrics*, **9**, 722.
Bulletin of the World Health Organization (1964). **30**, 407.

GAJDUSEK, D. C. (1957). *Pediatrics*, **19**, 543.
GITLIN, D. (1964). *Pediatrics*, **34**, 198.
GOOD, R. A., ROTSTEIN, J., and MAZZITELLO, W. F. (1957). *J. Lab. clin. Med.*, **49**, 343.
HITZIG, W. H., KAY, N. E. M., and COTTIER, H. (1965). *Lancet*, **2**, 151.
HUTCHISON, J. H. (1955). *Lancet*, **2**, 844 and 1196.
MARSHALL, W. C., WESTON, H. J., and BODIAN, M. (1964). *Arch. Dis. Childh.*, **39**, 18.
PETERSON, R. D. A., COOPER, M. D., and GOOD, R. A. (1965). *Amer. J. Med.*, **38**, 579.

Congenital Methaemoglobinaemia

BREAKEY, V. K. St. G., GIBSON, Q. H., and HARRISON, D. C. (1951). *Lancet*, **1**, 935.
EVELYN, H. T., and MALLOY, K. A. (1938). *J. biol. Chem.*, **126**, 655.
GERALD, P. S. (1958). *Blood*, **13**, 936.
GIBSON, Q. H. (1948). *Biochem. J.*, **42**, 13.

CHAPTER X

SPECIFIC INFECTIONS

TUBERCULOSIS

The incidence of infection by human type tubercle bacilli has fallen abruptly in Britain in recent years. This has been due to earlier diagnosis of adult type phthisis; to the detection by mass radiography of previously unknown sources of infection; and to the efficiency of modern anti-tuberculous drugs in rendering patients non-infective within a relatively short period. It would, however, be a grave error to regard the disease as having been defeated and cases still occur too frequently to permit of complacency. In some of the underdeveloped countries of the world tuberculosis remains a major public health problem and is the commonest cause of death. On the other hand, bovine tuberculosis which not so long ago was very common in the form of abdominal tuberculosis, cervical tuberculosis and disease of bone and joints has virtually disappeared from Britain. Indeed, the rather infrequent cases of tuberculosis affecting mesenteric or cervical lymph nodes, bones and genito-urinary tract are now almost invariably due to human type tubercle bacilli. The vast majority of cases of human tuberculosis are intrathoracic in their primary site and this form of the disease must, for a long time to come, be regarded as a major problem deserving of close study and understanding by the physicians of all countries.

INTRATHORACIC TUBERCULOSIS

Sources of Infection

By far the most usual source of tuberculous infection in infancy and childhood is the adult contact who suffers from "open" phthisis. In Britain the known case of adult tuberculosis is quickly rendered non-infectious by appropriate drug treatment and the danger is the undiagnosed or unsuspected adult (Miller, 1958). Infrequently, a child can be infected from a tuberculous domestic animal such as a dog, and this possibility should not be overlooked (Hawthorne et al., 1957).

Pathology

When a patient, of any age, inhales tubercle bacilli for the first time they produce a small caseous focus in the lung parenchyma (Wallgren, 1948). This is called "the primary focus" or Ghon's focus. It is usually single, occasionally multiple, and most often situated subpleurally, in 45 per cent of cases in the right upper lobe. From the primary focus, which is usually large enough to be visible to the naked eye, there is a peribronchial lymphangitis spreading towards the bronchopulmonary and tracheobronchial glands on the same side. These become enlarged and caseous, ultimately undergoing softening. Indeed, in primary tuberculosis the lung parenchyma lesion is small, almost trivial, while the regional lymph glands are heavily involved. This is in contrast to adult type phthisis, in which the tissues have earlier been sensitized by primary tuberculosis, and where the lung parenchyma may show extensive infiltration, caseation, cavitation and fibrosis while the regional lymphadenitis is slight or absent. The primary focus, lymphangitis and hilar adenitis constitute "the primary tuberculous complex". In more severe examples the disease may spread upwards to involve the paratracheal and the supraclavicular glands.

In the majority of cases the primary complex heals by calcification in the primary focus and regional lymph nodes. These are visible on radiographs but ultimately the calcium is absorbed so that little trace of the infection may remain. In others, especially infants and young children, the caseous hilar nodes exert local effects upon the adjoining bronchi which are thin-walled and pliable. Most often the enlarged glands completely obstruct a primary or secondary bronchus and the distal lobe or segment becomes airless. Histologically it shows resorption atelectasis and possibly low-grade tuberculous inflammation. Whereas in some cases the bronchial occlusion is brought about by extrinsic glandular compression, in many the caseous gland erodes its way through the bronchial wall, so that the mucous membrane is perforated and tuberculous granulation tissue can then be seen to fill the lumen. This frequent complication of primary tuberculosis was described by the author (Hutchison, 1949a; Veeneklaas, 1952; Gerbeaux and Masse, 1957). The right middle lobe is most often affected. This type of atelectasis or absorption collapse may completely resolve, but not infrequently it leaves behind bronchial narrowing and distortion, or a "dry" bronchiectasis which may become the seat of severe pyogenic infection many years later (Hutchison, 1951). In a few cases viable tubercle bacilli may lead to tuberculous endobronchitis and adult type phthisis in the already damaged lobe. Less frequent than complete bronchial occlusion ("stop-valve obstruction") is the situation which arises when the bronchial lumen is greatly narrowed although still patent during inspiration whereas during expiration, when the bronchi normally constrict, the lumen is completely blocked. This type of bronchial narrowing ("check-valve obstruction") allows the entry of air into the lobe during inspiration but prevents its egress during expiration. The result is over-distension and ballooning of the lobe with air—obstructive emphysema. This state may affect a lobe or the whole lung but never a segment. Very rarely involvement of the paratracheal glands has resulted in perforation of the trachea near its bifurcation, with rapid death from asphyxia.

Another infrequent complication of intrathoracic disease is tuberculous pericarditis (Chapter XIV) due to rupture of a caseous node in the left hilum into the pericardial sac. In other cases, however, the pericardium is infected by haematogenous spread.

Post-primary tuberculosis.—If the primary tuberculous complex fails to heal, some form of progressive tuberculosis must result. Any lesion which develops subsequent to the complete establishment of the primary complex is referred to as post-primary. This may arise from either haematogenous dissemination or bronchogenic spread.

Haematogenous Dissemination

For descriptive purposes it is convenient to describe three grades of severity, although all intermediate grades occur.

(1) **Silent bacillaemia.**—It can be presumed that some invasion of the blood stream by tubercle bacilli takes place in the course of every primary tuberculous infection. Thus, in many cases small *Simon foci* are later to be demonstrated radiologically as small areas of calcification in the upper zones of the lungs. Similar lesions in the spleen are known as *Duken foci*. These usually remain quiescent but they sometimes give rise to local tuberculosis in the years ahead, especially in the lungs. Similar tuberculomata sometimes develop in the subcortical region of the brain, and although tuberculous meningitis may develop during the course of acute miliary tuberculosis, in most cases this form of the disease arises from the rupture of one of these subcortical tuberculomata into the subarachnoid space (Rich and McCordock, 1929; Green and Mac-Gregor, 1937). Large intracranial tuberculomata which act as space-occupying lesions arise in similar fashion but are now rarely seen.

(2) **Acute miliary tuberculosis.**—This classical form of the disease arises from erosion of some part of the primary complex into a blood vessel and the discharge into the circulation of a large dose of tubercle bacilli. Like tuberculous meningitis this is most likely to occur within the first six months after the primary infection. All the organs of the body are studded with small miliary tubercles which are usually visible to the naked eye. Erosion of a caseous gland into a branch of the pulmonary artery explains those uncommon cases where the miliary spread is confined to the lungs.

(3) **Chronic disseminated tuberculosis.**—In this form of the disease which tends to occur some 3 or 4 years after the primary infection, the condition may appear to the clinician to be confined to one site, e.g. renal tract or bone and joint. The term "surgical tuberculosis" which has sometimes been applied to such cases is unfortunate and post-mortem examination reveals tuberculous lesions in other organs such as lungs, liver, spleen or lymph nodes. Of even later origin are haematogenous lesions of the male and female genital organs, and of the skin.

Bronchogenic Tuberculosis

(1) **Acute tuberculous pneumonia.**—This rapidly progressive form of pulmonary tuberculosis may be lobar or lobular in distribution. Once common as "galloping consumption", it has become rare and is almost confined to young infants. Cavitation, spontaneous pneumothorax and tuberculous empyema were common complications, but they have virtually disappeared in Britain since the advent of the anti-tuberculous drugs.

(2) **Chronic fibrocaseous phthisis.**—This is the common form of pulmonary tuberculosis in adults but it is exceedingly rare before puberty. In adolescence and early adult life it frequently arises as a direct spread from the primary tuberculous complex, usually within two years of the first infection. In older people the early lesion often appears as an infiltrative focus of activity under one clavicle, the *Assmann focus.* This probably arises from the reactivation of one of the Simon foci which resulted from bacillaemia during the primary tuberculous infection much earlier. It is probable that most cases of adult type phthisis are the result of endogenous exacerbation of pre-existing tuberculous foci, brought about by a change in the patient's immunity from inter-current disease, overwork, malnutrition and the like. Exogenous re-infection from another case may well favour a breakdown in the patient's immune state, but it is unlikely to be the direct and sole cause of fibro-caseous tuberculosis. The typical pathological changes, infiltration, caseation, cavitation, fibrosis and calcification, often associated with endobronchial tuberculosis, nowadays respond so well to drug therapy that the old lines of treatment by artificial pneumothorax and thoraco-plasty are rapidly becoming obsolete.

Clinical Aspects of the Primary Tuberculous Infection

The child with an intrathoracic primary infection may be symptomless or severely ill. When symptoms do appear they coincide with the development by the tissues of an allergic sensitivity towards tuberculo-protein. This takes about six to eight weeks to develop and may be demonstrated by means of a tuberculin skin test. In some patients spontaneous manifestations of this allergic state appear in the form of phlyctenular conjunctivitis or erythema nodosum, and these conditions should always be presumed to indicate tuberculous infection in children until they are proved to be otherwise caused. In some children, who are usually over the age of 5 years, the development of pleurisy with effusion (Chapter XIII) makes the diagnosis easy.

In most cases, the symptomatology tends to be non-specific and of a type common in other non-tuberculous ailments, e.g. loss of energy, lethargy, undue irritability, anorexia and a general loss of well-being. An irregular fever (99–100° F.) in the late afternoons is common. Less often there may be brisk sustained fever. Loss of weight or failure to gain are usual but not invariable. Local symptoms due to the effect on surrounding structures of pressure from caseous mediastinal glands are most severe in infants. Whereas in the school child cough may be relatively unimpressive, in the infant glandular pressure on the main bronchi frequently gives rise to spasmodic outbursts of coughing which closely simulate pertussis. In fact, the bronchi may be sufficiently narrowed by extrinsic pressure that a loud wheeze—"the asthmatoid wheeze" of Chevalier Jackson—may be heard. A diagnosis of asthma in the young infant should rarely be accepted before tuberculosis has been excluded. This type of "by-pass valve" bronchial narrowing is responsible in tuberculosis for what the older writers called "the wheezy wasting syndrome of infancy". Rarely, pressure on the trachea by caseous paratracheal glands can produce acute stridor. Pain in the chest is an infrequent complaint. Physical examination of the chest is rarely helpful unless there is absorption collapse or obstructive emphysema (*vide infra*). The diagnosis of primary intrathoracic tuberculosis must depend largely upon the ease with which the physician's suspicions are aroused. The good physician will always realize that the "sickly" child demands a precise diagnosis and that he must not be offered a "tonic" or some placebo. In some instances, of course, the child is brought to the physician because of known recent contact with a tuberculous adult. The possibility of such contact within or outside the family circle, should always be the subject of direct enquiry in the case of an unwell child in whom a satisfactory diagnosis has not been reached.

Diagnostic Tests

Tuberculin skin tests are, of all tests, the most useful in the diagnosis of primary tuberculosis. A positive reaction before the age of 3 years is evidence of active infection. After this age a positive test may only indicate previous infection not now necessarily active, but in an ill child it obviously merits further investigation. The most reliable test is the Mantoux intradermal reaction using suitable dilutions of Old Tuberculin (O.T.) or purified protein derivative (P.P.D.). The tuberculin jelly test is convenient in domiciliary practice although less reliable. When large numbers have to be tested the Heaf test, which makes multiple punctures with a test-gun through undiluted O.T., is useful (Miller, 1958). False negative results with all tests may be found in children who are overwhelmed by miliary tuberculosis and in those convalescent from measles. Apart from these exceptions a negative tuberculin test, properly performed with active material, excludes tuberculosis. It must be remembered, however, that these tests lose their value in children who have been immunized with B.C.G.

A chest radiograph may fail to reveal any abnormality in early primary tuberculosis. Most often, however, unilateral enlargement of the hilar glands is visible, but as this could be due to diseases other than tuberculosis the chest radiograph by itself cannot justify a diagnosis of primary tuberculosis. Only very rarely is the primary focus in the lung parenchyma visible, although it can be large enough to be so (Fig. 16). It is quite exceptional for the primary focus to cavitate (Figs. 17 and 18). When the primary complex heals by calcification it will become radiogically obvious (Fig. 19) although no longer responsible for symptoms. It must be stressed that the diagnostic value of the radiograph is limited in primary tuberculosis, in marked contrast to adult type phthisis where the lung parenchyma is heavily involved.

Gastric washings should be examined by direct staining, culture and guinea-pig inoculation. They are of limited usefulness in diagnosis in view of the time lag usually involved, but successful isolation of tubercle bacilli allows their sensitivities towards the anti-tuberculous drugs to be tested and this information is valuable.

The erythrocyte sedimentation rate, preferably by the Westergren technique, is not of direct diagnostic value, but a raised E.S.R. helps

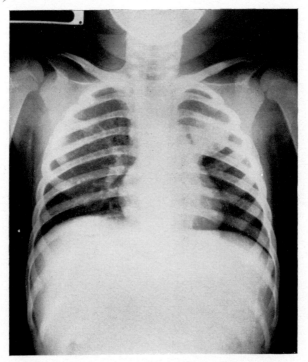

FIG. 16.—Radiograph of chest showing exceptionally large primary tuberculous focus in left upper lobe. Early calcification is present.

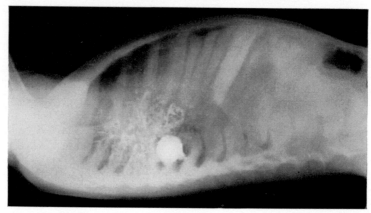

FIG. 18

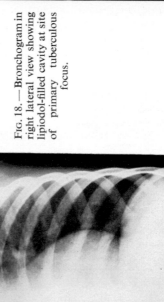

FIG. 17. — Chest radiograph showing tuberculous cavity in right lower lobe.

FIG. 18. — Bronchogram in right lateral view showing lipiodol-filled cavity at site of primary tuberculous focus.

FIG. 17.

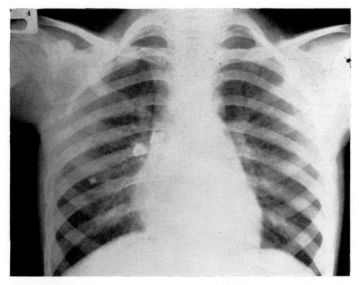

FIG. 19.—Healed primary tuberculous complex showing calcification in the primary focus and the hilar lymph nodes.

to confirm the presence of active disease and serial estimations are valuable in assessing progress during treatment.

Enough has been said to make it clear that a diagnosis of active primary tuberculosis can rarely be established on the basis of a single test, and certainly not on the X-ray appearances. However, when all the findings are weighed together—clinical history, possible adult contact, results of tuberculin tests, radiographs and E.S.R.—it is almost always possible to arrive at a correct diagnosis. The first test should be a skin test. Only if this is positive is further, and costly, investigation necessary. A wider recognition of this fact would save time and money on unnecessary X-rays, and it would avoid some regrettable errors.

Absorption collapse (atelectasis).—In 1920, Eliasberg and Neuland drew attention to the appearance of large homogeneous shadows in the chest radiographs of some children passing through their primary tuberculous infection. To this they gave the label "epituberculosis", and the condition was often regarded as a perifocal allergic reaction in tissues sensitive to tuberculo-protein. It has been explained above that the basic cause is the stop-valve type of bronchial obstruction, with absorption collapse due to compression or erosion of the bronchial wall by caseous lymph nodes (Figs. 20 and 21). Bronchoscopy frequently reveals tuberculous granulation tissue within the lumen (Hutchison,

1949*a*, *b*). Children so affected are <u>not</u> acutely ill, dyspnoeic or toxic. The physical signs are often remarkably slight, but an impaired resonance and diminished breath sounds over the affected lobe may be demonstrable. Infrequently the trachea or mediastinum is shifted towards the affected side. The prognosis of the primary infection itself does not appear to be worsened by this complication, although in some cases <u>bronchiectasis</u> remains as a sequel (Figs. 22 and 23), which can cause <u>trouble many</u> years later.

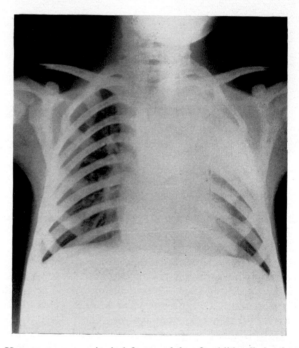

Atelectasis

FIG. 20.—Homogeneous opacity in left upper lobe of a child suffering from primary tuberculosis. This was previously called "epituberculosis".

Obstructive emphysema.—When the check-valve type of bronchial obstruction causes obstructive emphysema of a lobe or a lung, the child develops an "asthmatoid" <u>wheeze.</u> There is hyper-resonance to percussion but poor <u>air-entry</u> over the affected area. The radiograph, especially that taken during expiration, shows an area of increased translucency with depression of the diaphragm and mediastinal shift to the opposite side. It is easy for the unwary to make the mistake of misinterpreting the abnormality to be in the healthy lung (Fig. 24). In this condition, too, a good recovery can be expected.

CLINICAL ASPECTS OF EARLY POST-PRIMARY TUBERCULOSIS

It is proposed here to discuss only those post-primary lesions which commonly develop within six months of the primary infection, because chronic tuberculosis of the lungs, bones, joints and genito-urinary tract is best treated by the appropriate specialists.

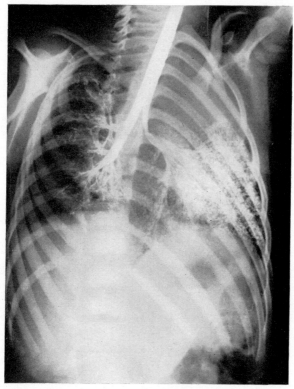

FIG. 21.—Bronchogram in same patient as FIG. 20 reveals failure of lipiodol to enter left upper lobe due to bronchial obstruction. Note also narrowing of lumen of left main bronchus.

Tuberculous meningitis.—This dreaded complication of primary tuberculosis tends to have an insidious type of onset with lethargy, fractiousness, anorexia, headache and vomiting. None the less, the mother can usually state the precise day on which the child became ill, and once begun the clinical picture unfolds inexorably and without remission. Rarely, the disease is heralded by a convulsion. A constant feature is constipation. It is not uncommon to obtain a history of recent trivial head injury or of an infection such as measles. In the

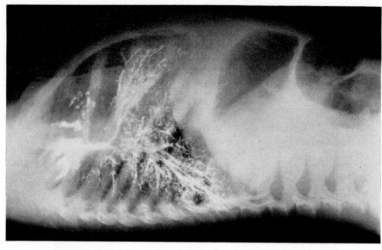

FIG. 23.

FIG. 22.—Chest radiograph showing bronchiectatic appearances in right upper lobe of a child under treatment for primary tuberculosis.

FIG. 23.—Bronchogram in right lateral view from same patient as Fig. 22 confirming presence of saccular bronchiectasis in right upper lobe.

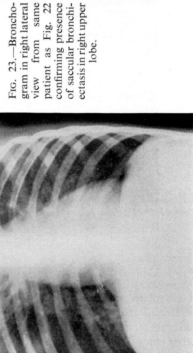

FIG. 22.

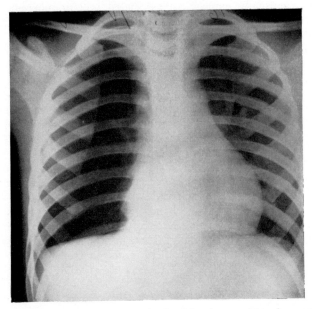

FIG. 24.—Chest radiograph taken in expiration. Note increased translucency on right side due to obstructive emphysema of right upper lobe. Lower lobe is collapsed against mediastinum which is displaced to left.

earliest stage of the disease, when correct diagnosis is vitally important, the child's consciousness is unimpaired and neurological signs are absent or minimal. Slight nuchal rigidity, or a full "boggy" fontanelle in an infant, are obviously most significant findings, but their absence in no way excludes the diagnosis. It is important also that the physician is not misled by the not infrequent association of tuberculous meningitis with signs of inflammation in the upper respiratory tract (Lincoln et al., 1960). An unusual degree of drowsiness or lethargy should always awaken the suspicion of the alert physician.

If this early stage of the disease is missed, when treatment is most successful, the intermediate stage inevitably ensues. By now there is obvious blurring of consciousness, nuchal rigidity is present, Kernig's sign may be positive, and focal neurological signs such as ophthalmoplegia, facial paralysis, hemiparesis and papilloedema ultimately appear. A most useful indication of increased intracranial pressure in the child whose fontanelle has not long closed is the "crackpot sound", obtained when the skull is held in the left hand and percussed by the middle finger of the right. It is due to starting open of the sutures. At this stage the patient often lies curled up on his side with his face averted from the light, and he resents interference. Choroidal tubercles (*vide infra*) usually indicate an associated miliary tuberculosis, but their presence is of such diagnostic value that careful ophthalmoscopy is an essential part of the examination of every excessively drowsy child. Most cases in the intermediate stage show a good response to treatment, although permanent neurological sequelae sometimes remain.

In the later or terminal stage of the disease treatment frequently fails to save the child's life, and the incidence of permanent brain damage such as hydrocephalus, blindness, deafness and mental deficiency is high. By now the child is comatose. There may be severe head retraction and opisthotonus or decerebrate rigidity. Paralytic squints, unequal or fixed pupils and other neurological signs are obvious. Disturbed vasomotor control is frequently reflected in a characteristic hectic flush on one side of the face, like the paint on the cheek of a toy soldier, and the palms of the hands may show a characteristic pink colour. Severe tissue wasting is a further distressing feature of the disease. Convulsions are common. There may be terminal hyperpyrexia, although earlier in the disease there is only a moderate rise in temperature.

Diagnosis

The cerebrospinal fluid shows an increase of globulin by the Pandy test. The total protein content is usually raised above 40 mg. per 100 ml. A low sugar content (below 45 mg. per 100 ml.) is very characteristic, but not invariable in the early stage of the disease. The cell count is raised to between 50 and 800 per cu. mm. and films show a marked preponderance of lymphocytes. The final proof is the isolation of tubercle bacilli. This entails a diligent search in Ziehl-Neelsen films of the spider-web clot which forms in the cerebrospinal fluid when it is allowed to stand overnight, or of the centrifuged deposit. Some of the fluid should also be cultured and inoculated into a guinea-pig. Other evidence of tuberculosis must also be sought. The Mantoux test is usually positive when 1/1,000 dilution of O.T. is used. Radiographs of the chest may also give valuable supporting evidence. The efficacy of modern treatment in early cases places a heavy responsibility upon the physician; and it is, of course, essential that prolonged drug treatment is not used in cases where the meningitis is non-tuberculous in aetiology.

Differential Diagnosis

Tuberculous meningitis is most likely to be mistaken for aseptic meningitis due to viruses such as those of the poliomyelitis, Coxsackie and ECHO groups. In these cases the onset is usually much more acute than in tuberculous cases, with brisk fever and obvious early rigidity of the neck and spine. The cerebrospinal fluid shows a lymphocytic pleocytosis in both types, but in viral cases there is no fall in sugar content, the protein content is less markedly raised, and a spider-web clot rarely if ever forms. There will be no other indications of tuberculosis in viral cases. A rare cause of lymphocytic meningitis is infection by *Leptospira canicola* (from dogs) or *Leptospira icterohaemorrhagiae* (from rats). In those cases proteinuria, conjunctival suffusion and sometimes jaundice should indicate the diagnosis. There is also a polymorphonuclear leucocytosis in leptospirosis. In older children tuberculous meningitis can simulate brain tumour, but the cerebrospinal fluid will reveal the true state of affairs.

Miliary tuberculosis.—When miliary spread is associated with meningeal involvement the clinical picture is that already described, but when the meninges are not involved miliary tuberculosis can be one of the most difficult diagnostic problems in medicine. The onset is insidious with lassitude, weakness, anorexia, malaise and fever. In some cases the temperature shows a rather characteristic tendency to be highest in the mornings. Loss of weight may be rapid and the most acutely ill patients quickly become cachectic. On the other hand, less acute examples of the disease are compatible with a remarkably good state of nutrition for many weeks. When the lungs are extensively involved dyspnoea may be obvious, in the absence of abnormal physical signs over the chest. In some patients gaseous abdominal distension may simulate typhoid fever. In infants and toddlers papulo-necrotic tuberculides may be seen over the face, trunk and limbs. These are small dusky red papules with a necrotic centre, best viewed under a hand lens. Splenomegaly of mild to moderate degree is common but not particularly helpful in diagnosis because it is a common finding in many of the diseases of childhood. The chest radiograph usually reveals the characteristic "snowstorm" appearances (Fig. 25), although these can be simulated by other diseases like malignant reticulosis (Chapter XI) and idiopathic pulmonary haemosiderosis (Chapter XIII), and they may be absent in fulminating cases.

Careful ophthalmoscopy is most important because choroidal tubercles are pathognomonic of miliary spread. They first appear as rounded yellow patches with ill-defined margins. They are often about the size of the optic disc but may be smaller. As they get older the centres become white and the margins become clearly defined by deposition of pigment. Under the influence of treatment the smaller lesions disappear completely whereas the larger ones are replaced by black pigment (Illingworth and Lorber, 1956). In the more chronic cases of miliary tuberculosis which run a slow course subcutaneous cold abscesses may develop, and in others tuberculous dactylitis may produce fusiform swellings of one or more fingers. The correct diagnosis rests upon a careful review of all the clinical evidence, including history of

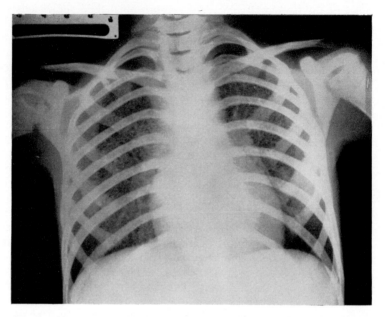

Fig. 25.—Chest radiograph showing diffused miliary mottling—"snowstorm" appearances—of miliary tuberculosis.

possible contact with a case of "open" tuberculosis, and here again the Mantoux test is usually of great value.

Chronic disseminated tuberculosis.—Whereas meningitis and miliary spread usually develop within the first six months after the primary tuberculous infection, tuberculous disease affecting bone and joint or the renal tract tends to develop within the next five years. These forms of tuberculosis have become uncommon in Britain but their diagnosis is rarely difficult. Bone and joint disease can be confirmed by tuberculin testing and synovial biopsy; renal involvement by pyelography and culture of the urine for tubercle bacilli.

Acute tuberculous pneumonia.—This form of "galloping consumption" was once common in children and young adults, but in Britain today is only rarely seen in very young infants. The infant is acutely ill with fever, dyspnoea, toxaemia and a productive spasmodic cough. There may be dullness on percussion with bronchial breath sounds and crepitations over affected areas of the lungs. Tubercle bacilli can often be seen in films made from material obtained by laryngeal swabbing or gastric lavage. The tuberculin skin tests are positive and radiographs show lobar or lobular areas of consolidation, sometimes with cavitation. In the pre-streptomycin era death was the inevitable outcome.

EXTRATHORACIC TUBERCULOSIS

Sources of Infection

Cervical and abdominal tuberculosis were once very common in Britain as a consequence of the ingestion of milk from tuberculous cows. They are now virtually unknown, although a rare case of infection in these sites by human tubercle bacilli is still encountered. Primary infection of the skin, conjunctiva, or within the mouth following tooth extraction, is less rare than is sometimes thought (Miller, 1953; Boyes et al., 1956). In these cases there is frequently a history of contact with an adult case of phthisis. Presumably the organisms find entry through a minor wound in the skin or mucous membrane.

Pathological Course

The primary tuberculous complex behaves in the same basic fashion whatever its site. In cervical tuberculosis the primary focus is in the tonsil, although it can only be seen under the microscope. There has often been preceding chronic sepsis in the tonsils. The affected cervical lymph nodes become caseous. They may later liquefy and coalesce, at the same time becoming adherent to the skin and surrounding tissues. If rupture occurs the classical "collar stud" abscess extending through a fascial plane, or one or more sinuses discharging through the skin may develop (Scrofula). In abdominal tuberculosis the primary focus is in the small intestine. This is a solitary microscopic lesion, not to be confused with the secondary tuberculous enteritis which may complicate advanced cases of adult type phthisis. Mesenteric lymph nodes are massively involved, and rupture into the peritoneal cavity leads to the once common picture of tuberculous peritonitis. The possibility of cutaneous, conjunctival or buccal primary tuberculosis should be considered when solitary but chronic enlargement of lymph nodes appears in unusual sites, e.g. pre-auricular, submandibular or inguinal. In all types of extrathoracic tuberculosis haematogenous spread may occur, although less acutely than in the intrathoracic disease. In the case of bovine infections, bone and joint lesions were at one time common complications which resulted in long periods of invalidism or crippling, even in death.

CLINICAL ASPECTS OF EXTRATHORACIC TUBERCULOSIS

The general symptoms tend to be common to all types of primary tuberculosis. They vary from none at all to listlessness, anorexia, undue fatiguability, low-grade fever and loss of weight. When the cervical glands are involved the first sign is a painless, firm, mobile mass at the angle of the jaw. Later the glands become matted together, adherent to the skin and no longer freely movable. Liquefaction is indicated by palpable fluctuation. Healing is by fibrosis and calcification which becomes radiologically visible. The differential diagnosis from other causes of cervical adenitis can be made by tuberculin skin testing.

Involvement of the *abdominal* glands (tabes mesenterica) is often diagnosed only by the exclusion of tuberculous disease elsewhere in the body in a child with positive tuberculin skin tests. Pain in the abdomen is too common a symptom during childhood to be very helpful in this disease. Subsequently the diagnosis may be confirmed in retrospect by the radiological demonstration of calcification within the abdomen. When tuberculous peritonitis ensues there is swelling of the abdomen. Ascites is often demonstrable and may be gross. In other cases there are palpable masses composed of omentum matted over caseating lesions. Wasting is sometimes extreme. At any time, partial or complete intestinal obstruction may complicate an already grim picture.

In *cutaneous, conjunctival or buccal tuberculosis* an enlarged lymph node is the usual presenting feature. A careful search will reveal the primary focus in the shape of an indolent, painless and relatively

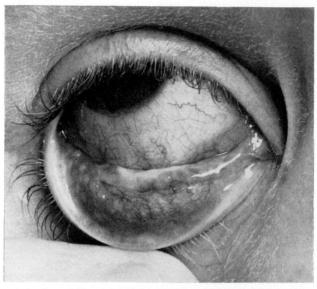

FIG. 26.—Indolent tuberculous ulcer on lower palpebral conjunctiva of a child whose sole complaint was an enlarged pre-auricular lymph node. Diagnosis was confirmed by biopsy.

inconspicuous ulcer, which alternates between healing and breaking down (Fig. 26). The diagnosis is confirmed by the positive tuberculin skin test and by microscopic examination of a piece of tissue removed from the margin of the lesion.

Treatment of Primary and Early Post-Primary Tuberculosis

It is now possible to bring about cure in every type of tuberculosis in childhood provided that (i) the disease is diagnosed at an early stage, and (ii) the tubercle bacilli in the lesions are sensitive to the drugs employed. In paediatric practice it is very rarely necessary to have resort to other than the following drugs in the dosage shown:

Streptomycin sulphate (intramuscular) 40 mg./Kg./day.
Isoniazid (oral) 10–20 mg./Kg./day.
Para-aminosalicylic acid P.A.S. (oral) 300 mg./Kg./day.

P.A.S. is much less effective than streptomycin or isoniazid and it is used in combination with one or both of these largely to prevent the emergence of drug-resistant strains of tubercle bacilli. In children it is usually sufficient to use two drugs in combination, and the dangers of the development of drug-resistance are small, in marked contrast to the situation which pertains in "open" cases of adult type phthisis. In certain circumstances detailed below the addition of corticosteroids to the anti-tuberculous drugs has some advantages. These hormones must on no account ever be used in tuberculous patients without concomitant anti-tuberculous drug therapy.

It is no longer necessary to confine children suffering from tuberculosis to bed for long periods, nor to banish them to inaccessible sanatoria in the country. When the child is fevered or feels ill he should obviously be in bed, but he can safely be allowed up, and outside in the fresh air as soon as he is afebrile and feeling well. Indeed, in many instances the child can be permitted to live his normal life and to attend school, provided his parents can be relied upon to give him his drugs regularly. It is, however, of the greatest importance that his progress be supervised by physicians who are familiar with the behaviour of primary tuberculosis. It should hardly be necessary to add that when the tuberculous child is also undernourished or is suffering from avitaminosis, an important part of the treatment would be their correction. In Britain, however, frank malnutrition and the deficiency diseases are now exceedingly rare.

Primary tuberculous infection.—When a child is ill with symptoms in the course of the primary infection, the need for anti-tuberculous drugs is not in doubt. They are invariably indicated when the primary infection is detected in the under three year old group, and in adolescents or young adults, because of the undoubted increased risk at these times of haematogenous and bronchogenic spread respectively. On the other hand, there has been doubt expressed as to the wisdom of using drugs in the pre-pubertal child of school age who is symptomless, and who may have been detected by routine tuberculin skin testing. The tuberculosis mortality rate in this group has always been very low. However, in recent years the weight of medical opinion has shifted towards the view that active and presumably recent primary tuberculosis should be treated with drugs irrespective of the patient's age and of the presence or absence of symptoms. The principal reason for this is the prevention of haematogenous lesions during the dangerous six months after primary infection, and of bronchogenic spread later in adult life. It is undoubted that the former aim can be achieved by this form of "chemoprophylaxis" (U.S. Public Health Service Tuberculosis Prophylaxis Trial, 1957), and probable also that the long-term benefits are substantial.

The ill and fevered child rapidly responds to a combination of streptomycin and isoniazid. After a period of 8–12 weeks, and indeed, in less severely ill patients from the outset excellent results will be obtained from isoniazid and P.A.S., both given orally. There are obvious advantages in dispensing with intramuscular injections as soon as possible. The treatment should be given for at least six months in children. In adolescents and adults it is wise to continue the drugs for $1\frac{1}{2}$ to 2 years, to protect against adult type phthisis. On the other hand, bronchial obstruction complicating primary tuberculosis is not greatly influenced by drug therapy. It may, in fact, first appear during the course of treatment. Occasionally absorption collapse or obstructive emphysema can be relieved by bronchoscopy. In an effort to prevent subsequent bronchiectasis (Figs. 22 and 23) some surgeons have advised thoracotomy and evacuation of the caseous gland which is eroding the bronchial wall, but this is not the generally accepted practice.

In the case of the symptomless child, discovered during routine testing to have recently converted to tuberculin positive, the infection may be cured and the risk of dissemination averted by chemoprophylaxis with isoniazid alone. While the use of one anti-tuberculous drug by itself is rightly to be condemned in the treatment of "open" phthisis, because of the near certainty that resistant strains of tubercle bacilli will emerge, in cases of "closed" primary infection this risk seems to be negligible, and the value of such chemoprophylaxis with isoniazid has been well established. It is *not* to be recommended in the case of ill children.

Streptomycin is administered as a single daily intramuscular injection. Isoniazid and P.A.S. are customarily given in two or four divided doses throughout the 24 hours. However, experience under carefully controlled conditions in South India has shown, at least in adult patients from a poverty-stricken area, that better results are obtained by the daily administration of a single large dose. The explanation seems to be that the efficacy of isoniazid is related to its peak serum level, and that this is more important than maintaining continuous inhibitory concentrations in the serum (Fox, 1962). It was, incidentally, re-affirmed that these adult patients did significantly better on P.A.S. and isoniazid than on isoniazid alone.

Tuberculous meningitis.—The advent of isoniazid in 1951 greatly simplified and improved the treatment of this most serious of tuberculous diseases. Spinal and cisternal blocks have become rare and intra-ventricular treatment is now mercifully rarely required. The results, however, still depend upon the stage of the disease at which treatment is started. Ninety per cent of patients who are conscious at the start of treatment may now be expected to recover (Lorber, 1956), whereas the recovery rate in comatose patients will hardly exceed 25 per cent (Lorber, 1954). In this disease the patient's life and reason depend upon his physician's diagnostic acumen. Once the diagnosis has been established beyond reasonable doubt, treatment should be started with intramuscular streptomycin and oral isoniazid. Some also add P.A.S. There is good evidence that the corticosteroids used *along with the anti-tuberculous drugs* are of benefit in that they diminish the risk of subarachnoid adhesions, allow the drugs easier access to the bacteria, and improve the patient's appetite and well-being. Some use them only when the child shows blurring of consciousness or neurological signs. A suitable drug and dosage would be prednisolone 15 mg. four times daily for 10 days; 10 mg. four times daily for 10 days; 5 mg. four times daily for 10 days; and 5 mg. twice daily for 10 days. There is still controversy as to the necessity for intrathecal treatment when isoniazid is being used. Some experienced workers still insist upon it (Lorber, 1954; Smith *et al.*, 1956), whereas others regard it as now unnecessary (Debré and Brissauld, 1956; Fyfe, 1959). Suitable intrathecal doses of streptomycin are 25 mg. for children under 3 years, 50 mg. under 12 years, and 100 mg. for older patients. It is often given daily until the cells in the cerebrospinal fluid have fallen to below 100 per c. mm. and then on every second or third day for some weeks. In the author's unit in Glasgow intrathecal treatment has been abandoned without deterioration in the results of treatment.

Miliary tuberculosis and acute caseous pneumonia.—The advent of isoniazid greatly improved the outlook in these forms of tuberculosis, because once it has been started in combination with streptomycin there is virtually no risk of tuberculous meningitis. This complication used to lead to many disappointments when streptomycin was the only drug available. The use of isoniazid has also abolished the later appearance of metastatic lesions in bones or kidneys. There is doubt about the value of corticosteroids. Their use undoubtedly improves the patient's early progress, and they may lessen residual scarring, but they have not been shown to alter significantly the ultimate results.

Summary

It can now be affirmed that, provided a child is given the opportunity of early diagnosis, death from tuberculosis should be rare. An exception is the infrequent case in which the tubercle bacilli are resistant to the commonly used three drugs. The source of such an infection is, of course, an adult whose disease has been so mismanaged that resistant strains of bacilli are permitted to thrive in the lesions. Even in these cases, however, reasonable hope of recovery can rest upon the use of less effective and more toxic agents such as cycloserine, ethionamide, pyrizinamide and viomycin.

RHEUMATIC FEVER

This disease, sometimes called juvenile rheumatism or the rheumatic infection, is not an infection in the usual meaning of the word. It has become a much less common cause of cardiac crippling than used to be the case in Britain and the other more prosperous countries of the world. The explanation lies in improved social conditions and nutrition, and to a lesser degree, in the ability of sulphonamide and penicillin to eradicate the β-haemolytic streptococcus from the upper respiratory tract.

Aetiology

It is generally accepted that rheumatic fever is causally related to infection by the β-haemolytic streptococcus although this organism cannot be recovered from the rheumatic lesions themselves. It is not proposed to consider the evidence for this statement in detail. It is sufficient to note the occurrence of streptococcal infections of the throat some one to three weeks before the majority of attacks or relapses of rheumatic fever. It should also be noted, however, that we do not know why only a small minority of individuals develop rheumatic fever after streptococcal infections. During the latent period between the streptococcal infection and the development of rheumatic fever presumably some kind of antigen-antibody reaction is initiated. Soon after this the titre of anti-streptolysin-O, one of several antibodies to extracellular streptococcal products, rises steadily, and it remains elevated for much longer than in people whose attack of tonsillitis or scarlet fever is not complicated by rheumatic fever (Wood and McCarty, 1954).

Several other factors have an impact on the aetiology and epidemiology. Thus, rheumatic fever is much more common among the poorer sections of the community who, until recently, lived in conditions of overcrowding than in the more prosperous families. It is less common in the tropics although both overcrowding and streptococcal infections are common. The frequency with which a family history of rheumatic heart disease, and sometimes of rheumatoid arthritis, can be obtained in cases of acute rheumatism has long been recognized (Wilson and Schweitzer, 1954). In fact this may at times be of positive diagnostic value. Other evidence which points towards a genetic predisposition to the disease in some individuals has been found in an apparent association of the susceptibility to rheumatic fever with the presence of mucopolysaccharide blood-group substances in the saliva (Glynn and Holborow, 1952), and with certain blood-groups (Buckwalter *et al.*, 1962).

Pathology

The lesions are found most often in the synovial tissues of joints and tendons, in subcutaneous tissues, and in the cardiovascular system, especially the wall of the left ventricle, the interventricular septum, the mitral and aortic valves, the left atrial appendage, the pericardium, and in the blood vessels of many organs. The typical microscopic lesion is the Aschoff body which starts as an oedematous node in the collagen structures, usually in or around a small blood vessel. The fully developed node consists of a necrotic centre surrounded by connective tissue cells, some multinucleated; the periphery consists of plasma cells, lymphocytes and some polymorphonuclears and eosinophils. On the cardiac valves, at the lines of apposition of the cusps, small firm white to yellow vegetations are formed. These are composed mainly of platelets and fibrin. Such vegetations are secondary to the development of Aschoff nodes within the cusps themselves, and it is the healing of the valvular damage by fibrosis which so often leads to permanent valvular incompetence, and/or stenosis. While the lesions in the heart are "proliferative" in nature, those affecting the synovial membranes, pericardium, and occasionally pleura, are "exudative" with resultant effusions. The pathological changes in the brain in cases of chorea have not been clearly defined and post-mortem studies have been infrequent.

Clinical Features

It is rare for rheumatic fever to occur before the age of five years, but when it does it often runs a malignant course. In older children the onset, frequently one to three weeks after an overt attack of streptococcal fever, is usually much less acute in its manifestations than in adults. Indeed, the constitutional and joint symptoms may be so slight that the physician may not be consulted until irreparable cardiac damage has resulted. In most cases, however, there are frank general symptoms such as fever, malaise, anorexia, undue tiredness and pallor. A common presenting symptom is abdominal pain which may even lead to laparotomy. Recurrent epistaxis is also common. Loss of weight is sometimes marked, especially when the heart is severely affected. Purpura is a rare phenomenon.

There is no specific laboratory test for rheumatic fever and it is convenient to describe the manifestations upon which the diagnosis must be based under the headings *major* and *minor*. The Cooperative Clinical Trial (1955) conducted by the Medical Research Council and the American Heart Association accepted two major manifestations or one major and two minor manifestations as justifying the diagnosis.

Major Manifestations

(i) *Arthritis.*—The polyarthritis of rheumatic fever renders the diagnosis easy when it results in the classical swelling, redness, pain and limitation of movement of the large joints, and when it flits from joint to joint. In children, however, arthritic manifestations are often mild, amounting perhaps to pain with only minimal objective evidence of joint involvement. In such cases the diagnosis of "growing pains" has frequently been made although this is an erroneous conception at any time. Occasionally, the disease presents as an acute arthritis confined, for a few days at least, to one joint such as the hip, when a wrong diagnosis of pyogenic arthritis can easily be made. And in some children involvement of the small joints of the hands or feet can make early differentiation from rheumatoid arthritis impossible. In most cases, however, a few days observation will allow the true situation to become clearer. It is important that a complaint of pains in the joints should always be taken seriously in children.

(ii) *Carditis.*—The appearance of abnormal signs in the heart of a child known previously to have been healthy is almost certain evidence of rheumatism. Undoubted signs of organic heart disease are: (*a*) cardiomegaly which is demonstrable clinically or radiologically; (*b*) a mid-diastolic murmur (Carey Coombs' murmur) at or just internal to the apex beat; (*c*) an early diastolic murmur of aortic origin down the left sternal border; (*d*) evidence of pericarditis (Chapter XIV); (*e*) a persistently raised sleeping pulse-rate; (*f*) prolongation of the P-R interval in the electrocardiograph or other more marked abnormalities; (*g*) signs of congestive cardiac failure.

It must be stressed that the Carey Coombs' murmur in active rheumatic carditis does not signify mitral stenosis, and it frequently disappears during the period of recovery. True mitral stenosis takes some years to develop after the acute attack. A common finding in rheumatic children is an apical systolic murmur. Its organic origin can be presumed when it extends throughout systole and when it is well propagated to the left axilla. It must be differentiated from the soft early or mid-systolic murmurs which are localized to the apical region and which are quite common in perfectly normal children. It is particularly important that a child is not confined to bed, or in any other way restricted, because of the chance finding of such an "incidental" cardiac systolic murmur. It should also be noted that severe cardiac crippling is rarely the sequel to a first attack of rheumatic fever, but that it indicates repeated attacks or continued rheumatic activity (Hutchison, 1955).

(iii) *Subcutaneous nodules.*—These are small firm nodules, most often found over bony prominences, e.g. occiput, olecranon, humeral condyles, knees, knuckles and malleoli, or in the tendon sheaths on the flexor aspects of the wrists or the dorsum of the feet. They are often better seen, blanching the skin when it is stretched by flexion of the joints, than palpated. They are of great prognostic significance because their presence always indicates active carditis and the likelihood of severe residual damage in the heart.

(iv) *Erythema marginatum* (Fig. 27).—This typical rash with map-like defined erythematous margins and white centres, and which changes shape continuously, is pathognomonic of rheumatic fever. However, it is lacking in any particular prognostic significance and, in fact, it may persist after all the other signs of rheumatic activity have vanished. It may appear over trunk or limbs.

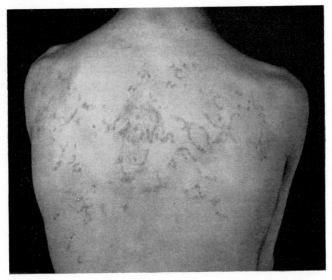

FIG. 27.—Erythema marginatum over the back of a rheumatic child. Note map-like outlines.

(v) *Sydenham's chorea.*—This major manifestation of the rheumatic state may occur in association with other manifestations like arthritis and carditis, but it frequently appears as a solitary and rather odd phenomenon. It is, in fact, the only major rheumatic manifestation which can affect the same child more than once, and sometimes several times, without the development of any of the other manifestations of rheumatism. For these reasons, and also because the E.S.R. and A.S.O. titre remain normal in uncomplicated chorea, the precise relationship of this disease to rheumatic fever has been the subject of an unresolved controversy. It is more common in girls. The clinical features fall into four broad groups.

(a) Involuntary, purposeless, non-repetitive movements of the limbs, face and trunk, e.g. grimacing, wriggling and writhing. The movements can be brought under voluntary control temporarily; they are aggravated by excitement; and they disappear during sleep. The first indication may be that the child begins to drop things, or her handwriting suddenly deteriorates, or she gets into trouble with her elders for "making faces". The movement results in a characteristic waxing and waning in the strength of the hand grip. Speech may become jerky and even unintelligible. Frequently the facial movements give rise to the so-called "society smile", and the out-stretched tongue may show undulating or jerky movements. The characteristic sustained knee-jerk, in which the leg rather slowly returns to its previous position after tapping the patellar tendon, is explained by the coincidence of a choreic movement with the physician's test. Sometimes the movements are confined to one side of the body (hemichorea).

(b) Hypotonia may result in muscular weakness. It also causes the characteristic posture of the out-stretched hands in which the wrist is slightly flexed, whereas there is hyperextension of the metacarpophalangeal joints. Rarely the child is unable to stand or even to sit up (chorea paralytica).

(c) Incoordination may be marked or only obvious when the child is asked to pick a coin off the floor.

(d) Mental upset is often an early sign. Emotional lability is almost constant. School work usually deteriorates. Infrequently the child becomes confused or even maniacal (chorea insaniens).

Minor Manifestations

(i) *Evidence of recent streptococcal infection.*—This may be based upon:

(a) Isolation of β-haemolytic streptococci from the throat swab.

(b) An A.S.O. titre above 200 units/ml.

(c) A reliable history of tonsillitis in the preceding month.

(ii) *Fever.*—This should have been above 101·3° F. per rectum on one occasion or above 100·3° F. on two occasions within 24 hours.

(iii) *Raised erythrocyte sedimentation rate.*

(iv) *Prolonged P-R interval.*

(v) *Previous evidence of rheumatic fever.* This should be based upon a reliable history of a previous attack or upon the existence of previous cardiac damage.

Differential Diagnosis

The difficulty which may be experienced in the distinction of rheumatic from pyogenic arthritis has already been mentioned. In the latter, polymorphonuclear leucocytosis is often but not always marked, a history of preceding sore throat is uncommon, and the condition remains confined to one joint. In rheumatoid arthritis there is often generalized lymphadenopathy or splenomegaly, and a much less rapid relief from salicylate than in rheumatic fever. The bone pains of acute leukaemia have been confused with the joint pains of rheumatic fever, but in the former there is usually a much more severe degree of anaemia, often haemorrhagic manifestations, and immature white cells are found in the blood films.

A most unfortunate mistake is to confuse the simple tic or habit spasm with chorea. In the former, rest in bed, which is essential in chorea, is the worst possible treatment. The movements in habit spasm are repetitive and, unlike those of chorea, always occur in the same sequence. It is possible to discern that they once had a purpose. They may be associated with other nervous disturbances, e.g. nail-biting, learning difficulties at school, or disharmony at home. In athetosis the movements are slower and more writhing than in chorea, and they appear in the first few years of life when chorea is unknown.

Treatment

The most important single therapeutic measure in rheumatic fever or chorea is rest in bed. In the absence of cardiac failure the child may be allowed to read and to feed himself, but he must not be allowed out of bed for any reason. The conditions which may be accepted as indicating the child's readiness to start getting up for gradually increasing periods are: (a) a normal E.S.R., (b) a normal sleeping pulse-rate, (c) a return of the haemoglobin level to normal, (d) a satisfactory gain in weight, (e) the absence of progression of the cardiac signs, (f) the disappearance of subcutaneous nodules, (g) the complete disappearance of chorea.

Elimination of any streptococci remaining in the upper respiratory tract should be ensured with benzylpenicillin, 250 mg. orally four times daily for seven days, or with a single intramuscular dose of a mixture of benzathine and soluble penicillin to a total of 1·25 mega units.

The value of salicylates in rheumatic fever has long been recognized. They abolish fever and joint manifestations rapidly, but their value in arresting carditis is doubtful. Those who claim they have value in carditis favour a dosage which will maintain the serum salicylate level between 30–40 mg. per 100 ml., but many would agree with Illingworth et al. (1954) that smaller doses prove equally effective. This eliminates the need for frequent estimations of the serum levels and the dangers of serious toxic effects. Aspirin is the most convenient and economic preparation. A dose of 2 grains (120 mg.) per Kg. body weight per day, divided into four or five equal doses, will rapidly abolish fever and joint pains. After this the dose may be reduced by one third and the aspirin continued until the E.S.R. has returned to normal. Children on salicylates must be carefully watched for signs of over-dosage such as over-breathing, tinnitus, deafness, nausea and vomiting. Avoidable fatalities have followed the careless use of this valuable group of drugs.

The other group which have been widely used in rheumatic fever in recent years are the corticosteroids. They have been the subject of a vast literature filled with conflicting findings and opinions. It must first be made clear that none of the presently available corticosteroids can supplant the time-honoured salicylates. They can undoubtedly lead to a more rapid relief of fever and arthritis, to disappearance of rheumatic nodules, and to a more rapid fall in the E.S.R. (Massell, 1954) than aspirin. On the other hand, the carefully controlled Cooperative Clinical Trial (1955) was unable to show that ACTH or cortisone had significant long-term advantages over aspirin, but Illingworth et al. (1957) concluded that cortisone and aspirin combined were more effective than either alone in combating carditis. Illingworth (1958) has expressed his opinion that it is wrong to treat any case of rheumatic fever with salicylate alone. Against this may be placed the undoubted efficiency of salicylates in relieving the child's subjective discomfort; also the serious side-effects which can accompany steroid therapy (Good et al., 1957). The latter include increased susceptibility to infection, osteoporosis, arrest of growth, sodium retention and heart failure, peptic ulceration, and diabetes mellitus. Minor side-effects such as moon-face, hirsutism and acne are almost invariable.

The author's present practice is to rely on aspirin alone, in the dosage given above, in first attacks of the disease. However, if cardiac signs progress on this regime, and also in all relapses, prednisolone is given in addition. The dosage schedule is 15 mg. four times daily for 10 days; 10 mg. four times daily for 10 days; 5 mg. four times daily for 10 days; and 5 mg. twice daily for 10 days. The aspirin is continued for at least two weeks thereafter in an effort to diminish the incidence of the "rebound phenomenon" as shown by a rise in the E.S.R. (Holt, 1956). In both types of regime it is essential that the cardiac state and the E.S.R. be regularly assessed as the best guides to progress.

Prevention of Relapses

It has been established that the prevention of further streptococcal infections reduces the risks of relapse in rheumatic children to very small proportions and drug prophylaxis has constituted a major advance in the management of this crippling disease. Sulphadiazine 0·5 gm.

twice daily is effective in this respect, but most physicians now follow the present fashion in preferring oral penicillin G or V, 250 mg. twice daily. This should be continued until the age of 18 years. Some parents and adolescent patients are, of course, careless and for them an alternative routine is a monthly intramuscular dose of 1·2 mega units of benzathine penicillin.

GLANDULAR FEVER (INFECTIOUS MONONUCLEOSIS)

Aetiology

It has been postulated that this disease is due to a virus, although none has been isolated. The author has seen an identical blood picture in cases of phenobarbitone idiosyncracy and it may be that "glandular fever" is more than a single disease. However, an infective cause must be presumed for most cases as epidemics have occurred in boarding schools and army barracks.

Clinical Features

The incubation period is thought to be 10–12 days. Children are usually less ill than adults and severe anginose cases with membranous pharyngitis are rare. The onset is acute with fever, malaise, headache and anorexia. The pharynx is inflamed but the young child may not complain of a sore throat. The fever may last only a few days, or for a few weeks. A characteristic finding in many cases and of diagnostic value is the presence of petechiae over the soft palate and other areas of the buccal mucosa. Generalized enlargement of the superficial lymph nodes is characteristic, although it may not develop for a week or more after the onset. Splenomegaly is almost invariable. In some cases jaundice and hepatomegaly occur. A rubelliform rash is not infrequent. In adults this can simulate the rash of secondary syphilis and diagnosis can be further confused by a false positive reaction in the Wassermann and Kahn tests. Rarely a child with glandular fever develops meningism and a lymphocytic reaction in the cerebrospinal fluid.

Diagnosis

The peripheral blood in glandular fever reveals a marked excess of mononuclear cells. Most of these are abnormal with deep blue staining cytoplasm which often contains vacuoles. The nucleus is frequently eccentric and the cell margin may appear to be lobulated, as if pseudopodia were forming. Some of the cells closely simulate lymphoblasts when the suspicion of leukaemia can be aroused. Proof of the diagnosis rests upon the Paul-Bunnell test for heterophil antibodies to sheep red cells. This becomes positive after one week. False positive results, such as may develop after an injection of horse serum, can be excluded by absorption techniques using guinea-pig kidney and beef red cells. A titre of 1 in 64 is considered to be diagnostic.

Differential Diagnosis

Glandular fever is diagnosed in children much more frequently than it exists. This is because polyglandular enlargement is a very common reaction in children to a wide variety of agents, e.g. viruses, toxoplasmosis, infective dermatitis etc. Furthermore, lymphocytosis is common in many childhood infections although abnormal monocytes are not seen. The diagnosis of glandular fever should probably not be accepted unless the Paul-Bunnell reaction is positive. It is not often that lymphatic leukaemia presents a diagnostic problem, but a marrow biopsy will resolve the issue in cases of doubt.

Treatment

There is no specific treatment. Rest in bed is indicated until the fever has disappeared and the lymphadenopathy has subsided. Relapses occasionally occur and convalescence should be gradual. Complete recovery is assured.

CONGENITAL SYPHILIS

This once common and tragic disease of infancy is now exceedingly rare in Britain. This is attributable to adequate antenatal care and the advent of penicillin. It is, however, still common in many parts of the world and every paediatrician must be able to recognize it promptly.

Aetiology

Treponema pallidum infects the foetus by passage across the placenta after the fourth month of pregnancy. The mother may have been recently infected or she may have had syphilis for years. The syphilitic foetus may be stillborn, or the infant may not develop frank signs of the disease until after the age of two weeks. Syphilis is not a common cause of early abortion.

Clinical Features

(a) *Early manifestations.*—These appear within the first eight weeks and they are associated with a general upset as shown by failure to thrive, fever, and increased susceptibility to secondary bacterial infections. One of the most characteristic manifestations is "snuffles" due to osteitis and osteo-chondritis of the nasal bones and cartilages. There is nasal obstruction with a purulent and blood-stained discharge. This is often associated with the so-called "eczema oris" (Fig. 28). When the nasal osteitis heals the collapse of the nasal bridge remains as the pathognomonic "saddle nose", a permanent stigma of the disease. The perioral eczema with fissuring at the angles of the mouth may also leave behind tell-tale radial scars called rhagades, which are a perman-

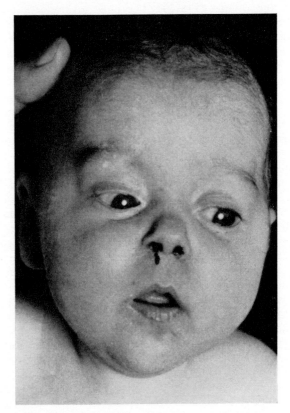

FIG. 28.—Syphilitic snuffles with blood-stained nasal discharge. There is early flattening of nasal bridge due to osteochondritis of nasal cartilages, and eczema around the mouth.

ent record of the disease. Rubbery discrete enlargement of the lymph nodes, especially in the occipital region, is very common. So also is hepatosplenomegaly. Hypoproteinaemic oedema and hypochromic anaemia are other common findings. A valuable aid to diagnosis is to be found in the typical coppery-coloured maculopapular rash. This may involve any part of the body, but on the palms and soles the skin is swollen, reddened and desquamating, giving rise to "washer-woman's skin" (Fig. 29). The fingers may show syphilitic paronychia. In many cases the cerebrospinal fluid shows an increased cell count, positive colloidal gold and Wassermann reactions. Obvious clinical signs of meningitis with bulging of the fontanelle and nuchal rigidity are uncommon but may precede hydrocephalus. Radiographs of the long bones almost invariably reveal a characteristic osteochondritis, periosteitis and osteitis (Fig. 30). The bone involvement may cause pain and lead to pseudoparesis of a limb. Later on at the toddling stage moist, flat perianal condylomata may be suggestive evidence of syphilis. Damage to the tooth buds may lead to the eruption subsequently of permanent upper central incisors which have a characteristic central notch—Hutchinson's teeth—and of six year molars with an extra cusp giving them a lobulated appearance—Moon's molars.

(b) *Late manifestations.*—These may lead to the diagnosis in children in whom there is no history of the early manifestations of infancy. The most common is interstitial keratitis which has a sudden onset about the age of 6–8 years, and involves one eye, then the other. There are pain, photophobia and lacrimation. The increased vascularity of the deeper layers of the cornea give it a salmon-pink discoloration. Permanent corneal opacity may follow. Chronic periosteitis of the tibiae may lead to an anterior thickening—"sabre-blade" tibiae. Gummata may cause perforations in the hard palate, nasal septum and vault of the skull. Ulceration of the skin may produce a foul-smelling sero-sanguineous discharge. Bilateral painless effusions into the knee joints is almost pathognomonic—Clutton's joints. Nerve deafness, optic atrophy and choroido-retinitis may develop. Neurosyphilis may be meningovascular in type, with intermittent but slowly progressive brain damage showing as cranial nerve palsies, hemiplegia, convulsions or intellectual impairment. Alternatively the parenchymatous type of neurosyphilis—tabo-paresis—leads to progressive dementia, delinquent behaviour, Argyll-Robertson pupils, extensor plantar responses, ataxia, loss of deep reflexes and death in a state of cachexia. The cerebrospinal fluid shows an increased content of globulin and cells, a paretic colloidal gold curve, and a positive Wassermann reaction.

Paroxysmal haemoglobinuria.—This rare late manifestation of congenital syphilis occurs in attacks which are precipitated by exposure to cold. An autohaemolysin unites with the erythrocytes in the cold peripheral capillaries, and the erythrocytes are then haemolyzed when they reach the warmer internal circulation by the complement normally present in the serum—Donath-Landsteiner reaction. In addition to haemoglobinuria, the patient complains of rigors, fever, lumbar or abdominal pain, and coldness or pain in the extremities. He may exhibit urticaria or jaundice. At the height of the attack there is haemoglobinaemia and methaemalbuminaemia; later there is hyperbilirubinaemia. Confirmation of the diagnosis can be obtained between

FIG. 29 (*see opposite*).—Soles of feet of syphilitic infant showing typical appearance of "washerwoman's skin".

FIG. 30 (*see opposite*).—Radiograph of legs of syphilitic infant showing osteitis, osteochondritis and periosteitis.

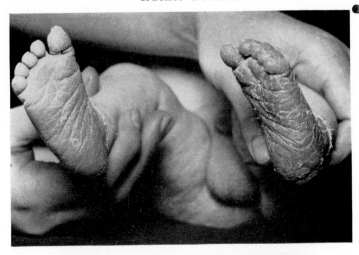

Fig. 29

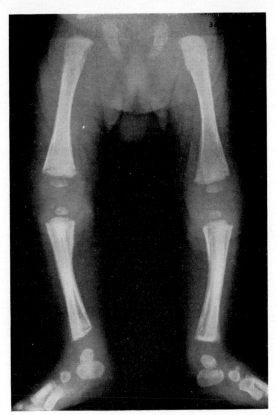

Fig. 30

attacks by means of the Donath-Landsteiner reaction (Sanford, 1933). The Wassermann reaction has sometimes reverted to negative by the time the attacks begin.

Diagnosis

It is important to appreciate that a syphilitic mother can give birth to a normal infant although, in those circumstances, the infant's serological reactions will be positive because maternal antibodies are transmitted from the mother across the placenta. A positive Wassermann or Kahn test is, therefore, never by itself proof of the presence of congenital syphilis during the first three months of life. After the age of six months, however, a continuing positive sero-reaction must be accepted as diagnostic of syphilis. A positive reaction in conjunction with any of the clinical or radiological signs of the disease is, of course, a clear indication for prompt anti-syphilitic treatment.

Treatment

Penicillin has replaced all of the formerly used preparations of arsenic, bismuth and mercury. It is extremely effective if started early in life, and there is no good reason for using the minimum effective dosage. A Jarisch-Herxheimer reaction is not less likely to occur with small doses. A suitable dose of benzylpenicillin is 100,000 units intramuscularly six-hourly for 21 days. This will result in complete cure and a negative sero-reaction in young infants. In children with late manifestations the sero-reaction may fail to revert completely and the effects of treatment, especially in tabo-paresis, are often disappointing. The pain in interstitial keratitis can be relieved by the two-hourly instillation of 0·5 per cent solution of hydrocortisone acetate. The pupils should be kept dilated with 1 per cent atropine sulphate drops. It is doubtful if any line of treatment influences the final outcome in the cornea.

TOXOPLASMOSIS

This protozoal disease is now recognized to be a not uncommon cause of illness in humans, and in its congenital form to be one of the causes of severe damage to the brain, eye and other organs.

Aetiology

The causal organism *Toxoplasma gondii* was first found in the gondi, a North African rodent, but is widespread in mammals, birds and even reptiles. It is an obligatory intracellular parasite, 4–7 microns in length and half this in width, with a crescentic shape.

Pathology

In man acquired infections are most often symptomless, but if a pregnant woman is infected during the last six months the parasites can cross the placenta to produce severe damage to the foetus. The parasites form pseudo-cysts in various tissues, e.g. brain, eyes, myocardium and lungs. These frequently calcify as healing takes place and the parasites die. It is believed that the formation of cysts is a response to the production of antibodies by the host.

Clinical Features

(*a*) **Congenital toxoplasmosis.**—In most instances the affected infant appears healthy at birth and lesions in the brain and eyes become manifest later on. Beattie (1957) has suggested that if the mother is infected long enough before full-term, sufficient antibody crosses the placenta to eliminate the parasites from the other tissues of the body. However, when the infection has been acquired late in pregnancy the infant may be born with severe manifestations. These include generalized purpura, often with thrombocytopenia (Fig. 31), hepatosplenomegaly, jaundice and erythroblastaemia which may mimic haemolytic disease of the newborn (Bain *et al.*, 1956).

The more typical manifestations cause the parents to seek medical advice, usually during the first year, because of delayed psychomotor development, convulsions or defective vision. The most characteristic finding is bilateral macular choroido-retinitis. Microphthalmia may also be present on one side. The nervous signs include mental retardation, spasticities, strabismus and convulsions. In over half the cases there is intracranial calcification (Fig. 32), either in the form of curvilinear streaks or as small calcified areas in the region of the basal ganglia. Microcephaly is frequently associated with internal hydrocephalus (Feldman, 1958). Apart from typical cases, the disease may be responsible for an unknown proportion of cases of mental retardation, epilepsy and cerebral palsy (Thalhammer, 1962).

(*b*) **Acquired toxoplasmosis.**—In Britain approximately 50 per cent of blood donors have positive serological tests for toxoplasmosis (Robertson, 1962), yet acquired toxoplasmosis is only infrequently recognized as the cause of illness. Rarely, acquired toxoplasmosis causes a severe illness such as encephalitis (Sabin, 1941), myocarditis (Potts and Williams, 1956), or peripheral neuritis (Robertson, 1962). More frequently in children, the illness is relatively benign with fever, generalized lymphadenopathy and splenomegaly (Cathie, 1954; Beverley and Beattie, 1958).

Diagnosis

The isolation of the parasites themselves may occasionally be achieved in active cases by inoculation of animals with cerebrospinal fluid, blood or tissue biopsy material. In routine work reliance is usually placed upon two serological tests. The more sensitive is the *dye test* of Sabin and Feldman (1948). This rests on the fact that antibodies

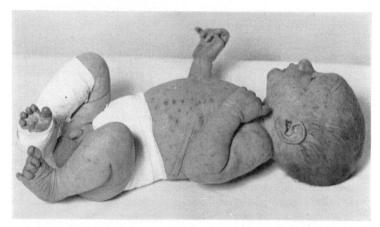

Fig. 31.—Infant suffering from congenital toxoplasmosis and showing generalized purpura present at birth.

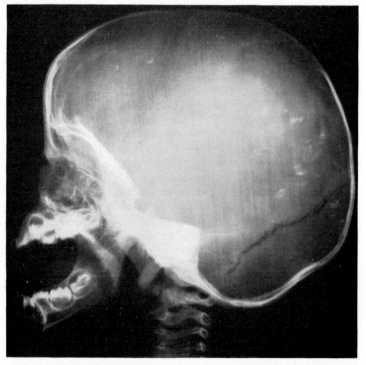

Fig. 32.—Radiograph of skull showing areas of intracranial calcification due to congenital toxoplasmosis.

from the patient so modify the cytoplasm of living toxoplasma that they no longer stain with methylene blue. The test becomes positive within two weeks of infection and high titres may be found. The test remains positive at diminishing titres for many years, so that a positive result does not indicate recent infection unless there is a very high or a rising titre. The *complement fixation test* takes longer to become positive and remains so for a shorter period. In congenital cases high titres in both tests are usual in the serum of both mother and infant, although sometimes the complement fixation test may be negative in the infant. The *intradermal skin test* is unreliable in young children.

Treatment

In congenital cases there has usually been irreversible damage to both brain and eyes before birth. Furthermore, drugs shown *in vitro* to be effective against toxoplasma are much less so when the parasite is in the cystic phase. None the less, in both congenital and acquired cases a three weeks' course should be given of pyrimethamine (Daraprim), 1 mg./Kg./day in divided doses, combined with sulphadiazine in customary dosage. Thalhammer (1962) has suggested serological tests as a routine procedure during pregnancy and a course of treatment during the eighth month in women with evidence of active infection. There is, of course, no information at present as to the possible deleterious effects of pyrimethamine on the foetus.

REFERENCES

Tuberculosis

BOYES, J., JONES, J. D. T., and MILLER, F. J. W. (1956). *Arch. Dis. Childh.*, **31**, 156.
DEBRÉ, R., and BRISSAUD, H. E. (1956). *Amer. Rev. Tuberc.*, **76**, 221.
ELIASBERG, H., and NEULAND, W. (1920). *Jb. Kinderheilk.*, **93**, 88.
FOX, W. (1962). *Lancet*, **2**, 413.
FYFE, W. M. (1959). *Arch. Dis. Childh.*, **34**, 334.
GERBEAUX, J., and MASSE, N. (1957). *Ann. Pédiat.*, **33**, 755.
GREEN, C. A., and MACGREGOR, A. R. (1937). *J. Path. Bact.*, **14**, 613.
HAWTHORNE, V. M., HANETT, W. F. H., LAUDER, I., MARTIN, W. B., and ROBERTS, G. B. S. (1957). *Brit. med. J.*, **2**, 675.
HUTCHISON, J. H. (1949*a*). *Quart. J. Med.*, **18**, 21.
HUTCHISON, J. H. (1949*b*). *Glasg. med. J.*, **30**, 271.
HUTCHISON, J. H. (1951). *Tubercle* (*Edinb.*), **32**, 271.
ILLINGWORTH, R. S., and LORBER, J. (1956). *Arch. Dis. Childh.*, **31**, 467.
LINCOLN, E. M., SABATO, V. R., SORDILLO, M. D., and DAVIES, P. A. (1960). *J. Pediat.*, **57**, 807.
LORBER, J. (1954). *Lancet*, **1**, 1149.
LORBER, J. (1956). *Brit. med. J.*, **1**, 1009.
MILLER, F. J. W. (1953). *Lancet*, **1**, 5.
MILLER, F. J. W. (1958). *Recent Advances in Paediatrics*, 2nd edit., edited by D. Gairdner, Chapt. 10. London: J. & A. Churchill.
RICH, A. R., and McCORDOCK, H. A. (1929). *Bull. Johns Hopk. Hosp.*, **14**, 273.

SMITH, H. V., VOLLUM, R. L., TAYLOR, L. M., and TAYLOR, K. B. (1956). *Tubercle (Edinb.)*, **37**, 301.
U.S. PUBLIC HEALTH SERVICE TUBERCULOSIS PROPHYLAXIS TRIAL (1957). *Amer. Rev. Tuberc.*, **76**, 942.
VEENEKLAAS, G. M. H. (1952). *Amer. J. Dis. Child.*, **83**, 271.
WALLGREN, A. (1948). *Tubercle (Edinb.)*, **29**, 245.

Rheumatic Fever

BUCKWALTER, J. A., NAIFEH, G. S., and AUER, J. E. (1962). *Brit. med. J.*, **2**, 1023.
COOPERATIVE CLINICAL TRIAL (1955). *Brit. med. J.*, **1**, 555.
GLYNN, L. E., and HOLBOROW, E. J. (1952). *J. Path. Bact.*, **64**, 775.
GOOD, R. A., VERNIER, R. L. and SMITH, R. T. (1957). *Pediatrics*, **19**, 95 and 272.
HOLT, K. S. (1956). *Arch. Dis. Childh.*, **31**, 444.
HUTCHISON, J. H. (1955). *Practitioner*, **174**, 400.
ILLINGWORTH, R. S. (1958). *Recent Advances in Paediatrics*, 2nd edit., edited by D. Gairdner, Chapt. 11. London: J. & A. Churchill.
ILLINGWORTH, R. S., BURKE, J. B., DOXIADIS, S. A., LORBER, J., PHILPOTT, M. G., and STONE, D. G. H. (1954). *Quart. J. Med.*, **23**, 177.
ILLINGWORTH, R. S., LORBER, J., HOLT, K. S., and RENDLE-SHORT, J. (1957). *Lancet*, **2**, 653.
MASSELL, B. F. (1954). *New Engl. J. Med.*, **251**, 183, 221, and 263.
WILSON, M. G., and SCHWEITZER, M. (1954). *Circulation*, **10**, 699.
WOOD, H. F., and McCARTY, M. (1954). *Amer. J. Med.*, **17**, 768.

Congenital Syphilis

SANFORD, A. H. (1933). *Proc. Mayo Clin.*, **8**, 115.

Toxoplasmosis

BAIN, A. D., BOWIE, J. H., FLINT, W. F., BEVERLEY, J. K. A., and BEATTIE, C. P. (1956). *J. Obstet. Gynaec. Brit. Emp.*, **63**, 826.
BEATTIE, C. P. (1957). *Trans. roy. Soc. Trop. Med. Hyg.*, **51**, 96.
BEVERLEY, J. K., and BEATTIE, C. P. (1958). *Lancet*, **2**, 379.
CATHIE, I. A. B. (1954). *Lancet*, **2**, 115.
FELDMAN, H. A. (1958). *Pediatrics*, **22**, 559.
POTTS, R. E., and WILLIAMS, A. A. (1956). *Lancet*, **1**, 483.
ROBERTSON, J. S. (1962). *Dev. Med. and Child Neurol.*, **4**, 507.
SABIN, A. B. (1941). *J. Amer. med. Ass.*, **116**, 801.
SABIN, A. B., and FELDMAN, H. A. (1948). *Science*, **108**, 660.
THALHAMMER, O. (1962). *Lancet*, **1**, 23.

CHAPTER XI

MALIGNANT DISEASE IN CHILDHOOD

Malignant disease has assumed a position of increased relative importance as a cause of mortality in childhood in Britain during the past 30 years. This is partly due to the defeat of the old killing infections by the sulphonamides and antibiotics, partly to a real increase in the incidence of certain types of malignant disease, e.g. leukaemia (Macgregor, 1961). The most common types of malignant disease in childhood in Britain in order of frequency are:

1. Leukaemia and other forms of malignant reticulosis, e.g. Letterer-Siwe disease, xanthomatosis etc.
2. Intracranial tumours, especially medulloblastoma and astrocytoma of the cerebellum and brain-stem.
3. Neuroblastoma arising from sympathetic nervous tissue within or without the adrenal medulla.
4. Nephroblastoma (Wilm's tumour of the kidney).
5. Retinoblastoma (Campbell et al., 1961).

Other less common tumours include those involving connective tissue, e.g. sarcoma, teratoma, Ewing's tumour of bone, and also tumours of the third and lateral ventricles, e.g. choroid papilloma. Primary hepatoma is rare in Britain although common in certain parts of Africa in association with malnutrition.

In the equatorial belt of Africa from the west to the east coast, and in New Guinea, the most common tumour of childhood is Burkitt's lymphoma (Burkitt, 1962). This most often begins as multiple tumours of the jaws or orbit with gross deformity. It may also present as an abdominal tumour in ovaries, kidneys, intestine, retroperitoneal tissues or testes. Infrequently, paraplegia may be the first sign. Generalized lymph node involvement and splenomegaly are rare. It has shown a remarkably good response to various cytotoxic drugs. Histologically it differs from lymphosarcoma as seen in the United Kingdom. Sheets of immature lymphoid cells are interspersed with non-malignant histiocytes which may contain erythrocytes, fat, nuclear debris and even phagocytosed tumour cells. It is clear that malignant disease is common also in African children, but that it tends to be very different in frequency distribution from that familiar to British paediatricians. Burkitt's lymphoma has, however, been reported in countries other than Africa such as Brazil, and infrequently in Britain and the United States. None the less, its remarkable geographical incidence in Africa suggested the possibility to Burkitt that it could be caused by an insect-transmitted virus.

The prognosis of malignant disease in childhood is very depressing. Campbell and his colleagues (1961) reported a mortality of 70 per cent in the Manchester area, and Macgregor (1961) gave a figure of 75 per cent in Scotland. Particularly high mortality figures are found in leukaemia, neuroblastoma, Wilm's tumour and lymphosarcoma. Many malignancies such as leukaemia and lymphosarcoma are incurable from the outset. Others like neuroblastoma and nephroblastoma are, unfortunately, associated with such non-compelling symptoms in the early stages that they have too frequently reached an advanced stage of the disease before the child is brought for treatment. None the less, recent advances in chemotherapy have improved the outlook to some extent. Intracranial tumours, on the other hand, are frequently so situated that complete surgical excision is impossible even at an early stage. Even an increased state of vigilance on the part of family doctors could achieve only a slight increase in the numbers of patients cured, and we must await new developments in therapeutics before this gloomy picture can change.

There has, however, been evidence to indicate a better understanding of the nature of carcinogenesis in recent years, although the picture is still a confused one. The evidence has come from different sources, e.g. statistical, cytogenetic and chemical. It now seems safe to assume that genetic or chromosomal change is a basic feature of the neoplastic process (Court Brown, 1962). A two-stage theory of carcinogenesis has been derived from work with chemical carcinogens, *initiation* which leads to a pre-neoplastic state, and *promotion* in which the abnormal cells proliferate. It can be postulated that the initiating agent can be some type of genetic damage, possibly itself acting upon cells which are already genetically abnormal. For example, it is known that certain types of individual with chromosomal abnormalities (e.g. Klinefelter's syndrome and mongolism) are especially prone to develop leukaemia. It is also known that most adults with chronic myeloid leukaemia have an abnormality involving deletion of material from the long arm of one of the small acrocentric chromosomes, probably 21, the so-called Philadelphia chromosome (Ph') (Tough *et al.*, 1961 and 1962). In these cases there is commonly a terminal acute leukaemic phase associated with the appearance of cells showing other and variable chromosomal aberrations. It is possible to look upon the chronic phase with its single Ph' chromosome as a pre-cancerous stage of initiation, whereas the terminal acute stage is the final malignant or promotion phase.

Particular thought has been given to the possible causal factors in acute leukaemia because this is the most common type of malignancy in childhood, it has a hopeless prognosis, and it has shown a true rise in incidence during the past 30 years. Stewart and her co-workers (1958) recorded some important findings from a survey of 1,694 deaths in young children from malignant disease. Among these were, (i) the risk of dying from leukaemia before the age of 10 years is twice as great as usual if the mother is over 40 years of age at the date of the child's birth, and the evidence suggests that childhood leukaemia and mongolism are influenced by a common factor rather than that one disease predisposes to the other, (ii) there is a causal relationship between prenatal exposure to X-rays and the subsequent development of malignant disease, (iii) X-ray films taken shortly after birth influence the distribution of childhood deaths from malignant disease, such exposure being more marked in respect of leukaemia than other cancers, (iv) children with leukaemia had a noticeable heavy incidence of acute pulmonary infections and severe injuries during the two years before they showed signs of the fatal disease. It must be stressed, however, that none of these associations appears to have great quantitative significance, and they can account for only a small number of childhood malignancies in relation to the increased incidence reported during the past 30 years.

Stewart (1961) has further shown that the recent increase in deaths from leukaemia has affected children between 1 and 5 years more than any other age-group below 70 years, and that this change has now brought the age-distribution of deaths from leukaemia more closely into line with the deaths from nephroblastoma and retinoblastoma. She has also produced some evidence to suggest that these young children with leukaemia associated with non-granular malignant cells—lymphoblasts, monoblasts or stem cells—have shown an especial proneness to pneumonia, an abnormal incidence of mongolism, and that occasionally two siblings have been affected with leukaemia. Stewart suggested that these are cases of *pre-zygotic* leukaemia, in which the "initiator" is the inheritance of a gene which produces pre-malignant changes in the ancestral cells of the reticulo-endothelial system. The "promoter" in these early cases of leukaemia is regarded as the cell stress of embryogenesis, which causes the genetically abnormal cells finally to lead to the formation of frankly malignant cells. Children who develop pre-zygotic leukaemia are more prone to pneumonia and other infections because they have genetically abnormal leucocytes. Before the advent of antibiotics these children, who nowadays develop leukaemia, would mostly have died of pneumonia etc. The arrival of these drugs is, therefore, a probable explanation for the spectacular increase in the early peak of leukaemia mortality. On the other hand, the leukaemia of older children which is much less common has not shown an increase in incidence. It is regarded by Stewart as *pre-natal* leukaemia. In this type the malignant cells may be lymphoblasts or myeloblasts and it is presumed that they arise from changes in the somatic cells of the body. These might, for example, be induced by exposure of the foetus to irradiation *in utero*.

An exciting possibility has been hinted at in recent years by the isolation of mycoplasmas (pleuro-pneumonia-like organisms) from tissue cultures inoculated with bone marrow from leukaemic patients (Fallon *et al.*, 1965). However, the relationship of mycoplasmas to leukaemia is not yet clear. If the mycoplasma has indeed come from the bone marrow it might not be related to the patient's disease; or it might represent infection due to failure of the patient's defence mechanisms; or it could form part of a sequence of events which is associated with the development of leukaemia.

Even more suggestive evidence of a viral aetiology has been obtained from cases of Burkitt's African lymphoma (Stanley, 1966), and it seems likely that the disease is transmitted by mosquitoes. Various agents have been associated with Burkitt's lymphoma including reovirus 3, herpes-like virus, and mycoplasma, the evidence being strongest in favour of reovirus 3.

LEUKAEMIA

In childhood leukaemia is nearly always of the acute variety. Chronic myeloid leukaemia does occasionally develop with a clinical picture similar to that seen in adult cases, but the author has never seen a case of chronic lymphatic leukaemia in a child. Between the ages of 1 and 5 years, when leukaemia is most common, the cell type is lymphoblastic in most cases; occasionally the cells are so undifferentiated as to merit the description of stem cells. Acute myeloblastic leukaemia is rare between the ages of 1 and 5 years, but oddly enough when leukaemia develops in the young infant or is congenital, and such cases are very infrequent, it is nearly always myelogenous. Monocytic, eosinophilic and megakaryocytic leukaemias are exceedingly rare. In all types there is a slight preponderance of boys over girls.

Pathology

In cases untreated by modern drugs there is extensive leukaemic infiltration in the liver, spleen, lymph nodes, bones, kidneys and many other tissues. In lymphoblastic cases leukaemic infiltration in the liver is markedly periportal in distribution, whereas in the myelogenous type infiltration of myeloblasts is extensive also in the sinusoids. Haemorrhage is a constant finding which may occur in many tissues and is, not infrequently, the actual cause of death. The other common feature is severe sepsis. In cases treated with antimitotic drugs or steroids severe monilial infection of the mouth, throat or oesophagus is common.

Clinical Features

Acute leukaemia is only rarely a difficult diagnostic problem, but the physician must obviously be sure of his diagnosis before imparting it to the parents who would not lightly forgive the hopeless prognosis when it was proved to be wrong. The disease has been well reviewed by Boggs *et al.* (1962).

The most common presenting features are rapidly progressive pallor and spontaneous haemorrhagic manifestations such as purpura, epistaxis, and bleeding from the gums. These are associated with increasing weakness, breathlessness on exertion, malaise, anorexia and fever. In some cases the onset takes the form of a severe oropharyngeal inflammation and enlargement of the cervical lymph nodes which does not respond to antibiotics. In other cases the onset is with bone pains due to leukaemic infiltration. The concomitant pallor, or purpura and ecchymoses, should obviate erroneous diagnoses like rheumatic fever or poliomyelitis. Physical examination most frequently shows polyglandular enlargement, splenomegaly and hepatomegaly, all of only moderate degree. In some patients, however, the signs are confined to pallor and haemorrhage of variable severity and distribution. Infrequently jaundice may develop or there may be evidence of involvement of the central nervous system. Ophthalmoscopy frequently reveals retinal haemorrhages. Proptosis may be the presenting feature in that rare form of myeloblastic leukaemia which has been called *chloroma*, because on cut-section the tumour tissue is green in colour. The enzyme responsible for the green colour is probably myeloperoxidase, a constituent of normal granulocytes as well as leukaemic cells. As the leukaemia progresses severe sepsis often develops, sometimes in the form of necrotic ulceration of skin or mucous membrane. A somewhat characteristic terminal event, often associated with extreme neutropenia, is a distressingly painful gangrenous ulceration of the lower rectum, perianal region, vulva and perineum. Alternatively severe haemorrhage into the brain, from the bowel, stomach or kidneys may lead rapidly to death.

When leukaemia is congenital or occurs in early infancy it is myeloblastic or myelocytic. The outstanding features are pallor, spontaneous haemorrhages, gross hepatosplenomegaly and often jaundice. The disease runs a rapid course in young infants.

Blood Picture

In addition to severe anaemia the peripheral blood films will show immature cells. These are most often lymphoblasts, less commonly myeloblasts and other granulocytic precursors, and sometimes precise nomenclature is impossible so undifferentiated are the cells. The total white cell count is often raised to between 20,000–30,000 per c.mm.; only rarely to a very high figure. More commonly the white cell count is within normal limits or abnormally low—*aleukaemic leukaemia*. Thrombocytopenia is almost invariably found. Reticulocytes are usually scanty. It is, however, rarely justifiable to base the diagnosis of leukaemia on the peripheral blood picture alone. Bone marrow biopsy will nearly always confirm the diagnosis beyond doubt, the films and sections showing gross leukaemic infiltration by immature or abnormal white cell precursors, diminution in erythropoietic activity and disappearance of megakaryocytes. Rarely, the differential diagnosis from aplastic anaemia cannot be made for some time.

Differential Diagnosis

The bone pains in leukaemia have on occasions led to diagnoses such as rheumatic fever, rheumatoid arthritis, poliomyelitis, undulant fever, and osteitis. A careful assessment of the history and clinical findings alone should serve to prevent these rather ridiculous errors. Infectious mononucleosis never produces the marked anaemia and thrombocytopenia of leukaemia, and the Paul-Bunnell reaction is never positive in leukaemia. Generalized lymphadenoma is not associated with the gross blood abnormalities of leukaemia. The distinction from lymphosarcoma also depends on the absence of a leukaemic blood picture but is, in fact, somewhat artificial as in lymphosarcoma frank leukaemia sometimes develops.

Prognosis

All forms of leukaemia are invariably fatal, but it is important to recognize that spontaneous remissions, usually of short duration, can occur. In most untreated patients death occurs within a few weeks to months of diagnosis.

Treatment

Remissions can be obtained in about 80 per cent of cases of lymphoblastic leukaemia with several drugs. It is rare to precipitate a remission in the much less common myeloblastic type. As a quick remission is often essential the initial drug is most often prednisolone, or one of the other corticosteroids. This should be supported by blood transfusion and a broad spectrum antibiotic. A suitable schedule of dosage is 15 mg. four times daily for 10 days; 10 mg. four times daily for 10 days; 5 mg. four times daily for 10 days; and 5 mg. twice daily as a maintenance dose which may be continued for some weeks or months (Hutchison, 1962).

It is common practice to start at the same time with one of several cytotoxic drugs which are also capable of initiating remissions of the leukaemia. There is some evidence that longer remissions can be obtained by a form of cyclic therapy which uses several drugs each for relatively short periods, before relapse occurs and the leukaemic process becomes resistant to the drugs (Zuelzer, 1964). The cyclic regime which has found favour in the author's unit comprises:

6-mercaptopurine, 2·5 mg./Kg./day for ten weeks,
followed by
methotrexate 0·125 mg./Kg./day for six weeks
followed by
cyclophosphamide 5 mg./Kg./day for six weeks.

This course is repeated for as long as the remission lasts. When the inevitable relapse ultimately occurs the cyclic therapy is discontinued and prednisolone is re-started in full doses as detailed above. At the same time the child is given vincristine sulphate intravenously in a weekly dose of 0·05 mg./Kg. until full remission is obtained. A return is then made to the maintenance cycle using the next drug in the sequence and omitting the drug to which resistance has developed. If vincristine fails to induce a remission intravenous methotrexate, 3 mg./Kg. every two weeks, may be substituted. Blood examinations should be performed at least twice weekly during the initial stages of treatment and in relapses. During cyclic maintenance therapy the blood should be checked every two weeks. Toxic effects of the drugs such as leucopenia, or oral ulceration and diarrhoea with methotrexate, may necessitate their temporary withdrawal. At times the need to distinguish between early relapse and drug toxicity may require marrow examination. It is now common to expect prolongation of life in lymphoblastic leukaemia for periods of up to two years, and occasionally much longer, but not, of course, complete recovery. These lengthy remissions are, nowadays, not infrequently complicated by intracranial or intraspinal involvements which present with meningismus, papilloedema, intense headaches, and focal neurological signs. It may be that small nests of leukaemic cells within the brain or spinal cord escape the cytotoxic effects of the drugs. Such neurological complications frequently occur when the leukaemia is in complete haematological remission, although malignant cells may be found in the cerebrospinal fluid. Dramatic but temporary relief can be obtained with small doses of radiation to the skull or with intrathecal methotrexate in 4 mg. doses given every few days for up to six doses.

Claims have been made that more satisfactory remissions can be obtained in the less common myelogenous leukaemia with methyl GAG (methylglyoxal-bisguanylhydrazone) in doses of 120 to 160 mg./square metre of body surface intravenously. The author has not had good results from this drug and severe toxic effects such as mucosal ulceration, diarrhoea or marrow hypoplasia are common.

Once a remission of the leukaemia has been obtained the child is happiest in his usual environment and going about his usual activities. The parents, who deserve the physician's deep understanding and support, should be dissuaded from trying to make the child's life artificially happy. Periods in hospital should be kept to a minimum.

LYMPHOSARCOMA

Lymphosarcoma in childhood is distinguished from lymphatic leuk-aemia principally by its tendency to localization, at least in the earlier stages, and by the usual absence of primitive cells from the peripheral blood and marrow. Reticulum cell sarcoma is much less common than lymphosarcoma and only distinguishable histologically.

Clinical Features

The mode of presentation depends upon the site of the tumour. There may be a mass of glands in the neck, or the tumour may arise in the nasopharynx with disturbances of speech, swallowing or breathing. When the tumour arises in the mediastinal lymph nodes, pressure symptoms such as suffusion and oedema of the face and arms, distended veins, respiratory difficulty and retrosternal pain can be most distressing. A fairly characteristic site is the ileum with abdominal pain and dis-tension, vomiting, and constipation or diarrhoea due to incomplete intestinal obstruction. A mobile soft mass may be palpable in the lower abdomen which also shows gaseous distension. In some cases intus-susception occurs with a resulting emergency situation. A plain radio-graph of the abdomen may reveal the distended loop of ileum proximal to the tumour, and this can be further defined with a barium suspension. We have seen a characteristic skin infiltration result in a discoloured and indurated zone over the chest or supraclavicular area. Infrequently a diffuse involvement of the bones results in generalized limb pains and a presenting anaemia when the diagnosis can be very difficult until radiographs reveal bone infiltration, or the bone marrow is sufficiently involved to show changes.

Prognosis

The disease is invariably fatal and it is rare for long remissions to be obtained from treatment.

Treatment

Great symptomatic relief and short remissions can be achieved by radiotherapy when the tumour is in the neck, nasopharynx or media-stinum. In other sites and when the disease is widespread, some relief and prolongation of life can be obtained from cytotoxic agents such as vincristine, cyclophosphamide, methotrexate or chlorambucil.

RETICULOSIS

This group includes malignant non-lipoid reticulosis (Letterer-Siwe disease), xanthomatosis (Hand-Schüller-Christian disease) and eosino-philic granuloma of bone. These diseases are now regarded by many pathologists as variants of the same basic granulomatous process in the reticulo-endothelial system, the differences between them being a function of age. Thus, in Letterer-Siwe disease of infants lipoid deposition within the reticulo-endothelial cells can occur when the disease process runs a long enough course, whereas in the Hand-Schüller-Christian syndrome of childhood the deposition of cholesterol is a constant feature and gives the cells their typical "foamy" appearance in histological preparations. In both these conditions the reticulo-endothelial hyperplasia is widespread and may involve almost every organ and tissue in the body. Eosinophilic granuloma of bone, on the other hand, tends to occur as a single lesion in older children or young adults. The lesion contains fibroblasts, giant cells and many eosinophils, but lipoid accumulation may also occur. Furthermore, biopsy specimens from early cases of xanthomatosis have been known to show identical appearances. The deposition of lipoid in this group is thought to be a secondary phenomenon, quite unlike the primary lipoid storage diseases such as Gaucher's disease, Niemann-Pick's disease and Tay-Sachs amaurotic family idiocy (Chapter XII). In both Letterer-Siwe disease and xanthomatosis a characteristic type of cavitation may develop in multiple lesions throughout the lungs, which can lead to a "honeycomb" appearance on radiographs of considerable diagnostic value (MacDonald and Shanks, 1954).

Another disease which can be regarded as a reticulosis is lymphadenoma. While this is much less common in childhood than in adults it occurs sufficiently frequently to be a practical problem in diagnosis to the paediatrician, and so merits a brief description in this chapter. Lymphadenoma (Hodgkin's disease) is a progressive disease of lymph nodes and lymphoid tissue throughout the body. The lymph node architecture is destroyed and replaced by large cells of the reticulo-endothelial system. Some of these cells become giant cells with one large or several smaller nuclei—Dorothy Reed or Sternberg cells. There are also many eosinophils and, in addition, lymphocytes which have survived from the original healthy lymph node. The disease runs a much more rapid and "visceral" course in children than in adults.

LETTERER-SIWE DISEASE

Clinical Features

This is a rapidly progressive disease of infancy and it may even be congenital (Hamilton, 1961). Fever, abdominal enlargement due to marked hepatosplenomegaly, and generalized lymphadenopathy are common features. In many cases there is a striking generalized purpuric rash (Fig. 33). In others there is a pseudo-seborrhoeic rash on the scalp forehead and neck. Anaemia, leucopenia and thrombocytopenia commonly develop. The chest X-rays may show the progressive development of honeycomb appearances and infiltrative lesions may appear throughout the bones of the skeleton. The diagnosis can be confirmed by biopsy of marrow, a skin lesion or an enlarged lymph node.

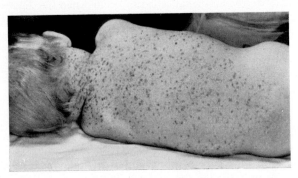

Fig. 33.—Purpuric rash in Letterer-Siwe disease. Note also cervical lymph node enlargement below ears.

Treatment

Remissions can sometimes be obtained with corticosteroids given in full doses. Complete recovery can occur but most cases prove rapidly fatal.

XANTHOMATOSIS YOUNG CHILDREN·

Clinical Features

The textbook picture of Hand-Schüller-Christian disease, which develops during the first six years of life, consists of the triad—diabetes insipidus, large defects in the membranous bones of the skull as visualized on radiographs, and exophthalmos. In practice this is a rare event. More often the picture is one of anaemia, hepatosplenomegaly, honeycomb lungs, numerous bone deposits which may cause spinal or limb pains, and involvement of the gums which become swollen and necrotic with resultant loosening of teeth. Various rashes may develop such as maculopapules, reddish-yellow lumps or yellow crusts on the scalp (xanthoma disseminatum). Otorrhoea due to mastoid involvement in the malignant process is common. The defects in the skull may become palpable as soft swellings. Hydrocephalus and papilloedema can develop. The blood cholesterol level is not abnormal.

Treatment

The prognosis is poor and treatment palliative. Radiotherapy may relieve pain or other distressing symptoms. Corticosteroids may precipitate partial remission. The diabetes insipidus can be controlled by daily intramuscular injections of 0·5 ml. pitressin tannate in oil, or by pituitary snuff 1 grain (60 mg.) per dose.

EOSINOPHILIC GRANULOMA OF BONE OLDER

Clinical Features

The patient is usually an older child or young adult with a solitary lesion. This most often presents as a painful swelling in the region of the skull, pelvis or on a limb. The author has seen a case present as an extradural tumour arising from the lower cervical vertebrae, with root pains and atrophic weakness of the muscles of the shoulder girdle and arm. The X-ray changes tend to be cystic in appearance, and when the skull is involved a map-like defect resembling that in Hand-Schüller-Christian disease is seen. The diagnosis is confirmed by a biopsy of the lesion.

Treatment

Complete local excision or deep X-ray therapy, according to the site of the lesion, yields excellent results. The long-term prognosis is good, although occasionally similar lesions appear elsewhere or the disease assumes a generalized form.

LYMPHADENOMA (HODGKIN'S DISEASE)

Clinical Features

The most common presentation is a painless mass of discrete, firm lymph nodes on one or both sides of the neck. Less frequently the mediastinal lymph nodes or abdominal viscera become first involved. In these cases there may be respiratory symptoms due to tracheal or bronchial compression, or oedema and congestion of the face due to pressure on the superior mediastinal great veins, or dysphagia. In other cases hepatosplenomegaly, jaundice and ascites appear. Lesions in the region of the spinal roots may result in pain or a lesion resembling herpes zoster. As the disease progresses increasing anaemia, leucopenia and thrombocytopenia may occur. At this stage the child is usually fevered, cachectic and very ill. Eosinophilia in the peripheral blood is rare. The textbook type of remitting Pel-Ebstein fever probably never occurs in childhood. Diagnosis is confirmed by lymph node biopsy.

Treatment

When only superficial lymph nodes are involved excellent remissions may be obtained by radiotherapy. When there is marked visceral involvement or when the condition ultimately becomes tolerant of X-rays, one of the nitrogen mustards is to be used, e.g. mustine, trillekamin, cyclophosphamide, TEM or thio-TEPA. Blood transfusion may be necessary for the correction of progressive anaemia. The disease is ultimately fatal.

NEPHROBLASTOMA
(EMBRYOMA OF KIDNEY: WILMS' TUMOUR)

This is the common neoplasm of kidney in childhood. It may be congenital but more often arises during the first four years. Hypernephroma which is common in adults does not occur in childhood. Nephroblastoma should be the most susceptible of cure of all childhood malignancies if only the diagnosis was made early enough.

Pathology

The tumour is often huge, but it remains encapsulated until a late stage when it ruptures into the renal pelvis, ureter, perirenal tissues or renal veins. Histologically a wide variation in pattern occurs. In some areas the tumour is composed of sheets of undifferentiated mesenchymal cells. In others, structures resembling renal tubules are present, and even glomerular-like structures may be found. Other features may be skeletal and smooth muscle fibres, squamous cells, even cartilage. Calcification is uncommon.

Clinical Features

The most usual mode of presentation is a large mass in the loin, which is first noted by the mother while bathing or dressing the child. The usual absence of pain or haematuria, unfortunately, allows the tumour to reach a massive size before detection. The mass feels smooth but hard and it is immobile on respiration. It extends well back into the renal angle and it never crosses the mid-line of the abdomen, although it may be of enormous size. The child's nutritional state remains remarkably good until the later stages when blood-borne metastases occur. These are especially frequent in the lungs and appear on radiographs as large, rounded "cannon-ball" opacities. By now the child is losing weight, is irritable and fevered, and has a raised E.S.R. *Palpation and handling of the tumour accelerate the spread into the blood-stream and should be kept to the absolute minimum required for diagnosis.* Intravenous pyelograms show distortion and often elongation of the pelvi-calyceal system.

Treatment

In recent years the results of treatment have been much more optimistic since the introduction of actinomycin D. Howard (1965) reported that the 2–5 year survival rate has increased from 11·5 per cent to 62 per cent on a therapeutic regime which consists of actinomycin D, nephrectomy and radiotherapy.

Actinomycin D is given intravenously in large doses—a total of 120 μg/Kg. body weight in eight equal injections on days 1, 2, 3, 4, 5, 7, 9 and 12. Nephrectomy is carried out on day 3. Deep X-ray therapy starts on day 26 and approximately 3,000 rads are given over a 28-day period. When pulmonary metastases are present segmental or lobar resection may also be worthwhile.

NEUROBLASTOMA (SYMPATHICOBLASTOMA)

This is one of the most common and highly malignant tumours of infancy and childhood. Congenital cases have been reported, and the main incidence is during the first five years. Neuroblastoma may arise wherever there is sympathetic nervous tissue, but the most common sites are the adrenal medulla, presacral area and the dorsal ganglia in the posterior mediastinum.

Pathology

The tumour is characterized by great vascularity and rapid growth. Blood vessel invasion is marked and explains the typical tendency to metastasise in bone. This is particularly frequent in the orbits and inner table of the skull, but the brain itself is rarely invaded. In young infants gross hepatic involvement is common, especially when the primary growth is in the right adrenal. The tumour cells occur in sheets, their nuclei tend to be spherical or polygonal, and mitoses are often numerous. In a minority of cases the cells grow in the form of rosettes, the centre of which is occupied by fine fibrils. These structures resemble the neuroblasts seen in the foetal adrenal during the formation of the medulla. In other cases even more embryonic cells are seen which do not form fibrils and these tumours are more accurately called *sympathicogoniomas*. In some neuroblastomas, especially of extra-adrenal origin, there is evidence in parts of differentiation into more mature tissue containing ganglion cells, but full maturation of a neuroblastoma into a benign ganglioneuroma probably does not occur. Multiple primary tumours have been reported in the same patient (Gross *et al.*, 1959).

Clinical Features

The child with a neuroblastoma is likely to be ill, miserable and fractious, anorexic, to lose weight and to be anaemic. The presenting sign may be proptosis (Fig. 34) due to an orbital metastasis, or this may only appear later in the illness (Fig. 35). When the inner table of the skull is involved there will be signs of increased intracranial pressure such as cerebral vomiting, a cracked-pot sound on percussion of the skull and papilloedema. In other cases, bone metastases cause a form of presentation with limb pains and pallor which simulates leukaemia until the peripheral blood is shown not to contain large numbers of immature white cells. Another mode of onset is with swelling of the abdomen due to an adrenal tumour, or to a mass growing upwards out of the pelvis which may have a dumb-bell shape. The neuroblastoma feels hard but

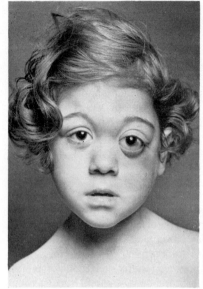

FIG. 34.—Proptosis with subconjunctival and periorbital haemorrhage as the presenting feature of adrenal neuroblastoma.

FIG. 35.—Gross proptosis and periorbital ecchymosis in late stage of illness from neuroblastoma.

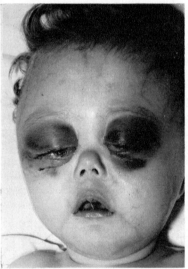

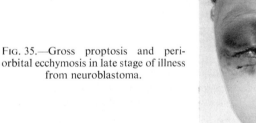

its irregular craggy surface contrasts with the usual smoothness of the renal tumour. Furthermore, it frequently extends across the mid-line, unlike the embryoma of kidney, and not infrequently calcification within the neuroblastoma can be visualized on radiographs. In young infants enormous hepatomegaly may be the principal finding, making differential diagnosis from a primary tumour of the liver difficult. Intravenous pyelograms may reveal the primary adrenal tumour by showing downward and lateral displacement of the kidney. The less common intrathoracic neuroblastoma appears on radiographs as a rounded shadow in the posterior mediastinum. It may invade the vertebral column and cause either local pain or pain referred down the nerve roots. Sometimes the diagnosis of neuroblastoma can be confirmed by demonstrating malignant cells in the bone marrow. Radiographs of the pelvis, skull and long bones may show areas of bone destruction and periosteal reaction. Final confirmation of the diagnosis is frequently made by biopsy of the tumour taken at laparotomy or thoracotomy.

Neuroblastoma is, of course, embryologically related to phaeochromocytoma and it is not surprising that it should produce pressor amines. Indeed, in some cases this is reflected clinically in the form of hypertension or excessive sweating. The demonstration of an excess of catecholamine metabolites in the urine is a useful method of differentiating neuroblastoma from nephroblastoma. In most cases of neuroblastoma there is a great excess of 3-methoxy-4-hydroxymandelic acid (HMMA or VMA). In a few cases the excretion of HMMA has not been greatly increased but in them another metabolite, 4-hydroxy-3-methoxy-phenylacetic acid (homovanillic acid or HVA), has been recovered from the urine in large quantities (McKendrick and Edwards, 1965). It is probable that neuroblastoma never exists with a normal excretion level of both HMMA and HVA. As metastases also produce catecholamines their serial determination in the urine can be used to measure the success of treatment.

Treatment

Spontaneous recovery from this highly malignant tumour is exceedingly rare, but its undoubted occurrence makes assessment of any form of treatment difficult. Complete surgical excision, the treatment of choice, is only rarely possible, but complete recovery has followed partial surgical removal with subsequent radiotherapy. These tumours are highly radio-sensitive and this form of therapy is worthwhile unless the skeleton is hopelessly riddled with metastases.

Bodian from Great Ormond Street reported several cures following massive daily doses (1,000–2,000 μg.) of intramuscular vitamin B_{12}, and the author has seen two recoveries associated with its use. However, the true value of vitamin B_{12} in neuroblastoma is very much open to doubt. There is more substantial evidence that radiotherapy in combination with both vincristine sulphate and cyclophosphamide results in a higher percentage of recoveries or prolonged remissions than any previous method of treatment, save complete surgical removal.

MALIGNANT TUMOURS OF THE BRAIN

Brain tumours are relatively common in young children. They are mostly situated below the tentorium in the posterior fossa of the skull. In contrast to adult experience supratentorial tumours are greatly in the minority. Unfortunately, both the cellular nature of these tumours and their situation make complete surgical extirpation only rarely possible and the prognosis is usually exceedingly gloomy.

Pathology

The most common tumour is the embryonic and highly malignant medulloblastoma. The astrocytoma is also fairly common, tends to become cystic, and shows variation in degrees of local malignancy. Both these tumours arise most often in the cerebellum or the brain stem. The ependymoma is also most often infratentorial and obviously inaccessible to the surgeon. Less common and not truly malignant tumours are hamartomas, haemangiomas, craniopharyngiomas and dermoids.

Clinical Features

Most infratentorial tumours cause early signs of increased intracranial pressure. These differ somewhat from the signs usually found in the adult, due to the fact that the recently united cranial sutures of the young child give way rather readily under pressure. Thus cerebral vomiting and headache, both more common in the morning, are less common and less intense in children. Papilloedema also tends to develop somewhat later. On the other hand, a valuable early sign due to starting of the sutures is the cracked-pot sound elicited by percussion of the skull with the middle finger of the right hand while the head is held in the left hand. Radiographs frequently show separation of the sutures and convolutional markings on the vault, sometimes called "paw marks" or "beaten silver" appearance (Fig. 36). In children under the age of 2 years there may occasionally be obvious enlargement of the head. Mental changes are late in appearance as a rule. There is increasing lethargy and apathy later leading to terminal coma.

Local Neurological Signs

These may be slight or absent, especially when the tumour is in the mid-line. The most common are *cerebellar signs* such as ataxia, nystagmus, head wobble, incoordination, rebound phenomenon, intention tremor, hypotonia and diminished deep reflexes. If the pyramidal tracts are also involved by extension of the tumour to the brain stem the plantar responses become extensor. External ophthalmoplegia may be due to increased intracranial pressure or to involvement of the cranial nuclei in the mid-brain or pons. When the tumour arises in the *brain stem* itself, increase in intracranial pressure may not develop. The child presents with various cranial nerve palsies and signs of involvement of the pyramidal tracts, e.g. exaggerated deep reflexes, ankle clonus, extensor plantar responses and possibly some spasticity of the limbs. Craniopharyngioma is situated in the *suprasellar region*. Signs of increased intracranial pressure are early. There may be optic field defects such as bitemporal heteronymous hemianopia due to pressure on the optic chiasma. Pressure on the pituitary gland may result in diabetes insipidus or dwarfism. The rare *pinealoma* causes downwards pressure on the mesencephalon. In addition to an early rise in intracranial pressure, this may result in dilatation of the pupils and a deficiency of upward

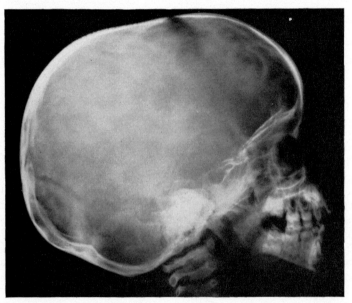

FIG. 36.—Radiograph of skull showing starting of sutures and convolutional markings due to increased intracranial pressure from cerebellar tumour.

gaze. Pressure on the nearby *hypothalamus* is one cause of premature puberty in males. This may also be caused by a primary neoplasm of the hypothalamus itself. Other manifestations of hypothalmic involvement are a disturbed sleep rhythm, irregular temperature control, hypertension, excessive appetite or profound anorexia.

Diagnosis

The special tests required are best performed by a neurosurgeon, who can immediately proceed to a craniotomy if untoward reactions occur. These tests include air ventriculography and encephalography, carotid or vertebral cerebral angiography, and in some supratentorial cases electroencephalography.

Treatment

Surgical removal of the tumour is only occasionally possible, e.g. in the case of cerebellar astrocytoma, but part of the tumour can usually be removed for histological examination. The craniotomy should be followed by intensive radiotherapy, which often results in excellent but temporary remissions. These usually last a few months, exceptionally for a year or two. Obstructive hydrocephalus can be relieved by a ventriculo-peritoneal drainage or other by-pass procedure.

RETINOBLASTOMA

This primitive tumour, formerly called "glioma of the retina", is confined to infants and young children. It is peculiar in showing a strong genetic influence and in some cases inheritance has been dominant in nature. Not uncommonly more than one sibling is affected. The condition is highly malignant and if left untreated causes death from spread along the optic nerve into the brain or from blood-borne metastases.

Clinical Features

The condition first appears in one eye, but in about one-third of cases both eyes are affected. In the earliest stage a small rounded pigment-free yellowish-white nodule appears on the retina. It is surrounded by smaller nodules. The tumour grows forward into the vitreous. In some cases the lens is pushed forwards and secondary glaucoma develops with a hard, painful and congested eyeball. After some months the tumour can be seen with the naked eye as a yellowish reflex behind the pupil. In fact, the parents may remark upon this "cat's eye" reflex in the dark. Ultimately there is proptosis and a fungating mass which bleeds readily protrudes between the eyelids.

Treatment

The best form of treatment is enucleation of the eyeball and removal of the optic nerve as far back in the orbit as possible. If the other eye becomes involved and the parents refuse permission for its removal some form of radiotherapy may be given, although this carries the risk of severe local damage. Local recurrences are not uncommon.

TUMOURS OF THE LIVER

Apart from secondary tumours of the liver such as neuroblastoma, certain primary tumours occur infrequently in Britain. They mostly present in infancy or childhood. *Carcinoma* (*hepatoma*) consists of neoplastic tissue in which there are closely packed hepatic cells showing varying degrees of differentiation. The *mixed hepatic tumour* shows sarcomatous change combined with hepatocellular, squamous or cholangiocellular carcinoma and osteoid or cartilage may also be present. In young infants *haemangioendothelioma* may act in a malignant manner with wild proliferation throughout the liver of new blood vessels. In *hamartoma* all the tissues normally found in the liver appear in a disorderly manner. The *mesenchymoma* is a highly malignant tumour composed of such mixed elements as angioma, fibroma and primitive mesenchymal tissues.

Clinical Features

The constant finding is progressive and massive hepatomegaly. Jaundice and ascites are less common. The hepatoma frequently metastasises to the lungs. Calcification may be radiologically demonstrable in the primary tumour but the diagnosis can only be confirmed by laparotomy and biopsy. A needle biopsy may lead to severe haemorrhage and should not be performed in cases of doubt.

Treatment

Complete surgical excision is only rarely possible. Radiotherapy can only be of temporary benefit. The prognosis is rarely optimistic.

SARCOMA BOTRYOIDES

This rare tumour is a highly malignant embryonic rhabdomyosarcoma which arises in the vagina or cervix. It causes urinary frequency, a foul-smelling bloody vaginal discharge and, ultimately, grape-like masses are to be found protruding into the vagina. Radical excision followed by radiotherapy is the only available treatment, but metastases in the lungs, lymph nodes and other tissues usually cause death.

CHORDOMA

This tumour arises from the primitive notochord. It is most common in the sacrococcygeal region where it invades bone and rectum. In addition to an obvious mass there is pain, paralysis of limbs and incontinence of faeces. When it arises in the cervical region it invades the base of the skull and may protrude into the nasopharynx. Radiographs will reveal gross bone destruction. The chordoma only rarely metastasises, but its local invasiveness usually makes surgical removal impossible.

REFERENCES

BOGGS, D. R., WINTROBE, M. M., and CARTWRIGHT, G. E. (1962). *Medicine (Baltimore)*, **41**, 163.

BURKITT, D. P. (1962). *Postgrad. med. J.*, **38**, 71.

CAMPBELL, A. C. P., GAISFORD, W., PATERSON, E., and STEWARD, J. K. (1961). *Brit. med. J.*, **1**, 448.

COURT BROWN, W. M. (1962). *Symposium: Genetics in Medicine*. Publications Dept., Royal College of Physicians of Edinburgh.

FALLON, R. J., GRIST, N. R., INMAN, D. R., LEMCKE, R. M., NEGRONI, G., and WOODS, D. A. (1965). *Brit. med. J.*, **2**, 388.

GROSS, R. E., FARBER, S., and MARTIN, L. W. (1959). *Pediatrics*, **23**, 1179.

HAMILTON, W. (1961). *Scot. med. J.*, **6**, 575.
HOWARD, R. (1965). *Arch. Dis. Childh.*, **40**, 200.
HUTCHISON, J. H. (1962). *Practitioner*, **189**, 436.
MacDONALD, A. M., and SHANKS, R. A. (1954). *Arch. Dis. Childh.*, **29**, 127.
MacGREGOR, A. R. (1961). *Scot. med. J.*, **6**, 34.
McKENDRICK, T., and EDWARDS, R. W. H. (1965). *Arch. Dis. Childh.*, **40**, 418
STANLEY, N. F. (1966). *Lancet*, **1**, 961.
STEWART, A. (1961). *Brit. med. J.*, **1**, 452.
STEWART, A., WEBB, J., and HEWITT, D. (1958). *Brit. med. J.*, **1**, 1495.
TOUGH, I. M., COURT BROWN, W. M., BAIKIE, A. G., BUCKTON, K. E., HARNDEN, D. G., JACOBS, P. A., KING, M., and McBRIDE, J. A. (1961). *Lancet*, **1**, 411.
TOUGH, I. M., COURT BROWN, W. M., BAIKIE, A. G., BUCKTON, K. E., HARNDEN, D. G., JACOBS, P. A., and WILLIAMS, J. A. (1962). *Lancet*, **2**, 115.
ZUELZER, W. W. (1964). *Blood*, **24**, 477.

CHAPTER XII

DISORDERS OF STORAGE

In this chapter various unrelated diseases are grouped together merely as a matter of convenience. The only common factor is a disturbance in one or more of the many storage mechanisms of the body. Thus, in obesity there is an excessive deposition of fat in the normal sites; whereas in the lipoidoses there is an abnormal intracellular accumulation of sphingolipids, and in gargoylism of mucopolysaccharides.

OBESITY

Aetiology

There is a large and often conflicting literature on the subject of obesity in children, especially in relation to its causation (Mayer, 1953; Steiner, 1955; Quaade, 1955; Bruch, 1957; Lloyd *et al.*, 1961). There is evidence of multifactorial inheritance in some cases (Börjeson, 1962), and fatness seems frequently to run in families. Some children eat excessive quantities of food, especially carbohydrates, but others actually eat less than the average child of the same age. However, as obesity must obviously result from an imbalance between appetite and physical activity, the small eaters must have a lower than average level of daily physical activity (Mayer *et al.*, 1956). In the common, simple, or exogenous type of obesity hormonal disturbances cannot be incriminated. There is some evidence, however, that in a few cases hypothalamic damage exists; this may explain the gross obesity seen in some retarded children who have suffered brain damage at birth. Bruch (1957) has stressed the part played by psychological factors in many obese children. Some react with over-eating and diminished physical activity when anxious or depressed. Others are obese because they are plied with food by their over-protective mothers, and Bruch has suggested that this maternal attitude is really a reaction arising from an incapacity to love and a deep-seated emotional rejection of the child. Other stressful environmental factors may be surgical operations, illness, and school difficulties. It is only right to point out, however, that some physicians find these explanations unconvincing.

Clinical Features

A precise definition of obesity is difficult, but in practice there is rarely any doubt as to its existence in the individual patient (Fig. 37). The excess fat is deposited in the region of the breasts, abdominal wall, hips, buttocks, thighs, and face. It is often stated that fat boys have a feminine type of body shape but this is only because in obesity, fat is distributed in the normal sites and in normal females these areas contain more fat than in normal males. It is uncommon for striae to appear on the skin in simple obesity although they may do so in gross cases. Obese children are nearly always taller than average, and some have suggested that this is due to an overproduction of pituitary growth hormone. In boys the genitalia are normal although they may look hypoplastic merely because they tend to get buried in the excess pubic fat. It is this misleading appearance which has often led to the erroneous diagnosis of Fröhlich's syndrome. In fact, this is an extremely rare condition and the author has not seen a case in 30 years of paediatric practice. Fat children are physically less active and agile than normal children. This disability, combined with the somewhat derisive nick-names like "Tubby", "Fatty", and "Lumpy", often results in a certain amount of unhappiness which, how-ever, need not be exaggerated.

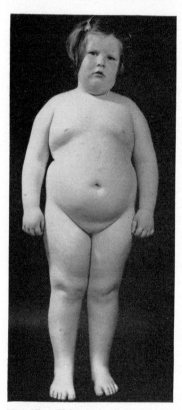

Fig. 37.—Girl aged 4 years with exogenous obesity who is also above average height for her age.

Treatment

The only way in which a fat child can safely be made to lose weight is by limitation of his food intake. A 1,200 calorie diet if strictly enforced will prove an effective, although often remarkably slow, method of treat-ment. The real difficulty is to ensure strict adherence to the diet, because so often the mother remains over-indulgent in spite of the physician's advice. Indeed, in severe cases of obesity it is necessary to admit the child to hospital for a period during which he can become accustomed and trained to his diet. Drugs are best avoided altogether in children. In less severe cases the child can at least be prevented from becoming more obese by a qualitative dietary limitation of carbohydrates such as bread, cakes, potatoes, steamed puddings and sweets. The problem, once more, is to obtain the mother's co-operation without which the physician's time is being wasted. It is this type of problem which has lead some paediatricians to doubt the value of any attempt at the treatment of obesity in young children. In older children who are themselves anxious to lose weight the outlook is much more optimistic.

LIPODYSTROPHIA PROGRESSIVA

This is a remarkable but rare condition in which, about the age of 6–8 years, there appears progressive loss of the subcutaneous fat from the face and neck. This process spreads downwards to involve the chest and trunk as far as the waist or the hips. The face ultimately has a gaunt and lined appearance, and the shoulder girdles and arms develop an emaciated look. The body contour and fat distribution is normal from the hips downwards, and the skin and muscles are unaffected. The disease is more common in girls, but its cause is quite unknown. Life expectancy is not shortened. There is no effective treatment.

THE LIPOIDOSES

This group includes Gaucher's disease, Niemann-Pick's disease and Tay-Sachs' disease. Gargoylism (lipochondrodystrophy) should probably not be included, as the principal substance stored in the cells in this disease is now demonstrated to be of a polysaccharide nature. In the lipoidoses there is an abnormal intracellular deposition of lipoid, often widely spread throughout many organs and tissues. In Gaucher's disease the lipoid is composed of cerebrosides, and in Niemann-Pick disease of sphingomyelin. In Tay-Sachs disease the ganglion cells of the brain are overloaded with gangliosides. Some workers consider that Tay-Sachs disease is closely related to Niemann-Pick disease, and it has been further considered that, in the brain, gangliosides might be the precursors of sphingomyelin. However, at the present time the chemical pathways of lipid metabolism are little understood and the pathogenesis of these diseases is obscure. They are all of rare occurrence, but they come into the differential diagnosis in paediatric practice sufficiently frequently to justify clinical description in a book devoted to the daily problems of the paediatrician.

GAUCHER'S DISEASE

Clinical Features

This disease appears to occur in two forms, *chronic* or *acute*. Both are inherited as autosomal recessive traits but the condition runs true to form in any single family. It is most often encountered in Jewish families.

The chronic form is the most common. It presents with gross splenomegaly. Hepatic enlargement may also be marked. There is also a progressive anaemia, and leucopenia and thrombocytopenia due to hypersplenism develop early in its course. Bone involvement may give rise to limb pains. Radiographs reveal a characteristic flaring outwards of the metaphyseal ends of the long bones with thinning of the cortex. This is most marked at the lower ends of the femora which have an Erlenmeyer flask appearance. These features develop in childhood or early adult life. In older patients especially the face, neck, hands and legs may show a characteristic brownish pigmentation, and the conjunctiva may show a wedge-shaped area of thickening with its base to the cornea (pinguecula). The serum cholestrol level is normal. The diagnosis can be confirmed by finding the typical lipid-filled cells which have a typical fibrillary appearance of the cytoplasm. These should be sought in material obtained by needle puncture of the bone marrow, spleen or lymph nodes. The disease runs a slow course but death is inevitable.

The acute form is a rare phenomenon confined to infancy. In addition to hepatosplenomegaly there is evidence of severe cerebral involvement which is rarely seen in the chronic form. There may be hypertonia, catatonia, trismus, opisthotonus, dysphagia, strabismus and respiratory difficulties. Death occurs by the age of 3 years.

Treatment

There is no curative treatment, but splenectomy is sometimes necessary to relieve hypersplenism.

NIEMANN-PICK DISEASE

Clinical Features

This disease is also more common in infants of the Jewish race and it too is inherited in autosomal recessive fashion. The infant's abdomen becomes greatly protuberant due to massive hepatosplenomegaly. Skin pigmentation is common and severe wasting is invariable. Deterioration in cerebral functions appears early and progresses to a state of idiocy, generalized muscular weakness and wasting. Anaemia of severe degree is an early sign but thrombocytopenia develops late, in contrast to its early appearance in Gaucher's disease. In some affected infants ophthalmoscopy reveals a cherry-red spot at the macula resembling the retinal appearances in Tay-Sachs disease. The mononuclear cells of the peripheral blood may have a vacuolated cytoplasm due to the deposition of lipid. The characteristic Niemann-Pick cell has a "foamy" appearance, with a waxy highly refractile cytoplasm due to lipid droplets. It can best be found by marrow or splenic puncture.

Treatment

None is available and death occurs in the first two years of life.

TAY-SACHS DISEASE

Clinical Features

This is the most common (infantile) form of amaurotic family idiocy. It is usually encountered in Jewish infants and appears to be transmitted in a recessive manner. Consanguinity is fairly commonly found. In this disease the deposition of lipoid is confined to the central nervous system and the symptoms are, consequently, neurological in character. They appear between the ages of 4–6 months as delay in psychomotor development, irritability, hyperacusis for sudden noises, spasticity, generalized weakness and muscle wasting. An outstanding feature is progressive loss of vision leading to complete blindness. The deep reflexes are exaggerated, at least to begin with, and the plantar responses are extensor. Ophthalmoscopy reveals primary optic atrophy and the diagnostic macular cherry-red spot on each side, surrounded by a greyish-white halo appearance. Convulsions may occur. Ultimately there are dysphagia, dementia, blindness, and a tendency to repeated respiratory infections due to the accumulation of mucus. The serum aldolase and glutamic-oxalacetic transaminase levels may be elevated. Death occurs before the age of 3 years.

There are several other forms of amaurotic family idiocy with a later onset than Tay-Sachs disease and it is likely that they are separate entities. In the late infantile form of Bielschowsky-Jansky the onset is about the age of 3–4 years. It is characterized by signs of cerebellar involvement but there is no cherry-red spot on the macula, only optic atrophy and increased retinal pigmentation. The juvenile form of Spielmeyer-Vogt begins at 5–10 years with loss of vision due to optic atrophy and with a reddish-black spot on the macula. Other signs include muscle rigidity, athetosis, tremor and convulsive attacks. The late juvenile form of Kufs usually starts after puberty. Retinal changes are usually absent but in addition to mental deterioration, convulsions, tremors, muscular rigidity and ataxia are seen. These types are not predominantly found in the Jewish race.

Treatment

None is available.

GARGOYLISM (HURLER'S SYNDROME)

The name "gargoylism" was suggested by Ellis *et al.* (1936) because of the peculiarly grotesque appearance of the affected children. The name is unfortunate in that it refers to an architectural feature in which man, beast or myth may be represented having only one feature in common—a large throat (gargouille) to shoot roof water clear of the walls—and that not a feature of this clinical syndrome.

Aetiology

In most cases gargoylism is inherited as an autosomal recessive characteristic. In fact, the disease may be reasonably regarded as an inborn error of metabolism, in which there is an abnormal intracellular deposition of certain acid mucopolysaccharides. Less commonly this metabolic error is inherited as a sex-linked recessive characteristic when all the affected children will, of course, be males. In this type of gargoylism corneal opacity rarely develops, but the children so affected are often deaf.

Pathology

At one time the material stored in many tissues was thought to be a lipid, hence the name "lipochondrodystrophy", but this was shown not to be the case by Henderson *et al.* (1952). The deposited substance is complex in nature but largely composed of polysaccharides. It appears as cytoplasmic vacuoles in the cells of many tissues, including the brain, liver, spleen and heart. The different genetic forms of gargoylism excrete different patterns of mucopolysaccharide in the urine, but the precise extent of this disease is not yet clearly defined (Terry and Linker, 1964). In the common autosomal recessive form of the disease the major component is chondroitin sulphate B, whereas in the rarer sex-linked recessive form heparitin sulphate and chondroitin sulphate B are present in the urine in roughly equal proportions. An even more rare atypical form excretes only heparitin sulphate in excess. The basic metabolic defect is still obscure and must await further elucidation of the complex biosynthesis and degradation of the mucopolysaccharides.

Clinical Features

The superficial appearances in a typical case of gargoylism allow of immediate diagnosis (Fig. 38). The head is large and scaphocephalic. The eyes are set wide apart and there are heavy supraorbital ridges and eyebrows. The nose is broad with a flattened bridge, and the lips are thick. The skin is dry and coarse. The corneae usually show a marked spotty type of opacity or cloudiness. The neck is short, there is a lumbo-dorsal kyphosis, and the protuberant abdomen often has an umbilical hernia. The spleen and liver are considerably enlarged. The hands tend to be broader than they are long. There is characteristic limitation of extension (but not of flexion) in many joints, most marked in the fingers. The fourth and fifth fingers may be short and curved towards the thumb. Genu valgum and coxa valga are common. There are also very characteristic radiological changes in the bones. The skull shows an elongated sella turcica, widened suture lines and an unduly large fontanelle. The long bones and phalanges are broader and shorter than normal and they are often bizarre in shape. The ribs too are excessively thick. The pelvis is distorted with abnormal acetabula. The vertebral bodies have an abnormal shape with concave anterior and posterior margins, and there is often a hook-like projection from the anterior

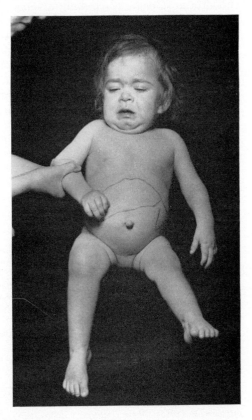

FIG. 38.—Typical case of gargoylism. Note grotesque features, large head, short neck, incomplete extension of fingers, and enlargement of spleen and liver.

border of the first or second lumbar vertebra which tends to be displaced backwards. Bone-age is usually retarded. Affected children are nearly always severely mentally retarded. They show diminished physical activity. This is partly due to excessive breathlessness on exertion when the heart is involved. Cardiomegaly, a precordial systolic murmur, and electrocardiographic evidence of left ventricular hypertrophy are commonly found. Death takes place before adult life, from congestive cardiac failure or intercurrent respiratory infection.

While the child with gargoylism somewhat resembles a cretin, there are very obvious clinical differences, e.g. corneal opacity, hepatosplenomegaly, limitation of extension of the interphalangeal joints, and characteristic radiological findings in the skeleton. There is also available a simple chemical test for the common autosomal recessive form of gargoylism based upon the fact that the urine of affected children contains a marked excess of chondroitin sulphate. In this test, described by Berry and Spinanger (1960), use is made of the fact that when chondroitin sulphate reacts with toluidine blue a metachromatic effect is observed which results in the development of a purple spot against a pale blue background. The diagnosis may also be confirmed by the demonstration of intracellular metachromatic lymphocyte inclusions (Muir *et al.*, 1963). In the rarer forms of Hurler's syndrome some complex laboratory tests have been used but these are beyond the scope of most hospital laboratories. Manley and Hawksworth (1966) have described a simple turbidity test which affords a means of screening the urine for excessive mucopolysaccharide content. They have also developed a technique whereby the urinary mucopolysaccharide pattern can be determined on Alcian Blue-stained cellulose acetate electrophoretic strips, thus permitting definition of the genetic pattern in individual cases.

Treatment

None is of any value.

REFERENCES

BERRY, H. K., and SPINANGER, J. (1960). *J. Lab. clin. Med.*, **55**, 136.
BÖRJESON, M. (1962). *Acta paediat.* (*Uppsala*), **51**, Suppl. 132.
BRUCH, H. (1957), *The Importance of Overweight.* New York: Norton & Co.
ELLIS, R. W. B., SHELDON, W., and CAPON, N. B. (1936). *Quart. J. Med.*, **5**, 119.
HENDERSON, J. L., MACGREGOR, A. R., THANNHAUSER, S. J., and HOLDEN, R. (1952). *Arch. Dis. Childh.*, **27**, 230.
LLOYD, J. K., WOLFF, O. H., and WHELEN, W. S. (1961). *Brit. med. J.*, **2**, 145.
MANLEY, G., and HAWKSWORTH, J. (1966). *Arch. Dis. Childh.*, **41**, 91.
MAYER, J. (1953). *Physol. Rev.*, **33**, 472.
MAYER, J., ROY, P., and MITRA, K. P. (1956). *Amer. J. clin. Nutr.*, **4**, 169.
MUIR, H., MITTWOCH, U., and BITTER, T. (1963). *Arch. Dis. Childh.*, **38**, 358.
QUAADE, F. (1955). *Obese Children.* Copenhagen: Dansk Videnskabs Forlag.
STEINER, M. M. (1955). *Pediat. Clin. N. Amer.*, **2**, 553.
TERRY, K., and LINKER, A. (1964). *Proc. Soc. exp. Biol.* (*N.Y.*), **115**, 394.

CHAPTER XIII

RESPIRATORY DISEASES

The rapid fall of mortality rates during infancy and early childhood in the past twenty-five years is largely attributable to the defeat of severe bacterial infections of the respiratory tract. The skill of the surgeon and the anaesthetist also has permitted us to approach the treatment of some intrathoracic abnormalities with greater confidence. On the other hand, our success in combating pneumococcal infections of the lungs seems to have resulted in an unexpected and disturbing capacity of staphylococci and Gram-negative bacilli to invade what must once have been unfamiliar territory. The clinician has still to learn the lesson that the indiscriminate use of anti-bacterial drugs carries danger for his patients. This problem is complicated by the fact that it is usually impossible to determine the microbial cause of respiratory infection at an early stage of the illness in the case of young children.

CONGENITAL ABNORMALITIES

The respiratory tract is infrequently the site of anatomical malformations in contrast to the nervous, cardiovascular and urinary systems (Norman, 1963).

Choanal atresia may be complete or partial, bilateral or unilateral (Diamant and Kinnman, 1963). Bilateral choanal atresia results in severe dyspnoea during feeds, dangerous attacks of apnoea, and thick gelatinous mucus in the nasal cavities. In partial cases the symptoms are similar but less severe. When the condition is unilateral the risk to life is much less. The most important feature is constant unilateral nasal obstruction and thick secretion which may cause excoriation of the skin of the nostril. Diagnosis can be confirmed by finding that a soft rubber catheter is arrested at the level of the choana about 30 mm. from the nostril. Furthermore, a dye such as gentian violet or methylene blue when instilled into the nostril will fail to appear on the posterior pharyngeal wall. Radiographs should also be taken after the nasal cavities have been cleared of secretion and replaced with contrast medium. Treatment is surgical. This may have to be performed during the neonatal period but it is frequently possible, even in bilateral cases, to avoid operation until an older age by tube-feeding for some weeks when the infant learns how to breathe through the mouth and take from a spoon.

Congenital laryngeal stridor is common and produces symptoms soon after birth in the form of inspiratory crowing with suprasternal indrawing. The respiratory difficulty is rarely severe enough to interfere with the infant's general well-being or nutrition. The common cause is an unusually long and curved epiglottis, which can be seen on direct laryngoscopy to become drawn down against the arytenoids during inspiration. Spontaneous recovery takes place within the first year. It has been usual to offer a good prognosis in this type of laryngeal stridor because it shows progressive improvement. However, Benians *et al.*, (1964) found that eight out of twenty-one cases were later associated with neurological abnormalities such as cerebral palsy, mental deficiency and convulsions. It would seem to be wise, therefore, to observe such infants' future development carefully. It is also important to exclude other causes of laryngeal stridor in the newborn such as goitre (Chapter XVIII), vascular rings (Chapter XV), chondromalacia of the larynx or trachea, intralaryngeal or tracheal webs and cysts, and subglottic haemangioma. An enlarged thymus was previously considered to be a cause of stridor—"thymic asthma"—but this is no longer accepted by those who appreciate how variable is the size of this structure in infants.

Agenesis of the lungs is rare. Complete absence of pulmonary tissue may be found in anencephalic monsters. When one lung or one lobe is absent the patient is usually symptomless, although the heart may be displaced into one hemithorax. In these cases there may or may not be a bronchial bud present. The diagnosis is frequently made during a routine medical examination and can be confirmed radiologically. Hypoplasia may also occur, sometimes in association with congenital heart disease or diaphragmatic hernia.

Sequestration of the lung may be intralobar, extralobar or complete, depending upon whether the segment of lung tissue which has no communication with the main bronchial tree is within a lobe of the lung, is outside the lung although still attached to it, or is completely separated from the lung (Potter, 1961). In the case of the extralobar and complete types the arterial blood supply is from the aorta and the venous return to the hemiazygous vein, whereas in the intralobar variety there may be a pulmonary artery with venous return by a pulmonary vein. The extralobar and complete sequestrations are most often on the left side, sometimes in association with a diaphragmatic hernia. Radiographic interpretation may be difficult without bronchography to demonstrate the absence of communication with the bronchial tree. Symptoms occur only if infection is superimposed. This is only common in the intralobar cases which are usually right-sided.

Congenital cystic disease of the lungs is a doubtful entity. The cysts are lined with bronchial epithelium. They may involve a lobe or both lungs. They are sometimes associated with polycystic disease of the kidneys. Solitary large cysts have also been described. The symptoms are usually dyspnoea and cyanosis as the cysts become distended with air due to a check-valve opening with the bronchus, or fever, malaise and cough when multiple cysts become infected. However, most cystic changes in the lungs are probably not congenital anomalies but secondary to mechanical obstructions of the small bronchi from various factors such as sepsis, artificial respiration etc. When a large solitary "tension cyst" is causing dyspnoea surgical removal of the lobe containing it is required.

Congenital lobar emphysema.—See page 217.

TUMOURS

Papilloma of the larynx is an uncommon cause of stridor in early childhood. In addition to hoarseness and feebleness of the voice, there may be alarming or even fatal attacks of dyspnoea and asphyxia. Direct laryngoscopy reveals multiple pink wart-like tumours which can be fairly easily taken off by forceps. Spontaneous recovery is usual about puberty. Repeated removal is often necessitated by the tendency to recurrence. In the presence of asphyxial attacks a tracheostomy may be required and it should then be maintained while the papillomata continue to recur.

Intrathoracic tumours are rarely primary in childhood. Primary malignant tumours of the thymus compress surrounding structures and result in cough, dyspnoea, stridor, venous distension, dysphagia and oedema of the face and arms. Teratomata or dermoid cysts arise in the anterior mediastinum and in lateral or oblique radiographs give the appearance of a circumscribed mass. Calcification frequently appears in these cysts. They too can cause mediastinal pressure effects. The ganglioneuroma is a solid, encapsulated benign tumour which may arise in the posterior mediastinum from one of the dorsal sympathetic ganglia. It may reach large size before giving rise to symptoms. The highly malignant neuroblastoma may also develop in this situation and metastasises rapidly (Chapter XI). The mediastinal lymph nodes are occasionally the site of origin of a lymphosarcoma. Radiographs in all these cases will reveal the mass to be in the posterior mediastinum. Bronchogenic carcinoma is excessively rare in childhood, but bronchial adenoma sometimes causes bronchial obstruction with obstructive emphysema (p. 217) or absorption collapse (p. 209). The diagnosis is suggested by haemoptysis which is not otherwise common in children. It should be confirmed by bronchoscopy and biopsy. The treatment of all intrathoracic tumours is surgical excision when this is possible. In malignant cases radiotherapy may prolong life.

INFECTIONS OF THE RESPIRATORY TRACT

Every year between October and March there is a high incidence of respiratory infection in both children and adults in the countries of the Western hemisphere. Indeed, respiratory illnesses account for more disability than any other infections. Every two or three years there is a virtual epidemic of bronchiolitis among infants (Nicol, 1957). The peak incidence of the respiratory infections in general is during the months December to February (Stuart-Harris, 1962). These infections tend to run through individual households and there is a higher attack rate among families of four or more persons. The attack rate is higher among the children than the adults and is especially severe on those under 3 years (Spence *et al.*, 1954).

The causal agents are a wide variety of viruses and bacteria, the former frequently preceding secondary invasion of the respiratory tract by the latter. A wide range of clinical patterns, from the trivial to the fatal, can be produced by many viruses, each of which may produce an essentially similar clinical illness. Classification of the acute respiratory diseases is difficult because the isolation of viruses is a slow business, requiring laboratory facilities which are not universally available. In fact, many of the viruses which cause respiratory disease have still to be identified. On the other hand, an anatomical classification cannot provide a satisfactory basis because a single virus can affect the respiratory mucous membrane, which is continuous from the nose to the alveoli, throughout the whole or any part of its extent. In clinical practice an anatomical diagnosis, such as nasopharyngitis, tracheitis or bronchitis, indicates merely the point of maximum impact by the infective agent. It gives no indication as to its identity or total distribution. Furthermore, some of the viruses (e.g. ECHO and Coxsackie) do not confine their ravages to the respiratory tract but may also invade the gastrointestinal tract, mesenteric lymph nodes, nervous system and meninges.

Several groups of viruses are known to cause respiratory disease and each group contains a bewildering variety of serologically identifiable types (Tyrrell, 1965). There are three main groups. The *myxoviruses* include the parainfluenza group, respiratory syncytial virus, and influenza viruses A, B, and C. The *adenoviruses* contain a large number of different types, some being regarded as "endemic", others as "epidemic". The *picornaviruses* are of two types: enteroviruses such as Coxsackie, ECHO and Coe virus; and rhinoviruses of many serological types. In children respiratory infections are most frequently related to adenoviruses, parainfluenza viruses and respiratory syncytial virus. The lower incidence of these viruses in adults (in whom the rhinoviruses are more common) is presumably attributable to the presence of antibodies arising from previous exposures in earlier life. On the other hand, adults seem to be as susceptible to the influenza viruses as children.

While the clinician need not, at present, know too much about the complex world of viruses, he should remember that none is vulnerable to the presently available antibiotics, and that the vast majority of children with respiratory infections will recover more safely without their use. On the other hand, their advent has enormously reduced the mortality from the respiratory illnesses in children when they are directed against the bacterial infections which may complicate the virus invasions. It is usually possible by a careful evaluation of the clinical features to hazard an informed guess as to when bacterial invasion has occurred. A major problem in young children is to isolate the causal bacteria at an early stage of the illness and thus to determine the antibiotic sensitivities. The existence of a good laboratory service within the area, however, will allow the clinician to be kept informed of the most frequent bacterial causes of respiratory illness and of the prevalent antibiotic sensitivities.

UPPER RESPIRATORY INFECTIONS

Aetiology

The vast majority of cases, including those in which tonsillitis is present, are due to the viruses already mentioned. A few cases of tonsillitis and pharyngitis are due to beta-haemolytic streptococci, but this is not true of the majority in whom throat swabs fail to yield pathogenic bacteria.

Clinical Features

Upper respiratory infections vary widely in their clinical presentations depending upon the area of maximum involvement, the age of the patient and the causal agent. Rhinitis with nasal obstruction and a mucopurulent discharge may seriously interfere with feeding in the infant, whereas a similar "common cold" in the toddler may result only in mild malaise, low-grade fever, and nasal discomfort. In most cases, however, the pharynx shows acute hyperaemia and some oedema. There may be cervical adenitis. The presenting features are often brisk fever, irritability and anorexia. A generalized convulsion may usher in the illness. Indeed, the existence of an upper respiratory infection is frequently discovered only by direct inspection of the throat because the young child rarely complains of sore throat. *The importance of careful inspection of the throat and tympanic membranes in every ill fevered child cannot be over-emphasized.* In other cases there is a tendency for inspiratory stridor to develop suddenly, usually during the night, so that the child awakens distressed and struggling for breath, and with a noisy barking cough. In this type of *laryngitis stridulosa* the morning usually sees the child much relieved, but careful medical supervision is required as in a few cases a severe and dangerous degree of laryngeal obstruction develops (see "acute laryngo-tracheo-bronchitis"). When the trachea is predominantly inflamed the outstanding symptom is a harsh cough, sometimes causing retrosternal pain, often worse during the night, and of a character which tends to alarm parents unduly. In other cases, the prominent complaints are abdominal pain and vomiting, presumed to be due to involvement of the mesenteric lymph nodes. The differential diagnosis from appendicitis may be difficult, but the viral infections are associated with higher fever and a flushed hot skin whereas consistent tenderness and muscle rigidity are often absent. In a few cases headache and neck stiffness may arouse the suspicion of meningitis. It is always wiser to perform a lumbar puncture than to risk leaving a pyogenic meningitis inadequately treated.

When the tonsils bear the brunt of the attack they are grossly hyperaemic and swollen. Small patches of yellow to white exudate may appear in the crypts—*acute follicular tonsillitis*. The lymph nodes at the angles of the jaw are usually enlarged and tender, and the child is, of course, briskly fevered, ill and miserable. While some of these cases are caused by beta-haemolytic streptococci they cannot be distinguished on clinical grounds alone from those of viral aetiology. Scarlet fever is, of course, to be regarded as no more than streptococcal tonsillitis accompanied by a rash. It is, nowadays, a relatively mild disease.

Treatment

In the great majority of cases simple measures will suffice. The sick room should be airy and with a temperature around 65° F. A good intake of fluids and glucose in the form of sweetened drinks must be encouraged. The diet should be light and palatable and the intake of calories is unimportant in a short illness. Tepid sponging is indicated if the rectal temperature rises above 103° F. and often promotes natural sleep. Sleeplessness in the baby can be treated with chloral hydrate 5 gr. (0·3 gm.) or elixir methylpentynol 125 to 250 mg. A useful sedative for the older child is quinalbarbitone $\frac{3}{4}$ to $1\frac{1}{2}$ gr. (50–100 mg.). Pain can be relieved with small doses of paracetemol, $\frac{1}{2}$–1 tablet thrice daily. Nasal obstruction which is interfering with feeding may be temporarily relieved by the instillation up each nostril before each feed of 2 drops of 1 per cent saline solution of ephedrine. Oily drops must never be used in infants because of the dangers of inhalation and consequent *lipoid pneumonia*, a grave condition once it has become established. The common practice of prescribing antibacterial drugs for every child with fever and respiratory signs is to be deplored. In most cases they can do no good, and their hurried use may mask an early meningitis, leading to inadequate or misdirected treatment. A throat swab should always be taken for culture when the pharynx is inflamed. When haemolytic streptococci are isolated the drug of choice is benzylpenicillin, 500,000 units given intramuscularly twice daily for three days and followed by oral penicillin G, 250 mg. four times daily for a further three to four days.

COMPLICATIONS OF UPPER RESPIRATORY INFECTION

The most common is spread to the lower respiratory tract in various forms—bronchitis, bronchiolitis, pneumonia—which are separately discussed. When chest radiographs are taken of children with upper respiratory infections, it is quite common to find areas of atelectatic pneumonitis or *aspiration pneumonia* which are segmental or lobar in distribution. While this condition may produce physical signs such as diminished resonance and air-entry, or a few crepitations, it is often only recognized radiologically. Indeed, this type of aspiration pneumonia is much more common than purely clinical diagnosis might suggest. Resolution is usual and may be assisted by postural drainage and forced coughing (see "Bronchiectasis"). The more local complications of upper respiratory infections are less common and much less dangerous since the availability of the antibiotics. It has already been stressed that it is not good practice to prescribe such drugs in every case of upper respiratory infection. Toxic effects are not unknown. It is more sensible to observe each child carefully until recovery takes place, or until a definite bacterial complication justifies the use of an anti-bacterial drug.

ACUTE OTITIS MEDIA

This is a relatively common complication, especially in young infants who lie supine for much of the day and in whom the Eustachian tube is short and straight. It can only be diagnosed by making inspection of the tympanic membranes through an electric auriscope part of the routine examination of every infant. Older children usually, although not invariably, complain of earache. Fever and malaise are usual and meningism may be present. In catarrhal otitis media the drum is red and injected. In suppurative cases it is seen to be bulging and it may pulsate. In neglected cases perforation of the drum occurs and it is then obscured by a profuse purulent discharge. Spread to involve the mastoid air-cells has become uncommon.

Treatment

Benzylpenicillin should be given intramuscularly in doses of 500,000 units every six hours. When the tympanic membrane is bulging myringotomy should be performed immediately and a specimen of pus sent for culture. In the presence of a perforated drum no ear-drops should be placed in the auditory canal. It is better to mop out the pus several times daily and to keep the canal closed with cotton wool. Most perforations heal rapidly on adequate antibiotic therapy. Chronic otitis media and mastoiditis and deafness should nowadays be exceedingly rare sequels to infections of the middle ear.

ACUTE SINUSITIS

Some degree of sinusitis occurs in most upper respiratory infections and most often recovers spontaneously. In older children acute empyema of a sinus may occasionally develop and cause severe pain. This is usually over the maxillary antrum or the frontal sinus. However, when the sphenoidal sinus is involved the pain is suboccipital in distribution and it may be over the temple and mastoid when the ethmoid cells are involved. Radiographs will then reveal opacity of the affected paranasal sinus.

Treatment

Ephedrine 1 per cent in physiological saline should be instilled up the nostril every four hours. An antibiotic should be prescribed according to the findings on culture of a nasal swab. This is most often benzylpenicillin. Surgical drainage is only rarely required.

ACUTE RETROPHARYNGEAL ABSCESS

This once common emergency has become rare. The child has severe difficulty in swallowing. He often assumes a characteristic position with his elbows on a table, head supported on his hands and neck hyperextended so as to widen the airway and relieve his respiratory difficulty. The mouth should be opened with a metal tongue spatula and the forefinger slid through the angle of the mouth over the back of the tongue and into the pharynx. A fluctuant mass can be readily palpated bulging forwards from the posterior pharyngeal wall. Lateral radiographs of the neck will also reveal the mass in the pharyngeal region. This method of examination also serves to exclude the rare case in which the abscess is secondary to tuberculosis of the cervical spine. Life can be in serious danger if a retropharyngeal abscess is allowed to rupture spontaneously, because the pus may flood into the larynx, burst into a blood vessel with severe haemorrhage, or even reach the mediastinum.

Treatment

Intramuscular benzylpenicillin should be started without awaiting the results of the preliminary throat swab. The abscess should be opened without general anaesthesia, preferably by a trained surgeon when time permits.

ACUTE PERITONSILLAR ABSCESS (QUINSY)

This is uncommon in childhood. It usually follows an acute streptococcal tonsillitis and is exceedingly painful. It interferes with swallowing, speech becomes "thick", and a characteristic sign is difficulty in opening the mouth. The tonsillar area is swollen, red and glistening, and palpation reveals a mass. The oedematous uvula is often displaced to the opposite side.

Treatment

Full intramuscular doses of benzylpenicillin should immediately follow a throat swab. If fluctuation is present it is better to incise the abscess than to let it rupture spontaneously.

ACUTE LARYNGO-TRACHEO-BRONCHITIS *Croup.*

Aetiology

This name is employed for a most dangerous illness in which inflammation and oedema of the epiglottis and arytenoids result in acute laryngeal obstruction. It is important to realize, however, that the trachea and primary bronchi are also severely involved and may be partially obstructed by mucosal oedema and tenacious purulent exudate. This disease can probably be caused by a variety of viruses. The parainfluenza myxoviruses have been particularly implicated (Chanock, 1956; Beale *et al.*, 1958), and secondary bacterial infection is common, especially by *Haemophilus influenzae*.

Clinical Features

Children of pre-school age are most at risk. The laryngeal stridor may develop very suddenly, with or without a preceding upper respiratory catarrh. Fever is usually high. The child looks anxious and distressed. He suffers increasing inspiratory difficulty and the sternomastoid and other accessory muscles of respiration can be seen to be in action. The voice is hoarse. After a short time inspiratory indrawing of the suprasternal and supraclavicular fossae appears and there is greyish cyanosis. Increasing hypoxia is also reflected in increasing restlessness which further exhausts the child. Tachycardia is marked. Treatment may become a matter of extreme urgency.

Treatment

On admission to hospital the first essentials are oxygen, high humidity, and a cool environment. These conditions can best be achieved in an oxygen tent fitted with a humidifier and capable of maintaining a temperature about 5° F. below that of the room. Suitable tents are the Humidair (Oxygenaire, Ltd.) or Croupette (Air Shields, Inc.). The patient should be propped up. It is wise to administer 20,000 units of diphtheria antitoxin without waiting for the results of throat swabs. Chloramphenicol should also be given intramuscularly (100 mg./Kg./day) in four divided doses to eradicate *H. influenzae*. Arrangements for tracheostomy should be kept in constant readiness. This life-saving procedure is more often performed too late than too early. It should be carried out in any patient in whom the respiratory difficulty worsens in spite of treatment and when there is diminishing air-entry over the lungs. Tracheostomy not only provides a safe airway, it greatly assists in tracheal aspiration using a plastic catheter and electric suction pump. The post-operative care must be in the hands of an experienced doctor and nurse. An adequate fluid intake is important, by mouth if possible. Sedatives should be used with caution and opiates are contra-indicated.

ACUTE BRONCHITIS

Aetiology

Most cases of acute bronchitis are due to an extension downwards of an upper respiratory viral infection, or they form part of the clinical spectrum of diseases such as measles, influenza, whooping cough or typhoid fever. Secondary bacterial infection by pneumococci, *H. influenzae* or staphylococci may aggravate the damage to the bronchial tree.

Clinical Features

The usual history is of a preceding upper respiratory illness with sudden worsening of fever, cough, malaise and anorexia. Most children are not very ill although infants may become dyspnoeic and toxic. The cough is initially unproductive but later sputum may be coughed up by the older child or vomited during spasms of coughing by the infant. Physical signs over the lungs consist of rhonchi and crepitations which vary considerably in severity and do not have a close correlation with the severity of the illness. Recovery usually begins after a week or thereabouts and serious sequelae such as bronchiectasis are rare.

Treatment

In the vast majority of cases the simple palliative measures described under "Upper Respiratory Infections" will be sufficient treatment, and spontaneous recovery can be expected. There is no evidence that the so-called expectorant mixtures have any useful effects and the use of cough suppressants is unwise and illogical. Antibiotics are rarely required but they should be used when the child is toxic or dyspnoeic. Sputum is usually unobtainable in young children for identification of the causal organism and a broad spectrum drug such as tetracycline (25 mg./Kg./day) should be given in divided doses. Oxygen is only rarely required for children with simple bronchitis.

ACUTE BRONCHIOLITIS OF INFANCY

Aetiology

This is a disease which is only seen in infancy. It occurs in epidemic form every two or three years during the period January to March.

The great majority of cases are due to respiratory syncytial virus which is, indeed, the most common cause of lower respiratory tract infections in infants and young children (Holzel et al., 1963; Elderkin et al., 1965; Field et al., 1966). This disease has also been called "capillary bronchitis", "acute interstitial pneumonitis" and "virus pneumonitis of infants". It is quite distinct pathologically and clinically from the bacterial pneumonias.

Clinical Features

There is normally a preceding history of upper respiratory catarrh and slight cough. The infant then becomes acutely ill with inspiratory difficulty, resulting in visible subcostal and intercostal recession, but there is also marked expiratory difficulty and wheezing or grunting. Severe spasms of coughing may so interfere with feeding as to lead to dehydration. This is further aggravated by tachypnoea and increased insensible loss of water from the lungs. Hypoxia is reflected in agitation and restlessness, and there may be cyanosis. Tachycardia is marked but the temperature rarely rises about 101° F. and may, in fact, be normal. Bilateral obstructive emphysema causes the chest to be in the inspiratory position and the percussion note is hyper-resonant. The breath sounds are diminished and there may be rhonchi or numerous crepitations. Cardiac failure may lead to hepatomegaly. Radiographs of the chest show increased lung markings due to interstitial infiltration. There may be a fall in the blood pH and a rise in the Pco_2 due to respiratory acidosis. The mortality rate is about 5 per cent.

Treatment

The infant should be propped in a Humidair or Croupette in a humid atmosphere containing 40 per cent oxygen. The relief of hypoxia frequently has a dramatic effect in relieving restlessness. An adequate fluid intake is important and if the infant refuses feeds 5 per cent glucose in quarter-strength physiological saline may be substituted. It is only rarely necessary to resort to intravenous fluids. Clothing must be light and non-restrictive. A broad spectrum antibiotic such as tetracycline, 25 mg./ Kg./day, is usually prescribed but rarely has a marked effect on the course of the illness. In the most gravely ill hydrocortisone may be given intramuscularly, 100 mg. in the first 24 hours with diminishing dosage over the next few days. It is extremely difficult to assess its value. Digitalization is only indicated if heart failure develops. In infants who recover, a tendency to wheeziness and cough may persist for some weeks after the acute illness, but permanent lung damage does not occur.

Strictly speaking, give no AB.

ACUTE BACTERIAL PNEUMONIA

An aetiological classification of the bacterial pneumonias would be of more practical value to the clinician, who is now armed with effective antibacterial drugs, than the traditional subdivision into broncho-pneumonia (lobular) and lobar pneumonia (alveolar). Unfortunately, sputum is rarely obtainable from young children and bacteria grown from the nose or throat are not necessarily those present in the lung. None the less, it is often possible from a knowledge of the epidemiology of the common pulmonary infections in a region, to hazard a shrewd guess as to the probable bacterial cause in the individual patient with pneumonia. This is also influenced by the age of the patient.

BACTERIAL PNEUMONIA IN INFANCY

Aetiology

In Britain today the most common cause of pneumonia during the first year of life is the *Staph. aureus.* In most cases these organisms have colonized the infant's nose in the maternity unit soon after birth. They are almost invariably penicillin-resistant and increasingly often also tetracycline-resistant. The bacterial pneumonia is frequently preceded by a viral infection of the respiratory tract which presumably damages the mucous membrane and permits its penetration by bacteria. Pneumococcal pneumonia which was the common type in the pre-antibiotic era has become relatively rare in the young infant. Occasional cases are due to streptococci, haemophilus and coliforms. The frequent association of staphylococcal pneumonia with fibrocystic disease of the pancreas is considered in Chapter XVI. Its importance in the neonatal period received attention in Chapter VI.

Pathology

The striking features in the staphylococcal cases are massive consolidation, destruction of tissue and abscess formation, and the frequent (PNEUMATOCOELES) appearance of emphysematous bullae. When these rupture into the pleural cavity the result is pyopneumothorax. In pneumococcal cases the lobular areas of consolidation rarely suppurate and empyema has become uncommon.

Clinical Features

There is frequently a preceding upper respiratory infection. The infant then becomes acutely ill, fevered, irritable and restless. Feeds are taken reluctantly. Dyspnoea is associated with inspiratory dilatation of the alae nasi and expiratory grunting. There may be subcostal recession. Cough is severe and may precipitate vomiting. Diarrhoea may occur. Meningism is relatively uncommon. Early in the illness there may be only a few crepitations over the lungs. In staphylococcal cases dullness on percussion over the affected areas, with bronchial or diminished breath sounds, becomes quickly obvious. The presence of consolidation can be confirmed radiologically. As the disease progresses radiographs frequently reveal emphysematous bullae (pneumatoceles) (Fig. 10), an appearance pathognomonic of staphylococcal pneumonia. Abscess formation may occasionally be demonstrable with fluid levels in the cavities.

Treatment

The mortality from bronchopneumonia in infancy is now very low, whereas in the pre-antibiotic days it was high and staphylococcal cases were invariably fatal. When staphylococcal pneumonia seems likely, and especially when pneumonia due to Gram-negative organisms cannot be excluded, a suitable antibiotic combination is cloxacillin, 50 mg./Kg./ day, and ampicillin, 50 mg./Kg./day, each given intramuscularly initially in four six-hourly doses. If the causal organism can be isolated from sputum or laryngeal swab the antibiotic can be more accurately chosen according to the bacterial sensitivities. A change to another antibiotic such as cephaloridine, 30 mg./Kg./day, fucidin 20 mg./Kg./day or erythromycin, 50 mg./Kg./day is indicated if a favourable response is not obtained within 72 hours. Severe dyspnoea or cyanosis is an indication for oxygen in an incubator or tent (Oxygenaire, Ltd.). Restlessness is often controlled by relief of hypoxia alone, but if sleeplessness is a problem chloral hydrate 5–7½ gr. (0·3–0·5 gm.) should be given. Good nursing is essential. The infant's position in the cot should be changed frequently and his head should be raised above his feet. An adequate intake of fluids must be ensured.

BACTERIAL PNEUMONIA IN THE OLDER CHILD

Aetiology

The great majority of cases are due to pneumococci which are invariably sensitive to benzylpenicillin. Although type-specific sera are available for many of the thirty-two types of pneumococci they are now rarely used.

Pathology

Post-mortem studies of pneumonia in older children are now fortunately exceedingly rare. The classical four stages of congestion, red hepatization, grey hepatization and resolution are well known. Complications such as empyema, pyopericardium, lung abscess and bacterial endocarditis are also rarely seen today. Abscess formation may, of course, occur in staphylococcal cases which complicate influenza, and in the infrequent example due to Friedländer's bacillus.

Clinical Features

The onset is sudden with high fever, malaise and cough. Pain in the chest or abdomen on the affected side is common, but rarely as severe as in adults. Meningism is not infrequent, especially when the upper lobes are involved. A rigor is not common in the child but a convulsion may herald the onset of the illness. Tachypnoea is the rule but severe dyspnoea or cyanosis is uncommon. Circumoral pallor, inspiratory dilatation of the alae nasi and an expiratory grunt frequently constitute a characteristic clinical picture. The heart rate tends to be less increased than the respiratory rate and ratios of 2:1 or 3:1 are found instead of the more usual 4:1. The movement of the affected side of the chest is diminished. Pleural friction is inconstant and usually transient. Dullness, bronchial breath sounds, pectoriloquy and fine crepitations are found in typical cases, but in many children the physical signs are remarkably slight in contrast to the segmental or lobar area of consolidation revealed by radiography. The white cell count is raised but in childhood is of little prognostic significance.

Treatment

The drug of choice is benzylpenicillin 500,000 units given intramuscularly two to four times daily for 3 to 4 days, after which oral penicillin G, 250 mg. six-hourly, may be substituted for a further few days. Good results can also be expected from oral sulphadimidine 150 mg./Kg./day in four divided doses. An adequate fluid intake is important. Sleeplessness can be relieved with quinalbarbitone $\frac{3}{4}$–$1\frac{1}{2}$ gr. (50–100 mg.). The so-called "expectorants" have no value. Oxygen is only infrequently required in older children suffering from pneumonia.

PRIMARY ATYPICAL PNEUMONIA

This disease became familiar to many physicians during the second world war. It is relatively rare in children and the same clinical pattern is not seen in infants at all. Many cases diagnosed as "primary atypical pneumonia" are, in fact, examples of aspiration pneumonia secondary to upper respiratory catarrh, but there are undoubtedly cases of primary viral pneumonia.

Aetiology

The clinical identity of primary atypical pneumonia can be distinguished by a rising titre of cold agglutinins (which will agglutinate human red cells in the cold) in the serum of affected individuals. Agglutinins are also commonly found against the streptococcus MG. Some cases are due to a virus-like agent (Eaton *et al.*, 1944; Goodburn *et al.*, 1963) which is now believed to be a mycoplasma (Chanock *et al.*, 1962). Some cases are really examples of psittacosis due to contact with sick parrots or budgerigars. Others have probably been due to *Rickettsia burnetii* which causes Q fever.

Pathology

There is infiltration of the bronchiolar walls, alveolar septa and interstitial tissues by mononuclear cells. The alveoli are often free of exudate but may be filled with a mixture of fibrin and mononuclear cells.

Clinical Features

The incubation period is 10 to 21 days. The onset is with headache, shivering, malaise and fever. Cough develops subsequently and blood-staining of the sputum may be observed. There may be remarkably few physical signs over the lungs, often only a few localized crepitations, but the radiograph shows patchy consolidation confined to one or two lobes (Fig. 39). Leucocytosis is absent. The somewhat delayed onset of

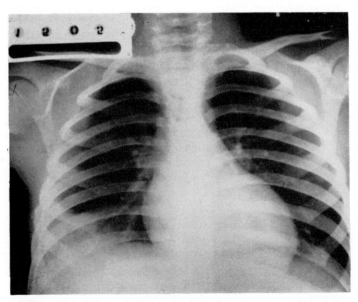

FIG. 39.—Primary atypical pneumonia showing characteristic patchy consolidation in right lower lobe.

cough contrasts with the situation in the much more common aspiration pneumonia, where cough has often preceded the constitutional upset.

Treatment

Spontaneous recovery usually takes place after an illness of 2 to 3 weeks' duration. Cases due to Eaton agent and *Rickettsia burnetii* respond favourably to large doses of tetracycline (50 mg./Kg./day).

LIPOID PNEUMONIA

This condition has been reported in young infants in whom oily nose drops have been used over long periods. It can also develop in debilitated infants given cod liver oil or castor oil by mouth. The lungs show interstitial fibrosis and cellular proliferation, and tumour-like paraffinomas may develop. The inhaled lipoid can be seen both in and outwith the cells and oil-laden cells are carried to the hilar lymph nodes. The principal clinical features are progressive dyspnoea and severe spasms of coughing. Radiographs show widespread opacity, most marked around the hila. Secondary bacterial infection may supervene. There is no specific treatment. Oily nose drops must not be prescribed for young infants.

(PNEUMOCYSTIS)

INTERSTITIAL PLASMA CELL PNEUMONIA

Aetiology

This type of lung infection is a common cause of death in early infancy in some central and northern European countries. It is, however, rarely seen in Britain or the U.S.A., except in association with such primary conditions as hypogammaglobulinaemia (Hutchison, 1955; McKay and Richardson, 1959), cytomegalic inclusion body disease (Baar, 1955), and various malignant reticuloses treated with corticosteroids, antimetabolites, irradiation and antibiotics (White *et al.*, 1961). The infective agent is a protozoan *Pneumocystis carinii* (Gajdusek, 1957; Bommer, 1961).

Pathology

The alveoli are filled with an apparently acellular exudate which shows a honeycomb appearance in sections. In the infants the alveolar septa are infiltrated by plasma cells, but these are conspicuous by their absence in cases associated with hypogammaglobulinaemia. When special staining methods are used the alveolar exudate is seen to be composed of parasites.

Clinical Features

The predominant feature is progressively severe dyspnoea and cyanosis which contrast with the paucity of physical signs over the lungs. Radiographs show a characteristic symmetrical ground glass opacity spreading outwards from the lung roots. Areas of lobular collapse may give a finely mottled appearance and emphysema is common. Interstitial emphysema or spontaneous pneumothorax may occur. The organism may be identified during life in material obtained by lung puncture.

Treatment

The prognosis is grave, but good results have recently been reported with pentamidine isethionate, 4 mg./Kg./day by intramuscular injection for ten days (Marshall *et al.*, 1964).

IDIOPATHIC PULMONARY HAEMOSIDEROSIS
(Ceelen's Disease)

Pulmonary haemosiderosis is a well-documented complication of mitral stenosis and left ventricular failure (Lendrum *et al.*, 1950). The idiopathic type (essential brown induration of the lungs) is a disease of previously healthy young children and is characterized by diffuse intra-alveolar haemorrhages throughout the lungs. It has been postulated that the cause may be an auto-immune mechanism.

Clinical Features

These have been reviewed by Wyllie *et al.* (1948), Browning and Houghton (1956), and Joseph *et al.* (1957). The prominent features are pallor, dyspnoea, cyanosis, fever and tachycardia. Jaundice may be present. Cough and haemoptysis are frequent. Cardiac failure may result in cardiomegaly, hepatosplenomegaly and gallop rhythm. Radiographs show generalized diffuse mottling throughout the lungs, the appearances simulating those seen in miliary tuberculosis, xanthomatosis or sarcoidosis. The intra-pulmonary haemorrhage, in which the blood is retained within the body, results in anaemia, erythroblastaemia, reticulocytosis and excess urobilinogenuria. These findings can easily be misinterpreted as due to haemolysis. The diagnosis should be confirmed by lung puncture or be demonstrating haemosiderin-laden phagocytes in the sputum.

Treatment

Anaemia can be corrected by blood transfusion and cyanosis relieved with oxygen, but the outlook is poor. Some benefit may be derived from corticotrophin or corticosteroids.

ABSORPTION COLLAPSE (ATELECTASIS) OF THE LUNGS

Resorption of air from a pulmonary segment or lobe is common in young children due to complete bronchial occlusion ("stop-valve"). The thin-walled bronchi and bronchioles can be compressed by enlarged lymph nodes in tuberculosis, measles, pertussis and malignant reticulosis. The narrow lumens can be blocked by mucopus, inhaled foreign bodies or stomach contents, and by mucosal oedema due to allergy in asthmatic subjects.

Pathology

The atelectatic portion of lung occupies a smaller volume than normal. This is in part filled by compensatory emphysema of the other lobes of the lung, in part by mediastinal shift to the affected side, by a rise in the level of the diaphragm and by some falling inwards of the chest wall.

Clinical Features

The symptoms will naturally depend upon the primary disease. It is important to remember that while the *inhalation of a foreign body* produces immediate respiratory distress with coughing, choking, gagging, stridor and cyanosis, it is possible for this short episode to pass unobserved in the case of a toddler. There may then be quite a long "silent" interval before secondary bacterial infection in the obstructed bronchus produces symptoms. Foreign bodies composed of vegetable matter, e.g. peanuts, result in early severe bronchitis with fever, cough and dyspnoea, whereas metallic or plastic substances may remain *in situ* for long periods without giving rise to obvious trouble. A segment of atelectasis may be obscured clinically by compensatory emphysema and the condition only becomes obvious when postero-anterior, lateral and oblique radiographs are examined. When a lobe or whole lung is collapsed there is diminished movement of the affected side of the chest with impaired resonance, diminished breath sounds and, possibly, tracheal or mediastinal shift towards the affected side. Collapse of an upper lobe can be distinguished from consolidation on the radiograph by the fact that in the former the lower border is convex (Fig. 40), whereas in the latter it forms a straight line. A collapsed lower lobe is visualized as a jib-shaped shadow (Fig. 41). The airless right middle lobe is seen in the lateral view as a triangular shadow of which the base is composed partly of diaphragm and partly sternum (Fig. 42). It may also be clearly defined as a triangular shadow when postero-anterior films are taken with the patient in the lordotic position.

Treatment

This largely depends upon the aetiology and often involves the use of a suitable antibiotic. Bronchoscopy is essential wherever there is a possibility of an inhaled foreign body, or if the atelectasis fails to respond to more conservative treatment. Postural drainage with percussion over the affected lobe is valuable. Rapid re-expansion must be achieved if bronchiectasis is to be avoided.

BRONCHIECTASIS

Aetiology

It is not proposed in a book chiefly concerned with clinical problems to discuss in detail the pathogenic mechanisms which can result in

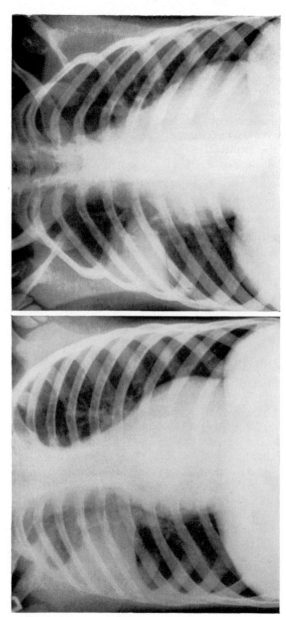

FIG. 40.—The radiograph on the left shows an opacity in the right upper lobe which from the convex lower border is due to atelectasis; the radiograph on the right shows a horizontal lower border to the opacity indicating consolidation.

bronchial dilatation. Two factors are commonly present, (i) bronchial occlusion, with absorption atelectasis, (ii) infection, which is usually due to pyogenic bacteria such as pneumococcus, haemophilus and staphylococcus, but may sometimes be tuberculous (Brock, 1950; Hutchison, 1951). The diseases most commonly preceding bronchiectasis are bronchopneumonia, measles, pertussis, fibrocystic disease of the pancreas, inhaled foreign body, tooth or tonsil fragment, or primary tuberculosis (Chapter X). There is also evidence to indicate that persistent infection with adeno-virus can lead to bronchiectasis (Macfarlane and Sommerville, 1957). A very few cases may be related to some congenital weakness in the bronchial walls. This is probably true in _Kartagener's syndrome_ in which situs inversus is associated with chronic sinusitis and bronchiectasis. (Absent frontal sinus)

Social Background

Bronchiectasis is nowadays much less common due to the use of antibiotics. It is mainly encountered in children from the poorer sections of the community who live in overcrowded conditions which expose them to repeated respiratory infections, and who, moreover, are less likely to receive an adequate convalescence after acute illnesses such as measles and pneumonia. A persistent cough is, also, less likely to receive adequate medical attention.

Clinical Features

The bronchiectatic patient of a bygone era reached a pitiful state in which his putrid breath made him a burden to his fellows and himself. Sputum was abundant and malodorous. Exertion precipitated distressing outbursts of coughing and dyspnoea. The fingers and toes were grossly clubbed. Cachexia was marked. Death finally resulted from empyema, brain abscess, cor pulmonale or amyloid disease.

The clinical presentation today is very different. The child is usually brought to the physician because of _persistent_ cough, dating often from an acute respiratory illness some months or years previously. In a few male cases the bronchiectasis is a feature of congenital hypogammaglobulinaemia (Chapter IX). In others it is part of the clinical spectrum of fibrocystic disease of the pancreas (Chapter XVI). Purulent sputum is obtainable but it is not usually abundant or maladorous. Haemoptysis,

FIG. 41 (_see opposite_).—Radiograph showing jib-shaped shadow behind the heart and indicating collapse of the left lower lobe.

FIG. 42 (_see opposite_).—Right lateral radiograph of chest showing triangular opacity with its base on lower sternum and diaphragm and indicating collapse of the right middle lobe.

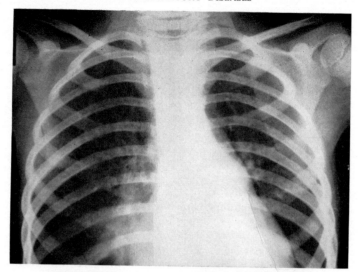

FIG. 41

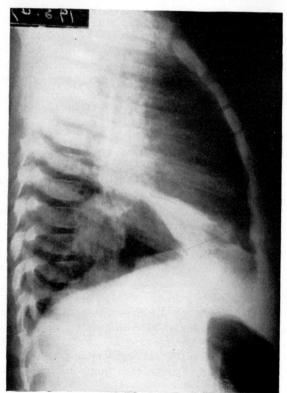

FIG. 42

to suffer from periodic episodes of fever and malaise, with aggravation of his cough, due to the retention of infected secretions within the bronchiectatic area of lung. None the less, his general condition is often remarkably good and clubbing of the fingers is often quite slight. Physical signs over the lungs are variable. There may be an impaired percussion note, diminished breath sounds and mediastinal shift to the affected side. After the dilated bronchi have been emptied of pus by postural drainage the breath sounds may become bronchial or amphoric with whispering pectoriloquy. In some cases there are numerous crepitations over the diseased lobe. Chronic sinusitis is an almost invariable accompaniment, although the causal relationship of the one to the other is not clear.

Radiographs may reveal the cavities in the saccular type of bronchiectasis whereas in the more common cylindrical type there are only heavy linear markings or, sometimes, no obvious abnormality. A persistent area of atelectasis as revealed by a jib-shaped shadow is also good evidence that bronchiectasis has developed. Confirmation of the diagnosis and estimation of the extent of the process can be obtained from well-planned bronchography. Bronchoscopy is frequently informative and imperative when there is a suspicion of foreign body. The sputum should be cultured from time to time to assist in the choice of suitable antibiotics. The most common predominating organism is *H. influenzae*. When staphylococci are isolated the probability is that there is fibrocystic disease of the pancreas. In male children it is wise always to measure the gamma globulin level in the serum.

Treatment — as for CF.

Surgical treatment is now less frequently advised than formerly. This is because some cough and sputum frequently persist after successful resection of the bronchiectatic area due to chronic bronchial catarrh in the non-bronchiectatic parts of the lungs. Furthermore, conscientiously followed medical treatment with efficient supervision usually permits the child to live a normal life, to attend school regularly and to grow into a useful adult, even although established bronchiectasis is irreversible. The most important measure is postural drainage, performed twice daily. The child should lie prone with his head and chest over the side of the bed and supported by his hands on the floor. Vigorous coughing, assisted by gravity, produces sputum and empties the dilated bronchi. Percussion over the affected lobe helps to dislodge tenacious mucopus. Following the postural drainage the child should be encouraged to breathe slowly and deeply for ten minutes. Febrile episodes should be treated promptly with antibiotics chosen according to the results of sputum cultures and bacterial sensitivities, e.g. tetracycline (25 mg./Kg./day) or ampicillin (50 mg./Kg./day). The dangers of blood dyscrasia make chloramphenicol unsuitable for repeated use. Good results may also be obtained with streptomycin 250 mg. or neomycin 250 mg. in aerosol form four or five times each day. Sepsis in the teeth, tonsils or paranasal sinuses should receive attention. Some parents require education in the constituents of a balanced diet, in the need for adequate sleep in childhood, and in the importance of protecting the child from avoidable exposures to infection in crowded places of entertainment etc.

Lobectomy should only be considered after medical treatment has been tried for at least two years, and after the most thorough investigation as outlined above. The operation is only advisable when the bronchiectasis is confined to one, or at most two, lobes and when the remainder of the bronchial tree is reasonably free from infection.

SINO-BRONCHITIS ("THE CATARRHAL CHILD")

The catarrhal child is one of the common and unsolved problems of paediatrics (Fry, 1961). Very little is really known about the aetiological factors in this type of child and this is reflected in the widely different methods which physicians employ in his management. It is important to realize that frequent "head colds" are the normal experience of children during the age-period 3 to 8 years. Three to six such colds a year is not out of the way, but in most children recovery is complete between colds. It can be assumed that these colds are caused by a considerable variety of viruses and that in this fashion a child develops immunity. The "catarrhal child" is one who retains some of his symptoms between the acute episodes, sometimes in the form of persistent rhinitis, nasal obstruction and sinusitis; frequently in the form of an unproductive barking cough with wheezy rhonchi and/or crepitations over the lungs. These children are also prone to attacks of acute otitis media, although acute mastoiditis is now a rarity. Chronic otitis media and otorrhoea are also relatively uncommon nowadays and mostly confined to children from the poorest home conditions. Bronchiectasis seems rarely to complicate sino-bronchitis. In most affected children spontaneous recovery takes place after the age of 7 to 8 years, but the proportion of such children who suffer from chronic bronchitis in adult life is not known. It is unlikely to be large (Scottish Health Services Council, 1963).

Management

Many catarrhal children seem to possess parents who worry unduly. At least, so it has seemed to the author who has been only too familiar with the problem, but recognizes from experience that at the end of the day the child will "outgrow" his susceptibility to respiratory catarrh.

On the other hand, from the parents' viewpoint the physician must frequently appear comparatively impotent when called upon to bring immediate relief. Perhaps his most useful role is to take the time to explain the nature of the problem to the parents and to reassure them as to its relatively benign nature and good long-term prognosis. Some parents also need assurance that they themselves are in no way to blame for the child's repeated, but not severe, illnesses. In particular, parents frequently seek relief from their unspoken fears that the child may have tuberculosis, asthma or some other grave disorder. They must be dissuaded from over-protecting the child by keeping him indoors whenever the weather is inclement, by over-clothing him, and by keeping him unnecessarily away from school. In acute febrile episodes an automatic resort to antibiotics is certainly unwise. Indeed, the treatment may then prove more dangerous than the disease. They are only indicated when pathogenic bacteria are isolated from the throat swab or sputum, or if the child remains highly fevered and ill after three days. In most cases relief can be obtained from rest in bed for a few days, and if there is nasal obstruction from the short-term use of 1 per cent ephedrine nose drops. The so-called expectorants are of no value.

Sooner or later the parents will raise the question of removal of tonsils and adenoids, if this has not already been discussed with them by their medical adviser. The more experienced the physician the more familiar he will have become with the disappointment of parents who have found little change in their child's catarrhal state after this operation. It is, after all, hardly reasonable to expect that the extirpation of some superficial lymphoid tissue can greatly influence infection by adenoviruses or bacteria in the paranasal sinuses or bronchial tree. None the less, tonsillectomy accounts for a third of all the admissions of children to British hospitals. Fry (1961) estimated that 20 to 30 per cent of catarrhal children had their tonsils and adenoids removed, although in his own practice the figure was 3 per cent. There is, undoubtedly, a failure by many physicians to appreciate the naturally good prognosis in sino-bronchitis, and a tendency too easily to succumb to the parents' pressure that "something must be done". There are, of course, certain clear indications for removal of the tonsils and adenoids; (i) recurrent attacks of acute follicular tonsillitis, especially if associated with quinsy, (ii) recurrent attacks of acute otitis media, (iii) persistent or recurrent visible enlargement of the cervical lymph nodes. The mere size of the tonsils is not a reliable guide to the degree of chronic infection. The operation should rarely be performed before the age of four years. In children with any form of organic heart disease it should be "covered" by intramuscular penicillin to obviate the risk of bacterial endocarditis. It should never be forgotten that tonsillectomy is an operation which can, and occasionally does, result in the death of a child who was not previously in any danger of his life.

EMPHYSEMA IN CHILDHOOD

During infancy and childhood *obstructive emphysema* is the most common type. It may involve one lobe when a primary bronchus is partially obstructed to a degree which permits the entry of air into the alveoli, but obstructs its egress during expiration ("check-valve"). This is seen in primary tuberculosis (Chapter X) but may also be caused by an inhaled foreign body. A special variety called *congenital lobar emphysema* occurs in the newborn due to a defect in the bronchial cartilage (chondromalacia). It results in respiratory distress within a few days or weeks of birth (Fig. 43). In lobar obstructive emphysema

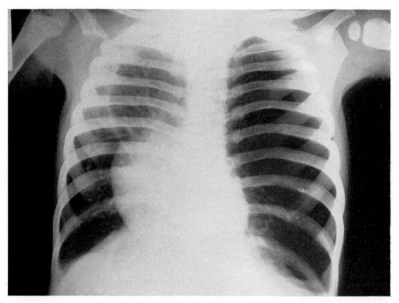

FIG. 43.—Congenital obstructive emphysema of left upper lobe. Note herniation across the mid-line and compression collapse of the left lower lobe.

the lobe is over-distended with air. There is usually an "asthmatoid" wheeze at the open mouth, hyper-resonance over the affected side of the chest, and diminished breath sounds. The mediastinum is displaced towards the opposite side and the ribs may even be separated. The radiograph confirms this and shows increased translucency in the emphysematous lobe which may in fact herniate across the mid-line.

Check-valve obstruction in the bronchioles results in generalized bilateral obstructive emphysema. This can occur temporarily in acute bronchiolitis, or in a chronic form which can lead to cor pulmonale in fibrocystic disease of the pancreas (Chapter XVI). Generalized emphysema is uncommon in asthma during childhood. Radiographs reveal hypertranslucency in both lung fields, flattening and diminished excursions of the diaphragm, and the ribs tend to be horizontally placed instead of being "tiled".

Bullous emphysema is seen most often in staphylococcal pneumonia (Fig. 10) when multiple bullae or pneumatoceles develop. If these rupture into the mediastinum a rapidly fatal *interstitial emphysema* without or with spontaneous pneumothorax results. *Subcutaneous emphysema* with palpable crackling under the skin may arise from interstitial emphysema or from perforation of the trachea, pharynx or oesophagus. It may also complicate the operation of thoracocentesis. Interstitial emphysema and spontaneous pneumothorax may also complicate attempts at resuscitation of the newborn by tracheal intubation and the administration of oxygen under pressure (Chapter I).

Treatment

This obviously depends upon the cause. In congenital lobar emphysema immediate lobectomy is a remarkably safe and successful operation.

SPONTANEOUS PNEUMOTHORAX

Aetiology

This may complicate asphyxia neonatorum, especially when intratracheal intubation has been employed. It is, however, most frequently seen in staphylococcal pneumonia with bullous emphysema. It is an occasional complication of tracheostomy and of thoracocentesis. It does not occur in primary tuberculosis.

Clinical Features

When the pneumothorax is not so large that it produces a positive intrapleural pressure the lung falls away from the chest wall ("relaxation collapse") and there will be no symptoms directly referable to the pneumothorax. A tension pneumothorax with a strongly positive intrapleural pressure ("compression collapse") causes severe pain, dyspnoea, cyanosis and circulatory collapse. There is hyper-resonance over the affected side and the breath sounds are distant or inaudible. The mediastinum and trachea may be displaced to the opposite side. In an "open" pneumothorax which is in communication with a bronchus, the breath sounds may be amphoric with whispering pectoriloquy. When there is fluid as well as air in the pleural cavity gurgling or splashing may be heard as the child's position is moved. The radiograph usually confirms the diagnosis, although in the infant there may be difficulty in distinguishing pneumothorax from a large diaphragmatic hernia or giant emphysematous bulla. Screening and a drink of gastro-grafin usually resolve the difficulty.

Treatment

Direct treatment of the pneumothorax itself is only urgently required when there is tension and acute respiratory embarrassment. A suitable cannula or catheter should be inserted into the pleural cavity and plastic or rubber tubing led from the needle to below the level of the chest and under water. In the infant a Birmingham patent needle and cannula makes a satisfactory instrument for the purpose. If air continues to collect and bubble out from the end of the tubing, negative pressure drainage should be instituted. Occasionally when a broncho-pleural fistula complicates a pyopneumothorax open thoracotomy is required.

PLEURISY WITH EFFUSION

Aetiology

In childhood serous effusions into the pleural cavity are usually tuberculous and they develop within 8 to 12 weeks of the primary infection (Chapter X). Rarely the primary cause may be acute rheumatism, neoplasm or hydatid cyst. In tuberculous cases it is frequently possible to isolate tubercle bacilli from the fluid by culture or guinea-pig inoculation. Sometimes a clear sterile effusion complicates pneumococcal pneumonia treated with sulphonamides and represents an abortive empyema; it is uncommon when penicillin is given in adequate dosage. Hydrothorax is seen in nephrosis and cardiac failure; it is not, of course, inflammatory in origin.

Clinical Features

The onset is often insidious with general loss of weight and slight fever. It may be more acute with pain in the chest, hypochondrium or shoulder. Pleural friction may be audible but is usually transient. When fluid has collected in the pleural space there is marked dullness to percussion and the affected side of the chest shows diminished movement. In large effusions the mediastinum is shifted towards the opposite side, and even the intercostal spaces may be filled in. In such cases there may be dyspnoea at rest. Above the fluid level the percussion note may have a "boxy" quality—skodaic resonance—due to compensatory emphysema of the uncollapsed portion of the lung. Auscultation may reveal greatly diminished breath sounds and vocal resonance. In children, however, the breath sounds are sometimes well heard and bronchial in quality, so that consolidation is wrongly suspected. The curved upper line of dullness with its highest point in the axilla (Ellis's S-shaped line), and Grocco's triangle of dullness over the opposite paravertebral region are, in practice, of no diagnostic value. The postero-anterior radiograph shows a uniform opacity with a curved upper border. When air is also present the fluid line is horizontal. Lateral and oblique films are necessary to define interlobar effusions. Thoracocentesis is necessary to confirm the diagnosis and to determine the nature of the fluid. In tuberculous cases the fluid is straw-coloured and the cells are mostly lymphocytes, whereas in hydrothorax the cells are mostly of endothelial origin. The tuberculin skin test is, of course, of great diagnostic value.

Treatment

In all tuberculous cases a course of anti-tuberculous drug treatment is necessary, as described in Chapter X. The pleural fluid should be emptied as far as possible, and it may be replaced on several occasions by streptomycin sulphate 250 mg. The prognosis is excellent. In other diseases the prognosis is that of the primary condition.

EMPYEMA

Aetiology

The aetiology of empyema has vastly altered in the thirty years since the author began the practice of medicine. Whereas empyema used to be either pneumococcal (usually metapneumonic) or streptococcal (usually synpneumonic), the great majority of cases today are staphylococcal in origin, and they are mostly encountered within the first year of life. Rarely a pneumococcal empyema is seen in an older child in whom the diagnosis of lobar pneumonia has been delayed for one reason or another. This changed situation in Britain and the United States has been reviewed by Hoffman (1961) and Ravitch and Fein (1961).

Clinical Features

When an empyema complicates an acute staphylococcal pneumonia in an infant, or chronic lung sepsis in fibrocystic disease of the pancreas, it is only part of the continuing septic process, so that the patient's temperature may show no significant alteration from its previous pattern. The physical signs in the chest are essentially those described in pleurisy with effusion, and the frequency with which bronchial breath sounds are heard in young infants can readily mislead the physician into thinking that they indicate consolidation alone. It is not always easy to detect the shift of the mediastinum which accompanies fluid in the pleural cavity in the case of a gravely ill, dyspnoeic infant. Radiography should be used to help in diagnosis, and thoracocentesis should always be performed on mere suspicion of pleural pus. A neglected empyema can lead to alarmingly rapid deterioration and death.

Treatment

In staphylococcal empyema in infants the organism is nearly always resistant to benzylpenicillin. The drugs of choice are methicillin, 100 mg./Kg./day or cloxacillin, 50 mg./Kg./day in four intramuscular doses. Methicillin should also be given intrapleurally in 100 mg. doses to replace the pus aspirated through a large bore needle every day or on alternate days. This regime is often sufficient to bring about recovery. However, if the pus is very thick, or if there is a pyopneumothorax, diagnosis should be followed by intercostal drainage by a polyethylene catheter under negative pressure. In pneumococcal cases in older children the drug of choice is benzylpenicillin, 500,000 units intramuscularly six-hourly. The pleural pus should also be removed by frequent aspirations through a needle, to be replaced on each occasion with 250,000 units of benzylpenicillin. Unpleasant manoeuvres like thoracocentesis in children should always be performed under sedation, such as can be achieved with rectal thiopentone in suitable dosage for weight. When pneumococcal pus is too thick to come through a needle, many thoracic surgeons now prefer pleurectomy to rib resection and drainage. It is imperative to avoid chronic empyema because of the severe bronchial damage which may ensue. For this reason the wise physician does not continue with repeated needle aspirations unduly long in unresponsive cases.

BRONCHIAL ASTHMA

A great deal has been written of this affliction and it has been approached through many channels, but like most "psychosomatic" disorders its satisfactory treatment continues to elude us. Even our understanding of its aetiology is incomplete and many of the ideas which have been expressed have revealed more of the writer's lack of scientific method than of the aetiology of asthma.

Aetiology

The existence of an allergic basis to true bronchial asthma cannot be doubted. Rarely, attacks can be traced to exposure to one allergen, but in most cases there appears to be a plethora of possible antigens. One of the difficulties in interpretation lies in the fact that symptomless and apparently normal individuals may quite commonly react to skin tests with a variety of foreign proteins. It is also certain that psychological disturbances of a quite ordinary kind can precipitate attacks of asthma in some individuals, although psychotherapy has proved to be disappointing in the management of the great majority of patients. A genetic influence is also clear enough in the frequency with which a family history of asthma, or other allergic conditions such as eczema and hay-fever, can be obtained. Many children with asthma have earlier suffered from atopic eczema and they may continue to suffer from flexural eczema—the prurigo-asthma syndrome. On the other hand, the role of reflex irritation from nasal polyps and the like has probably been exaggerated. Removal of such sources of irritation do not often greatly benefit the asthma. Asthmatic attacks are often precipitated by intercurrent respiratory infections. In some children this may well be a manifestation of sensitization to bacterial antigens, but the picture is confused by our not infrequent inability to distinguish true asthma from asthmatic bronchitis where the sole aetiological role may be played by viruses and bacteria. This difficulty is particularly great in the young infant in whom a diagnosis of asthma is frequently impossible until time has elapsed.

Clinical Features

The typical acute asthmatic attack is rarely seen before the second birthday. It frequently starts during the night when the child is awakened by expiratory respiratory distress. He looks frightened as well as distressed. He can be heard to wheeze with each forced expiration, and he may show some cyanosis. The chest is held in the full inspiratory position and the prolonged expiratory phase can be seen to involve the use of the accessory muscles of respiration. The percussion note is hyper-resonant and there is diminution of the areas of cardiac and liver dullness. Air entry to both lungs is greatly reduced so that the breath sounds are almost inaudible in some patients. The expiratory phase on auscultation is longer than the inspiratory phase and there may be many rhonchi. Crepitations are more common in very young children. The sputum is composed of sticky mucus. Microscopic examination reveals many eosinophils and mucus in the shape of spirals. The blood may also show a mild eosinophilia.

Many asthmatic children become completely free from bronchospasm between attacks. In others, expiratory difficulty and wheezing become established as a more or less permanent disability. The sternum may become unduly prominent with the development of Harrison's sulci through the years. In some children chronic respiratory infection still further aggravates the situation. Occasionally bronchial obstruction from tenacious mucus results in segmental or lobar atelectasis. This usually expands spontaneously and bronchiectasis is a rare complication.

Asthma rarely endangers life during childhood and hypertrophic vesicular emphysema does not develop.

Status asthmaticus can be dangerous. This is the name given to an acute attack which continues for several days at a time and is unusually unresponsive to treatment.

Treatment

(a) *The acute attack.*—In the fully developed attack the most useful routine measure is an intramuscular injection of 1/1,000 solution of adrenalin B.P., 0·3 to 0·5 ml. This may require to be repeated at half-hourly intervals to maintain relief from bronchospasm. Adrenalin is dangerous when given into a vein, so the plunger of the syringe must always be pulled back slightly before the injection is made to ensure that the needle has not entered a vein. If adrenalin fails to provide relief aminophylline 125 to 250 mg. may be injected intravenously in 5 to 10 ml. of water over a period of 10 minutes. This drug can cause syncope but the risk is small provided it is given slowly, and it is often most effective. Acute attacks of asthma can frequently be aborted if treated at the first sign of "tightness of the chest" with oral ephedrine hydrochloride ½–1 gr. (30–60 mg.). Alternatively, isoprenaline sulphate may be used, either as 10 mg. in tablet form sublingually or as a 1 per cent solution which is sprayed into the pharynx from an all-glass nebulizer during a forced inspiration. This is only practicable in older children. In status asthmaticus which has not responded to the treatment outlined above *the use of corticosteroids on a short-term basis* can be life-saving. It is doubtful if these potent drugs should be used outwith hospital. Indeed, we have been impressed by the frequency with which the emotional effect of hospitalization has itself resulted in the termination of an attack. Suitable oral dosage of prednisolone or prednisone is 15 mg. four times in the first 24 hours, 10 mg. four times in the second 24 hours, 10 mg. twice in the next 24 hours, and 5 mg. twice for another 24 hours. In dire emergency hydrocortisone sodium succinate may be given intraveneously in six-hourly doses of 50 to 100 mg. for 24 hours, to be followed by an oral steroid for another two or three days. As an attack of asthma begins to subside a sedative should be prescribed, such as quinalbarbitone ¾–1½ gr. (50–100 mg.). In this emergency the physician must show the equanimity which Osler stressed, and he must try to calm the anxious and alarmed parents.

(b) *Long-term management.*—Perhaps the most important consideration in this chronic problem is its psychological management. This can best be carried out by the child's family physician with his knowledge of the home background, its strengths and its weaknesses. The nature of the affliction should be carefully explained to the parents who should be brought to recognize that the child must live with his asthma and come to terms with it. Over-protection, avoidable absences from school, and an introspective attitude on the part of the child should be positively discouraged. Asthmatic children are often of high intelligence and do well at school in spite of periodic short absences. The author has frequently observed marked improvement in children whose parents are able to afford and willing to permit their education at a good boarding school. Sedatives and tranquillizers should not be given regularly. Anti-histamines such as promethazine hydrochloride (Phenergan) 25 mg. twice or thrice daily, or mepyramine maleate (Anthisan) 50 mg. twice or thrice daily are frequently prescribed. While they may control the hay-fever which some asthmatic children have, they do little for the bronchospasm. Ephedrine hydrochloride $\frac{1}{2}$ to 1 gr. (30–60 mg.) thrice daily is useful in chronic asthma, especially during bad spells. It loses its effectiveness after a few weeks and is better given intermittently rather than continuously.

Corticosteroids have been used on a long-term basis in some severely disabled children. The incidence of side-effects such as slowing of growth, obesity, osteoporosis, peptic ulcer, diabetes mellitus and acne renders the decision to institute such treatment a very onerous one. It can only be justified on very rare occasions and should rarely be taken by a single physician on his sole responsibility. It is, moreover, extremely difficult to withdraw steroids after prolonged use. Desensitization of the patient to those substances (house dust, feathers, animal hairs, various foods etc.) towards which he reacts when applied intradermally by scratch or injection has been much practised. Suitable testing sets are obtainable from several pharmaceutical firms who also supply the desensitizing solutions. It is often difficult to separate the psychological effects of frequent injections and medical interviews from the pharmacological effects of such treatment, but the author has not been impressed by its efficacy. On the other hand, deep breathing exercises supervised by a trained physiotherapist and preferably in a class with other children are of undoubted value in chronic asthmatics. So also is participation, under adequate supervision, in competitive games such as swimming, field sports and football. When asthma first makes its appearance in the pre-school child there is a strong possibility that he will "outgrow" his disability before or about the time of puberty. A more cautious prognosis is indicated when asthma has its onset at a later age.

REFERENCES

BAAR, H. S. (1955). *J. clin. Path.*, **8**, 19.

BEALE, A. J., McLEOD, D. L., STACKIW, W., and RHODES, A. J. (1958). *Brit. med. J.*, **1**, 302.

BENIANS, L. C., BENSON, P. F., SHERWOOD, T., and SPECTOR, R. G. (1964). *Guy's Hosp. Rep.*, **113**, 360.

BOMMER, W. (1961). *Germ. med. Mth.*, **6**, 291.

BROCK, R. C. (1950). *Thorax*, **5**, 5.

BROWNING, J. R., and HOUGHTON, J. D. (1956). *Amer. J. Med.*, **20**, 374.

CHANOCK, R. M. (1956). *J. exp. Med.*, **104**, 555.

CHANOCK, R. M., HAYFLICK, L., and BARILE, M. F. (1962). *Proc. nat. Acad. Sci.* (*Wash.*), **48**, 41.

DIAMANT, A., and KINNMAN, J. (1963). *Acta. paediat.* (*Uppsala*), **52**, 106.

EATON, M. D., MEIKLEJOHN, G., and VAN HERICK, W. (1944). *J. exp. Med.*, **79**, 649.

ELDERKIN, F. M., GARDNER, P. S., TURK, D. C., and WHITE, A. C. (1965). *Brit. med. J.*, **2**, 722.

FIELD, C. M. B., CONNOLLY, J. H., MURTAGH, G., SLATTERY, C. M., and TURKINGTON, E. E. (1966). *Brit. med. J.*, **1**, 83.

FRY, J. (1961). *The Catarrhal Child.* London: Butterworth & Co.

GAJDUSEK, D. C. (1957). *Pediatrics*, **19**, 543.

GOODBURN, G. M., MARMION, B. P., and KENDALL, E. J. C. (1963). *Brit. med. J.*, **1**, 1266.

HOFFMAN, E. (1961). *Thorax*, **16**, 128.

HOLZEL, A., PARKER, L., PATTERSON, W. H., WHITE, L. L. R., THOMPSON, K. M., and TOBIN, J. O'H. (1963). *Lancet*, **1**, 295.

HUTCHISON, J. H. (1951). *Tubercle (Edinb.)*, **32**, 271.

HUTCHISON, J. H. (1955). *Lancet*, **2**, 844 and 1196.

JOSEPH, R., JOB, J-C., and GENTIL, C. (1957). *Arch. franç. Pédiat.*, **14**, 1.

LENDRUM, A. C., SCOTT, L. D. W., and PARK, S. D. S. (1950). *Quart. J. Med.*, **19**, 249.

MACFARLANE, P. S., and SOMMERVILLE, R. G. (1957). *Lancet*, **1**, 770.

MCKAY, E., and RICHARDSON, J. (1959). *Lancet*, **2**, 713.

MARSHALL, W. C., WESTON, H. J., and BODIAN, M. (1964). *Arch. Dis. Childh.*, **39**, 18.

NICOL, C. G. M. (1957). *Mth. Bull. Minist. Hlth. Lab. Serv.*, **16**, 192.

NORMAN, A. P. (1963). *Congenital Abnormalities in Infancy.* Oxford: Blackwell Scientific Publications.

POTTER, E. L. (1961). *Pathology of the Fetus and Infant*, 2nd edit. Chicago: Year Book Publishers.

RAVITCH, M. M., and FEIN, R. (1961). *J. Amer. med. Ass.*, **175**, 1039.

SCOTTISH HEALTH SERVICES COUNCIL (1963). *Bronchitis.* (Report of a Sub-Committee of the Standing Medical Advisory Committee). Edinburgh: H.M. Staty. Office.

SPENCE, J., WALTON, W. S., MILLER, F. J. W., and COURT, S. D. M. (1954). *One Thousand Families in Newcastle-upon-Tyne.* London: Oxford Univ. Press.

STUART-HARRIS, C. H. (1962). *Brit. med. J.*, **2**, 869.

TYRRELL, D. A. J. (1965). *Common Colds and Related Diseases.* London: Edward Arnold.

WHITE, W. F., SAXTON, H. M., and DAWSON, I. M. D. (1961). *Brit. med. J.*, **2**, 1327.

WYLLIE, W. G., SHELDON, W., BODIAN, M., and BARLOW, A. (1948). *Quart. J. Med.*, **17**, 251.

CHAPTER XIV

ACQUIRED DISEASES OF THE HEART

The most common cause of acquired heart disease in childhood is, of course, acute rheumatism (Chapter X). Apart from causing death during childhood from extensive myocardial involvement leading to congestive cardiac failure, the rheumatic process may result in severe valvular deformities which from mechanical reasons give rise to trouble in adult life, e.g. mitral stenosis and incompetence and/or aortic stenosis and incompetence. It is, of course, common to find mitral and aortic regurgitation singly or together in children who have active rheumatic endocarditis in addition to myocarditis. On the other hand, acquired stenosis of the mitral or aortic valves is very rare in childhood, because several years must elapse before constriction of the valve rings can develop. It is not proposed to devote space to the diagnosis of individual valvular lesions because the acute rheumatic manifestations have already been dealt with in Chapter X and the chronic lesions come more often within the orbit of the general physician or the cardiologist. It remains to state, however, that rheumatic fever has shown a greatly reduced incidence in the more prosperous countries of the world in recent years. It is, therefore, likely that chronic rheumatic disease of the heart valves will occupy less of the internist's time in the future.

Other acquired diseases of the heart are rare in childhood but sufficiently important as causes of death or severe illness to justify adequate description.

ACUTE MYOCARDITIS

Aetiology

There are several widely different causes of myocardial disease in childhood. Diphtheritic myocarditis was once a common cause of death, signs appearing usually in the third week of illness, but in Britain today is virtually unknown. Physicians of an earlier era used to talk of "toxic myocarditis" as a factor in causing death in a large number of the common infectious diseases of that day, e.g. scarlet fever, pneumonia, influenza, poliomyelitis and meningococcal septicaemia. The existence of such a condition is open to doubt and the modern physician deals with these varied infections without much anxiety as to the state of the patient's myocardium. Myocardial involvement in acute nephritis, on the other hand, has been increasingly recognized as a not uncommon cause of cardiac failure in childhood. Indeed, the author has been led to the diagnosis of acute glomerulonephritis on several occasions by finding that a child who was in obvious cardiac failure also had systemic hypertension (Chapter XVII).

A separate fairly clearly defined clinical entity has been called "idiopathic myocarditis" or "Fiedler's myocarditis". This disease may occur at any age, but is most often seen in the first seven years. Cases have been reported in the neonatal period and the peak incidence appears to be between 1 and 2 years. In recent times there have been reports that such cases are due to infection by Group B Coxsackie viruses (Javett et al., 1956; Van Creveld and De Jager, 1956; Woodward et al., 1960; Boles and Hosier, 1963). These enteroviruses can cause a variety of diseases including also meningo-encephalitis, pericarditis and hepatitis. In fact, all of these conditions have been found in young children who have died of acute myocarditis.

Clinical Picture

The symptoms of abdominal pain, fever, anorexia, dyspnoea and cough develop suddenly in a young child who has previously been perfectly well. He quickly becomes seriously ill with pallor, cyanosis of peripheral type, and frequently diarrhoea and vomiting. The signs of congestive cardiac failure which predominate are cardiac enlargement, gallop rhythm without a murmur, crepitations over the lungs, and increasing hepatomegaly. Oedema is often slight or absent. The chest X-ray shows generalized cardiac enlargement and often, bilateral pleural effusions. The electrocardiograph (ECG) shows abnormalities of a non-specific character in the S-T segments and T waves. The erythrocyte sedimentation rate is moderately raised but the ASO titre is normal.

Differential Diagnosis

At the onset of the illness the severe abdominal pain may simulate acute appendicitis. There is usually less muscular rigidity in myocarditis, and enlargement of the liver should direct attention to the heart. It is often impossible during life to exclude other causes of cardiac failure in early childhood such as endocardial fibro-elastosis, anomalous left coronary artery (Chapter XV) and glycogen storage disease of the heart (Chapter IX). Acute myocarditis is more likely when the child has been in good health prior to the onset of the illness and when his nutritional state is obviously good. Later confirmation of the diagnosis may be obtained by isolation of the Coxsackie virus. "Acute benign pericarditis" also enters the differential diagnosis; indeed the two diseases are often caused by the same virus and may co-exist.

Treatment

The prognosis is grave and many cases end fatally. Some, however, show a marked response to treatment. The child should be propped up in bed and given oxygen in a tent. Digitalization should be achieved with oral or intramuscular digoxin (paediatric lanoxin elixir, B. W. & Co.) 0·08 mg./Kg./day in four divided doses. After 24 to 48 hours a maintenance dose of 0·02 mg./Kg./day may be given in two equal doses. An oral diuretic such as chlorothiazide 25 mg./Kg./day should also be given in four divided doses. A broad spectrum antibiotic such as tetracycline 25 mg./Kg./day should be administered to protect the very ill child from intercurrent bacterial infection. Corticosteroids have been recommended but they cannot be free from risk of aggravating the cardiac failure by producing water and salt retention. Perhaps their use should be confined to patients who do not show a rapid response to more conservative treatment. The course of the disease should be controlled by regular radiographic and electrocardiographic observations, especially as some patients show undue susceptibility to digoxin. None the less, digitalization should be maintained for many weeks after recovery from the acute attack.

ACUTE PERICARDITIS

Aetiology

Until a few years ago acute pericarditis in children indicated rheumatic fever, with the exception of a few less acute cases which were tuberculous in origin. Within the past decade or thereabouts both these varieties of pericarditis have become quite uncommon. Indeed, in the past few years the author has seen pericarditis associated with rheumatoid arthritis (Chapter XXVI) as frequently as with rheumatic fever. In the former, of course, endocarditis and myocarditis are usually absent. "*Acute benign idiopathic pericarditis*" has become relatively more common. Many of these cases are due to Group B Coxsackie viruses (Weinstein, 1957; Woodward *et al.*, 1960). Septic pericarditis was once a common complication of pneumonia and left sided empyema, and of pyaemia due to a variety of pyogenic organisms. It has been almost abolished by the modern antibacterial drugs. Finally, pericarditis may develop in the child dying from uraemia. This is thought to be chemical irritation of the pericardial endothelium.

Clinical Features

While these vary to some extent according to the aetiology, certain features are common to all types of pericarditis. One of the most characteristic is pain. This may be severe in rheumatic or viral cases, and is often slight in tuberculous cases. The pain is most often retrosternal, but it may be in the upper abdomen or in the left shoulder. The ease with which the abdominal pain may be misinterpreted as due to appendicitis has been stressed by Boles and Hosier (1963). Other general features are dyspnoea, fever, and a tendency on the part of the child to lean forwards. The most valuable diagnostic sign is, of course, pericardial friction which may have a double or triple rhythm and which, in any event, is not synchronized to the heart sounds as are murmurs. It is best heard with the patient leaning forwards and with the stethoscope placed firmly against the chest wall. It is not heard in every case, nor is its presence indicative of the amount of fluid in the pericardial sac. The area of cardiac dullness is usually demonstrably increased upwards as well as to the left and right. A common finding is dullness and bronchial breath sounds at the inferior angle of the left scapula (Ewart's or Bamberger's sign). Its cause has been variously attributed to pleural effusion, pulmonary compression by the pericardial sac and "rheumatic pneumonia". When there is a lot of fluid in the pericardial sac with cardiac tamponade the heart sounds are distant and muffled, the neck veins are visibly distended, hepatomegaly develops and the pulse pressure is reduced due to inadequate cardiac output. There may be pulsus paradoxicus in which the systolic blood pressure is reduced during inspiration. This may be palpable at the radial pulse but is best demonstrated with a sphygmomanometer. The heart shadow on radiography is usually much enlarged with a short wide supracardiac shadow—"water-bottle" shape. Fluoroscopy reveals much diminished cardiac pulsation. The heart shadow in pericarditis frequently fluctuates rapidly in size, a useful distinguishing feature from gross cardiac enlargement due to rheumatic pancarditis, in which cardiomegaly only recedes very slowly if ever. The characteristic electrocardiographic changes are low voltage, elevation and convexity of the S-T segment in all three standard leads, and T wave inversion.

Diagnosis

In rheumatic pericarditis there is almost invariably a loud apical systolic murmur in addition to pericardial friction. The child is pale, toxic in appearance, and may have other manifestations such as arthritis or nodules. The A.S.O. titre is usually raised. It is unusual to find a large volume of fluid in pericarditis of rheumatic origin and paracentesis is rarely indicated. On the other hand, in tuberculous cases large collections of straw-coloured lymphocytic exudate with cardiac tamponade are the rule in the early stages of the disease. The Mantoux test will be positive and there may be other signs of intrathoracic or disseminated tuberculosis. Septic pericarditis is associated with gross suppuration elsewhere. Cardiac tamponade is common and a large volume of pus may be found in the pericardial sac. In viral pericarditis there are, of course, no signs of disease in other systems of the body. The heart sounds are usually pure, if muffled, and if there is a systolic murmur it is soft and unimpressive. There is frequently a history obtainable of a recently preceding upper respiratory infection.

Treatment

General measures include bed rest with the head and back supported. Cyanosis demands the use of an oxygen tent. An ice-bag placed over the precordium may be old-fashioned but is often extremely soothing. Anti-rheumatic treatment with a combination of salicylates, corticosteroids and penicillin (Chapter X) should be given in rheumatic pericarditis, although the child is likely to be left with a severe permanent cardiac disability from the associated myocarditis and endocarditis. Tuberculous cases require the energetic use of streptomycin, isoniazid and PAS (Chapter X). Whenever there is a cardiac tamponade the fluid should be removed from the pericardial sac by paracentesis. This is especially often a problem in tuberculous cases. The prognosis in tuberculous pericarditis, once very poor, is now quite good although constrictive pericarditis may develop in some instances. Patients with septic pericarditis must have intensive antibiotic treatment according to the sensitivities of the causal bacteria. It is essential also to empty the pericardial sac either by paracentesis or thoracotomy. There are no specific drugs available for Coxsackie virus infections. It should be stressed that in large pericardial effusions from any cause paracentesis can be life-saving, whereas digitalization is ineffective.

CHRONIC CONSTRICTIVE PERICARDITIS
(Pick's Disease)

This is a rare condition in paediatric practice. The majority of cases seen by the author have been undoubtedly tuberculous in origin. We have seen it follow a proven Coxsackie virus pericarditis on one occasion. In many adult cases, however, the primary cause cannot be determined.

Clinical Features

These are due to impaired ventricular filling, diminished stroke volume and increased pressure in the veins and right atrium. The neck veins are visibly distended. This distension may increase during inspiration and decrease during expiration, in contrast to the normal state of affairs. Pulsus paradoxicus is also found. Gross ascites and hepatomegaly tend to contrast with the mild degree of oedema found in the legs. The heart sounds are pure but feeble. There may be protodiastolic triple rhythm. Fluoroscopy reveals a small heart with absent or greatly diminished pulsations. The diagnosis can sometimes be confirmed by the demonstration of pericardial calcification. The electrocardiograph shows low voltage and T wave inversion.

Treatment

The only measure which can relieve the fully developed case is radical pericardiectomy. These patients are particularly likely to develop cardiac arrest during the induction of anaesthesia. The results are good to moderate in those who survive the operation.

BACTERIAL ENDOCARDITIS

This is not a common disease in childhood. The customary sub-division into "acute" and "subacute" forms is not really satisfactory and cases are better classified according to their bacterial cause. The majority are due to *Streptococcus viridans*, but many organisms can cause the disease, e.g. staphylococci, β haemolytic streptococci, pneu-mococci and coliforms. Staphylococcal cases are more common in children than in adults. The vast majority of infections are superimposed upon pre-existing rheumatic or congenital heart disease, the latter forming a much higher proportion than is the case in bacterial endo-carditis in adults. It is well known that the bacteraemia which must precede bacterial endocarditis is sometimes related to the extraction of teeth or the removal of tonsils, but in most cases there is no such defined preceding event. In the young infant a rather different category of bacterial endocarditis is occasionally encountered. This forms but part of a generalized pyaemic process with other septic foci such as osteitis, empyema and pyoderma. There is no underlying cardiac malformation in these infants and the endocarditis is only one factor in causing death.

Pathology

The typical finding is of large crumbling vegetations on the valve cusps along the lines of apposition. These are composed of fibrin, leucocytes and bacteria. In some cases the process is not found on the valves. For example, in cases complicating patent ductus arteriosus the vegetations are commonly found on the wall of the pulmonary artery opposite to the site of entry of the duct—bacterial endarteritis. In cases complicating ventricular septal defect the vegetations may be on the right-hand surface of the ventricular septum or on the wall of the right ventricle—mural endocarditis. The bloodstream carries off small portions of these vegetations to result in embolism in many organs, e.g. lungs, kidneys, brain and spleen.

Clinical Features

The diagnosis should be suspected whenever a child with rheumatic or congenital heart disease develops fever, leucocytosis, an alteration in the character of the cardiac murmurs, and embolic phenomena such as splenomegaly, haematuria, petechiae and subungual flame-shaped haemorrhages. Osler's nodes, raised tender red spots on the fingertips, are uncommon in children. Clubbing of the fingers is of diagnostic significance in the absence of preceding cyanotic congenital heart disease. In cases due to *Strept. viridans* fever is not usually above 102° F. and progressive muddy pallor is common. In staphylococcal cases high fever, 102–104° F., is the rule and the disease runs a rapid course. In mural endocarditis of the right ventricle pulmonary embolism may cause pain in the chest, dyspnoea, haemoptysis and clinical and radiographic signs of infarction. The diagnosis can be confirmed by isolation of the organism in blood cultures, which should be taken at least three times daily as soon as the diagnosis is suspected. When blood cultures are repeatedly negative the clinician is posed with a difficult problem, but in the child acutely ill with cardiac and embolic signs treatment should rarely be delayed for longer than 72 hours.

Treatment

An antibiotic, bactericidal rather than bacteristatic, chosen according to the bacterial sensitivities should be given by the intramuscular or intravenous routes in large doses for at least six weeks. *Strept. viridans* is usually sensitive to benzylpenicillin and a suitable dosage is 1 mega unit four times daily. In more resistant cases even larger doses should be given and, in addition, streptomycin sulphate 50 mg./Kg./day should be given intramuscularly in two divided doses. In staphylococcal cases the drug of choice is still benzylpenicillin for sensitive organisms. In cases of penicillin-resistance suitable drugs are methicillin (Celbenin) 100 mg./Kg./day and cloxacillin (Orbenin) 50 mg./Kg./day in four daily intramuscular doses. Drugs such as ampicillin, tetracycline and chloramphenicol are required in the rare cases caused by Gram-negative organisms.

Prevention

Minor surgical procedures such as dental extraction or tonsillectomy should always be "covered" with penicillin in children known to have organic disease of the heart. A mixture of benzyl, procaine and ben-ethamine penicillins has proved satisfactory, e.g. one intramuscular dose of Triplopen 1·25 mega units on the morning of operation.

DISORDERS OF CARDIAC RHYTHM

The cardiac arrhythmias are less common and usually of less serious import in children than in adults.

SINUS ARRHYTHMIA

In this phenomenon the heart rate increases during inspiration and slows during expiration. The condition has been related to increased vagal activity. It is commonly found in perfectly healthy children, although it is considerably over-stating the case to suggest that sinus arrhythmia in itself indicates a normal heart.

EXTRASYSTOLES

Ectopic cardiac beats arise from impulses which have their origin outwith the sino-atrial node, e.g. the atria, the atrioventricular node or the ventricles. They do not, in themselves, carry serious significance. Indeed they may occur in apparently healthy children. In present-day Britain enquiry as to cigarette smoking is not superfluous in the case of the older child. Extrasystoles may also complicate organic disease of the heart or the action of digitalis. They may cause the child to become aware of his heart action but are more often symptomless. In the case of ventricular extrasystoles the premature beat is followed by a compensatory pause which fully compensates for the preceding short diastole. In atrial or nodal ectopic beats the following compensating pause is not marked. The diagnosis should be confirmed by electrocardiography. Extrasystoles which occur in a healthy heart are usually abolished by exercise, whereas they are rendered more frequent when the myocardium is diseased. Treatment should be directed towards the underlying cardiac disease. Ectopic beats in healthy children do not require treatment unless they are producing anxiety when phenobarbitone $\frac{1}{2}$ gr. (30 mg.) twice daily may provide some relief.

PAROXYSMAL TACHYCARDIA

This is most often seen in supraventricular form in young infants who do not exhibit any other signs of heart disease. Early diagnosis is important to avoid death from cardiac failure, especially as the long-term prognosis is excellent. The condition is rare in older children but in about 10 per cent of cases is then associated with the Wolff-Parkinson-White syndrome in which, between attacks of tachycardia, there is a short P-R interval and a wide QRS complex so that the total P-S duration remains normal. Ventricular tachycardia is very uncommon in children.

Clinical Features

The young infant with paroxysmal tachycardia early develops congestive cardiac failure. He looks anxious and ill with dyspnoea, restlessness, subcostal recession, greyish cyanosis, and reluctance to feed. Cardiomegaly and hepatomegaly are marked. There may be facial or generalized oedema. Crepitations over the lungs may be due solely to cardiac failure or in part to the respiratory infection which sometimes seems to precipitate the tachycardia. The heart rate is over 280 per minute. There may be a systolic murmur which disappears after the attack has been brought under control. Radiographs show an enlarged heart and passive congestion of the lungs.

In older children cardiac failure ultimately develops if the paroxysm lasts long enough. Accurate diagnosis of the nature of the tachycardia can only be reached by electrocardiography.

Treatment

In paroxysmal tachycardia in infants the drug of choice is digoxin given orally or intramuscularly as 0·1 mg./Kg./day divided into four daily doses. After the tachycardia has been controlled a maintenance dose of 0·025 mg./Kg./day in two equal doses should be continued for at least six months to prevent recurrences which are liable to be precipitated by minor infections. The long-term prognosis is excellent, and the immediate effects of digitalization are most impressive and gratifying.

In older children vagal stimulation may be tried before resort is made to digitalis. There are several methods, e.g. pressure on one carotid artery as high in the neck as possible, pressure on the eyeballs, the Valsalva manoeuvre, or the induction of vomiting with 1–2 teaspoonfuls (4–8 ml.) of syrup of ipecacuanha.

In the rare cases of ventricular tachycardia reflex stimulation and digitalis should be eschewed. The drug of choice is procainamide given intramuscularly, 50 mg. at once and 50 mg. every two hours until the attack ceases. Hypotension is an indication for withdrawal of treatment. In an emergency the drug may be given intravenously under continuous electrocardiographic control.

ATRIAL FLUTTER AND ATRIAL FIBRILLATION

These serious arrhythmias are rarely seen in children and they are almost invariably associated with grave rheumatic or congenital lesions. In flutter there is a regular tachycardia, and in fibrillation an irregular irregularity. The diagnosis should be confirmed by electrocardiography. Congestive failure is the rule because the heart is already seriously damaged. The drug of choice in each case is digoxin in the dosage recommended above. When the heart rate has been slowed and if sinus rhythm does not return spontaneously quinidine may be tried. After a test dose of 25 mg. by mouth, 100 mg. should be given every two hours until normal rhythm is restored. The dose may need to be increased to 200 mg. two-hourly. Toxic effects such as nausea, vomiting and tinnitus necessitate withdrawal of the drug. After normal rhythm has been restored the digoxin may be slowly withdrawn but a maintenance dose of quinidine, 200–400 mg. four times daily, should be continued for some months. These children, however, rarely have long to live after such an episode.

HEART BLOCK

In childhood, heart block is often congenital and it is then usually complete. In some cases there are cyanotic or acyanotic congenital anomalies; in others no cardiac abnormality can be detected. Incomplete heart block may also be unassociated with detectable cardiac disease, but in most cases there is a discoverable cause, e.g. rheumatic, diphtheritic or viral myocarditis; congenital anomalies such as atrial septal defect or Ebstein's anomaly; and digitalis over-dosage.

INCOMPLETE HEART BLOCK

In first-degree block the P-R interval on the electrocardiogram is longer than is normal for the age of the patient (Nadas, 1963). In second-degree block some P waves fail altogether to be followed by ventricular QRS complexes. In the Wenckebach phenomenon there is progressive lengthening of the P-R intervals until finally a QRS complex is missed. In other cases the block may involve every third, fourth or fifth complex in a regular manner.

COMPLETE HEART BLOCK

In third-degree block there is a complete dissociation of the contractions of the ventricles and the atria. In children the ventricular rhythm is usually set at about 40 per minute, rising rarely more than 20 after exercise. The electrocardiograph shows, of course, that P waves have a rhythm which is totally unrelated to that of the QRS complexes. Stokes-Adams attacks are very rare in children and the prognosis of heart block is that of the primary cardiac condition. Some affected children with congenital heart block seem likely to have a normal life-expectancy.

Treatment

Specific treatment is required only for the underlying cardiac disease. In its absence no attempt should be made to alter the cardiac rate or rhythm.

CARDIAC FAILURE IN INFANCY

Aetiology

Congestive cardiac failure in infancy is not at all uncommon. It may be due to paroxysmal tachycardia when the long-term prognosis is excellent. Various congenital anomalies can result in heart failure in the early days or weeks of life, especially aortic valve atresia, hypoplastic aortic arch, transposition of the great vessels, patent ductus arteriosus with or without coarctation of the aorta, and ventricular septal defect with pulmonary hypertension. Other causes include endocardial fibro-elastosis, viral myocarditis and glycogen accumulation disease of the heart.

Clinical Features

Breathlessness on exertion takes the form of slowness with feeds. The infant becomes dyspnoeic with subcostal recession. The precordium may become unduly prominent. There is sleeplessness, restlessness and often pallor and cyanosis. Venous congestion is not readily detected in the infant, but hepatomegaly is marked and easily found. The heart is usually grossly enlarged, tachycardia is present, and there is often a loud murmur. Oedema is a late sign. It appears first in the face of the young infant, then in the genitalia and lumbosacral area before the feet. Crepitations over the lungs may be misinterpreted as due to respiratory infection; indeed such an infection may be the precipitating cause of the cardiac failure and it is important that the physician recognize the true significance of the other signs of heart disease.

Treatment

The infant should be nursed with the head well raised above the feet. Cyanosis and restlessness are indications for oxygen given by tent. Digoxin should be administered in the doses recommended on p. 234. The first one or two doses can be given intramuscularly. If oedema is marked chlorothiazide 25 mg./Kg./day is given in four divided doses by mouth. When diuretics are being given the serum potassium level should be tested frequently and the electrocardiograph carried out at regular intervals. Hypokalaemia should be treated with oral potassium chloride 0·5 gm. twice daily. Oedema may also be reduced by replacing the infant's usual milk formula with a low sodium dried milk such as Edosol (Trufood) which contains 1 mg. sodium per reconstituted fluid ounce.

CARDIAC FAILURE IN OLDER CHILDREN

The clinical picture of cardiac failure in older children is very much the same as that with which we are familiar in adults and a detailed description is unnecessary. Pure left heart failure is uncommon in childhood but may occur in renal hypertension, aortic stenosis, coarctation of the aorta, mitral stenosis and patent ductus arteriosus. It is characterized by pulmonary oedema and rales, left sided hydrothorax, gallop rhythm, cardiac asthma and pulsus alternans. Pure right heart failure is more common in the form of increased venous pressure, hepatomegaly, peripheral oedema and right hydrothorax. It may be caused by pulmonic stenosis, atrial septal defect, transposition of the great vessels and anomalous pulmonary venous drainage. However, in children the most common form of congestive cardiac failure involves both ventricles. It may be due to most of the causes mentioned above, to myocarditis, most often rheumatic, to paroxysmal tachycardia, or to pericarditis. The treatment is along the lines so well tried in adults.

REFERENCES

BOLES, E. T., and HOSIER, D. M. (1963). *Amer. J. Dis. Child.*, **105**, 70.

JAVETT, S. N., HEYMANN, S., MUNDEL, R., PEPLER, W. J., LURIE, H. I., GEAR, J., MEASROCH, V., and KIRSCH, Z. (1956). *J. Pediat.*, **48**, 1.

NADAS, A. S. (1963). *Pediatric Cardiology*, 2nd edit. Philadelphia: W. B. Saunders.

VAN CREVELD, S., and DE JAGER, H. (1956). *Ann. paediat. (Basel)*, **187**, 100.

WEINSTEIN, S. B. (1957). *New Engl. J. Med.*, **257**, 265.

WOODWARD, T. E., McCRUMB, F. R. Jr., CAREY, T. N., and TOGO, Y. (1960). *Ann. intern. Med.*, **53**, 1130.

CHAPTER XV

CONGENITAL ABNORMALITIES OF THE HEART

Incidence, Aetiology and Classification

The cardiovascular system comes only after the nervous system in the frequency with which developmental abnormalities occur. It is, perhaps, insufficiently appreciated by physicians who see only older children and adults with heart disease that 70 per cent of all infants born with cardiac malformations fail to reach their first birthday. Remarkable although surgical advances in the correction of cardiac anomalies have been in recent years, it must be realized that the vast majority of such cases are still inoperable. The main efforts of the paediatric cardiologist and the surgeon are now being directed towards the malformations which so often cause death during early infancy. It should be stated also that the marked fall in the incidence of rheumatic fever in the more prosperous countries has now resulted in the fact that congenital heart disease is more common than rheumatic heart disease.

The aetiological factors in congenital heart disease are only vaguely perceived at the present time. It is known that certain environmental factors operating in early pregnancy can result in malformations, e.g. rubella, irradiation, and drugs such as thalidomide. In most cases, however, no specific cause can be detected. Genetic influences seem not to be of great importance, although the relatives of affected children are more often similarly abnormal than would be expected to occur by chance. The risk of a sib of an index patient also having congenital heart disease is of the order of 1 in 50 as against a frequency of about 1 in 100 in the community at large. There are, however, single families in which the risk is much higher. In addition, cardiac malformations are well recognized to be the frequent accompaniment of several syndromes, e.g. mongolism (Fallot's tetralogy, ventricular septal, and ostium primum defects), arachnodactyly (defects of the aorta), polydactyly (ventricular septal defects), Turner's syndrome (coarctation of the aorta), triphalangeal thumbs (atrial septal defects in the Holt-Oram syndrome).

No classification of congenital heart disease can be entirely satisfactory. It is convenient to subdivide the malformations into those which cause central cyanosis, largely due to shunts of blood from the right to the left side of the heart, and those in which cyanosis is absent. The separation is not absolute. Thus, less severe lesions such as Fallot's tetralogy may not cause cyanosis during the early months of life. On the other hand, some anomalies such as patent ductus arteriosus or ventricular septal defect, where there is a left-to-right shunt, may later cause cyanosis if pulmonary hypertension causes a reversal of the shunt through the defect—*cyanose tardive*. The physician must be careful in every child with central cyanosis that he does not fall into the trap of making a diagnosis of congenital heart disease in the rare case of congenital methaemoglobinaemia (Chapter IX). In this metabolic disorder there is, of course, no abnormality in the heart. The possible combinations and variations of cardiac malformations are so numerous that precise diagnosis frequently demands an extremely high standard of clinical expertness, plus complicated ancillary investigations such as cardiac catheterization, dye dilution studies and angiocardiography and aortography. For details of these methods the reader is referred to the excellent textbooks by Keith *et al.* (1958), Kjellberg *et al.* (1959), Taussig (1960), Nadas (1963) and Gasul *et al.* (1966). In this chapter attention is confined to the more common malformations which, naturally, comprise the great majority of cases encountered in practice. The paediatrician must be able to recognize these, to realize when a case is unusual, and refer to a paediatric cardiologist all patients for whom detailed investigation and surgery seem likely to offer hope of cure.

(A) CYANOTIC CONGENITAL HEART DISEASE

TRANSPOSITION OF THE GREAT VESSELS

This is the most common type of cyanotic congenital heart disease, but as few patients survive beyond their first birthday it is infrequently encountered in cardiac units which do not regularly admit young infants.

Anatomy

The aorta arises from the right ventricle and the pulmonary artery from the left. The venae cavae and the pulmonary veins drain normally into the right and left atria respectively. There is occasionally stenosis of the valve between the left ventricle and the pulmonary artery. Life could not be maintained if this situation were to exist alone, but there is a left-to-right shunt through a ventricular septal defect, atrial septal defect, patent ductus arteriosus or some combination of these.

Clinical Features

Affected infants fail to thrive and are usually markedly cyanosed from birth. Dyspnoea may be present at rest with subcostal recession, and it is always obvious during feeds. Finger clubbing may develop early in life. The precordium is seen to be prominent and palpation reveals an excessively forceful cardiac impulse in the left parasternal area. Thrills are absent. There may be no murmurs but a loud systolic murmur is often best heard at the left lower sternal border. The pulmonic second sound is not remarkable. Cardiac enlargement of gross degree develops rapidly. The characteristic cardiac silhouette in postero-anterior or oblique radiographs shows an enlarged heart with a narrow supracardiac shadow, rather like an egg lying on its side (Fig. 44). The lungs are engorged. In the left anterior oblique view, however, the supracardiac shadow may appear wide.

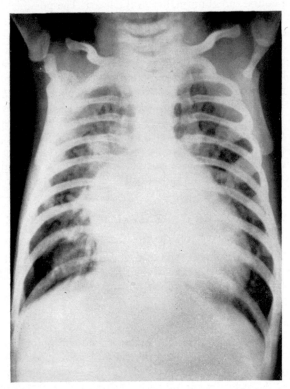

Fig. 44.—Radiograph in transposition of great vessels. Note enlarged egg-shaped heart, narrow supracardiac shadow and engorged lungs.

The electrocardiograph shows right axis deviation with right ventricular or biventricular hypertrophy, and there may be a P pulmonale. Cardiac catheterization will reveal that the catheter leaves the right ventricle by the aorta. The pulmonary artery blood has an oxygen concentration above that in the aorta. Various other shunts can be demonstrated according to their site. The diagnosis can also be confirmed by angiocardiography.

Prognosis

Most infants go into cardiac failure in the early months of life with increasing dyspnoea, cyanosis, cardiomegaly and hepatomegaly. This is frequently precipitated by intercurrent respiratory infection.

Treatment

Without surgical treatment 85 per cent of infants with transposed great arteries die in the first six months of life. Until recently none of the surgical operations devised had proved very successful, although the Blalock-Hanlon procedure, whereby an atrial septal defect is created or enlarged, has been a valuable palliative measure capable of prolonging life beyond early infancy. In the past few years some highly gratifying results have been reported from an operation devised by Mustard (1964) of Toronto, and later modified at Great Ormond Street (Aberdeen et al., 1965). A patch of pericardium is so inserted into the atria that the systemic venous blood is directed via the mitral valve to the left ventricle and thence via the transposed pulmonary artery to the lungs. Pulmonary venous blood is correspondingly routed via the tricuspid valve to the right ventricle and into the transposed aorta. This complicated procedure obviously requires the use of a heart/lung machine and the palliative Blalock-Hanlon procedure must be an essential preliminary to permit the infant to survive to an age when the major operation becomes practicable. The ideal surgical manoeuvre would be repositioning of the transposed great arteries but the necessary transfer of the coronary arteries has not yet been achieved.

Total Anomalous Pulmonary Venous Drainage

This is a less common defect which also ends fatally before the end of the first year of life in many cases.

Anatomy

All the pulmonary veins, as well as the venae cavae enter the right atrium. There must, of course, be an atrial septal defect for life to continue at all. There are several possible anatomical variations. Most commonly the pulmonary veins form a common vessel which empties into a persisting left superior vena cava, less often into the right superior vena cava. The pulmonary veins may also unite to form a common trunk which drains directly into the right atrium or into the coronary sinus. Rarely the pulmonary veins drain into the inferior vena cava or even the portal vein.

Clinical Features

These infants fail to thrive, are cyanotic, and become dyspnoeic on slight exertion. They are extremely prone to respiratory infections.

P.P.P.—9

Cardiac pulsation is forceful over the left parasternal area, that is over the right ventricle and its outflow tract. The precordium may bulge. Auscultation often reveals triple or quadruple rhythm and there is usually a blowing systolic murmur. The electrocardiograph shows right axis deviation, severe right ventricular hypertrophy and a P pulmonale. Radiographs show right atrial and right ventricular enlargement with engorged (pleonaemic) lungs. In the common type of anomaly with a

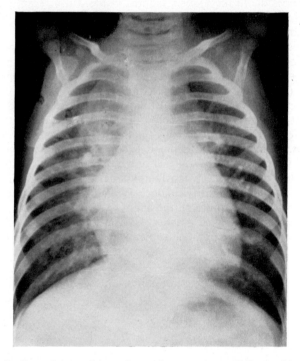

Fig. 45.—Radiograph in total anomalous pulmonary venous drainage with persisting left superior vena cava. Note "cottage-loaf" or "figure-of-eight" heart due to broad supracardiac shadow. The lungs are engorged.

persisting left superior vena cava the supracardiac shadow is very broad giving rise to the so-called "cottage-loaf", "figure-of-eight" or "snow-man" heart (Fig. 45). Cardiac catheterization reveals the same oxygen concentration in the right atrium, right ventricle, pulmonary artery and femoral artery; the pressures in the right ventricle and pulmonary artery are above normal. The diagnosis can also be confirmed by selective angiocardiography when the opaque medium is injected into the pulmonary artery.

Prognosis

Most affected infants develop right heart failure early with progressive dyspnoea, cardiomegaly and hepatomegaly.

Treatment

The most common type of operation is based upon an anastomosis of the common pulmonary venous trunk to the back of the left atrium. After the age of one year this type of correction carries a low mortality and gives good results, but the same operation in early infancy is associated with a considerable mortality.

FALLOT'S TETRALOGY

This is the most common type of cyanotic congenital heart disease in children over the age of 1 year.

Anatomy

The classical tetrad consists of pulmonary stenosis (rarely atresia), ventricular septal defect with right-to-left shunt, dextroposition of the aorta which receives blood from both ventricles, and right ventricular hypertrophy. There are many variations depending upon the degree and type of pulmonic stenosis, the size of the ventricular septal defect and the degree of over-riding of the aorta. In most instances the pulmonic obstruction is infundibular, there being a long, narrow separate infundibular chamber; in others it is a valvular stenosis. In some cases there is a right-sided aortic arch, a matter of importance to the cardiac surgeon. ~25% of cases.

Clinical Features

Cyanosis is usually marked from early childhood, although it is often absent in the first few months of life. It may be quite slight in some less severely disabled children. Cyanosis is associated with stunting of growth, clubbing of the fingers and polycythaemia. Affected children usually show marked breathlessness on exertion and they take frequent rests in a very characteristic squatting position. The most severely affected infants with severe pulmonic stenosis have episodes of deep cyanosis, dyspnoea, unconsciousness and convulsions. The heart is not enlarged and the apex beat may be difficult to locate. Right ventricular pulsation, however, can be readily felt over the left parasternal area where there is also a systolic thrill. In most cases a loud systolic murmur is heard down the left sternal border but this may be slight or absent when pulmonic stenosis is severe. The second pulmonic sound is often quiet and may be single. The characteristic radiographic appearances (Fig. 46) show a small heart with concavity in the region of the pulmonary artery, and with the apex raised above the left diaphragm (*coeur en sabot*). The lungs are oligaemic due to diminished pulmonary blood flow. The electrocardiograph shows marked right axis deviation and right ventricular hypertrophy. Cardiac catheterization reveals a high right ventricular pressure, and the presence of an infundibular chamber or a valvular stenosis can be demonstrated. The catheter may leave the right ventricle through the over-riding aorta. Angiocardiography shows simultaneous filling of the pulmonary artery and the aorta.

[handwritten margin notes: ① RV = LV pressure at all times. ② i̇.e - Systolic gradient + V. low PA pressure. ③ LA bld. fully saturated, but O₂ satn. of Ao. blood ↓ by R→L shunt.]

Prognosis

Fallot's tetralogy is not compatible with long life and the child gets progressively more limited in his exercise capacity. The severely affected infants who have anoxic episodes require early operation to

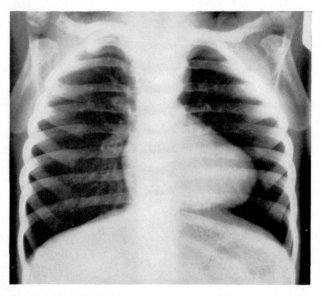

FIG. 46.—Radiograph in Fallot's tetralogy. The apex of the heart is raised above the diaphragm, there is an absence of the pulmonary conus and the lung fields are excessively translucent due to diminished blood flow through the pulmonary arteries.

ensure survival. There is a peculiar tendency to the development of brain abscess in this disease. It often follows a respiratory infection, but the mechanism of its production is not understood. It should be suspected whenever an affected child develops neurological manifestations. These may, also, be due to severe anoxia or thrombosis, e.g. sudden hemiplegia. Their investigation necessitates lumbar puncture, air ventriculography and electroencephalography.

Treatment

Complete or major alleviation of the cyanosis and dramatic improvement in exercise capacity can be expected from the Taussig-Blalock operation in which the subclavian artery is anastomosed to the pulmonary artery, or from Pott's operation of anastomosis of the aorta to the main pulmonary artery. In those cases where the pulmonic stenosis is valvular excellent results have followed valvotomy. The optimum time for these operations is between the ages of 4 and 5 years, although in severely affected infants having anoxic attacks emergency surgery may be required much earlier. These operations are, of course, palliative and it is increasingly becoming the practice to carry out a complete correction of all the defects by open heart surgery using a heart-lung by-pass machine. This may be attempted initially or some time after the performance of a palliative operation, when the left ventricle has become accustomed to handling a larger return of oxygenated blood from the lungs.

TRICUSPID ATRESIA

This is a relatively rare condition, but it must be considered in the differential diagnosis of every child with cyanotic congenital heart disease.

Anatomy

The basic defect is the absence of communication between the right atrium and the right ventricle, so that all blood entering the right atrium from the venae cavae must cross an atrial septal defect to mix in the left atrium with blood from the pulmonary veins. There are several variations. Most often there is a patent ductus arteriosus which diverts some of the blood entering the aorta from the left ventricle into the lungs. In some cases there is a ventricular septal defect allowing some blood from the left ventricle to enter the underdeveloped right ventricle; in these cases there is sometimes a pulmonary stenosis. In other cases the great vessels are transposed and there is then always a large ventricular septal defect. The pulmonary valve which, in such cases, forms the exit from the left ventricle may or may not be narrowed. If there is a substantial pulmonary blood flow cyanosis may be slight.

Clinical Features

As a rule cyanosis is marked from birth with dyspnoea on feeding, failure to thrive, and early clubbing of the digits. Anoxic attacks of unconsciousness may occur. The heart is frequently but little enlarged and the pulsation often felt in the left parasternal region arises from the left ventricle. There is a loud systolic murmur at the left sternal border.

The second pulmonic sound may be quiet and single. The cardiac contour on radiographs may simulate that seen in Fallot's tetralogy, but oblique films will reveal underdevelopment of the right ventricle. The important diagnostic clue is to be found in the electrocardiograph which shows left axis deviation and left ventricular hypertrophy. This may be associated with a P pulmonale due to high pressure in the right atrium.

Prognosis

Few affected infants survive for more than 1 year. Cardiac failure occurs with progressive dyspnoea, hepatomegaly and oedema.

Treatment

The surgical operations devised for tricuspid atresia have all had the objective of improving pulmonary blood flow. None is very successful. Arterial shunts such as the Taussig-Blalock procedure, sometimes combined with enlargement of the atrial septal defect, give better results with children over a year old, whereas in early infancy the most successful operation is probably that devised by Glenn in which the superior vena cava is anastomosed to the right pulmonary artery.

OTHER TYPES OF CYANOTIC CONGENITAL HEART DISEASE

These are numerous although each occurs infrequently. In *transposition of the venae cavae* the systemic veins, as well as the pulmonary veins, open into the left atrium. This results in a functional abnormality similar to that described in tricuspid atresia. In *single ventricle* the child is underdeveloped and unduly dyspnoeic. Cyanosis is variable in degree. Cardiomegaly is gross. A systolic thrill and murmur are found, sometimes also a mid-diastolic murmur. The electrocardiograph may show a left ventricular hypertrophy pattern. In *persistent truncus arteriosus* a common arterial trunk drains both ventricles. The pulmonary arteries may arise from the common truncus or the blood flow to the lungs may depend entirely on the bronchial arteries, so that the degree of oxygen unsaturation is very variable. There may also be pulmonary hypertension in some patients. Thus, cyanosis may be severe or slight. Cardiomegaly is marked. A systolic or continuous murmur may be found. The second pulmonic sound is single. The chest X-ray may show absence of a pulmonary conus but a large aortic shadow. The electrocardiograph shows left ventricular or biventricular hypertrophy. Precise diagnosis in these anomalies is often impossible without cardiac catheterization or angiocardiography.

In *Ebstein's anomaly* the posterior and septal cusps of the tricuspid valve arise from the wall of the right ventricle near the apex so that part of the right ventricle is, in fact, incorporated within the right atrium. There is, in addition, tricuspid incompetence. The child is dyspnoeic on exertion, cyanosed to a variable degree, and poorly developed. Death ultimately takes place from right heart failure. The neck veins are distended and C and V waves may be observed. Auscultation reveals triple or quadruple rhythm, and there may be both presystolic and soft systolic murmurs. The radiograph shows a huge right atrium and on fluoroscopy cardiac pulsations may be seen to be diminished. The lung fields are often oligaemic. The electrocardiograph shows a large notched P wave and some degree of right bundle branch block. These patients are subject to atrial extrasystoles and to attacks of paroxysmal tachycardia. Cardiac catheterization is dangerous but intracardiac electrocardiography may be required to establish the diagnosis.

(B) ACYANOTIC CONGENITAL HEART DISEASE WITH LEFT-TO-RIGHT SHUNTS

VENTRICULAR SEPTAL DEFECT

Ventricular septal defects may be thought of as small in size and relatively benign (*Maladie de Roger*), or as large and associated with a reduction in life expectancy. The latter may, furthermore, exist with or without peripheral pulmonary hypertension (pulmonary vascular obstruction) associated with intimal and medial thickening in the pulmonary arterioles. The causes of this serious type of pulmonary hypertension are not fully understood. In some cases it may be the consequence of a torrential pulmonary blood flow due to a large left-to-right shunt and resulting in damage to the pulmonary vasculature. In many infants, however, it probably represents a persistence of the high pulmonary vascular resistance which is normal in the foetus. Severe pulmonary hypertension causes severe symptoms to develop in early infancy and constitutes one of the common causes of cardiac failure in that age-period.

Clinical Features

(*a*) **Maladie de Roger.**—The child is symptomless and normally developed. The heart is normal in size or minimally enlarged. A palpable systolic thrill in the left parasternal area is associated with a harsh systolic murmur maximal at the fourth left interspace. The electrocardiograph is normal or shows slight left ventricular preponderance. The condition may be complicated by bacterial endocarditis, but the risk can be minimized by the use of penicillin-prophylaxis before dental extractions, tonsillectomy etc. Most patients seem to remain trouble-free for many years.

(*b*) **Large ventricular septal defects without pulmonary hypertension.**—The child is often underdeveloped and sooner or later develops undue dyspnoea on exertion. There is often marked susceptibility to respiratory infections. The heart is enlarged with a forceful apex beat. A systolic thrill and loud pansystolic murmur are maximal at the left sternal border at the level of the fourth interspace. Radiographs show left or biventricular enlargement and engorged (pleonaemic) lungs. The electrocardiograph shows left ventricular hypertrophy. Cardiac catheterization reveals a higher concentration of oxygen in the blood in the right ventricle than in the right atrium, and the catheter may be induced to traverse the septal defect to enter the left ventricle. In some cases the pressures in the right ventricle and pulmonary artery may be elevated due to the large volume of blood being shunted across the defect from the powerful left ventricle. However, in this "dynamic" type of pulmonary hypertension there is no true pulmonary vascular obstruction.

(c) **Large ventricular septal defect with peripheral pulmonary hypertension (Eisenmenger's syndrome).**—In this type of case symptoms are usually present from early infancy with failure to thrive, dyspnoea on exertion such as feeding, and repeated respiratory infections. When the pulmonary hypertension is severe, and especially if there is some overriding of the aorta, the right-to-left shunt so occasioned may cause constant or intermittent cyanosis to be present. Cardiomegaly is gross and palpation reveals not only a powerful apical thrust but excessive pulsation over the right ventricle and its outflow tract in the left parasternal area. There may be no thrill but a pansystolic murmur is invariably heard on auscultation. The second heart sound at the pulmonic area is loud and booming and closely split. There may be an apical mid-diastolic murmur. Radiographs confirm the presence of biventricular hypertrophy, enlargement of the pulmonary artery, and engorgement of the lung roots with translucent peripheral lung fields. Fluoroscopy reveals hyperdynamic cardiac action and the main pulmonary arteries at the lung roots show vigorous pulsation ("hilar dance"). The electrocardiograph indicates biventricular hypertrophy or right ventricular hypertrophy and there may be tall P waves due to enlargement of both atria. Cardiac catheter studies will show high pressures in the right ventricle and in the pulmonary arteries.

Prognosis

Infants with ventricular septal defects and pulmonary hypertension frequently die in congestive cardiac failure with hepatomegaly, pulmonary crepitations and oedema, or from respiratory infection. On the other hand, when they can be carried through the difficult period of infancy with the help of digitalization, antibiotics, and possibly palliative surgery, there is frequently a remarkable improvement during early childhood. This is often to be explained on the basis that hypertrophy of the ventricular muscle produces, in effect, an infundibular stenosis which protects the pulmonary vasculature and reduces the volume of blood shunted from left-to-right. However, if this compensatory process should go too far and raise the right ventricular pressure high enough to reverse the shunt from right-to-left, cyanosis makes its appearance and the situation is then analogous to that in Fallot's tetralogy. Most patients with large ventricular septal defects, with or without pulmonary hypertension, get into difficulties and few are likely to reach middle age. In some cases, however, spontaneous closure of sizeable ventricular defects has been documented (Evans *et al.*, 1960; Nadas *et al.*, 1961).

Treatment

Small ventricular septal defects should be left alone and these patients should be encouraged to undertake full physical activities in all respects. Large ventricular septal defects without severe peripheral pulmonary vascular obstruction but with cardiomegaly should be closed surgically on heart-lung by-pass. In childhood the mortality rate should not exceed 10 per cent. The major hazard of this operation is complete heart block. In infants who are seriously ill with pulmonary hypertension the Dammann-Muller operation should be considered. The pulmonary artery is constricted sufficiently to reduce the high pulmonary blood-flow in the hope that protection of the pulmonary vasculature may make a later operation possible for closure of the ventricular septal defect.

ATRIAL SEPTAL DEFECT

There are two embryologically distinct types. The more common is a failure to close of the ostium secundum which is in the upper part of the interatrial septum. This defect is not uncommonly associated with partial transposition of the pulmonary veins, so that one or both veins from the right lung enter the right atrium. Much less common, but more serious and arising at an earlier stage of embryogenesis, is failure of the ostium primum in the lower part of the septum to close. The base of this defect commonly involves the mitral and tricuspid valves so that one or both may be rendered incompetent. There is, furthermore, a high ventricular septal defect in many of these cases (persistent atrioventricular canal).

Clinical Features

(*a*) **Ostium secundum defect.**—These children are usually symptomless save for undue susceptibility to respiratory infections. Girls are more often affected than boys and they frequently have a somewhat characteristic slender asthenic body build. The sternum may be unduly prominent with accompanying Harrison's grooves. The heart varies in size from normal to very large, but right ventricular pulsation is excessive over the left parasternal area. A soft systolic murmur is best heard at the second or third left interspace and the second pulmonic heart sound is wide and fixedly split. When there is an associated pulmonic stenosis, which is common, a systolic thrill is palpable over the pulmonic area and the systolic murmur is loud and harsh. An apical mid-diastolic murmur may be heard when the atrial septal defect is large with a greatly excessive pulmonary blood-flow. The X-ray shows a large pulmonary conus and pleonaemic lungs. Fluoroscopy may reveal right atrial and ventricular enlargement and a "hilar dance".

The electrocardiograph shows partial right bundle branch block (RsR¹pattern). There may be prolongation of the P-R interval or right ventricular hypertrophy. An increased oxygen concentration is demonstrable in the right atrium during cardiac catheterization; a figure above 95 per cent suggests the presence of an anomalous pulmonary vein which has, in fact, been entered by the catheter from the right atrium. The catheter frequently crosses the atrial septal defect into the left atrium, but this can happen in a normal heart through the foramen ovale and is not by itself a significant occurrence. The precise site of the atrial septal defect can be determined by angiocardiography although this information is not essential before operation.

(*b*) **Ostium primum defect.**—The child in this case usually fails to grow normally from infancy. There may be episodes of cardiac failure and respiratory infections are often severe. Cardiomegaly is associated not only with a powerful right ventricular thrust in the left parasternal area, but also with a displaced heaving apex beat due to left ventricular hypertrophy. When there is mitral incompetence a pansystolic murmur is heard at the apex and propagated into the axilla. A palpable systolic thrill is usually detected. There may be an apical mid-diastolic murmur. The pulmonic second sound is loud and widely split. Fluoroscopy usually shows enlargement of both ventricles, an enlarged pulmonary artery and a "hilar dance". The most characteristic electrocardiographic changes are left axis deviation, partial right bundle branch block and right ventricular hypertrophy. When mitral incompetence is marked, however, there may be evidence of hypertrophy of the left or of both ventricles. Heart block may be present when there is a persistent atrioventricular canal. The vectorcardiograph is of diagnostic value. In the frontal plane the QRS loop advances in a clockwise direction in ostium secundum defects, whereas in ostium primum defects it moves in a counter-clockwise direction.

Prognosis

In ostium secundum defects of large size increasing cardiomegaly is associated with increasing limitation of exercise tolerance. This can be aggravated by the late development of peripheral pulmonary vascular obstruction. An increased susceptibility to rheumatic fever may lead to superimposed mitral stenosis (Lutembacher syndrome). Patients with smaller defects may, however, live to a good age. In ostium primum defects the expectation of life is considerably curtailed.

Treatment

Surgical closure of ostium secundum defects is indicated under hypothermia in every case in which there is cardiac enlargement. The mortality rate is now very low. The repair of ostium primum defects necessitates the use of a heart-lung bypass machine, but it should always be attempted in view of the poor prognosis.

PATENT DUCTUS ARTERIOSUS

In the typical case the blood flow is from the aorta through the ductus to the pulmonary artery, and the lungs are pleonaemic. In a minority of cases the patent duct is associated with pulmonary vascular obstruction, which is itself probably a persistence of the foetal state. This entirely alters the picture and, indeed, in severe cases the blood flow may be right-to-left through the ductus with consequent cyanosis. This type of peripheral pulmonary vascular obstruction must be distinguished from the "dynamic" pulmonary hypertension commonly found in the larger pulmonary arteries in cases of patent ductus arteriosus and due only to the torrential flow of blood reaching them from the aorta. The former situation is irreversible whereas "dynamic" pulmonary hypertension can be completely relieved by simple ligation of the ductus.

Clinical Features

In the vast majority of cases a patent ductus arteriosus produces no cardiac symptoms during childhood. In a few, failure to thrive with or without episodes of congestive cardiac failure occur in early infancy. However, even the child without symptoms is frequently rather underdeveloped for his age, and the dramatic growth spurt and increase in physical activity which is seen after successful ligation of the ductus reveal in retrospect a degree of previous incapacity. The diagnostic physical sign is a continuous murmur, loudest during systole but also extending through diastole, maximal at the pulmonic area and well conducted under the left clavicle. It is associated with a systolic thrill at the second left interspace. The pulses are collapsing in type due to a large pulse pressure. The heart may or may not be enlarged, but fluoroscopy reveals an overactive pulmonary artery with a marked "hilar dance". There may also be enlargement of the left ventricle (Fig. 47). The electrocardiograph is often normal but may show some left ventricular preponderance. In young infants the diastolic component of the murmur is not always audible.

When the patent ductus is complicated by peripheral pulmonary hypertension a vastly different clinical picture presents itself. The child is markedly underdeveloped, highly susceptible to respiratory infections and unduly breathless on exertion. Cardiomegaly is marked with a very large pulmonary artery and the presence of combined ventricular enlargement can be demonstrated both on radiographs and electrocardiographs. The lung roots show severe engorgement but the periphery of the lung fields on radiographs are characteristically clear and translucent. The typical continuous murmur is no longer audible, being

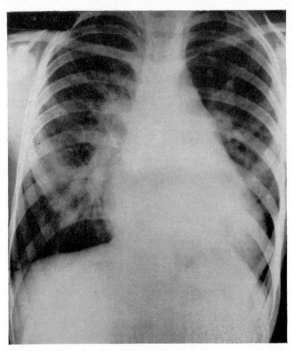

FIG. 47.—Radiograph in patent ductus arteriosus. Enlarged pulmonary conus and pulmonary arteries at hila. Lung fields are engorged. There is also enlargement of the left ventricle.

replaced by a pansystolic bruit and a soft diastolic murmur. The second pulmonic sound, which tends to be obscured in a typical case of patent ductus, is now loud and booming. A systolic thrill is not always palpable. On the other hand, a large pulse pressure and collapsing pulses are still the rule. When the shunt is reversed from right-to-left the presence of cyanosis makes differentiation from transposition of the great vessels with patent ductus a difficult matter without cardiac catheterization.

In typical cases cardiac catheterization is unnecessary, but it should always be performed if there is any suspicion of an accompanying defect or of pulmonary hypertension. There will be a rise in oxygen concentration in the pulmonary artery and the duct may be crossed by the catheter.

Differential Diagnosis

If an aneurysm of the sinus of Valsalva ruptures into the right ventricle there will be a continuous murmur and collapsing pulse, but its differentiation from a patent ductus will be suggested by the sudden appearance of these signs, and possibly cardiac failure, in a previously healthy person. A congenital aorto-pulmonary fenestration can only be distinguished from patent ductus at thoracotomy. The most difficult problem is to differentiate a patent ductus with pulmonary hypertension from a large ventricular septal defect with pulmonary hypertension. The only safe rule is to perform cardiac catheterization and also retrograde aortography in every case of left-to-right shunt with signs suggestive of pulmonary hypertension.

Prognosis

Even in simple patent ductus arteriosus cardiac enlargement sooner or later develops. Death takes place from cardiac failure or bacterial endocarditis before middle age. When pulmonary hypertension complicates the picture death is likely to occur in infancy or early childhood from cardiac failure or pneumonia.

Treatment

Every case of uncomplicated patent duct should be treated surgically by ligation. Recanalization of the duct is rare with modern surgical techniques. The operation is best performed before serious schooling begins. It may have to be carried out in infancy if cardiac failure, failure to thrive or significant cardiac enlargement form part of the picture. The presence of "dynamic" hypertension in the larger pulmonary arteries is a clear indication for operation. On the other hand, the presence of peripheral vascular obstruction makes the operation a hazardous one and it may fail to help the patient. Against this must be set the fact that without surgery the patient's expectation of life is very short. It has been the author's practice in such cases to advise operation in spite of the risks involved unless cyanosis due to a right-to-left shunt is already established.

(C) ACYANOTIC CONGENITAL HEART DISEASE WITHOUT SHUNTS

PULMONIC STENOSIS

This defect occurring alone is usually due to fusion or malformation of the semilunar cusps. Infundibular stenosis in which there is a narrow infundibular chamber between the valve and the right ventricular cavity may also occur alone, but is more often associated with other anomalies (see Fallot's tetralogy). Uncomplicated pulmonic stenosis is a common condition.

Clinical Features

Most affected children are symptomless and they are often well developed with somewhat highly coloured cheeks and lips. Slight cyanosis is seen only in a few very severe cases. Palpation reveals a powerful right ventricular thrust over the left parasternal area, and a systolic thrill at the second left interspace. At this area there is a harsh systolic murmur of ejection type which is conducted into the neck, under the left clavicle and through to the back. The second pulmonic sound is quiet and usually single because the low pressure in the pulmonary artery makes the valve closure inaudible. Radiographs reveal post-stenotic dilatation of the pulmonary artery and translucent oligaemic lung fields. The electrocardiograph shows right ventricular hypertrophy; there may be a P pulmonale and partial right bundle branch block. Cardiac catheterization demonstrates a high right ventricular pressure, with a steep pressure gradient between the ventricle and the pulmonary artery. Withdrawal tracings differentiate clearly between valvular and infundibular stenosis.

Prognosis

Mild degrees of pulmonic stenosis are compatible with long life, but the more severe cases end in cardiac failure before middle age.

Treatment

Surgical correction under direct vision should be advised in all cases where the pressure gradient across the pulmonary valve is more than 50 mm. Hg. The mortality rate is now extremely low.

AORTIC STENOSIS

In most cases there is fusion of the cusps of the aortic valve. Less commonly there is a fibrous ring around the left ventricular outflow tract (subaortic stenosis).

Clinical Features

This defect is more common in boys. Most are symptomless but in a few anginal pain develops on effort. The danger of sudden death during exertion is well known although it is, in fact, an uncommon event. Affected children are usually well grown. The maximal cardiac impulse is at the apex beat although the heart is not commonly enlarged. A systolic thrill is palpable at the second right interspace and also along the carotid arteries and in the suprasternal notch. A harsh systolic murmur is best heard in the aortic area, and there may be a short soft diastolic murmur. The pulse is anacrotic and of small volume. The pulse pressure is low. The heart may appear quite normal in radiographs. The electrocardiograph often shows left ventricular hypertrophy in these cases. The pressure gradient across the aortic valve can be obtained by left heart catheterization through the brachial artery, but this is only indicated in the presence of marked electrocardiographic changes and when operation is considered to be a possibility.

Treatment

Most children with aortic stenosis are likely to live well into middle age. This makes an operation which may leave the patient with the more severe disability of aortic regurgitation of doubtful wisdom. Surgery is probably only to be advised at the present time in the most severe cases with anginal symptoms. It is probably wise, however, in this congenital lesion to depart from the usual practice in other acyanotic congenital defects and to forbid arduous competitive games.

Coarctation of the Aorta

This is a relatively common anomaly and one so amenable to surgical correction that *palpation of the femoral arteries should form part of the physical examination of every patient of any age.* The common site of narrowing of the aorta is just beyond the origin of the left subclavian artery and of the ligamentum arteriosum. The earlier classification into "adult" and "infantile" types should be abandoned. The latter is but one variant of the "aortic arch syndrome" (see below).

Clinical Features

In a few cases coarctation of the aorta results in congestive cardiac failure in early infancy (see Chapter XIV). In the vast majority the child is well developed and symptomless. The murmur, which is discovered during routine medical examination or during an intercurrent illness, is systolic in time. It is well heard at the aortic area, in the suprasternal notch, and in both interscapular areas. The apex beat is forcible due to left ventricular hypertrophy but it may not be displaced for many years. *The femoral pulses are absent or only weakly felt.* A marked blood pressure difference can be shown between the arms and legs, and in time hypertension is established in the upper extremities, head and neck. In adolescence dilated and tortuous collateral vessels may be visible around the scapulae.

Radiographs may show no abnormality during childhood but ultimately left ventricular enlargement develops. An overpenetrated film may reveal a notch in the aortic shadow at the site of the coarctation, and the aortic arch above with some dilatation of the aorta below this notch produces an outline somewhat like the figure three (3). Notching of the inferior borders of the ribs by the enlarged intercostal arteries is seen in adolescents. The electrocardiograph may reveal left ventricular hypertrophy. The length of the narrowed segment can be visualized by retrograde aortography.

Prognosis

Some patients survive into late middle age. Some die suddenly from a cerebrovascular accident. Most die in cardiac failure before the age of 40 years. A few develop rheumatic carditis or bacterial endocarditis.

Treatment

Surgical resection of the narrowed segment of the aorta with direct anastomosis or the insertion of a graft is now so safe and satisfactory that operation should be advised in all cases. This is best performed between the ages of 4 and 7 years. In young infants with cardiac failure operation should be avoided if digitalization and other measures prove successful (Chapter XIV). However, in some cases surgical intervention has to be undertaken; the results are most gratifying in those infants who do not also suffer from other more serious defects.

THE AORTIC ARCH SYNDROME

A wide variety of related anomalies, all incompatible with life, may affect the aortic arch. The most severe, often causing cardiac failure during the first week of life, is aortic atresia or extreme stenosis. There may also be hypoplasia of the aortic arch, the left ventricle and the left atrium. In other cases extensive hypoplasia of the aortic arch is associated with a widely patent ductus arteriosus through which blood flows from the pulmonary artery into the aorta below the narrowed arch. Endocardial fibro-elastosis is a common accompaniment of the aortic arch syndrome. Other associated defects commonly found are mitral atresia or stenosis, ventricular septal defect, and transposition of the great vessels.

Clinical Features

These babies are early in trouble with severe dyspnoea, hepatomegaly, gross cardiomegaly and oedema. Cyanosis is common and in cases with a right-to-left flow through a patent duct the lower half of the body may show a more severe degree than the head and arms. Cardiac murmurs are inconstant as are the electrocardiographic changes. Precise diagnosis is usually impossible even after cardiac catheterization or angiocardiography. Indeed, these infants are often too ill to permit these investigative procedures. The femoral pulses, however, are usually absent or feeble.

Treatment

The response to medical measures is usually poor and transient. Thoracotomy is worthwhile in all but the most desperate of cases because in a very small number, where the hypoplastic part of the aorta does not involve the origins of the great vessels to the head and neck, surgery can prove successful. The parents must, of course, be told frankly of the slender hopes to be pinned on this type of surgery.

VASCULAR RINGS

Several aberrations can occur in the formation of the large arteries in the superior mediastinum. Amongst the most common are double aortic arch, right aortic arch with left ligamentum arteriosum, anomalous right subclavian artery and anomalous innominate artery. In all these situations the trachea and oesophagus may be compressed by vessels which run normally in front of them and abnormally behind them.

Clinical Features

The symptoms vary considerably in severity. The typical picture is an underdeveloped infant with feeding difficulties and with constant laryngeal or tracheal stridor. When symptoms are delayed until later infancy dysphagia may be obvious. There may be repeated severe respiratory infections. The diagnosis is confirmed by fluoroscopy during a barium swallow, when indentations of the oesophagus by the aberrant vessels can be visualized. It is frequently possible to identify the precise anomaly by this technique. Further information may be sought from a lipiodol tracheogram.

Treatment

Thoracotomy and division of the aberrant vessel when this is surgically possible provides complete relief in the great majority of cases.

ANOMALOUS LEFT CORONARY ARTERY

When the left coronary artery arises from the pulmonary trunk the myocardium is perfused with venous blood at low pressure and serious trouble arises early in life. An anomalous right coronary artery, on the other hand, seems not to shorten life.

Clinical Features

After some months of extra-uterine life the infant begins to have attacks of severe pallor, sweating and pain which are probably anginal in nature. They tend to occur during the exertion of feeding. The heart is found to be grossly enlarged but murmurs are absent. The electrocardiograph shows the changes which in the adult are associated with anterior myocardial infarction, namely, a QR pattern with inverted T waves in leads I and aVL, and in leads V5 and V6 deep Q waves, elevated S-T segments and inverted T waves. Selective angiocardiography into the pulmonary artery may outline the anomalous left coronary artery.

Treatment

Death usually occurs before the age of one year. The only available treatment is directed towards congestive cardiac failure (Chapter XIV).

(D) ENDOCARDIAL FIBRO-ELASTOSIS

This is a common disease of infancy. The aetiology is obscure although the changes are presumed to be present from birth. These consist of a fibro-elastic thickening which involves the endocardium and subendocardial tissues. They are most marked in the left atrium and left ventricle where the endocardium has a thickened and milky appearance. The disease may occur alone and is also seen in combination with those anatomical abnormalities which involve the aortic valve and arch. The condition behaves functionally like constrictive pericarditis (Chapter XIV) causing impairment of left ventricular filling, diminished systolic ejection and narrowing of the pulse pressure.

Clinical Features

Symptoms may appear at any time during infancy and the general features of congestive cardiac failure have been described in Chapter XIV. Murmurs are frequently faint or absent. Fluoroscopy reveals an enlarged heart with poor pulsation. The electrocardiograph usually shows left ventricular hypertrophy and T wave inversion.

Treatment

Apart from the treatment of cardiac failure nothing can be done. It is doubtful if recovery is ever possible.

REFERENCES

ABERDEEN, E., WATERSTON, D. J., CARR, I., BONHAM-CARTER, R. E., and SUBRAMANIAN, S. (1965). *Lancet*, 1, 1233.
EVANS, J. R., ROWE, R. D., and KEITH, J. D. (1960). *Circulation*, 20, 1044.
GASUL, B. M., ARCILLA, R. A., and LEV, M. (1966). *Heart Disease in Children.* Philadelphia: J. B. Lippincott.
KEITH, J. D., ROWE, R. D., and VLAD, P. (1958). *Heart Disease in Infancy and Childhood.* New York: Macmillan Co.
KJELLBERG, S. R., MANNHEIMER, E., RUDHE, U., and JONSSON, B. (1959). *Diagnosis of Congenital Heart Disease*, 2nd edit. Chicago: Year Book Publishers.
MUSTARD, W. T. (1964). *Surgery*, 55, 469.
NADAS, A. S. (1963). *Pediatric Cardiology*, 2nd edit. Philadelphia: W. B. Saunders.
NADAS, A. S., SCOTT, L. P., HANCK, A. J., and RUDOLPH, A. M. (1961). *New Engl. J. Med.*, 264, 309.
TAUSSIG, H. B. (1960). *Congenital Malformations of the Heart*, 2nd edit. Cambridge, Mass.: Harvard Univ. Press.

CHAPTER XVI

ALIMENTARY DISEASES

Disorders of the alimentary system are amongst the most common in paediatric practice. They are often highly dangerous to life, being at the same time readily amenable to surgical or medical correction. They demand of the doctor early and accurate diagnosis because the course of the illness is frequently rapid. For surgical details the reader is referred to the excellent textbooks by Benson *et al.* (1962), Mason Brown (1962) and Swenson (1962).

CONGENITAL ABNORMALITIES

HARE-LIP AND CLEFT PALATE

The diagnosis of these abnormalities is obvious. They vary widely in degrees of severity, and may occur singly or together, unilaterally or bilaterally. The reader is referred to surgical texts for details (Veau and Borel, 1931). Only the most severe degrees of cleft palate interfere with sucking and necessitate feeding by spoon, pipette or tube in the early days of life. Hare-lip should be repaired during the first three months of life. Cleft palate can be improved by early orthodontic measures but plastic repair of the gap in both hard or soft palate is best delayed until the age of 15 to 18 months. Speech therapy should be started soon after successful operation to prevent the cleft palate type of speech. These children are subject to nasopharyngitis and otitis media. The resultant loss of hearing may interfere with their education. Furthermore, the mean I.Q. of children with cleft palate is somewhat below that of the population as a whole (Illingworth and Birch, 1956). These aspects must receive attention in addition to the purely surgical problems.

MICROGNATHIA (PIERRE ROBIN SYNDROME)

The primary abnormality is hypoplasia of the mandible. A secondary effect is glossoptosis due to backward displacement of the attachments of the genioglossi to the mandible. This allows the tongue which falls backwards and downwards, to obstruct the oropharynx. There is commonly a post-alveolar cleft of the soft and hard palate.

Clinical Features

In all cases the infant has a typical "shrew face" with a grossly receding chin. The severity of the symptoms is related to the degree of glossoptosis (Forrest and Graham, 1963). The principal difficulties are severe inspiratory stridor, cyanotic attacks, sternal recession and feeding difficulties. Death commonly occurs from bronchopneumonia or inhalation of vomitus. Micrognathia, however, becomes progressively less of a handicap if the infant can be brought through the early months of life. In some cases, unfortunately, there are other anomalies such as cardiac defects, macrostoma or accessory auricles.

Treatment

The effects of glossoptosis should be minimized by nursing the infant in the prone position. In the worst cases tracheostomy should be performed to relieve the respiratory obstruction. Little benefit can be obtained from attempts at traction on the tongue or from the use of a mandibular brace. Repair of a cleft palate is unlikely to bring about improvement. "Orthostatic" feeding is often helpful, whereby the infant is fed in the upright position with the teat pressed against the upper alveolus and held sufficiently away from the lower alveolus to make him strain forward with his lower jaw to grasp the teat. Sometimes resort must be had to prolonged tube-feeding.

OESOPHAGEAL ATRESIA

This defect is frequently correctable provided the diagnosis is reached before aspiration pneumonia and severe electrolyte imbalance have developed. The various anatomical types are described in surgical texts. In the most common there is a blind upper oesophageal pouch and the lower part of the oesophagus forms a fistulous communication with the trachea at its bifurcation (Waterston et al., 1963).

Clinical Features

The diagnosis should be suspected whenever there is a history of hydramnios in the mother. The first clinical sign is the accumulation of excess mucus in the mouth and pharynx, and the condition must be suspected in every infant who requires an undue amount of pharyngeal suction after birth. *In these cases no feeds must be offered until the diagnosis has been confirmed or excluded.* If a feed is given it will result in acute respiratory distress with cyanosis, choking and vomiting. The signs disappear quickly after the early feeds but as aspiration pneumonia develops, usually in the right upper lobe, respiratory distress becomes permanently established up to the time of death. *The diagnosis should, of course, be established before a feed is given.* This can be done quite easily by passing a sterile rubber catheter (English No. 8). If atresia is present the catheter will stick about 5 to 7 cm. from the gums. The size of the upper oesophageal pouch can be assessed by taking radiographs with a radio-opaque catheter *in situ*. The use of contrast media for this purpose is unnecessary and dangerous to the lungs. The most difficult diagnosis is in the rare case where there is a tracheo-oesophageal fistula without atresia. Suspicion should be aroused by respiratory difficulty during feeds and early chest signs. The fistula is usually extremely difficult to detect by bronchoscopy, oesophagoscopy or fluoroscopy. In some such infants auscultation over the lungs during a feed may reveal the gurgling sounds as milk runs through the fistula into the trachea.

Treatment

Surgical correction in one or more stages, with or without gastrostomy, is now possible in most cases but this is an operation for the experienced paediatric surgeon. The paediatrician's duty is to present the infant to the surgeon as soon after birth as possible, and so to organize the neonatal unit in the maternity hospital that there is no possibility of these infants being offered feeds before the diagnosis is confirmed.

DIAPHRAGMATIC HERNIA

Herniation of abdominal contents through the diaphragm (excluding hiatus hernia) is uncommon, but as it creates a neonatal emergency which is extremely amenable to surgical repair its recognition is important. Most often the hernia occurs through the posterolateral portion of the diaphragm (foramen of Bochdalek) usually on the left side. There may or may not be a thin covering sac of peritoneum. In *eventration of the diaphragm* the abdominal contents in the thorax are covered by a fibrous sheet and an emergency situation is rather less likely. Much less frequently the bowel herniates through a defect in the anterolateral part of the diaphragm, or retrosternally through the foramen of Morgagni (Bonham Carter *et al.*, 1962).

Clinical Features

The acute emergency which arises in the great majority of infants is due to the lung being prevented from expanding by the intestine, spleen and other abdominal organs. Furthermore, the entry of air into the intestine after birth causes the heart to be displaced and the opposite lung to be embarrassed. There is rapidly increasing dyspnoea and cyanosis. The heart may be found on the right side, simulating dextrocardia, and there may be diminished breath sounds, or bowel sounds on auscultation. The percussion note varies according to the intestinal contents, fluid or gas producing dullness or tympanicity. There may be a suspiciously empty and scaphoid abdomen. The diagnosis can be confirmed by plain radiographs and without the use of contrast media (Fig. 48). When the hernia is through the foramen of Morgagni, however, a neonatal emergency does not occur. The symptoms have a later onset with respiratory problems and, often, a puzzling radiographic picture. The diagnosis can, however, be made by barium meal.

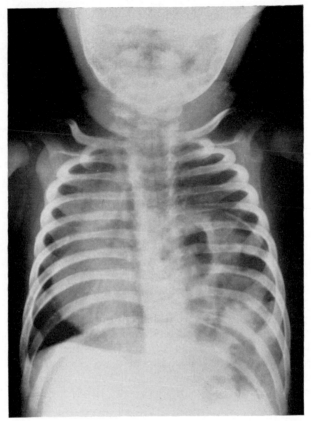

Fig. 48.—Congenital diaphragmatic hernia on left side. Note bowel and gas shadows in left hemithorax.

Treatment

When asphyxial signs develop in the newborn the essential measure after diagnosis is endotracheal intubation and inflation of the lungs by intermittent positive pressure. This can save the infant's life until operation for full repair of the diaphragmatic defect can be arranged within the next hour or two. Under no circumstances should oxygen be given through a face mask because distension of the gut will aggravate the infant's distress. In some infants, unfortunately, death occurs from other associated congenital anomalies.

HIATUS HERNIA

In this condition a pouch of stomach slides up into the chest through a lax oesophageal hiatus in the diaphragm and the cardia is situated above instead of below the diaphragm. The oesophagus is, in consequence, shortened. This is a congenital abnormality, often demonstrable in the first weeks of life, and unrelated to the acquired type of hiatus hernia of adult life. The primary cause of symptoms is regurgitation of stomach contents and acid up the oesophagus due to an incompetent sphincteric mechanism at the cardia (*chalasia cardia*). This results in peptic ulceration of the oesophagus. The common "sliding hernia" must be distinguished from the para-oesophageal hernia in which a portion of the stomach enters the chest through the hiatus, but in which the cardia remains in its normal situation below the diaphragm. The latter responds considerably better to a surgical repair than the more common sliding hernia. There is also a somewhat odd association in some cases of hiatus hernia with pyloric stenosis.

Clinical Features

These have been fully discussed in recent years by Burke (1959), Carré (1959), Carré and Astley (1960) and Carré (1960). Vomiting and failure to thrive date from the early weeks of life. The vomiting may sometimes be projectile, and the vomitus usually contains much mucus. Frequently there is altered blood in the vomit, a point of great diagnostic significance. Constipation is common when vomiting is severe. These symptoms tend to lessen in severity when solid foods are added to the diet. A major hazard in this disease is the development of an oesophageal stricture from fibrosis and cicatrization in the ulcerated oesophagus. This should be suspected when weaning on to solid foods fails to bring about some amelioration of symptoms, and especially if there is any dysphagia. In such cases there may be marked emaciation. In other instances a severe iron-deficiency anaemia can result from repeated haematemeses. Although a typical clinical history and positive tests for occult blood in the stools provide strong presumptive evidence, the diagnosis must always be confirmed by barium swallow and fluoroscopy carried out by an experienced paediatric radiologist. It is almost always possible to demonstrate the intrathoracic loculus of stomach (Fig. 49), and the presence of an oesophageal stricture can also be visualized.

Treatment

In two cases out of three a satisfactory response can be expected by keeping the patient in an upright position day and night. This is best done in a specially constructed padded wooden or plastic box with suitable straps to retain the infant in a sitting position. Vomiting can be made less likely by thickening the feeds with one of the pre-cooked infant cereals, although breast feeding should never be abandoned for this purpose. An alkali such as Aludrox 30–60 minims (2–4 ml.) can be given with each feed. Complete functional recovery occurs in

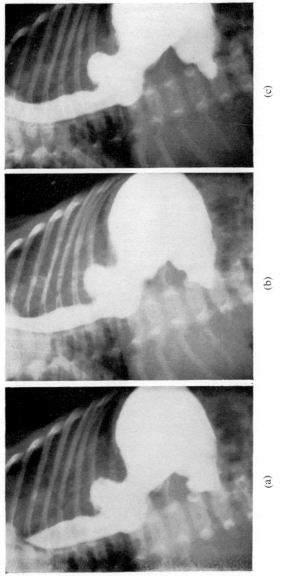

(a)   (b)   (c)

Fig. 49.—Ba. swallow appearances in hiatus hernia, showing pouch of stomach above the diaphragm.

favourable cases by the age of 2–3 years or earlier. Surgical treatment should be reserved for cases in which there are repeated haematemeses and in which oesophagoscopy shows severe peptic ulceration. Unfortunately, it is sometimes only partially successful in relieving the oesophageal regurgitation due to chalasia cardia. An established oesophageal stricture should be treated by repeated bougienage under direct oesophagoscopic vision. In the worst cases it may be necessary to undertake resection and reconstruction of the lower third of the oesophagus with transverse colon.

DUODENAL OBSTRUCTION

The most common cause is atresia of the duodenum, usually situated distal to the ampulla of Vater. Rarely a web is stretched across the lumen with a small hole in the centre through which fluid can still pass. Another rare cause of incomplete duodenal obstruction is an annular pancreas which constricts the second part of the duodenum. The duodenum is more frequently partially obstructed by folds of peritoneum in the presence of malrotation of the bowel. This causes the weight of the ascending colon, which has failed to reach its normal position in the right lumbar gutter, to tighten the peritoneal reflection across the lower portions of the duodenum.

Clinical Features

In complete duodenal obstruction vomiting starts within a few hours of birth and bile-staining is present in nearly every instance. The abdomen is not distended although there may be some fullness in the epigastrium just before a vomit. Dehydration develops rapidly and there is a metabolic alkalosis due to the loss of chloride ions in the vomits. When the obstruction is incomplete the symptoms develop more slowly and may suggest pyloric stenosis. The presence of bile in the vomits is an important differentiating point. A straight radiograph in the upright position will show air confined to the stomach and dilated proximal duodenum (Fig. 50) when the obstruction is complete, and the diagnosis should thus be confirmed within a few hours of birth. In partial obstruction the use of a radio-opaque medium such as lipiodol or gastrografin may help in reaching a diagnosis. Barium should not be used in the newborn because it is very irritating to the lungs if aspirated.

Treatment

Surgical intervention should be performed before severe electrolyte and acid-base disturbances have developed. Pre-operative intravenous half-strength physiological saline may be required (60 ml./Kg./day).

The operation of choice is duodenojejunostomy, but in high duodenal obstruction gastro-enterostomy may be unavoidable.

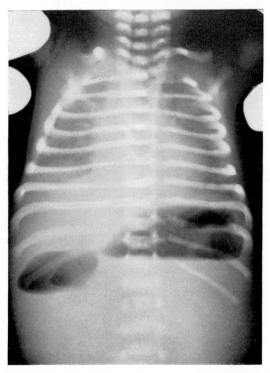

FIG. 50.—Straight radiograph with infant in erect position in duodenal atresia. Gas visible in stomach and dilated duodenum; none below the level of the duodenum.

INTESTINAL OBSTRUCTION

The most common variety is due to jejunal or ileal atresia. Infrequently herniation with strangulation of small bowel occurs through a congenital defect in a mesentery, or a congenital peritoneal fold can create such an opening for small bowel. Another common cause of intestinal obstruction is *meconium ileus* which presents in the neonatal period as one form of the clinical picture of fibrocystic disease of the pancreas (p. 293). Here the terminal ileum is obstructed by grey inspissated meconium. The colon in these cases is hypoplastic—"microcolon". Small bowel obstruction can cause perforation during foetal life. This leads to *meconium peritonitis* and intraperitoneal calcification. The perforation has usually closed spontaneously before birth but if it has not, bacterial peritonitis rapidly develops after birth with massive pneumoperitoneum.

Clinical Features

The typical findings, which develop within a few hours of birth, are repeated bile-stained vomiting, increasing abdominal distension, and (in complete cases) absolute constipation. A history of hydramnios in the mother is an important diagnostic pointer. Radiographs taken in the erect and supine positions reveal numerous dilated loops of bowel

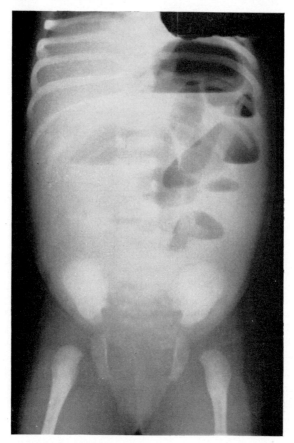

Fig. 51.—Straight radiograph with infant in erect position in intestinal atresia. Observe dilated loops of small bowel and fluid levels.

which often contain fluid levels; these shift with changes of position (Fig. 51). In meconium ileus, gas bubbles in the inspissated meconium may be visualized (Fig. 52). The existence of meconium peritonitis will be shown by numerous areas of calcification in the lower abdomen, whereas in bacterial peritonitis erect radiographs will show gas under

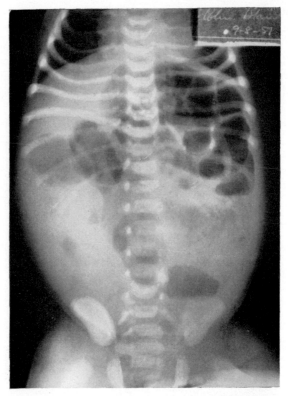

FIG. 52.—Straight radiograph with infant in supine position in intestinal obstruction due to meconium ileus. Small bowel shows dilated loops. Note air bubbles in inspissated meconium in left lower quadrant.

both sides of the diaphragm. A useful diagnostic clue in meconium ileus may lie in the history that previous children have had fibrocystic disease of the pancreas. Diagnosis of the precise cause of the intestinal obstruction in the newborn is not always possible, but as laparotomy is always indicated this is relatively unimportant.

Treatment

The key to successful surgery is early diagnosis. Severe electrolyte disturbance such as hypokalaemic alkalosis, and aspiration pneumonia render the prognosis grave. Intravenous fluid therapy before, during and after operation demands expert management. Overhydration is very dangerous and the intake of 5 per cent dextrose in quarter-strength physiological saline, diluted plasma 50:50 with 5 per cent dextrose, or blood should not exceed 60 ml./Kg./day plus the losses from gastric

(ie - 30 mls. /lb.)

suction (Peonides *et al.*, 1963). After operation hypokalaemia may have to be corrected by the addition of potassium chloride (10–20 mEq/l.) to the infusion fluids. Antibiotics are required if chest signs appear. Operative details should be sought in surgical texts. In atresia the usual procedure is resection and decompression of the dilated proximal bowel with end-to-end anastomosis. The results are remarkably good in experienced hands. Unfortunately, some infants die of other associated congenital anomalies which are not always obvious pre-operatively. The results of treatment in meconium ileus, by resection, enterostomy, irrigation of the bowel through an enterotomy, or Mikulicz type of resection are much less satisfactory. The survivors will later develop other manifestations of fibrocystic disease of the pancreas.

IMPERFORATE ANUS

This is a relatively common emergency. In female infants there is frequently an associated recto-vaginal fistula and in males a fistula to the bladder or urethra. Less often there is a small anteriorly placed perineal fistula or one involving the scrotum. Imperforate anus is also sometimes associated with other anomalies such as oesophageal atresia.

Clinical Features

Testing the patency of the anus should form part of the routine examination of every infant at birth so that a delayed diagnosis ought never to occur. If the diagnosis is missed and there is no fistula the infant will rapidly develop bile-stained vomiting and abdominal distension. Meconium will not be passed. In the presence of a fistula the signs of large bowel obstruction will be less severe or absent but meconium will be seen to exude from the vagina, urethra or perineum. When there is no fistula radiographs should be taken after the infant has been held head downwards for 3–4 minutes with a lead marker on the perineum; the films will then outline the gas in the blind rectal pouch and its distance from the skin can be estimated.

Treatment

Anoplasty or an abdominoperineal operation will be necessary according to the length of the gap. Colostomy is best avoided but may be the operation of choice when the infant is in poor condition. Post-operative difficulties such as constipation and faecal incontinence are common and regular rectal wash-outs may be required over long periods in childhood.

HIRSCHSPRUNG'S DISEASE

After years of confusion it has now been established that the primary defect in this disease is a congenital absence of the ganglion cells of the

myenteric parasympathetic nerve plexus of Auerbach from a segment
of the colon. This extends upwards from the internal anal sphincter for
a variable distance. In most cases the aganglionic segment involves only
the rectum and lower part of sigmoid colon and there is gross hypertrophy and distension of the remaining length of the colon. There may
also be extensive mucosal ulceration. Rarely the entire colon may be
devoid of ganglion cells (Zuelzer and Wilson 1948; Swenson *et al.*, 1949;
Bodian *et al.*, 1951).

Clinical Features

These vary considerably in severity. In many instances symptoms
appear during the neonatal period with severe constipation, gross
abdominal distension and even bile-stained vomiting. Indeed, Hirschsprung's disease must enter into the differential diagnosis in every case
of intestinal obstruction during infancy (p. 266). More often the clinical
course is a series of episodes of incomplete large bowel obstruction and
absolute constipation does not occur. Even during the most acute episodes of abdominal distension the passage of a finger or a rectal tube
will produce faeces and gas. Vomiting and anorexia soon lead to a state
of marasmus. In some cases diagnostic difficulties may arise from severe
diarrhoea due to the development of an "ulcerating" colitis, but the
true situation should always be suggested by the gross abdominal distension. Few children survive infancy without treatment and in them
the picture is one of severe constipation, gross distension, anorexia and
stunting of growth. In typical cases the examining finger will reveal an
empty rectum but this is not invariable. In older infants a barium
enema carefully performed by an expert radiologist will reveal the
narrow aganglionic segment of bowel (Fig. 53). In the newborn, however, these appearances have not had time to develop. The most important diagnostic test, because it can also reveal the length of the aganglionic segment, is rectal biopsy (Swenson, 1959).

Treatment

The results of modern surgical techniques have completely transformed the outlook for these infants since 1948, although problems with
post-operative incontinence have not been completely solved. The curative operation is usually delayed until a colostomy has allowed the gross
distension to subside. The most commonly performed operations are
rectosigmoidectomy by the pull-through technique of Swenson, or the
operation devised by Duhamel (1960) which retains part of the circumference of the rectum.

MECKEL'S DIVERTICULUM AND DUPLICATION OF THE BOWEL

These two conditions are considered together because they may produce very similar symptoms. They are, however, embryologically quite

separate. *Duplications* of the gastro-intestinal tract are extremely rare and they may occur at any level and to any extent. Most involve only a small part of the bowel and have also been called "enterogenous cysts". They always arise from the mesenteric border of the bowel, in contrast to Meckel's diverticulum which is invariably anti-mesenteric. Like Meckel's diverticulum they may contain heterotopic acid-secreting

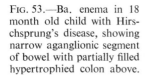

Fig. 53.—Ba. enema in 18 month old child with Hirschsprung's disease, showing narrow aganglionic segment of bowel with partially filled hypertrophied colon above.

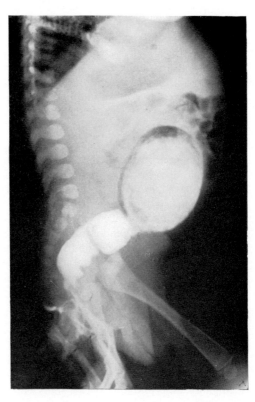

gastric mucosa. Rarely enterogenous cysts are found in the posterior mediastinum where they produce symptoms by bronchial compression. They are then often associated with developmental anomalies of the cervical and upper dorsal vertebrae. Very rarely a mediastinal duplication penetrates the diaphragm to end in the small bowel. *Meckel's diverticulum* is a remnant of the vitelline duct, always arising from the anti-mesenteric border of the terminal ileum. There is sometimes a fibrous cord attachment to the umbilicus. Very infrequently a persistence of the omphalomesenteric duct results in an umbilical faecal fistula.

Clinical Features

The most common cause of a previously unheralded massive intestinal haemorrhage during infancy is peptic ulceration occurring in a Meckel's diverticulum or duplication of bowel. This appears first as melaena and later as red currant jelly stools. Haematemesis only occurs in the rare cases of duplication of the stomach or duodenum. A less common effect of such peptic ulceration, which is due to the acid produced by the heterotopic gastric mucosa, is perforation leading rapidly to generalized bacterial peritonitis. This is, of course, a highly dangerous possibility. Intestinal obstruction with strangulation and gangrene of bowel can also complicate a Meckel's diverticulum, either because it starts off an intussusception, or because bowel becomes twisted around the fibrous remnant of the vitelline duct. Lastly diverticulitis may develop but it cannot be distinguished pre-operatively from appendicitis.

Treatment

All these emergencies demand early surgical intervention. Haemorrhage must, of course, be treated first by blood transfusion, and as repeated massive bleeding is uncommon time is well spent on restoring the blood volume and red cell mass before operation is undertaken. Intestinal obstruction causes severe electrolyte disturbances, and as extensive resection of gangrenous bowel may be necessary the pre- and post-operative management of these patients with intravenous fluids, gastric suction and antibiotics, often demands a very high standard of skill from clinicians and laboratory workers.

INTESTINAL POLYPS

The common type of *juvenile polyp of the colon* is situated most often in the rectum. Unlike polyps found in the adult it is not pre-malignant. Symptoms are usually delayed until after the first year of life. There may be a passage of bright red blood per rectum or a polyp may prolapse through the anus and appear as a shiny bluish mass. Rectal polyps may be palpated with the finger, or they may be situated where only the sigmoidoscope can reveal their presence. Rarely, a barium enema is necessary to visualize a polyp high in the colon. The usual treatment is removal of the polyp through a sigmoidoscope. Opinions are divided on the need to remove a high polyp when laparotomy and colotomy are required.

A rare type of polyposis involving the jejunum, duodenum and sometimes even the stomach is seen in the *Peutz-Jeghers syndrome*. There is frequently a positive family history. The clue to correct diagnosis is the presence in affected children of small pigmented areas like freckles which are characteristically distributed on the lips, buccal mucous membrane, gums, palate, face, palms and soles. The abdominal symptoms vary from attacks of incomplete intestinal obstruction due to recurrent intussusceptions, to frank haematemesis and melaena. The diagnosis can be confirmed by barium meal. These unfortunate children have repeated operations for the reduction of intussusceptions, but resections should be avoided if possible. Anaemia must also be treated. This condition is not pre-malignant.

In marked contrast to the Peutz-Jeghers syndrome is *familial polyposis of the colon*, which is well known to lead to cancer at an early age. It is, however, quite rare for this inherited disease to cause symptoms before puberty. The diagnosis is confirmed by sigmoidoscopy and barium enema by the double contrast technique. As the disease is transmitted as a Mendelian dominant the children of affected adults must come under suspicion as having a 50/50 chance of developing the disease. Detailed investigation should probably not be undertaken unless and until symptoms such as rectal bleeding develop. The only treatment is early and total colectomy, although the rectum may be preserved if polyps there are few in number.

CONGENITAL HYPERTROPHIC PYLORIC STENOSIS

In spite of its name this condition is probably not congenital. It develops in most cases during the second or third week of life. The pathogenesis is unknown but there is a clear genetic influence and several cases may occur in one family through one or more generations. There is marked hypertrophy of the circular muscle fibres of the pylorus and severe narrowing of the pyloric canal. The disease has a male:female sex incidence of 4:1, and it affects the first-born more frequently than later offspring.

Clinical Features

Vomiting usually starts during the second or third week of life and rapidly becomes projectile in character. The vomitus is never bile-stained but occasionally may contain altered blood. Visible gastric peristalsis can be observed during a feed, the appearance having been likened to a golf ball moving under the skin from the left hypochondrium downwards and to the right. Palpation in the right side of the epigastrium *with a warm hand* will almost always reveal the thickened pyloric muscle as a small hard tumour. A barium meal is only necessary in the 1–2 per cent of cases in which the pyloric tumour cannot be found *during the course of a test-feed*. It will show much delay in gastric emptying time and outline the narrow and elongated pyloric canal. If diagnosis is delayed the infant becomes marasmic but remains very eager for feeds. The urinary chlorides are greatly diminished and the loss of chloride ions in the vomit causes a metabolic alkalosis with a raised plasma CO_2 level. Rarely, convulsions occur due to alkalotic tetany. Dehydration may also become severe in neglected cases.

Treatment

There has long been a controversy between the supporters of surgical and medical methods of treatment respectively (Jacoby, 1962). Provided experienced surgeons are available most British paediatricians now opt for surgical treatment, which should have a mortality rate considerably under 1 per cent. An exception may be made in the few infants first seen over the age of ten weeks provided they are still in reasonably good condition. The infant must be protected from the risks of infection by as short a stay in hospital as possible and by isolation in a cubicle. The operation devised by Ramstedt should be performed within 24 hours of admission to hospital. If dehydration and alkalosis are marked this should be corrected pre-operatively with 5 per cent dextrose in half-strength physiological saline, 150 ml./Kg./day, by continuous intravenous infusion. In practice the use of parenteral fluids is rarely required in the United Kingdom today and it is only rarely necessary to estimate the plasma electrolytes and bicarbonate. Either local or general anaesthesia may be used. Oral fluids should be started four hours after operation. Two-hourly feeds of breast-milk or half-cream dried milk, $\frac{1}{2}$ fl. oz. (15 ml.), are given initially. Half-strength physiological saline is offered freely by mouth every two hours, alternating with the milk feeds. Every 12 hours the milk feeds are increased by $\frac{1}{2}$ fl. oz. (15 ml.) per feed. After 48 hours the infant can go on to four-hourly feeds of 2 fl. oz. (60 ml.) with added sucrose, and the saline supplements can be omitted. The bottle-fed infant can be discharged from hospital on the fourth or fifth post-operative day and his feeds continue to be increased at home until they meet his full caloric requirements. Breast-fed infants may safely be allowed home 48 hours after operation to breast-feed in the normal manner.

When medical treatment is employed a long period of supervision is required. The infant should be fed his full caloric requirements. If a feed is vomited he should immediately be offered another which will frequently be retained. Gastric lavage with half-strength physiological saline should be performed daily, and the same electrolyte solution should be offered between feeds. An anti-spasmodic such as atropine methylnitrate (Eumydrin), 2 drops of 0·6 per cent alcoholic solution, should be given orally 15–20 minutes before every feed. After some weeks vomiting ceases and weight gain becomes satisfactory in most cases.

The physician must be prepared to call for surgical help if the response to medical treatment is not satisfactory and before the infant has become marasmic or dehydrated. The author employs medical treatment very infrequently.

ACQUIRED DISEASES

Acute Stomatitis

The great majority of cases of acute aphthous or of ulcerative stomatitis in young children are due to a primary infection by the virus of herpes simplex. In most cases this primary infection is subclinical, but it can cause a severe stomatitis in some children. The common type of herpes febrilis can only develop in persons who have earlier had a primary infection.

Clinical Features

The child with acute stomatitis is acutely ill with fever (102–105° F.), malaise, anorexia and toxaemia. Feeding and fluid intake may be severely interrupted by the inflammation and pain in the lips, buccal mucous membrane, gums, palate and pharynx. Numerous vesicles may form and when they rupture leave greyish sloughs and ulcers. The submandibular lymph nodes are often greatly enlarged. Spontaneous recovery can be expected in 8–10 days. This disease can be difficult to distinguish from *herpangina* which is due to one of the group A Coxsackie viruses, but in the latter the lips, gums and tongue usually escape.

Treatment

There is no specific drug therapy, but potassium chlorate 1 gr. (60 mg.) thrice daily for a few days sometimes seems to afford relief. Sedation and frequent mouth washes help to relieve discomfort and permit the swallowing of fluids. Life is rarely endangered. *Gentian violet.*

Recurrent Parotitis

Acute suppurative parotitis due to *Staph. aureus* is only rarely seen in severely debilitated children. Recurrent non-suppurative parotitis, probably due to *Strept. viridans*, is a somewhat characteristic disease of older infants and young children. It may be unilateral or bilateral. The first attack of the disease may closely simulate mumps (epidemic parotitis), but recurrences continue throughout childhood. Each attack subsides in about 2–3 weeks and the disease usually stops spontaneously about the time of puberty. Individual attacks are probably shortened by antibiotic therapy. In a few cases sialectasis develops when parotidectomy may be required. This is a difficult operation, endangering the facial nerve, and should be reserved for the experienced surgeon.

Peptic Ulcer

Gastric and duodenal ulcers are less rare in childhood than has often been imagined and they may be increasing in frequency (Barger,

1958; Fällström and Reinand, 1961). Peptic ulceration is also a recognized complication of steroid therapy. The author has twice in recent years seen perforation of a duodenal ulcer complicate the treatment of rheumatic fever with steroids combined with aspirin. The acute peptic ulcer which sometimes occurs in severe illnesses and extensive burns is to be regarded as a different problem.

Clinical Features

Symptoms tend to be less "typical" in children than in adults. None the less, abdominal pain relieved by food and wakening the child at night should suggest the diagnosis. So also should a history of periodicity. Heartburn and vomiting are not uncommon. There is frequently localized epigastric tenderness on palpation. The faeces may give a positive reaction for blood with orthotolidine. As in the adult, some children first present with brisk haematemesis or melaena. The diagnosis is at its most difficult in the young infant. In some the first evidence is copious bleeding with oligaemic shock. In others a sudden collapse with acute respiratory distress indicates perforation of a peptic ulcer; the diagnosis once suspected can quickly be confirmed by straight radiographs which will reveal free gas in the peritoneal cavity.

In less acute cases the ulcer crater can be revealed by fluoroscopy after the ingestion of lipiodol in infants or barium in older children.

Treatment

Perforation must obviously be closed by the surgeon as rapidly as possible, and severe haemorrhage requires rapid blood transfusion. In older children rest in bed, a bland diet, antacids and anti-cholinergics will promote healing although remissions and relapses are likely to persist into adult life. In severe cases a combination of vagotomy and pyloroplasty is probably preferable to partial gastrectomy during childhood, but every effort should be made to avoid any type of operative interference.

Infantile Gastro-enteritis

The disastrous epidemics of this disease which used to occur in British cities every autumn have totally disappeared. Cases are now seen in small numbers throughout the year, and small epidemics still occur in infant wards and nurseries. Occasional outbreaks in maternity units have earned it the name "epidemic diarrhoea of the newborn". The disease is, however, still a major cause of infant mortality in many of the less fortunate countries of the world.

Aetiology

The majority of cases are due to various specific strains of entero-pathogenic E. coli. These are now usually classified according to the

Kauffmann (1947) antigenic scheme. The most important are O·111 : B4; O·55: B5; O·26: B6; O·119: B14; and O·128: B12. In routine laboratory work it is usual to identify only the somatic (O) antigen. The entero-pathogenic *E. coli* rarely cause symptoms in older children and adults, although they readily become short-term carriers (Stevenson, 1952). Bacteria of the *Salmonella* and *Shigella* groups may also cause gastro-enteritis. In many cases, however, no pathogens can be isolated. Some of these may be due to viruses (Buddingh and Dodd, 1944; Light and Hodes, 1949) although the evidence is far from conclusive.

Pathology

Death in gastro-enteritis is due mainly to severe electrolyte distur-bances and to hypovolaemia. There is frequently minimal inflammatory change in the stomach and small bowel. The liver may show severe fatty change. Aspiration pneumonia, suppurative otitis media and mastoiditis, once common findings at autopsy, are now rarely seen.

Clinical Features

The onset is sudden with diarrhoea and vomiting. The stools are large in volume, watery in consistency and usually grass-green in colour. When the infant's weight has previously been known a sudden loss of about 0·2 Kg. (½ lb.) often precedes other clinical manifestations. Vomiting may be frequent or slight. Dehydration develops rapidly due to the losses of body water and electrolytes (sodium, chloride and potassium) in the stools and vomits. The mildly dehydrated infant has lost between 2·5 and 5 per cent of his body weight. He is fretful and sleepless with a slightly depressed fontanelle. Thirst is marked and feeds are taken eagerly, although they are often vomited. In more marked degrees of dehydration weight loss varies between 5 and 10 per cent of body weight. Irritability is more marked, and the fontanelle, eyes and abdomen are visibly sunken. The skin wrinkles abnormally when lifted between the thumb and forefinger. The extremities feel cold and may be cyanosed. At this stage the losses of cations (sodium and potassium) in excess of anion (chloride) in the stools have produced a severe metabolic acidosis. This may be reflected in the presence of rapid, pauseless, acyanotic breathing (air hunger). Thirst is usually extreme, although repeated vomiting is likely to interfere with the in-take of fluids. If the loss of weight should exceed 10 per cent of body weight the infant's condition becomes critical, due to oligaemia and peripheral circulatory failure. The body skin is cold and ashen, the face has a wizened Hippocratic look, the extremities are deeply cyanosed, and the desire to suck has been lost. The corneae are glazed and the eyeballs are often rolled upwards. The fontanelle is deeply sunken and there is usually visible over-riding of the sutures. Even at this stage of dehydration recovery is possible if rapid emergency steps can be taken to restore the blood volume, and to return towards normal the electrolyte losses and the acid-base equilibrium. Unfortunately, the situation may be complicated by thrombosis in the superior longitudinal sinus with convulsions and spasticity.

The clinical picture so far described, and that most commonly seen, can be called *"hypotonic dehydration"* because the losses of electrolytes in the stools and vomits exceed the loss of body water, which comes mostly from the extracellular compartment. It is important to recognize the less common but highly dangerous type of *"hypertonic dehydration"*. This clinical state occurs if the loss of body water, mostly from the intracellular compartment, exceeds the loss of electrolytes so that a state of hyperelectrolytaemia develops. It is usually associated not only with some diarrhoea and vomiting but also with a marked reluctance to take feeds by mouth. The resultant diminished fluid intake, while insensible water loss continues from skin and lungs, causes a disproportionate loss of water over electrolytes. This state may, indeed, arise from any infection, enteral or parenteral, which causes marked anorexia and reluctance to feed. The clinical manifestations of dehydration described above tend to be much less striking in this type of dehydration because it is so largely intracellular, and its recognition rests largely upon the estimation of the serum electrolyte levels. These infants commonly develop convulsions and unconsciousness due to hypernatraemia, and permanent brain damage is a considerable hazard. The most important safeguard against the development of hypertonic dehydration would be an increased recognition by physicians that an infant's diet and his fluid intake coincide; and that if he is anorexic for any reason it is essential to ensure an adequate fluid intake in the form of quarter or fifth strength physiological saline.

Biochemical Changes

In *hypotonic dehydration* haemocentration and hypovolaemia are reflected in abnormally high levels of haemoglobin, red cells, packed-cell volume and serum proteins, provided the infant has not previously been anaemic or severely undernourished. Metabolic acidosis is shown by a lowered plasma bicarbonate and in uncompensated cases by a lowered blood pH. Diminished glomerular filtration rate explains the high blood urea. The serum electrolyte levels do not accurately indicate the extent of the losses in the stools and vomits, and they are not usually seriously abnormal until the state of dehydration is corrected when hypokalaemia is often marked, reflecting the large losses of intracellular potassium in the stools and urine.

In *hypertonic dehydration* there is little haemoconcentration but markedly raised levels of serum sodium and chloride. Metabolic acidosis may also be severe. The considerable hypertonicity of the interstitial fluid due to high electrolyte concentrations causes a shift of water out of the cells with resultant intracellular dehydration.

In both types of dehydration periodic estimations of the serum electrolytes can be a valuable guide to treatment.

Treatment

When dehydration is mild it is possible, and indeed preferable, to treat the infant in his own home. Milk feeds should be withdrawn and replaced by half-strength physiological saline, 90 ml./lb./day (200 ml./Kg.), given in small quantities every two hours during the day and every four hours during the night. Milk feeds, either human or half-cream dried, should be re-started after 24 hours, $\frac{1}{2}$ fl. oz. (15 ml.) four-hourly. The feeds can be increased by $\frac{1}{2}$ fl. oz. (15 ml.) per feed every 24 hours. At the same time the half-strength saline is correspondingly reduced. Sucrose is only added to the feeds after the stools have become formed.

When hypotonic dehydration is severe, admission to hospital for parenteral fluid therapy is indicated. This should always be given by the intravenous route. Various electrolyte solutions are suitable for such treatment; their precise composition is less important than accurate supervision of the fluid intake, the daily weight measurement, and the blood chemistry such as pH, plasma CO_2, blood urea, serum potassium, sodium and chloride. The most commonly used fluid is 5 per cent dextrose in half-strength physiological saline. In the first four hours the dehydrated infant should receive 20–30 ml. per lb. body weight (45–65 ml./Kg.). Thereafter an adequate fluid intake is 60–90 ml./lb. (130–200 ml./Kg.) per day. In the newborn, however, a much smaller fluid intake is indicated (30 ml./lb. or 65 ml./Kg.) because of the severe risks of over-hydration. It is also a safe precaution in the case of very small infants to change over to quarter-strength saline once the urinary output is again satisfactory to avoid the danger of chloride over-dosage. When there is very severe dehydration, with imminent danger to life, the most useful solution for rapid reconstruction of the plasma volume consists of a mixture of equal parts of citrated plasma and 10 per cent dextrose in water. In emergency 20 ml. per lb. (45 ml./Kg.) can be given fairly rapidly by syringe, to be followed by slow infusion. On the other hand, when the blood chemical findings indicate a severe metabolic acidosis, a useful initial infusion is 1/6 molar sodium lactate 15 ml./lb. (30 ml./Kg.) given by syringe and repeated if necessary four hours later.

When the acid-base state can be estimated frequently by the Astrup micro-method, metabolic acidosis can be corrected more rapidly by periodic intravenous doses of 8·4 per cent sodium bicarbonate (1 ml $=$ 1 mEq.). Taking the extracellular space as equivalent to 35 per cent of the body weight, suitable individual doses of 8·4 per cent sodium bicarbonate can be calculated on the following formula:

$$\text{body weight in Kg.} \times 0.35 \times \text{base deficit in mEq./litre.}$$

The acid-base state should be re-assessed shortly after each intravenous dose of sodium bicarbonate.

After a period of 24–36 hours on intravenous fluids the diarrhoea and vomiting have usually subsided and milk feeds may be gradually introduced in the manner outlined above. The volume of intravenous fluid intake, is, of course, correspondingly reduced. In severe cases, it will usually be found when dehydration has been overcome and the urinary output is again adequate, that the marked losses of intracellular potassium which have taken place in both stools and urine are reflected in a reduced serum potassium level and in characteristic changes in the E.C.G. In most cases this can be corrected with potassium chloride, 1–2 gm. per day, given orally with feeds. When the hypokalaemia is severe, and especially if oral feeds must be delayed because of continued vomiting, a more rapid correction can be achieved by adding potassium chloride, 10–20 mEq/l. to the infusion fluid. As a rise in serum potassium above 8 mEq/l. carries the risk of cardiac arrest, intravenous therapy must be carefully monitored by frequent serum estimations and E.C.G's. More detailed descriptions of electrolyte replacement can be obtained in the M.R.C. Memorandum No. 26 (1952).

The treatment of hypertonic dehydration requires the extremely careful use of intravenous solutions. An excess of electrolytes, especially of sodium, can seriously aggravate the hypernatraemia. On the other hand, dextrose in water can lead to water intoxication. It is recommended that 5 per cent dextrose in quarter strength or fifth strength physiological saline be given in the volumes suggested above but that the serum sodium, potassium and chloride levels be frequently measured.

In any type of severe dehydration, and particularly when there is peripheral circulatory failure, the administration of oxygen in a tent is a valuable measure.

Drugs

The use of antibiotics, preferably under laboratory guidance, has also greatly reduced the mortality from gastro-enteritis. These should be given orally in most cases. Suitable drugs and dosages are neomycin 50 mg./Kg./day; colistin sulphate 150,000 units/Kg./day; polymyxin B 100,000 units/Kg./day; and streptomycin 1–2 gm. per day, each in four divided doses. In very severe cases with much vomiting colistin, streptomycin, tetracycline and chloramphenicol are suitable drugs for parenteral administration. It should be stressed that castor oil, mercury preparations and other laxatives can only aggravate losses of water and electro-lytes from the stools. Their use is completely contra-indicated.

INTUSSUSCEPTION

Aetiology

In older children and adults intussusception is uncommon but almost always has an obvious local cause, e.g. Meckel's diverticulum, polyp or carcinoma. The common age-group for intussusception, however, is 3–9 months when a discoverable local cause is the exception. In recent years evidence has been collected to suggest a causal relationship with infection by the adenoviruses and possibly also herpes simplex virus (Gardner, 1961; Gardner *et al.*, 1962). Other contributory factors may be bottle feeding and the misuse of laxatives (Knox *et al.*, 1962). The disease also shows a geographical and seasonal variation in its incidence.

Pathology

Intussusception is the invagination of one part of the bowel into another. The most common variety is ileo-colic.

Clinical Features

In the typical case diagnosis is easy. The infant, usually plump and healthy, starts to have recurring spasms of intense abdominal colic which causes him to draw his legs up on the abdomen, to scream with pain, and to become white and shocked with a clammy skin. He remains playful and happy between these attacks in the early hours of the illness, but if diagnosis is delayed for over 24–36 hours he begins to vomit persistently and to become dehydrated. Blood and mucus are passed per rectum. Careful and gentle palpation will reveal a sausage-shaped mass somewhere along the line of the colon. This can be difficult to define when it is in the right hypochondrium, and in late cases bimanual examination with a finger in the rectum may be necessary to palpate the mass which is now in the pelvis. The abdomen is usually scaphoid, but in late cases the distension of intestinal obstruction will sooner or later develop. The child usually has a low-grade fever. In some cases, how-ever, the clinical course of the illness is less striking and the diagnosis less easy. For example, the early passage of blood and mucus after an initial faecal stool may simulate bacillary dysentery, a misdiagnosis which can have disastrous consequences. Whenever there is doubt a barium enema must be carefully performed, because it is capable of revealing an intussusception with certainty.

Treatment

The standard method of treatment is by operative reduction of the intussusception. This is probably the safest method outwith large paediatric centres. In some clinics, however, reduction of the intussusception by means of a barium enema has now become the preferred method of treatment (Zachary, 1955). This demands close co-operation between surgeon and radiologist, and the former must always be prepared for an immediate operation if the attempt at reduction should fail. The irreducible intussusception necessitates resection of gangrenous bowel. The mortality rate from intussusception in the best paediatric centres is now almost negligible.

ACUTE APPENDICITIS

This most common of the surgical emergencies of childhood can be one of the most difficult to diagnose early and tragedies still occur, probably more frequently than is necessary. In toddlers and infants especially the inflamed appendix can rupture and lead to generalized peritonitis within a matter of hours. In other cases atypical features may lead to a delay in diagnosis until a palpable appendix abscess has formed. It behoves the doctor to supervise the child with abdominal pain with great diligence.

Clinical Features

The onset is sudden with para-umbilical colicky pain. This is almost invariably followed by vomiting. The pain migrates to the right iliac fossa where it assumes a constant aching character. The temperature rarely rises above 102° F. The child looks ill to the experienced eye. Gentle palpation of the abdomen, which should start in the left lower quadrant with a warm hand, will reveal consistent tenderness and involuntary rigidity in the right iliac fossa. The examination of a fractious toddler often demands great patience and gentleness. Constipation is the rule, but diarrhoea may be quite severe when an appendix lying low in the pelvis is in contact with the sigmoid colon. In doubtful cases a rectal examination is essential. It may reveal an area of consistent tenderness or the fluctuant mass of a pelvic abscess. Leucocytosis is a useful finding but its absence does not exclude the diagnosis. The urine should always be examined for protein, pus cells and sugar. The onset of generalized peritonitis is indicated by a sudden deterioration in the child's condition, generalized abdominal tenderness and rigidity followed later by distension due to paralytic ileus, dehydration, ketosis, high fever and a rising pulse rate.

Differential Diagnosis

Many diseases can simulate acute appendicitis, e.g. pneumonia, pyelonephritis, diabetic ketosis, the periodic syndrome, typhoid fever and simple constipation. In most instances the problem can be resolved on the basis of a careful history and physical examination, which must include chemical and microscopical examination of the urine. A most difficult problem can be presented by *non-specific mesenteric adenitis*, which is probably due to adenovirus infection, and in which the prominent features are abdominal pain, vomiting and tenderness. There is usually a history obtainable of a preceding upper respiratory infection. The abdominal pain is not well localized as it is in appendicitis, and true involuntary muscle rigidity can be shown with patience to be absent. The temperature is frequently above 102° F. Leucocytosis is absent.

Treatment

It is always safer to remove the appendix in cases where real doubt exists. In difficult cases, however, a few hours of unhurried observation in hospital, where an hourly pulse rate can be measured, will frequently resolve the diagnostic uncertainty. The reader is referred to surgical textbooks for operative details.

ULCERATIVE COLITIS

Aetiology

The cause of this unpleasant disease is unknown. It is, fortunately, uncommon in children. No specific infective agent has been isolated. On the other hand, the presence of severe psychological disturbances in most affected children such as abnormal parent-child relationships, social maladjustments, or school difficulties, has led many to regard the disease as a psychosomatic problem. In some cases evidence of an allergy towards milk has been found. Others have suggested that the disease is one of the so-called "auto-immune diseases".

Pathology

The mucous membrane of part or all of the colon and sometimes of the terminal ileum becomes hyperaemic, oedematous and ulcerated. In some areas oedema may give rise to pseudopolypoid nodules. The ulceration may extend through the muscularis; indeed perforation of the colon is by no means unknown. Fibrosis and cicatrization can lead to stenosis. Cirrhosis of the liver is sometimes also present.

Clinical Features

The onset is sudden with diarrhoea and the frequent passage of small stools containing blood and mucus. There may be abdominal pain and, when the rectum is severely involved, tenesmus. Anorexia and loss of weight lead to a state of cachexia. Hypochromic anaemia, partly due to loss of blood, is almost invariably present. Hypoproteinaemic oedema may develop. Fever is slight or absent. The diagnosis requires first the exclusion by repeated tests of other causes of bloody diarrhoea such as amoebiasis, bacillary dysentery and gonococcal proctitis. It is confirmed by the typical appearances on sigmoidoscopy and barium enema.

The latter shows loss of the normal haustrations in the colon and the so-called "lead-pipe" appearance. In some areas pseudopolypoid appearances may be visualized.

Treatment

The basis of medical treatment is rest in bed when symptoms are acute, low-residue high protein diet, and an adequate intake of vitamins. Anaemia should be corrected by blood transfusion. Psychiatric advice and treatment is often helpful and should always be sought. Remissions can frequently be obtained by daily colonic instillations of hydrocortisone sodium succinate 100 mg., or prednisolone disodium phosphate 20 mg. in 100 ml. of isotonic buffered solution. This is preferable to the systemic use of corticosteroids, as the adrenal cortex is less markedly suppressed and side-effects are uncommon. Sulphasalazine, 0·5–1·0 gm. six-hourly, has been claimed a useful antibacterial in this disease, but the author has been unimpressed by its value in children. When symptoms are unrelieved by medical treatment or if relapses are frequent, the surgeon must be consulted before the child's general condition has deteriorated severely. Colectomy with ileostomy, or even with preservation of the rectum in carefully selected cases, is an unhappy mutilation of a growing child but it may be unavoidable if his life is to be saved.

CHRONIC CONSTIPATION, ACQUIRED MEGACOLON AND ENCOPRESIS

These inter-related conditions are common in children over the age of 3 years, and they can present the physician with a most difficult problem in treatment. Many cases of chronic constipation are due to atony of the bowel wall, consequent upon long-continued misuse of laxatives by parents who are obsessed by the desirability of a daily bowel movement, an obsession greatly encouraged by intensive advertising by the manufacturers of patent medicines. In other instances the parents' obsessional or coercive attitude to toilet training in infancy has resulted in the child associating the act of defaecation with a long succession of unhappy episodes. In some of these children persistent constipation and dyschezia cause a dilatation and hypertrophy of the rectum and sigmoid colon. This type of "acquired" megacolon is to be distinguished from Hirschsprung's disease by the fact that symptoms do not start for some years after birth, the rectum is always full of hard faeces, and there are no acute episodes of partial intestinal obstruction. The barium enema reveals a grossly dilated rectum which tapers to a cone at the anal junction, "terminal reservoir" appearance. There is no narrow aganglionic segment as in Hirschsprung's disease. Most cases of encopresis or faecal soiling in children are secondary to acquired megacolon. A small number, however, are due to more acute psychological disturbances.

Treatment

The major difficulty in management is often the obsessive attitude of the parents. They must be brought to realize that constipation is not, in itself, a major hazard to health, and that repeated laxatives in larger and larger doses defeat their own object. Indeed, the complete withdrawal of laxatives and the institution of a weekly saline rectal wash-out for a period, will frequently abolish the encopresis and allow the bowel to regain some spontaneous rhythmic activity. In the worst cases the treatment may have to be initiated by manual disimpaction of faeces under general anaesthesia. The diet should be rich in fruit and roughage such as vegetables and cereals. Psychotherapy is frequently indicated. It is of great value in encopresis of recent origin related to obvious psychological difficulties, but less successful in acquired megacolon of long standing. In some children an associated enuresis complicates the problem. The ultimate prognosis is good but the physician must be prepared for a prolonged period of supervision.

INFECTIVE HEPATITIS

Aetiology

In children most cases are caused by virus A acquired by inhalation or ingestion. Syringe-transmitted homologous serum jaundice due to virus B is relatively uncommon during childhood. The incubation period in virus A infections is 24–30 days, whereas in virus B infections it extends to 90–120 days after the injection or transfusion.

$A \rightarrow {}^3/_{52}$

$B \rightarrow {}^3/_{12}$

Pathology

The principal features are centrilobular parenchymal necrosis of variable severity and periportal cellular infiltration with polymorphonuclears, plasma cells, lymphocytes and macrophages. Bile stasis is also found. Complete recovery is the rule, but in rare cases acute hepatic necrosis (acute yellow atrophy) causes death. Cirrhosis of the liver is probably a rare sequel.

Clinical Features

The relative mildness of infective hepatitis in most children must not lull the physician into an over-casual approach to what can occasionally be a fatal disease. Jaundice is usually preceded by some days of anorexia, nausea, vomiting and upper abdominal pain. Fever may be absent or quite high. When jaundice develops the stools become clay-coloured. The urine contains an excess of urobilinogen and bile pigments. Pruritus is not a common complaint in children. The liver is enlarged and tender, and the spleen may become palpable. Liver function tests reveal abnormal results, e.g. raised levels of serum glutamic-oxaloacetic and glutamic-pyruvic transaminases, positive zinc sulphate turbidity, thymol turbidity and colloidal gold reactions, and raised plasma alkaline phosphatase.

Differential Diagnosis

In the pre-icteric stage appendicitis may be simulated, but sensitive tests (Fouchet or Ictotest) will usually reveal bile in the urine. True involuntary muscle rigidity does not occur in hepatitis. *Leptospiral jaundice* due to *L. canicola* from dogs or *L. icterohaemorrhagiae* from rats is rare in the United Kingdom. It is characterized by conjunctival suffusion, herpes labialis which may even become purpuric, proteinuria, and sometimes by lymphocytic meningitis. The diagnosis can be confirmed by inoculation of guinea-pigs with the patient's blood early in the illness or by a specific agglutination test on the serum (Hutchison *et al.*, 1946).

Prevention

The course of the illness can be modified by intramuscular gamma globulin given soon after exposure and not later than six days before the onset of symptoms. The dose level is 0·06–0·12 mg./Kg.

Treatment

The patient should be kept in bed until bile pigments have disappeared from the urine and the appetite has returned to normal. Thereafter convalescence takes 2–3 weeks. In the acute stage of nausea light diet with an abundant intake of glucose and fluids is required. Later a diet rich in protein and low in fat is advised. Vomiting can be relieved with one of the anti-histamine group which is used for motion sickness. Constipation should be treated with a saline laxative.

Acute liver failure is a rare emergency in childhood. If the hepatitis seems to be getting more severe in spite of bed rest corticosteroids should be tried. Suitable dosage with prednisolone is 40 mg./day for 10 days, 20 mg./day for 10 days and 10 mg./day for 10 days. However, if to persistent vomiting are added mental confusion or abnormal neurological signs, protein must be completely withdrawn from the diet. Glucose, 25 per cent solution, should be given by intragastric drip or by slow infusion into the inferior vena cava (at least 500 gm. per day). Hypokalaemia should be corrected with potassium chloride, 10 mEq. to each 500 ml. of 25 per cent glucose solution. Some add insulin, 10 units with each 50 gm. of glucose, to promote the deposition of glycogen in the liver. Neomycin 50 mg./Kg./day should be given orally to reduce the ammonia-producing bacterial flora of the gut. Intravenous vitamin B complex (Parentrovite) is indicated on theoretical grounds. Vitamin K_1, 10 mg./day should be given intravenously. The value of intravenous sodium glutamate is doubtful.

CIRRHOSIS OF THE LIVER

Aetiology

Hepatic cirrhosis is uncommon in children in the United Kingdom and the histological differentiation into "portal" and "biliary" types tends to be less well defined than in adults. A pathological picture similar to that of Laennec's portal cirrhosis may follow neonatal hepatitis, blood group incompatibility, the de Toni-Fanconi syndrome, and it may be the form of presentation of Wilson's hepatolenticular cirrhosis (Kerr *et al.*, 1961). Infective hepatitis may also lead to hepatic cirrhosis. Other rare causes of cirrhosis of the liver include galactosaemia, Gaucher's disease, Niemann-Pick disease and xanthomatosis. Although congenital syphilis can cause a pericellular cirrhosis in stillborn infants it is doubtful if it ever causes postnatal hepatic cirrhosis. Pure biliary cirrhosis is seen invariably in congenital biliary atresia and a focal type is very common in fibrocystic disease of the pancreas. In India hepatic cirrhosis is a common disease of children in the age-group 1–3 years. It is not yet clear whether most of these cases are the sequel to infective hepatitis or the result of chronic malnutrition. In Jamaica a form of cirrhosis called *veno-occlusive disease of the liver*, in which there is occlusion of the small hepatic veins, is due to the toxic effects of an alkaloid in bush tea (Jelliffe *et al.*, 1957). Kerr *et al.* (1961) have described a condition which they call "congenital hepatic fibrosis", in which liver function is well preserved although thick bands of fibrous tissue divide up the liver. Jaundice is rare in spite of gross hepatomegaly. This is probably a variant of congenital cystic disease of the liver. There is often a familial incidence.

Clinical Features

The child usually presents with abdominal swelling due to enlargement of the liver which has a firm edge, sometimes smooth, often nodular. Anorexia, lack of energy and slowing of growth are common complaints. Splenomegaly develops if there is portal hypertension. In most cases jaundice makes its appearance sooner rather than later. Spontaneous bleeding is usually due to hypoprothrombinaemia. Orthochromic anaemia is common. When ascites develops the outlook is grave; it is usually associated with hypoproteinaemia and portal hypertension. The latter may result in massive gastro-intestinal haemorrhage. In other cases death occurs from hepatic encephalopathy with flapping tremor, mental confusion, extensor plantar responses and coma. Spider naevi and "liver palms" are uncommon in children, but clubbing of the fingers may develop. Hypersplenism may produce leucopenia and thrombocytopenia (Banti's syndrome). Various derangements of liver function can be demonstrated biochemically, e.g. raised direct bilirubin levels, hypoalbuminaemia, and raised serum gamma globulin. In hepatic encephalopathy the blood ammonia level is high. Diagnosis should be confirmed by liver biopsy either through a special needle or at laparotomy.

Treatment

Specific treatment is available only for the few cases due to metabolic errors such as Wilson's disease or galactosaemia. Life can be prolonged with a high protein diet, plus a liberal intake of the B vitamins and oral vitamin K_1, 10 mg. per day. Ascites should be treated with chlorothiazide and a low sodium diet. Hypokalaemia may require supplements of potassium chloride. In resistant cases diuresis may be improved by giving (along with chlorothiazide) an aldosterone antagonist such as spironolactone, 25 mg. four times daily. Paracentesis abdominis should be avoided whenever possible. When signs of hepatic failure supervene protein should be completely eliminated from the diet and the therapeutic regime already described for this emergency should be started. Both the parents and the child require sympathetic handling in this chronic and incurable disease.

PORTAL HYPERTENSION

Aetiology

In contrast to the situation in adults, only a small minority of cases of portal hypertension in children are due to cirrhosis of the liver. Most are extrahepatic and due to thrombosis in the splenic or portal veins (Shaldon and Sherlock, 1962). This may follow umbilical sepsis in the neonatal period or replacement transfusion via the umbilical vein (Oski et al., 1963), although Thompson and Sherlock (1964) failed to find a case of portal vein thrombosis in a prospective study of 493 children who had required catheterization of the umbilical vein in the neonatal period. It may also follow a ruptured appendix, osteitis or pyaemia. Congenital abnormalities of the portal vein are rare. Most of the cases with cavernous changes in the porta hepatis represent the results of recanalization in a previously thrombosed portal vein; they are not true malformations.

Clinical Features

Frequently the first trouble is a massive haemorrhage from oesophageal varices with haematemesis and melaena. The enlarged spleen may so diminish in size after such a haemorrhage that the cause of the haemorrhage is temporarily obscured. However, the characteristic physical finding is a greatly enlarged firm spleen. This may have been noted for some time before the first haemorrhage. Thrombocytopenia and leucopenia may also be found, but they are not of much diagnostic assistance. Less severe chronic bleeding can result in a marked hypochromic anaemia. Ascites may occur as a result of hypoproteinaemia caused by haemorrhage but it is uncommon. Liver function tests and liver biopsy findings are normal in the common case of extrahepatic origin. The oesophageal varices can usually be demonstrated on a barium swallow or by oesophagoscopy. The site of the obstruction in the portal circulation should, however, be determined by the technique of splenoportal venography (Steiner *et al.*, 1957).

Treatment

Every effort should be made to postpone surgical intervention until the child is as old as possible and the veins which may have to be used are as large as possible. Indeed, in many cases portacaval anastomosis is technically impossible and lienorenal anastomosis rarely functions satisfactorily in children. Most children can be managed by blood transfusions repeated as and when they bleed and without spending long in hospital. Oesophageal tamponade with a Sengstaken tube is rarely advisable in children. Splenectomy alone is, of course, an illogical procedure and should never be performed nowadays. In older children shunting operations to relieve the portal hypertension are frequently very successful. In a few, however, repeated massive haemorrhages have to be dealt with by partial oesophagectomy and gastrectomy, a formidable procedure of only temporary value.

MALABSORPTION SYNDROMES

The great majority of cases of steatorrhoea in paediatric practice are due to coeliac disease or fibrocystic disease of the pancreas. Steatorrhoea occurs, of course, in obstructive jaundice, but its importance is overshadowed by the primary disease, e.g. biliary atresia, choledochal cyst etc. There are, however, several very rare causes of steatorrhoea, e.g. a-betalipoproteinaemia (Salt *et al.*, 1960), congenital absence of bile salts (Ross *et al.*, 1955), regional ileitis, extensive resection of bowel, intestinal lymphangiectasia etc. It is important that every case of malabsorption in a child be fully investigated because rational therapy depends upon accurate diagnosis, not always an easy problem. The stools should always be examined microscopically for evidence of infestation with *Giardia lamblia*. This can alone cause malabsorption and it is very readily eradicated with mepacrine 100 mg. twice daily for 5–7 days.

COELIAC DISEASE

Aetiology

A great advance was made when Dicke (1950) showed that children with coeliac disease lost their symptoms when wheat and rye flour were removed from the diet. It soon became apparent that the harmful substance was in the protein, and in particular the gluten, fraction of wheat and rye flour. Weijers and Van de Kamer (1960) have shown that the noxious component of gluten lies in the gliadin fraction. It has been suggested that coeliac disease is an inborn error of metabolism, in which an enzyme defect in the cells of the intestinal mucosa results in the defective splitting of the glutamine-containing peptides of gliadin into aminoacids. The abnormal presence of these peptides in the blood could damage the metabolism. They could act through an immunological mechanism, because it has been shown that the sera of patients with coeliac disease contain antibodies to a proteolyzed fraction of wheat gluten in higher incidence and titre than normal sera (Taylor *et al.*, 1961).

Pathology

The histological features have been defined mainly from a study of specimens obtained by duodenal or jejunal biopsy (Doniach and Shiner, 1957; Booth *et al.*, 1962). The most typical appearance is called total villous atrophy. The mucosa is flat and devoid of normal villi but the underlying glandular layer is thickened to measure more than 300 μ and shows marked cellular infiltration. The absence of villi has been confirmed by electron microscopy. In other cases, however, there is "subtotal villous atrophy" in which short, broad and thickened villi appear to be present. These vary in height from 150–300 μ in contrast to normal villi in the range 320–510 μ. The electron microscope has shown that, in fact, there are no villi at all but that the surface of the mucosa is composed of a series of ridges, convolutions and whorls. These appearances appear to be pathognomonic of coeliac disease.

Clinical Features

Symptoms do not develop until gluten-containing foods are introduced into the infant's diet. In most cases the first symptoms are noted in the last three months of the first year of life, but the child is usually not brought to the physician until the second year. A considerable number of milder cases go undetected for much longer and even into adult life.

The first change is in the child's personality when he becomes fractious and miserable. Anorexia is associated with failure to gain weight. The stools are characteristically of porridgy consistency, pale, bulky and foul-smelling, but in some children this feature is not very marked. In others, however, the illness may start with vomiting and watery diarrhoea to simulate an enteral infection. A constant feature of coeliac disease is slowing of growth; indeed a normal height virtually excludes the diagnosis. The abdomen becomes distended as a result of carbohydrate fermentation and this contrasts with the child's wasted buttocks and thighs (Fig. 54). The bones become osteoporotic and ossification is delayed; this is the result of calcium deprivation because the dietary calcium combines with the excess fatty acids in the gut to form insoluble calcium soaps. In the worst cases malabsorption of protein can lead to hypoproteinaemic oedema.

Various other defects in absorption may become clinically manifest. Iron-deficiency anaemia is common. There is usually diminished absorption of folic acid as revealed by a lowered serum folate level, but a frank megaloblastic anaemia is seen only infrequently in older coeliac children who have not been adequately treated. Clinical signs of deficiency of vitamin B complex, such as angular stomatitis or glossitis, are also rarely seen in childhood. Although deficiency of vitamins A and D is probably always present rickets is quite rare (due to lack of growth) and xerophthalmia is almost unknown. However, coeliac rickets sometimes develop in the untreated case during the growth period at 5–7 years; it may also develop as a consequence of treatment with a gluten-free diet if supplements of vitamin D are omitted while active growth continues. Rarely in the older child with untreated coeliac disease hypocalcaemic tetany develops.

Diagnostic Tests

There is a wide variety of tests and only those which we have found most useful are discussed. Fat balance studies on a diet containing a known amount of fat (30–40 gm./day) will show diminished absorption (under 90 per cent). A simpler technique is to determine the daily fat output in the faeces on a similar diet. A daily output in excess of 4 gm. in a child indicates steatorrhoea. The xylose absorption test, suitably modified for young children, is extremely reliable. A 24 hour collection of urine after the oral ingestion of 5 gm. of d-xylose should contain at least 25 per cent of the dose; less than this indicates malabsorption. An oral glucose tolerance test after 1·5 gm. glucose per Kg. body weight will show a "flat" curve, whereas an intravenous glucose tolerance test will give normal results. The bones of the hand and forearm, or of the legs, will show osteoporosis, and there may be considerable delay in skeletal maturation. A barium meal and follow-through examination provides very reliable evidence of malabsorption, although the changes from normal are not confined to coeliac disease. These changes, with the modern barium suspensions, are marked coarsening of the mucosal pattern of the small bowel, jejunal dilatation and, in many cases, delay in the passage of the barium through the small bowel to the colon. We have found the barium meal in the hands of an experienced radiologist to be an extremely reliable "screening" test for malabsorption, and one particularly suitable in out-patients. The most reliable test of all in the diagnosis of coeliac disease is duodenal or jejunal biopsy (Cameron et al., 1962; Hubble, 1963). It carries a small risk of haemorrhage or perforation of the bowel and its performance demands a certain amount of expertise.

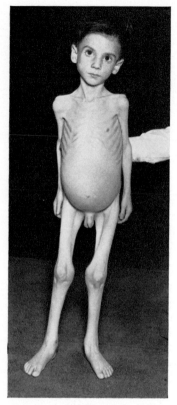

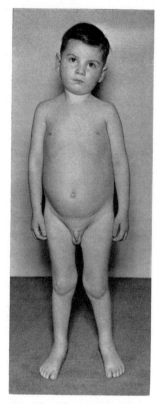

FIG. 54.—Seven-year-old boy with untreated coeliac disease. Note gaseous abdominal distension and gross tissue wasting.

FIG. 55.—The same boy as in Fig. 54 after nine months treatment on gluten-free diet.

Treatment

Coeliac disease is to be regarded as a gluten-induced enteropathy and the results of treatment with a gluten-free diet are impressive (Fig. 55). This is first apparent as a striking improvement in personality soon to be followed by rapid growth, while the stools more slowly return to normal. Strict supervision is essential and the child's height and weight should be recorded at regular intervals. Satisfactory results must also require a high sense of responsibility on the part of the parents.

In the United Kingdom a gluten-free diet is one from which, in effect, all wheat flour has been excluded. The parents should be supplied with a comprehensive list of the many foodstuffs which contain gluten and are, therefore, forbidden; also a list of the gluten-free foods which are freely permitted. Bread and biscuits made from gluten-free wheat starch are commercially available. It is also possible to home-bake gluten-free bread, biscuits and cakes with recipes supplied by hospital dietetic departments. An adequate intake of vitamins, and especially of vitamin D, is important. This is best given in a water-miscible preparation such as Paladac (P. D. & Co.), 60 to 120 minims (4–8 ml.) daily. The child should also receive an adequate daily ration of fruit. A suitable prescription for iron-deficiency anaemia is:

Ferrous sulphate 3 gr. (180 mg.)
Dilute hypophosphorous acid ½ minim (0·03 ml.)
Dextrose 15 gr. (1 gm.)
Chloroform water to 60 minims (4 ml.)
Label: 60 minims thrice daily with food.

When the anaemia fails to respond to oral iron it should be treated with iron-dextran complex (Imferon-Benger) given intramuscularly. When the serum folate level is low, or if there is megaloblastic anaemia, folic acid should be prescribed in a dose of 5 mg. twice daily. If the serum vitamin B_{12} level is low, and this is uncommon, the child should receive in addition intramuscular cyanocobalamin 100 μg. weekly until the anaemia has been corrected, followed by 100 μg. once per month.

The gluten-free diet should be continued for at least five years when gluten-containing foods may again be gradually introduced into the diet. Some children prove to be always intolerant to gluten and probably should remain permanently on a gluten-free diet. The abnormal intestinal mucosa returns towards normal with successful treatment but it relapses if the diet is broken or relaxed too soon.

FIBROCYSTIC DISEASE OF THE PANCREAS

Aetiology

This common disease of infancy and childhood (Bodian *et al.*, 1952) was at first thought to be primarily a pancreatic disorder (Andersen, 1938). It was later called "mucoviscidosis" when the abnormality of the mucous glands was recognized (Farber, 1944), but it is now known to be a genetically determined disease affecting all the exocrine glands of the body including the liver (Claireaux, 1956) and the sweat glands (di Sant'Agnese *et al.*, 1953; Schwachman *et al.*, 1955). The probable mode of inheritance is an autosomal recessive and the familial incidence is of great diagnostic significance (Andersen and Hodges, 1946). Koch (1960) studying the families of adult cases has suggested an autosomal dominant inheritance with a fairly high penetrance, but he seems not to have considered the possibility of partial forms of the disease in heterozygotes. The pathogenesis of the disease is obscure but Roberts (1959) working in the author's hospital, has suggested a persistent over-secretion of all the cholinergic glands, e.g. pancreas, mucous and salivary glands. Although the sweat glands are supplied by sympathetic nerve fibres they are anomalous in that they are induced to secrete by acetylcholine and not by adrenalin.

Pathology

The pancreas is abnormal in over 90 per cent of cases. A constant change is fibrosis with atrophy of the exocrine parenchyma. Cystic dilatation of acini and ducts is common but not invariable. The islet tissue, however, is rarely involved. The earliest change in both pancreas and salivary glands is an absence from the cells of zymogen granules, a feature which favours Robert's theory of pathogenesis. The mucous glands throughout the body, including Brunner's glands in the duodenum, are grossly distended and they secrete an abnormal viscid mucus. The sweat glands appear normal histologically but they secrete sweat with an abnormally high concentration of electrolytes. A characteristic feature of the disease is the widespread bronchiolitis. This is due to the *Staph. aureus* which grows best in a salt-rich medium. The bronchiolitis results in generalized obstructive emphysema, multiple abscesses, and even pyopneumothorax. The bronchial ciliated columnar epithelium often undergoes squamous metaplasia. The liver shows a focal type of biliary cirrhosis, most marked under the capsule; it may lead to portal hypertension.

Clinical Features

The widespread pathological changes in this disease can obviously lead to an extremely varied symptomatology. None the less, the symptoms tend to occur in a more or less ordered fashion and the diagnosis is not often unduly difficult. In about 10 per cent of cases the illness presents in the neonatal period in the form of meconium ileus (p. 266). Very rarely the biliary cirrhosis is of such degree as to cause obstructive jaundice and death from hepatic failure during the first month of life. The most common presentation, however, is in the form of an intractable respiratory infection dating from the early weeks or months of life. Indeed, fibrocystic disease of the pancreas should always be suspected when a respiratory infection in infancy fails to respond promptly to adequate antibiotic therapy. Some rather typical features in these cases are the slight rise in temperature which contrasts with the obvious dyspnoea and subcostal recession; the distressing spasms of coughing which cause vomiting and interfere with feeding; and the inspiratory position of the chest wall with active use of the accessory muscles of respiration arising from the generalized emphysema. Auscultation sometimes reveals numerous fine crepitations, at other times only a few rhonchi. In the early stages of the disease radio-

à. "T.B.W." pattern (Hodson)

graphs of the chest may show only increased translucency of the lung fields; later heavy interstitial markings appear; then multiple soft shadows representing small lung abscesses. In other cases there may be lobar consolidation, empyema or pyopneumothorax. In children who survive the early months of life the respiratory picture becomes that of bronchiectasis with purulent sputum, areas of bronchial breathing and crepitations, increasing emphysema, and clubbing of the fingers. Sputum culture in such cases will show the predominant organism to be the *Staph. aureus.* ± *Pseudomonas aeruginosa.*

In a minority of cases the respiratory infection is less prominent than the presence of semi-formed, greasy, bulky and excessively foul-smelling stools. This feature coincides with the introduction of mixed feeding. After the first year of life, indeed, the history of abnormal and frequent stools occurring in association with abdominal distension and general-ized tissue-wasting may simulate coeliac disease. The differential diagnosis can, however, almost always be made on clinical grounds alone. In pancreatic fibrosis a careful history will elicit that symptoms first appeared in the early weeks of life, whereas coeliac disease rarely presents before the age of nine months. The excellent, often voracious, appetite in pancreatic fibrosis contrasts sharply with the unhappy anorexia of the coeliac child. Chronic respiratory infection of some degree, usually severe, is an invariable accompaniment of pancreatic fibrosis but it is not a feature of coeliac disease. Iron-deficiency anaemia is common in coeliac disease whereas there may be an increased absorption of iron in pancreatic fibrosis (Davis and Badenoch, 1962). Furthermore, the diagnosis of pancreatic fibrosis may be suggested by a history that previous siblings have died of the same disease.

If the affected infant survives the first year, childhood seems often to bring with it a period of improvement in the chest condition. All too frequently, however, the approach of puberty is associated with cor pulmonale. Less commonly biliary cirrhosis and portal hypertension lead to massive gastro-intestinal haemorrhage. It has also been recently recognized that some affected persons can live to adult life. The disease may then take a familiar form such as chronic staphylococcal bronchiec-tasis and emphysema in association with steatorrhoea. In other cases its clinical manifestations are unfamiliar in paediatric practice, e.g. severe peptic ulceration with emphysema and hypotension (Koch, 1960), or pulmonary infection, steatorrhoea, choroiditis, vitreous opacities and enlarged submandibular salivary glands (Marks and Anderson, 1960).

Diagnostic Tests

The most useful are designed to reveal the absence of pancreatic enzymes or the excessive concentration of sodium and chloride in the sweat. A useful "screening test" in infants is the determination of tryptic activity in the stools by the use of serial dilutions (Emery, 1952). A high tryptic activity excludes pancreatic fibrosis, but in the absence of such evidence the diagnosis must be confirmed by more delicate tests such as the demonstration of absent or grossly diminished trypsin in the duodenal juice obtained by duodenal intubation (Andersen and Early, 1942). There are various methods of testing the sweat electrolytes. The "finger print" method is a useful screening test for out-patients (Schwachman and Gahm, 1956; Knights et al., 1959). If this test is positive a firm diagnosis must subsequently be based upon quantitative estimation of the sodium and chloride concentrations in the sweat obtained by enveloping the patient in a plastic bag (Schwachman et al., 1955), or by means of pilocarpine iontophoresis (Gibson and Cooke, 1959). Diagnostic levels of sodium and chloride are 70 mEq/l. in each case.

Treatment

The most important factor is control of the staphylococcal lung sepsis; indeed upon the success of these efforts depends the prognosis. In most cases the permanent administration of suitable antibiotics is unavoidable. The organism is usually resistant to benzylpenicillin, and as it readily becomes resistant to other antibiotics the sensitivity tests should be repeated at intervals. In practice it usually becomes necessary to change from one antibiotic to another as time goes on. Suitable antibiotics for long-term oral use are tetracycline (25 mg./Kg./day), cloxacillin (50 mg./Kg./day), ampicillin (50 mg./Kg./day), and erythromycin (50 mg./Kg./day). Chloramphenicol is too toxic for prolonged treatment. The recently introduced oral antibiotic fucidin seems particularly valuable for short-term use in exacerbations of lung infection. It is given in a daily dosage of 20 mg./Kg./day in four divided doses. It is also possible to give antibiotics in the form of aerosols, e.g. streptomycin 250 mg. or neomycin 250 mg. four times daily. When the sputum is viscid and the child suffers from distressing outbursts of coughing, relief may often be obtained by the use of a Humidair (Oxygenaire, Ltd.) or Croupette (Air Shields, Inc.) into the humidity chamber of which is put 10 per cent propylene glycol in 3 per cent sodium chloride solution. The child can spend the night in such a tent which can contain air or oxygen. After a week or two the sodium chloride, which is bactericidal in this concentration, can be removed from the aerosol so that the bronchial mucous membrane is not unduly irritated. It is often helpful if the child can continue the aerosol therapy at home using a vacolyser pump and inhaling 10 per cent propylene glycol in water with an antibiotic several times each day. We have not found N-acetylcysteine to be as effective a substance for aerosol treatment. Physiotherapy is an important adjunct to the management of the pulmonary disease. It should include properly planned postural drainage and deep breathing exercises.

The diet should be rich in protein (at least 6 gm. per Kg.) and low in

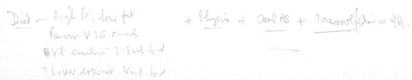

fat. Extra salt is required because of losses in the sweat; indeed in hot climates 2–3 gm. of sodium chloride per day should be given in addition to dietary salt to prevent salt-losing crises. Pancreatin should be given as Pancrex V (Paines & Byrne) 1–3 gm. daily with food. A water miscible vitamin preparation should also be prescribed, e.g. Abidec (P. D. & Co.) 15 drops daily.

The services of a surgeon may be required at several stages of the disease, e.g. for meconium ileus in the neonatal period, for lobectomy in bronchiectasis, or for portacaval anastomosis if portal hypertension is severe.

FERMENTATIVE DIARRHOEA (DISACCHARIDE INTOLERANCE)

In health the starch, sucrose and lactose in the human diet are broken down and absorbed from the small intestine in the form of glucose, glucose + fructose, and glucose + galactose respectively. If this fails to happen because of a deficiency of the enzymes maltase, sucrase or lactase there is an excess in the intestine of carbohydrates which are acted upon by bacteria, so that fermentative diarrhoea occurs with the passage of highly acid stools (Weijers and van de Kamer, 1963). Other features include failure to thrive, abdominal distension and irritability. The symptoms are relieved if the offending sugar is removed from the diet, and aggravated if the intake is increased, so that a careful history will often point to the diagnosis. Lactase deficiency leads to persistent diarrhoea from birth because both human and cow's milk contain lactose. Delay in the onset of symptoms suggests sucrose or maltase deficiency because sucrose or starch may not be added to the diet for a period. Apart from the cases in which lactase or sucrase deficiency are present from birth and presumably genetic in origin, disacchararide intolerance may occasionally be acquired following an acute diarrhoeal episode or in coeliac disease.

The diagnostic confirmation of a disaccharide intolerance can be obtained from several laboratory tests (Cornblath and Schwartz, 1966). Firstly the pH of the fresh stool is less than 5·5. Secondly the stools have a high lactic acid content. Thirdly the results of loading tests, performed only when the diarrhoea has been controlled by removing all disaccharides from the diet and replacing them with monosaccharides, will define the specific enzyme deficiency. The sugar under test such as lactose or sucrose is given in 10 per cent solution in a dose of 2 gm./Kg. body weight in the fasting state. The total blood sugar and true blood glucose levels are then measured at times 0, $\frac{1}{2}$, 1, $1\frac{1}{2}$, 2 and $2\frac{1}{2}$ hours. A rise in blood sugar of at least 50 mg. per 100 ml. is to be expected in the normal subject. If this fails to happen with a lactose or sucrose load a deficiency of lactase or sucrase respectively may be suspected. The test is then repeated with 1 gm./Kg. each of glucose + galactose in the case of suspected lactase deficiency or with glucose + fructose in suspected sucrase deficiency when a normal rise in blood sugar is to be expected. Its absence would suggest the existence of the even less common monosaccharide malabsorption syndrome (Cornblath and Schwartz, 1966), where only fructose can be absorbed. Finally, a jejunal biopsy can be performed and the specimen examined for specific enzyme activities, in addition to histological study. The diarrhoea in such infants and children can be abolished by the total exclusion from the diet of the offending carbohydrate after its precise identification.

INTESTINAL PARASITES

Parasitic worms are relatively uncommon in British paediatric practice, with the exception of threadworms, and their incidence is highest where personal hygiene is poor.

CESTODES (Tapeworms)

The only common form of cestodiasis in Britain is caused by *Taenia saginata* (the beef tapeworm), infection being acquired from imperfectly cooked beef. The adult worm lives in the intestine of man (definitive host), is about 20 feet long, and has about 2,000 segments each containing a lateral genital pore which alternates irregularly and a branched uterus. The head is pear shaped with four suckers but no hooklets. The ova are passed in the stools and eaten by the ox. *Taenia solium* (the pork tapeworm) infects man when he eats poorly cooked pork. The adult worm is about 10 feet long, has about 1,000 segments with branched uteri and regularly alternating lateral genital pores. The head is globular with four suckers and a rostellum carrying two rows of hooklets. The ova are eaten by the pig after the segments are passed in the host's faeces. *Diphyllobothrium latum* is common in Finland and it is acquired by eating badly cooked fish or caviare. The adult worm is about 30 feet long, has about 8,000 segments with a central uterus and ventral genital pore, and the head is olive shaped with suction grooves on ventral and dorsal aspects but without hooklets. The ova are swallowed by various crustacea and subsequently by fish. The larvae of these worms form in the muscles of the ox, pig or fish (intermediate hosts), and when eaten by the definitive host grow into adult worms.

Clinical Features.—Infection by *diphyllobothrium latum* can cause a megaloblastic anaemia in a small minority of people. Otherwise tapeworm infection is only recognized when segments are passed in the stools. Infrequently the human being swallows the ova of *Taenia solium* and the cysticerci develop in his muscles, eyes, subcutaneous tissues or brain —*cysticercosis*. Symptoms include epileptic seizures, and at a later stage the calcified dead larvae can be demonstrated radiologically in the muscles. This disease is not seen in children in the United Kingdom.

Treatment.—The child should be admitted to hospital and kept in bed on a completely fluid fat-free diet for 48 hours. After a dose of magn. sulph. on the evening before, he should be given 0·6 gm. mepacrine (0·3 gm. for children under 5 years) by mouth next morning, to be followed two hours later by another dose of magn. sulph. The bright yellow staining of the worm by mepacrine makes identification of the scolex (head and neck) fairly easy if the stools are carefully examined. If the head is not dislodged from the intestinal mucosa by this somewhat rigorous regime the treatment can be repeated some months later if fresh segments reappear in the stools.

Taenia Echinococcus (Hydatid Cyst)

The definitive host of *Taenia echinococcus* is the dog, wolf or jackal. Man may become the intermediate host by swallowing the ova from the dog and this is especially likely in sheep-rearing countries such as Australia. The adult worm in the dog is very small, ¼ inch, but the ingested ovum swallowed by man liberates a six-hooked onchosphere. This penetrates to the tissues, usually the liver but sometimes lung, bones, kidneys or brain to form a hydatid cyst. This has a three layered wall—an outer layer of host fibrous tissue, a laminated middle layer, and an inner germinal layer which produces many daughter and grand-daughter cysts.

Clinical Features.—These are largely due to local pressure effects. The liver may be greatly enlarged and there may be a palpable rounded swelling over which the classical "hydatid thrill" can be elicited. This is done by placing one hand over the swelling and percussing sharply with the fingers of the other hand. Eosinophilia may be marked. The diagnosis can be confirmed with the Casoni test. Erythema and oedema develop around the site of an intradermal injection of filtered hydatid fluid which is usually obtained from the cyst of a sheep.

Treatment.—The only measure is surgical excision. The cyst must never be tapped as leakage of hydatid fluid into the tissues can cause shock or death. The outlook is grave if suppuration occurs within the cyst. Spontaneous recovery can occur if the cyst dies, inspissates and calcifies.

NEMATODES

These are round, elongated, non-segmented worms with differentiation of the sexes.

Ascaris lumbricoides (Roundworm)

The male adult is about 8 inches (20 cm.) in length, the female about 12 inches (30 cm.), and they are light brown in colour. Their habitat is the small intestine. The ova are not embryonated when passed in the faeces but they become infective in soil or water. When swallowed by man the hatched larvae penetrate the intestinal wall and pass via the liver and lungs to the trachea, oesophagus, stomach and intestine where they grow into mature worms.

Clinical Features.—In most cases the existence of infestation is only recognized when a mature roundworm is vomited or passed in the faeces. Very rarely the worms are so numerous as to cause intestinal obstruction. When very large numbers of ova are swallowed the passage of many larvae through the lungs can result in fever, cough, radiological changes and eosinophilia. Ova may be found in the faeces under the microscope.

Treatment.—The drug of choice is piperazine as detailed under the treatment for threadworms. An alternative is hexylresorcinol (Crystoids) which must be given in capsule form because of its tendency to burn the tongue and buccal mucosa. The dose is 100 mg. per year of age up to 10 years, given in the morning on an empty stomach. It is not suitable for very young children. Toxic drugs like santonin and oil of chenopodium are no longer used.

Oxyuris vermicularis (Threadworm; Pinworm)

The male worm is about 3 mm. in length, and the female which looks like a small piece of thread, is about 10 mm. The female lives in the colon; the eggs are laid when the female passes out of the anus and they contaminate the child's fingers who may then re-infect himself. The ova after ingestion hatch in the small intestine. The male worm also fertilizes the female in the small intestine, after which the male dies while the female migrates to the caecum. It is common for this infestation to affect all members of a family because the ova can be found on many of the objects in a household. The initial infection may also be acquired from contaminated water or uncooked foodstuffs.

Clinical Features.—The most common symptom is pruritus ani. Vaginitis may also occur, but the author is sceptical of the claim that threadworms can cause abdominal pain, restlessness or irritability. In most instances the mother has observed the small thread-like worms on the child's perianal skin or in the faeces. To detect ova a glass rod is tipped with a small square of cellophane; this is then rubbed gently over the perianal region after which the cellophane is placed between a glass slide and a coverslip and examined under the microscope.

Treatment.—The child's hands must be kept clean and the nails short to minimize the risks of re-infection. The perianal skin must also be kept clean and at night pyjama trousers should be worn to prevent scratching of the skin with the fingers. It is wise to treat all members of the family. An effective drug is elixir of piperazine citrate (500 mg. per teaspoonful) in a daily dose of 1 teaspoonful for children under 2 years, 2 teaspoonfuls for children under 5 years, 3 teaspoonfuls for children under 13 years, and 4 teaspoonfuls for adults. The drug should be given for two 7-day courses with a week intervening. An effective alternative is viprynium embonate in a single dose of 5 mg./Kg. body weight (available as 50 mg. tablets or a suspension containing 10 mg. per ml.).

Hookworm (*Ankylostoma duodenale; Necator Americanus*)

There are two types of hookworm, *ankylostoma duodenale* being most commonly found in Egypt, India, Ceylon, Queensland and the Southern U.S.A., while *necator americanus* is found in the Americas, the Philippines and India. Ankylostomiasis is sometimes encountered in immigrants to the United Kingdom. The male and female worms live chiefly in the jejunum. The worm attaches itself to the intestinal mucosa by its teeth and sucks blood. The ova, passed in the faeces, hatch out in water or damp soil and the larvae penetrate the skin of the feet. They reach the heart and lungs by the blood stream, penetrate into the bronchi, are coughed up the trachea and then pass down the oesophagus to mature in the small intestine.

Clinical features.—The larvae produce vesicular or pustular lesions on the feet ("ground itch") which heal in a week or two. Months later the child may present with a severe microcytic hypochromic anaemia. It may be of sufficient severity to lead to cardiac enlargement and congestive failure. Its differentiation from other causes of iron-deficiency anaemia (Chapter XIX) is indicated by the finding of a marked eosinophilia, and ova can be found in the stools. Pica (dirt eating) may be a feature.

Treatment.—The drug of choice is tetrachloroethylene which should be given only after a 12-hour period of fasting. It should be stored in a cool dark place. The adult dose is 4 ml., and for children 0·2 ml. for each year of life to a maximum of 4 ml. It can be dispensed in 30–60 ml. of a saturated solution of sodium sulphate. An alternative is bephenium hydroxynaphthoate, a quaternary ammonium compound, given before breakfast in a single dose of 1·25 gm. bephenium ion for children under 10 Kg., and 2·5 gm. for those of larger size.

Trichinella spiralis (Trichiniasis)

The male and female adult worms have their habitat in the small intestine. Man is infected by eating raw or partially cooked pork sausages or ham. The encysted trichinella in the pig's striated muscle are then digested in man's intestine to liberate larvae which grow into adult worms. The adult worms produce ova which hatch into embryos. These migrate by the blood stream or lymphatics to striated muscles where they coil up and become encysted. The disease is uncommon in the United Kingdom although a considerable outbreak occurred in 1941 during the Second World War.

Clinical features.—The incubation period is from 5 to 15 days. There may be preliminary diarrhoea and vomiting but after a week or so the migration of embryos is associated with fever, swelling of the face and eyelids, headache and muscular pains. Splinter haemorrhages may be seen under the nails. Encephalitic or meningitic signs sometimes develop. The absence of proteinuria excludes nephritis and the diagnosis is suggested by the presence of a marked eosinophilia. Sometimes the larvae can be found in the blood in the early weeks of the illness in which muscular pains and weakness can last for some months. Later in the disease muscle biopsy of the pectoralis major, biceps or gastrocnemius may reveal the encysted worms. The disease carries a small mortality rate from myocarditis or encephalitis.

Treatment.—Apart from purging during the invasive stage of gastrointestinal symptoms to drive out the adult worms, only palliative measures are available. If systemic manifestations are severe, relief may be obtained with corticosteroids. Good results have recently been reported in animals from thiabendazole, 50 mg./Kg. body weight.

GIARDIA LAMBLIA

Giardiasis or lambliasis is the only common protozoan intestinal parasitic infection in the United Kingdom, apart from the non-pathogenic *Entamoeba coli*. Indeed, it is not completely certain how pathogenic is *Giardia lamblia*, but in severe infestations it appears to result in fat dyspepsia with semi-formed bulky stools and abdominal distension or discomfort. The parasite may appear as a trophozoite with eight flagella or as an ovoid cyst, and its normal habitat is the upper small bowel.

Treatment.—The infection is easily eradicated with mepacrine, 0·1 gm. daily in two doses for infants, 0·2 gm. daily for children, for a period of five days.

REFERENCES

ANDERSEN, D. H. (1938). *Amer. J. Dis. Child.*, **56**, 344.
ANDERSEN, D. H., and EARLY, M. V. (1942). *Amer. J. Dis. Child.*, **63**, 891.
ANDERSEN, D. H., and HODGES, R. G. (1946). *Amer. J. Dis. Child.*, **72**, 62.
BARGER, A. J. (1958). *Amer. J. Roentgenol.*, **80**, 426.
BENSON, C. D., MUSTARD, W. T., RAVITCH, M. M., SNYDER, W. H., and WELCH, K. J. (1962). *Pediatric Surgery*. Chicago: Year Book Publishers.
BODIAN, M. M., CARTER, C. O., and NORMAN, A. P. (1952). *Fibrocystic Disease of the Pancreas*. London: Wm. Heinemann (Medical Books).
BODIAN, M. M., CARTER, C. O., and WARD, B. C. H. (1951). *Lancet*, **1**, 302.
BONHAM-CARTER, R. E., WATERSTON, D. J., and ABERDEEN, E. (1962). *Lancet*, **1**, 656.
BOOTH, C. C., STEWART, J. S., HOLMES, R., and BRACKENBURY, W. (1962). *Intestinal Biopsy*. (Ciba Foundat. Study Group No. 14). London: J. & A. Churchill.
BURKE, J. C. (1959). *Brit. med. J.*, **2**, 787.
BUDDINGH, G. J., and DODD, K. (1944). *J. Pediat.*, **25**, 105.
CAMERON, A. H., ASTLEY, R., HALLOWELL, M., RAWSON, A. B.. MILLER, C. G., FRENCH, J. M., and HUBBLE, D. V. (1962). *Quart. J. Med.*, **31**, 125.

CARRÉ, I. J. (1959). *Arch. Dis. Childh.*, **34**, 344.
CARRÉ, I. J. (1960). *Arch Dis. Childh.*, **35**, 569.
CARRÉ, I. J., and ASTLEY, R. (1960). *Arch. Dis. Childh.*, **35**, 484.
CLAIREAUX, A. E. (1956). *Arch. Dis. Childh.*, **31**, 22.
CORNBLATH, M., and SCHWARTZ, R. (1966). *Disorders of Carbohydrate Metabolism in Infancy*, Chap. 12. Philadelphia: W. B. Saunders Co.
DAVIS, A. E., and BADENOCH, J. (1962). *Lancet*, **2**, 6.
DICKE, W. K. (1950). M.D. Thesis, Utrecht.
DI SANT'AGNESE, P. A., DARLING, R. C., PERERA, G. A., and SHEA, E. (1953). *Pediatrics*, **12**, 549.
DONIACH, I., and SHINER, M. (1957). *Gastroenterology*, **33**, 71.
DUHAMEL, B. (1960). *Arch. Dis. Childh.*, **35**, 38.
EMERY, J. L. (1952). *Arch. Dis. Childh.*, **27**, 67.
FÄLLSTRÖM, S. P., and REINAND, T. (1961). *Acta Paediat. (Uppsala)*, **50**, 431.
FARBER, S. (1944). *Arch. Path.*, **37**, 238.
FORREST, H., and GRAHAM, A. G. (1963). *Scot. med. J.*, **8**, 16.
GARDNER, P. S. (1961). *Brit. med. J.*, **2**, 495.
GARDNER, P. S., KNOX, E. G., COURT, S. D. M., and GREEN, C. A. (1962). *Lancet*, **2**, 697.
GIBSON, L. E., and COOKE, R. E. (1959). *Pediatrics*, **23**, 545.
HUBBLE, D. (1963). *Brit. med. J.*, **2**, 701.
HUTCHISON, J. H., PIPPARD, J. S., GLEESON-WHITE, M. H., and SHEEHAN, H. L. (1946). *Brit. med. J.*, **1**, 81.
ILLINGWORTH, R. S. and BIRCH, L. B. (1956). *Arch. Dis. Childh.*, **31**, 300.
JACOBY, N. M. (1962). *Lancet*, **1**, 119.
JELLIFFE, D. B., GERRIT BRAS, and MUKHERJEE, K. L. (1957). *Arch. Dis. Childh.*, **32**, 369.
KAUFFMANN, F. (1947). *J. Immunol.*, **57**, 71.
KERR, D. H. S., HARRISON, C. V., SHERLOCK, S., and MILNES WALKER, R. (1961). *Quart. J. Med.*, **30**, 91.
KNIGHTS, E. M., BRUSH, J. S., and SCHROEDER, J. (1959). *J. Amer. med. Ass.*, **169**, 1279.
KNOX, E. G., COURT, S. D. N., and GARDNER, P. S. (1962). *Lancet*, **2**, 692.
KOCH, E. (1960). *Germ. med. Mth.*, **5**, 40.
LIGHT, J. S. and HODES, J. L. (1949). *J. exp. Med.*, **90**, 113.
MARKS, B. L. and ANDERSON, C. M. (1960). *Lancet*, **1**, 365.
MASON BROWN, J. J. (1962). *Surgery of Childhood*. London: Edward Arnold.
MEDICAL RESEARCH COUNCIL (1952). *The Treatment of Acute Dehydration in Infants*. (Memorandum No. 26.) London: H.M. Staty. Office.
OSKI, F. A., ALLEN, D. M., and DIAMOND, L. K. (1963). *Pediatrics*, **31**, 297.
PEONIDES, A., YOUNG, W. F., and SWAIN, V. A. J. (1963). *Arch. Dis. Childh.*, **38**, 231.
ROBERTS, G. B. S. (1959). *Lancet*, **2**, 964.
ROSS, C. A. C., FRAZER, A. C., FRENCH, J. M., GERRARD, J. W., SAMMONS, H. G., and SMELLIE, J. M. (1955). *Lancet*, **1**, 1087.
SALT, H. B., WOLFF, O. H., LLOYD, J. K., FOSBROOKE, A. S., CAMERON, A. H., and HUBBLE, D. V. (1960). *Lancet*, **2**, 325.
SCHWACHMAN, H., LEUBNER, H., and CATZEL, P. (1955). *Advanc Pediat.*, **7**, 249.
SCHWACHMAN, H., and GAHM, N. (1956). *New Engl. J. Med.*, **255**, 999.
SHALDON, S., and SHERLOCK, S. (1962). *Lancet*, **1**, 63.
STEINER, R. E., SHERLOCK, S., and TURNER, M. D. (1957). *J. Fac. Radiol. (Lond.)*, **8**, 158.
STEVENSON, J. S. (1952). *Brit. med. J.*, **2**, 123.
SWENSON, O. (1962). *Pediatric Surgery*, 2nd edit. New York: Appleton-Century Crofts.
SWENSON, O. (1959). *New Engl. J. Med.*, **260**, 972.
SWENSON, O., NEUHAUSER, E. B. D., and PICKETT, L. K. (1949). *Pediatrics*, **4**, 201.

TAYLOR, K. B., TRUELOVE, S. C., THOMSON, D. L., and WRIGHT, R. (1961). *Brit. med. J.*, **2**, 1727.

THOMPSON, E. N., and SHERLOCK, S. (1964). *Quart. J. Med.*, **33**, 465.

VEAU, V. E., and BOREL, S. (1931). *Division Palatine.* Paris: Masson et Cie.

WATERSTON, D. J., BONHAM-CARTER, R. E., and ABERDEEN, E. (1963). *Lancet*, **2**, 55.

WEIJERS, H. A., and VAN DE KAMER, J. H. (1960). *Pediatrics*, **25**, 127.

WEIJERS, H. A., and VAN DE KAMER, J. H. (1963). *Acts Paediat. (Uppsala.)*, **52**, 329.

ZACHARY, R. B. (1955). *Arch. Dis. Childh.*, **30**, 32.

ZUELZER, W. W., and WILSON, J. L. (1948). *Amer. J. Dis. Child.*, **75**, 40.

CHAPTER XVII

DISEASES OF THE URINARY TRACT

BRIGHT'S DISEASE

The classification of the various forms of what, as a matter of convenience, we may call Bright's disease has long been a confused subject. This has been reflected in the different interpretations which physicians and morbid anatomists have put upon the words "nephritis" and "nephrosis" and their subdivisions. Three main problems account for our difficulties, (i) our incomplete knowledge in respect of causation, (ii) our ignorance regarding the natural history of these diseases, and (iii) our inability often to reconcile the finer subdivisions of the histologist with the clinical features as they are encountered during the life of the patient. The position is, fortunately, becoming less confused as clinicians have shown more interest in the natural history of Bright's disease in its various forms, and as renal biopsy has made it possible to study the pathological changes in the kidneys at various stages during the life of the patient. Ellis (1942) in his classification of nephritis into Types I and II made the important observation that acute glomerulonephritis and hydraemic nephritis with massive oedema and proteinuria are to be regarded as two distinct diseases. This was confirmed by Davson and Platt (1949), although there is a rare case, usually an adult, in which Type I does seem to progress into the clinical picture of Type II. The traditional concept of acute (non-embolic) focal nephritis is also of doubtful validity as a clinical concept although it certainly exists as a histological entity; it is better regarded as a mild form of acute glomerulonephritis—Type I (Payne and Illingworth, 1940). Embolic nephritis is, of course, a different form of focal nephritis seen in bacterial endocarditis.

Other types of renal disease such as lower nephron nephrosis, diabetic glomerulosclerosis, polyarteritis nodosa, disseminated lupus erythematosus, and chronic pyelonephritis can simulate the various clinical pictures of glomerulonephritis, but to simplify the problem of semantics they are not included here under the title "Bright's disease". We have adopted a simple classification of Bright's disease based essentially on the more complicated classification of Volhard and Fahr (Fig. 56). It makes no assumptions regarding causation but it can point the way to rational investigation and treatment. Its over-simplification of a complicated problem is probably acceptable until further advances in our knowledge make it inadequate in paediatric practice.

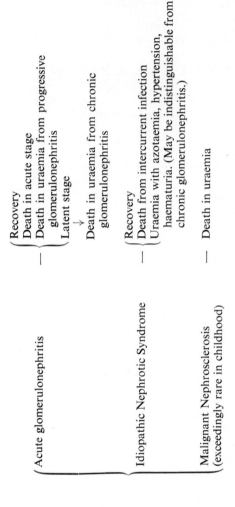

Bright's Disease

Acute glomerulonephritis
— Recovery
Death in acute stage
Death in uraemia from progressive glomerulonephritis
Latent stage
→ Death in uraemia from chronic glomerulonephritis

Idiopathic Nephrotic Syndrome
— Recovery
Death from intercurrent infection
Uraemia with azotaemia, hypertension, haematuria. (May be indistinguishable from chronic glomerulonephritis.)

Malignant Nephrosclerosis (exceedingly rare in childhood)
— Death in uraemia

FIG. 56—Classification and possible course of Bright's disease

ACUTE GLOMERULONEPHRITIS
(acute haemorrhagic nephritis: Type I)

Aetiology

In over 80 per cent of cases there is a history of a preceding infection 7–21 days before the onset of renal manifestations. In the vast majority this infection is due to one of the Lancefield group A beta-haemolytic streptococci, most often type 12. It has been presumed that during the latent period of 7–21 days an antigen-antibody reaction takes place between the streptococcal endotoxin and the cells of the glomerulus. Apart from the cases due to streptococcal tonsillitis, otitis media or impetigo, a few cases appear to be provoked by viral illnesses and in such cases haematuria, frequently recurrent, may be the only overt manifestation (Bodian *et al.*, 1965). Nephritis is also commonly seen in Henoch-Schönlein purpura (Chapter XIX) which often follows non-streptococcal illnesses.

A distinct form of the disease is *hereditary nephritis*, usually accompanied by *perceptive nerve deafness*. In this peculiar malady the disease takes a severe and progressive form in males with death from uraemia before the age of 40 years, whereas affected females rarely die of renal failure. In some but not all families with signs of hereditary nephritis and perceptive deafness *hyperprolinaemia* has also been found (Scriver *et al.*, 1964; Kopelman *et al.*, 1964). This results not only in an "overflow" excess aminoaciduria in respect of proline, but also to an excess of hydroxyproline and glycine despite normal plasma concentrations of these aminoacids, that is, a "renal" type of aminoaciduria. It must be stressed, however, that hereditary nephritis is extremely rare, whereas acute glomerulonephritis following streptococcal infections is an exceedingly common disease.

Pathology

In the acute stage the glomeruli show cellular proliferation of the endothelial cells of the capillaries and also of the epithelial cells of the tufts and Bowman's capsule. There is also polymorphonuclear infiltration. In the worst cases there may be fibrinoid necrosis of the tufts and afferent arterioles. In cases which fail to resolve and progress rapidly, crescents appear due to proliferation of the capsular epithelial cells; some glomeruli become completely hyalinized, and interstitial fibrosis may be marked; the tubules frequently show dilatation. In chronic glomerulonephritis which develops after a long latent stage, and is rare in childhood, there is extensive loss of glomeruli; scar tissue is profuse, and the arterioles show degenerative arteriosclerotic changes. The histological changes in hereditary nephritis are variable but glomerulonephritis of focal distribution is common, and there may be lipid-containing "foam cells" between the renal tubules.

Clinical Features

In the typical case, a child of school age, the onset is abrupt with fever, malaise, headache, vomiting and the passage of red or brown coloured urine. The preceding tonsillitis, scarlet fever or other infection has usually resolved by this time. Examination reveals mild oedema, most obvious in the face, and hypertension of moderate severity. Urinary output is reduced and the specific gravity is raised. There is proteinuria (under 2 gm./litre) and macroscopic haematuria. Microscopy shows red cells and casts. There may be slight cardiomegaly associated with abnormal T waves on the electrocardiogram, and radiographs of the lungs frequently show opacities caused by pulmonary oedema. In many cases, however, constitutional upset is slight and both oedema and hypertension may be absent. Haemolytic streptococci are frequently isolated from the throat swab and in most cases the A.S.O. titre is raised (above 200 units/ml.). The blood urea is frequently raised but a normal level (20–40 mg. per 100 ml.) need not invalidate the diagnosis.

Complications

Oliguria is almost invariable but, fortunately, it rarely goes on to *complete anuria* in children. When this occurs the blood urea may reach high levels and death occurs from uraemia with metabolic acidosis, hyperkalaemia and severe anaemia. A more common emergency is *left ventricular failure*. Although the cause of cardiac failure in acute nephritis is not simply the hypertension, its presence in a child who is in cardiac failure is almost diagnostic of acute nephritis. The outstanding features are orthopnoea and reluctance to lie flat in bed, combined with restlessness. There will be cardiac enlargement, triple rhythm, possibly an apical systolic murmur, tachycardia and crepitations at the lung bases. Hepatomegaly and venous over-filling develop later. *Hypertensive encephalopathy* is heralded by marked hypertension, severe headache and vomiting. Later there is mental confusion, loss of vision, convulsions or coma. In most cases there are no changes in the ocular fundi.

Course and Prognosis

The prognosis of acute glomerulonephritis in childhood is excellent. Provided cases of "hydraemic nephritis" (nephrotic syndrome) are excluded, complete recovery can be expected in about 90 per cent. A few patients (1–2 per cent) die in the acute stage from anuria, cardiac failure or encephalopathy. A few enter a progressive phase with persisting proteinuria, haematuria, casts and azotaemia; death occurs some months from the onset. About 10 per cent enter a "latent" phase during which they feel well but continue to have persistent proteinuria with red cells and casts in the urine and a raised Addis count. These patients ultimately enter the terminal stage of chronic glomerulonephritis ("secondarily contracted kidney"). This is characterized by excessive thirst and polyuria, malignant hypertension with retinopathy, normocytic orthochromic anaemia, and pale urine of fixed specific gravity. Death occurs from uraemia with high blood urea, metabolic acidosis, hypocalcaemia, hyperphosphataemia, hyponatraemia and hyperkalaemia. This type of chronic glomerulonephritis is in practice rarely seen during childhood. A similar clinical picture can, however, develop in chronic pyelonephritis which is by no means rare in children. Indeed, it is our experience that in the child chronic renal failure is almost invariably due to causes other than chronic glomerulonephritis, e.g. chronic pyelonephritis, bladder neck obstruction, bilateral renal hypoplasia.

Treatment

Complete rest in bed is essential until the E.S.R. has returned to normal. This period varies from 4–8 weeks. Proteinuria and a raised Addis count may persist for some months longer, but further bed rest is not to the benefit of the patient and in due course the urine returns completely to normal. The intake of fluid, sodium and protein should be restricted during the acute stage although physicians vary in the rigidity with which they apply these restrictions. The author's practice is to limit fluids to 30–40 fl. oz. (900–1,200 ml.) per day, one half of which is milk, until oedema and hypertension disappear. The calorie intake is augmented with boiled sweets. Fruit juices should be avoided at this stage because of their potassium content. The blood pressure and urine should be tested daily. If hypertension is severe or increases, phenobarbitone $\frac{1}{2}$ gr. may be given twice or thrice daily. The loss of oedema is best assessed by daily weighing, whereas measurement of the daily urinary output is not always accurate in young children. When diuresis has occurred and hypertension subsided, cereals, potatoes, vegetables, rice, bread, biscuits and fruit may be allowed. When haematuria has become microscopic the protein intake is increased by the addition to the diet of eggs, fish, chicken, etc. Penicillin should be prescribed at the start of treatment to eradicate any surviving haemolytic streptococci, e.g. oral penicillin G. 250 mg. four times daily, or intramuscular benzylpenicillin, 500,000 units twice daily for 5–7 days. Diaphoresis and purgation are no longer practised although a laxative may be required if the patient is constipated. Most children can be allowed back to school four weeks after being allowed up.

Complications sometimes require emergency measures. In the rare case of *anuria* or severe oliguria with a rapidly rising blood urea, some modification of Bull's regime is required. Protein must be completely withdrawn and replaced by 40–50 per cent dextrose in water given by intragastric drip via a pernasal or peroral polyvinyl tube. The daily fluid intake in this form is restricted to the amount lost in the breath and in the sweat, minus the water derived from the oxidation of body fat. In a child 500 ml. per day is a reasonable assessment. To this should be added the volume of fluid lost in stools, vomits and urine during the preceding 24 hours. This obviously requires accurate record keeping and charting. If severe vomiting makes an intragastric drip impracticable the fluid should be given into the inferior vena cava. Penicillin is given intramuscularly to reduce the risk of respiratory infection. If hyperkalaemia is marked (over 8 mEq/l.) an ion-exchange resin in the sodium phase, 15 gm. thrice daily by mouth, should be given. Severe anaemia may require the slow transfusion of blood, 20 ml./Kg. Metabolic acidosis can be combated by adding a 40 ml. ampoule of molar sodium lactate to each 500 ml. of intravenous fluid. It is also customary to add ascorbic acid and vitamin B complex (Parentrovite) to the gastric or intravenous fluid. Once the urinary output has been re-established and the blood urea has started to fall rapidly the intragastric or intravenous fluid can be discontinued. Fruit juices and carbohydrates such as jellies, porridge, bread and biscuits are given by mouth. At this stage of recovery hypokalaemia may call for extra potassium as fruit juice and potassium chloride 2–4 gm. per day, and hyponatraemia can be corrected by adding salt to the food. The need for peritoneal dialysis or the artificial kidney is fortunately very rare in childhood. Their use should be confined to centres specializing in this form of "rescue operation".

A much more common emergency is *left ventricular failure*. The child should be propped up on pillows. Restlessness is best relieved by morphine 1/6 gr. (10 mg.). Venesection and the withdrawal of 300 ml. of blood is often very effective. Digitalization should be carried out with digoxin 0·08 mg./Kg./day in four divided doses, the first one or two being given intramuscularly; after 24–36 hours the dosage is reduced to 0·02 mg./Kg./day. When there is orthopnoea aminophylline 0·25 gm. should be given intravenously over a period of ten minutes. Recovery is often rapid with effective treatment.

The initial treatment of *hypertensive encephalopathy* is venesection (300 ml. blood), lumbar puncture (15 ml. cerebrospinal fluid), and an intramuscular dose of 25 per cent magnesium sulphate (0·4 ml./Kg./ dose). Magnesium sulphate is an effective hypotensive agent which can be repeated in four hours, but it must not be used if the blood urea is over 100 mg. per 100 ml. If convulsions are severe and repeated they can be controlled with 3–5 ml. of paraldehyde given intramuscularly. It is only rarely necessary that resort must be had to one of the newer hypotensive drugs. They must be used with great caution, the blood pressure being recorded every ½ hour. We have used pentolinium tartrate (Ansolysen) in an initial intramuscular dose of 1·25 mg. The frequency and size of the subsequent doses depend upon the initial response. The effective dose, given every 6–8 hours, varies between 1·25 and 10 mg.

THE NEPHROTIC SYNDROME

This is a clinical syndrome in which gross proteinuria and hypo-albuminaemia are always present. Oedema and hyperlipaemia are usually severe. Hypertension, azotaemia, hypogammaglobulinaemia and haematuria sometimes develop in the course of the illness.

Aetiology

A nephrotic clinical picture may be associated with a variety of diseases, e.g. diabetic glomerulosclerosis, disseminated lupus erythematosus, renal vein thrombosis, amyloidosis, quartan malaria and syphilis. It may also be caused by certain drugs, e.g. troxidone, penicillamine, mercury and gold. In children, however, the vast majority of cases are "idiopathic", unrelated to other conditions, and not preceded by streptococcal or other infections. The condition, whatever its primary cause may prove to be, is now recognized as a glomerular disturbance, not the tubular degeneration which the term "nephrosis" was originally intended to suggest by Muller. Animal experiments have indicated that nephrosis can be due to auto-immunity (Heymann, 1961), but antibodies to kidney protein have not yet been demonstrated in the human.

Pathology

The histological changes in idiopathic nephrosis have been profitably studied by electron microscopy, (Joekes et al., 1958; Blainey et al., 1960; Vernier et al., 1961). These and the appearances under the light microscope have been examined in biopsy specimens at various stages in the disease. In the early stages the glomeruli show minimal changes under the light microscope such as proliferation of the cells of the glomerulus, leucocytic infiltration and adhesions of the tufts to Bowman's capsule. The electron microscope, however, shows fusion of the epithelial cell foot processes so that the basement membrane is covered by a continuous layer of cytoplasm. As the disease advances light microscopy shows marked cellular proliferation in the glomerulus and gross thickening of the basement membrane. Finally, the lumina of the capillaries become obstructed by hyaline material and the glomerulus assumes a dense hyalinized and fibrotic appearance. These late appearances closely simulate those in chronic glomerulonephritis. The electron microscope reveals marked accumulation of hyaline material on the true basement membrane. It should be noted that the severity of the proteinuria seems to be directly related to the process of fusion of the epithelial cell foot processes.

Clinical Features

Although the nephrotic syndrome is seen at all ages the majority of cases occur in pre-school children. The first manifestation is oedema which causes swelling of the face, legs and abdomen. Gross ascites is the rule; indeed in some children peripheral oedema may be relatively slight while ascites is massive in amounts. In most, generalized oedema is gross enough to mask the severe underlying tissue wasting which is also a feature of the disease. Hypertension is typically absent, but it tends to develop after a period of months or years when glomerular failure appears. Proteinuria is also very heavy; at least 10 gm. may be lost each day. Haematuria is usually absent until the terminal stage of the disease. In a few cases, however, haematuria is present at the onset and it invariably indicates a poor prognosis. In the phases of gross oedema and proteinuria the child is anorexic and miserable. Spontaneous remissions sometimes occur and they are associated with a dramatic improvement in well-being. Until the final stages of the illness the blood urea and renal function tests give normal results.

Biochemical Features

The most characteristic changes in the blood are, (i) gross reduction in the total serum proteins (normal 6·5 to 8·0 gm. per 100 ml.), (ii) disproportionate reduction in serum albumin (normal 3·5 to 4·5 gm. per 100 ml.) with inversion of the albumin/globulin ratio, (iii) reduction in gamma globulin (normal 12 per cent of the total serum proteins), (iv) normal or elevated alpha 2 and beta globulins, (v) high serum cholesterol (normal 180 to 250 mg. per 100 ml.). It has been shown by the use of tracer doses of specific plasma proteins labelled with ^{131}I that the protein fractions albumin and gamma globulin, which are of the lowest molecular weight, are lost in the urine in large amounts. On the other hand, the beta-lipoproteins of high molecular weight, which are responsible for the hyperlipaemia in nephrosis, are not excreted in the urine (Metcoff and Janeway, 1961). The cause of these disturbances in protein metabolism is not clear but they have serious consequences. In addition to the diagnostic biochemical changes already described, nephrotic patients retain excessive amounts of sodium and water while at the same time excreting intracellular potassium derived from tissue breakdown. This may be due to the excess elaboration of aldosterone by the adrenal glands and this hormone has been reported to appear in excessive amounts in the urine of oedematous subjects (Leutscher and Johnson, 1954). These hormonal and electrolyte changes may well be secondary to the heavy loss of albumin in the urine with diminishing plasma volume leading to an increased production of antidiuretic hormone by the posterior pituitary gland. This, in turn, could lead to an increased content of body water with dilution of the electrolytes in the body fluids, which would have the effect of stimulating the excretion of aldosterone. These suggestions are put forward to indicate that the chemical changes in the nephrotic syndrome are most complex. Renal oedema is not to be thought of as due simply to hypoalbuminaemia and diminished osmotic pressure in the plasma.

Complications

Many children with the nephrotic syndrome died of intercurrent pyogenic infections in the pre-antibiotic era. This susceptibility was presumably due to the low serum gamma globulin level of this disease. The most typical infection is primary pneumococcal peritonitis, although pneumonia and staphylococcal cellulitis are also common. It used to be a common observation that a severe infection occasionally resulted in a remission of the nephrosis and this was the basis of such methods of treatment as protein-shock with T.A.B. vaccine, and malaria.

Course and Prognosis

The antibiotics have brought about an abrupt fall in the mortality figures from nephrosis in childhood, and they are probably being further reduced by the therapeutic use of corticosteroids. The prognosis is much better than in the nephrotic syndrome in adults. Indeed, complete recovery may be expected with proper management in 60–70 per cent of cases (Lawson et al., 1960; Arneil, 1961). Death from intercurrent infection should now be infrequent. Most deaths are from uraemia after a long course of oedema and massive proteinuria with or without remissions, spontaneous or induced by treatment. The prognosis and response to treatment can often be forecast by a study of material obtained by renal biopsy. A good result can be expected when the glomeruli show only minimal changes on light microscopy, whereas marked hypercellularity ("proliferative glomerulitis") and thickening of the basement membrane indicate a poor prognosis. Clinical indications of a poor prognosis are the presence of haematuria, hypertension and azotaemia.

Treatment

Before the introduction of corticosteroids there was no satisfactory form of therapy. This was reflected in the wide variety of methods, most of which are better forgotten, e.g. intravenous infusions of plasma, human serum albumin, salt-free dextran, and gum acacia; diuretics; thyroid; malaria; ion-exchange resins; and paracentesis. Fortunately, it is now possible in the majority of nephrotic children (in contrast to adults) to induce diuresis and complete or partial remission of proteinuria with any of the newer steroids such as prednisolone, prednisone, triamcinolone, and dexamethasone which are comparatively free from sodium-retaining or potassium-losing effects. As relapses also respond favourably the nephrotic child now rarely has to spend long periods in hospital and he can usually attend school and live a normal existence for most of the time.

At the start of treatment fluid intake should be reduced to 30–40 fl. oz. (900–1,200 ml.) per day and sodium intake should not exceed 2 gm. per day. These restrictions can be removed as soon as the oedema has disappeared. In the author's experience the steroid of first choice and least side-effects is prednisolone. A suitable scheme of dosage is:

Prednisolone 15 mg. four times daily for 10 days,
            10 mg. four times daily for 10 days,
             5 mg. four times daily for 10 days,
             5 mg. twice daily maintenance dose.

We usually withdraw treatment after 6–10 weeks because longer courses increase the risks of serious side-effects such as arrest of growth and osteoporosis, peptic ulcer, diabetes mellitus, and convulsions with or without hypertension. There is little evidence that continuous steroid therapy improves the ultimate prognosis. The remission, as shown by sudden diuresis, rapid loss of proteinuria, reversal towards normal of the blood chemistry and fall in the E.S.R., commences between 10 and 14 days after the start of treatment. The same sequence of events is to be expected from subsequent courses of steroid when relapses of the nephrotic picture take place. Unfortunately, the prevention of relapses remains an unsolved problem. The development of resistance to steroid therapy in the course of time often indicates a poor prognosis, although in some such cases good remissions have again been obtained from the use of another steroid (e.g. triamcinolone) in place of the preparation (e.g. prednisolone) previously employed (Lorber, 1962). Other workers have used a different regime involving large doses of cortisone given for several days in each week over long periods (Lange et al., 1958; Mitchell, 1960). We have not achieved such satisfactory results with this method.

When a case of nephrosis is no longer responsive to steroid therapy it is often possible to remove oedema by the use of modern diuretics, thereby making the patient more comfortable and able to get out and about. This line of treatment will not significantly reduce the protein-uria or improve the blood chemistry. A suitable drug regime is chloro-thiazide 2–4 gm. per day in four divided oral doses. After seven days an aldosterone antagonist is started, e.g. spironolactone (Aldactone A) 25 mg. four times daily. The daily intake of water and sodium must be reduced and the serum potassium level must be watched for evidence of hypokalaemia.

In the light of the poor prognosis of the steroid-resistant case of the nephrotic syndrome, and on the theory that the disease has an immuno-logical basis, attempts are now being made to treat such patients with drugs known to suppress an immune response. Drugs which have been or might be tested are inhibitors of purine synthesis such as 6-mercapto-purine or azathioprine (Shearn, 1965), inhibitors of pyrimidine synthesis such as methotrexate, or the safer alkylating agents cyclophosphamide or chlorambucil. At the present time such drug trials should be confined to specialized renal units in large hospitals because the risks are considerable and suitable cases few in number.

Infection must be immediately combated with an appropriate antibiotic at any time in the course of nephrosis. The author does not use prophylactic antibiotics during courses of steroid therapy, believing that careful supervision is a safer policy.

PYELONEPHRITIS

The term "pyelitis" although in common use is best abandoned. The renal pelvis can hardly be inflamed while the renal parenchyma escapes. It is difficult to write concisely on the subject of pyelonephritis although it is one of the common diseases of paediatric practice. Much remains unknown about its aetiology and natural history. It may involve only a short sharp illness; or years of vague ill-health which terminate in death from chronic renal failure may follow upon a long forgotten or unrecognized initial infection of the renal tract. Pyelonephritis in the newborn has been discussed in Chapter VI.

Aetiology

The most common infecting organism is *E. coli*, and the highest incidence of the disease is in the first two or three years. Less frequently the organisms are the *Streptococcus faecalis, Proteus vulgaris, Staphylococcus aureus, Streptococcus pyogenes* or *Pseudomonas pyocyanea*. Rarely the urinary tract is infected by one of the Salmonella group. Renal tuberculosis has become rare in the U.K. There has long been controversy as to the route by which the organisms reach the kidney. Haematogenous spread undoubtedly occurs, especially in the newborn, but the present tendency is to attach more importance to ascending infection via the urethral lumen or the lymphatics. There is good evidence that infection often invades the kidneys via the ureters and vesico-ureteric reflux is now recognized to be a common accompaniment of pyelonephritis (Hutch *et al.*, 1963; Rosenheim, 1963). It has, of course, always been recognized that urinary stasis due to congenital anomalies of the renal tract or to acquired causes of obstruction such as calculi predisposes to infection. Indeed, these conditions most often present with pyuria and their existence must always be suspected when pyuria proves resistant to treatment or when relapses occur.

Pathology

In the acute stage the inflammation may vary from little more than leucocytic infiltration under the pelvic epithelium to almost complete destruction of the kidney with multiple interstitial abscesses. If the infection is allowed to become chronic, extensive scarring and irregular contraction of the kidney may occur. At this stage of chronic pyelone-phritis there may be little evidence of active bacterial infection, but there can be extensive loss of nephrons and arteriosclerotic changes in the renal arterioles may be severe. Indeed, the disease may now closely mimic chronic glomerulonephritis and it is important to realize that the most common cause of chronic renal failure with hypertension in child-hood is, in fact, chronic pyelonephritis. It is for this reason that hospital physicians have become increasingly aware of the need for intensive treatment in every case of acute pyelonephritis and for a careful follow-up period of at least one year.

Clinical Features

Pyelonephritis occurs four times as frequently in girls as in boys, with the exception of the first six months of life. The equal sex incidence in young infants is explicable on the basis of the equal sex incidence of the major congenital anomalies of the urinary tract which soon becomes infected. The higher female incidence after the early months of life has been attributed to the short female urethra.

The onset of the acute stage is usually sudden with fever, pallor, toxaemia, anorexia, vomiting and tachycardia. Urinary infection is one of the few causes of rigor in young children. A bowel upset, constipation or diarrhoea, commonly precedes the acute symptoms. In the young infant meningismus or convulsions are common, whereas symptoms pointing to the renal tract are often absent. In some cases, however, the mother may have observed that there is frequency of micturition or that the infant screams during the act of urination. Attacks of screaming and drawing up of the legs can simulate an abdominal emergency. In less acute cases during infancy there may be persistent vomiting and failure to thrive, and diseases such as hiatus hernia, pyloric stenosis or idiopathic hypercalcaemia may be wrongly suspected.

In older children frequency and dysuria make diagnosis easier although their absence does not exclude the diagnosis. In untreated cases of acute pyelonephritis the high fever usually subsides spontaneously after 7–10 days but the child remains apathetic, anorexic, has a somewhat characteristic muddy pallor and fails to gain weight. In a few cases death may occur quite rapidly from a combination of toxaemia, dehydration and uraemia.

Diagnosis

In older children symptoms referable to the urinary tract may make the diagnosis comparatively easy, but many children and nearly all infants do not have any symptoms pointing to the urinary tract. There can be no doubt that pyelonephritis escapes clinical diagnosis in a high percentage of patients, and it will continue to do so until doctors make urine analysis part of their routine investigation of every ill infant or child. *The diagnosis must be based upon examination of the urine including microscopy* (Hutchison, 1965). In most cases all doubt is rapidly dispelled by the presence of proteinuria and numerous pus cells in an uncentrifuged specimen of urine. In a few the pyuria may be intermittent so that more than one specimen of urine has to be examined. In others the pus cells are relatively scanty (under 5 per high power field) and the diagnosis remains in doubt. When there is clinical suspicion of renal infection a white cell count should be performed by a more accurate quantitative method, such as that described by McGeachie and Kennedy (1963). The causal organism and its antibacterial sensitivities must also be determined by culture, *within one hour of its collection*, of a midstream specimen of urine. In doubtful cases a bacterial count can be done using the simplified stroke-plate method of McGeachie and Kennedy (1963); bacterial counts over 100,000 organisms per ml. indicate undoubted infection. There can be no question that the use of these or similar quantitative methods of urinary investigation can lead to a correct diagnosis in most of the doubtful cases seen in hospital practice. The collection of mid-stream specimens of urine is practicable in most infants, after cleansing of the penis or vulva with pHisoHex or Cetavlon. Catheterization is only required with a few small female infants. In males a sterile test-tube can be tied on to the penis when a mid-stream collection proves difficult.

Differential Diagnosis

In older children acute appendicitis can simulate pyelonephritis and the pelvic appendix in particular can produce urinary frequency and discomfort. Mistakes will be few if the urine is always examined microscopically before resort to surgery. In young infants the presence of meningismus may necessitate lumbar puncture to exclude pyogenic meningitis.

Course and Prognosis

In the majority of cases of acute pyelonephritis complete recovery occurs with adequate treatment. Failure to achieve a sterile urine or recurrences of pyuria should suggest the probability of some congenital or acquired cause of urinary stasis. The author's experience agrees with that of Smellie *et al.*, (1964) that about one-third of children in their first attack of pyelonephritis have a developmental anomaly in the renal tract, whereas in children with a history of previous attacks such anomalies can be found in two-thirds of the cases. This is an indication for full urological investigation by plain radiographs, intravenous pyelography, and possibly cystoscopy, retrograde pyelography, micturating cystography and even renal biopsy. Recurrent pyuria is particularly common in girls and is discussed below. Inadequately treated pyelonephritis can cause prolonged and vague ill-health with pallor, anorexia, failure to grow, febrile episodes and slow renal destruction. In some cases the picture of terminal chronic pyelonephritis develops with hypertension, thirst, polyuria, retinopathy and azotaemia. In cases which run a slow course renal osteodystrophy may develop (see p. 324). In rare cases chronic pyelonephritis is unilateral, being superimposed upon a hypoplastic or duplex kidney. In a few such cases renal hypertension has been relieved by nephrectomy and every case of hypertension encountered in childhood should be regarded as an indication for detailed urological investigation.

Treatment

General nursing measures include a large fluid intake, tepid sponging when there is high fever, and a laxative if the patient is constipated. Drug treatment should be based upon laboratory determination of the sensitivity of the causal organisms. The sulphonamides are effective in most cases and can be started while awaiting the results of urine culture. Another drug can be substituted later in resistant cases. A suitable soluble sulphonamide is sulphadimidine in a dose of 150–200 mg./Kg./day in four divided oral doses. Its use should be associated with a good fluid intake, and an alkaline diuretic such as sodium bicarbonate or citrate may also be given, 15–45 gr. (1–3 gm.) four times daily. In sulphonamide-resistant cases a variety of other drugs can be used according to the bacteriological findings, e.g. nitrofurantoin 8 mg./Kg./day, tetracycline 25 mg./Kg./day, ampicillin 50 mg./Kg./day all given orally, and streptomycin 50 mg./Kg./day or colistin methosulphonate 150,000 units/Kg./day given intramuscularly in 2 and 4 doses respectively. Chloramphenicol 100 mg./Kg./day is also valuable but it must never be used for long periods or in repeated courses. In difficult infections there is still a place for mandelamine, 250 mg. four times daily by mouth.

In view of the dangers of continued low-grade pyelonephritis it is the author's practice to continue the appropriate drug, e.g. sulphadimidine or nitrofurantoin, in half the above dosage for six months after the acute infection has been dealt with. The patient is thereafter kept under observation with periodic urine tests for another six months. Any recurrence or resistance to treatment demands full urological investigation. Remediable renal abnormalities should be treated surgically. When the developmental anomaly is not amenable to surgery continuous antibacterial treatment will greatly reduce the risk of relapses (Normand and Smellie, 1965).

RECURRENT PYURIA IN GIRLS

Recurrent attacks of urinary infection—previously called "pyelitis"—is a common and difficult problem in girls. It must be regarded seriously because it can lead to chronic pyelonephritis with renal scarring and to trouble during pregnancy or even to renal failure in adult life. Clinically the girl suffers from frequent and painful micturition, bed wetting, episodes of fever and malaise, or from chronic ill-health without much in the way of urinary symptoms. Every girl suffering from chronic or recurrent pyuria must be fully investigated by intravenous pyelography, micturating cysto-urethrography, endoscopy and, on occasions, by renal biopsy. In some cases the cause will be found in some frank developmental or acquired anomaly, such as hydronephrosis, duplex kidney or calculus, for which effective surgical treatment may be available. In the majority, however, a normal intravenous pyelogram is found. It is in such cases that micturating cystograms show bilateral ureteric reflux. The patient is examined preferably under an image intensifier. The precise significance of vesico-ureteric reflux without accompanying dilatation of the renal pelves is not clear. Some workers, observing a degree of trabeculation of the bladder, have considered that it indicates mild obstruction at the bladder neck. Whatever its mechanism it must have considerable importance in the causation of pyelonephritis.

The treatment of affected girls is still open to controversy. A trial of conservative measures should certainly be the initial approach. This consists of the long-term use of an appropriate antibacterial drug combined with "triple micturition", which means that at each voiding the child empties her bladder three times at intervals of 3–4 minutes to allow it to refill from the reflux up the ureters. In recent years, however, there has been an increasing tendency to advise surgical measures for these unfortunate children. This may take the form of a reflux-preventing operation such as vesico-ureteroplasty (Politano and Leadbetter, 1958), or a "Y-V" plastic procedure at the bladder neck (Williams and Sturdy, 1961). The results of carefully supervised medical treatment are often very satisfactory and surgical intervention should not be lightly advised. These operations demand considerable expertise and they are not wholly free from undesirable complications such as urinary incontinence. It is as yet too early to assess whether or not surgical treatment is more successful than medical measures in preventing the development of irreversible pyelonephritic scarring of the kidneys.

RENAL CALCULUS

Aetiology

The great majority of renal calculi found in children in the U.K. are secondary to infection of the renal tract, especially by *Proteus vulgaris* which by maintaining a high urinary pH favours the deposition of phosphate in combination with calcium, ammonium and magnesium. The typical example is the "staghorn" calculus which fills the renal pelvis and calyces. Calculus formation is especially likely when there is an obstruction in the renal tract, e.g. at the pelvi-ureteric or vesico-ureteric junction. Very rarely calcium phosphate or oxalate stones are a manifestation of primary hyperparathyroidism or hypervitaminosis D. They may also occur after prolonged immobilization, as from chronic osteitis. *Cystinuria*, one of Garrod's original inborn errors of meta-bolism, is a rare cause of renal stone. In this condition there is a defect in the tubular reabsorption not only of cystine but also of lysine, arginine and ornithine. In spite of the passage of the typical hexagonal crystals in the urine only a minority of cystinurics form calculi (Stanbury *et al.*, 1965). This condition must not be confused with the quite separate metabolic error called cystinosis (see below). Another ex-ceedingly rare cause of renal lithiasis, also an inborn metabolic error, is *primary hyperoxaluria*. In some cases in addition to calcium oxalate calculi extrarenal deposits may occur—*oxalosis* (Stanbury *et al.*, 1965). This rare type of very dense nephrocalcinosis and nephrolithiasis can be distinguished from the common calcium oxalate stones by the con-tinuous high urinary excretion of oxalate, which sufferers from primary hyperoxaluria always show. In certain parts of the world, e.g. India, endemic urolithiasis leads to the formation of vesical calculi. This used to be seen in England 100 years ago, and an undetermined dietary deficiency has been postulated.

Clinical Features

The majority of children present as cases of pyuria. Classical renal colic with haematuria is relatively uncommon in childhood. In a few instances, and especially in primary hyperoxaluria, the infant or child has appeared before the physician already in a state of chronic renal failure, sometimes also associated with renal osteodystrophy. The presence of a renal calculus is confirmed by straight radiography which should invari-ably precede intravenous pyelograms in which a renal calculus can be obscured. In confirmed cases it is wise to determine the urinary output of calcium, cystine and oxalate so that metabolic upsets are not overlooked.

Treatment

This consists of sterilization of the urine by appropriate drug therapy and removal of the calculus when this is practicable. In unilateral cases nephrectomy may be necessary when the renal parenchyma has been severely damaged, provided always that the opposite kidney has been shown to be healthy. The urine should be kept acid in reaction with ammonium chloride in children who have suffered from phosphate stones. The formation of stones can be discouraged in cystinurics by alkalinizing the urine with sodium bicarbonate and ensuring a really large fluid intake. There may be a place for the use of D-penicillamine in the prevention of cystine stones (Milne, 1964). There is, unfortunately, no effective treatment for primary hyperoxaluria.

DEVELOPMENTAL ANOMALIES OF THE RENAL TRACT

THE UPPER URINARY TRACT

One of the most common abnormalities is hydronephrosis due to obstruction at the pelvi-ureteric junction from kinking or aberrant blood vessels, or due to a stricture at the uretero-vesical junction. In the latter situation a ureterocele, which has distinctive pyelographic and cystoscopic appearances, may develop. It is, in effect, a cystic dilatation of the terminal intravesical portion of the ureter, the "cyst" being lined with ureteric epithelium and covered by vesical epithelium. Another common anomaly, which may be bilateral or unilateral, is duplex kidney with double ureters. These two ureters may join before entering the bladder, both may enter the bladder or one may open ectopically into the urethra or vagina resulting in urinary incontinence. One half of a duplex kidney frequently becomes infected or hydronephrotic. A single ureter may also end ectopically. An ectopic kidney is also encountered. It may lie in the pelvis, or both kidneys may be situated on the same side—crossed ectopia. In "horseshoe" kidney an isthmus of renal tissue joins the two kidneys below the level of the inferior mesenteric artery. Ectopic kidneys like duplex kidneys often become the site of infection, hydronephrosis or calculus. Megaureter is the term employed to denote a grossly dilated but not apparently obstructed ureter, a condition often leading to pyelonephritis and nephrolithiasis. Diverticula of the ureters are exceedingly rare; they may remain trouble-free or cause obstruction and hydronephrosis.

Clinical Features

Most developmental anomalies of the upper urinary tract come to light during the investigation of children who have presented with urinary infections and pyuria. Their early recognition and surgical correction is necessary to prevent chronic pyelonephritis and calculus formation. In some children hydronephrosis causes an aching pain in the loin or recurrent attacks of poorly localized abdominal pain. There is occasionally a soft palpable mass in the loin. In other cases haematuria may be the first symptom. An ectopic ureter is very rare; it should be suspected when there is a history of dribbling incontinence in spite of acts of micturition at normal intervals. The existence of the various anomalies is usually first noted on intravenous pyelograms. Precise diagnosis may require cystoscopy, retrograde pyelography and micturating cystography. Considerable experience may be needed in the interpretation of some radiographic appearances.

Treatment

Although nephrectomy or heminephrectomy is sometimes unavoidable, every effort should be made to preserve functioning renal tissue by plastic procedures at the pelvi-ureteric or uretero-vesical junctions. Extensive pyelonephritis on one side or in one half of a duplex kidney is an indication for excision of the diseased tissue. In megaureter good results are often obtainable by medical treatment alone. An ectopic ureter, once identified, can be implanted into the bladder, or in the case of duplex kidney removed with enormous relief to the patient.

CYSTIC DISEASE OF THE KIDNEYS

This is a miscellaneous group of disorders which are distinct from the common familial fibrocystic disease of the kidneys of adults. There is a type of bilateral polycystic disease of the kidneys which is seen in young infants and which may affect siblings. It may co-exist with cystic disease of the liver but it does not occur in families affected by the adult type. It produces palpable renal masses and hypertension, and leads to early death from urinary infection or uraemia. There are various histological types of unilateral cystic disease which present usually in the form of a painless renal mass. The treatment is nephrectomy. In these cases the ureter is often aplastic and there is an absence of secretion in intravenous pyelograms. Congenital solitary cysts, unilateral or bilateral, can usually be excised with conservation of the kidney.

RENAL AGENESIS AND HYPOPLASIA

Bilateral renal agenesis is incompatible with life. It is often but not invariably associated with characteristic facial abnormalities which permit of a firm diagnosis at birth. These include large abnormally low-set ears, marked epicanthic folds, broad space between the eyes, micrognathia, flattening of the nose and a crease on the chin (Potter, 1946). There are frequently abnormalities in other systems, especially hypoplasia of the lungs. The presence of unilateral agenesis is sufficiently frequent to make an intravenous pyelogram essential before nephrectomy is performed for any reason. In these cases there may also be an absence of the ureter and half of the trigone, or the ureter may end blindly when it is catheterized.

Bilateral hypoplasia of the kidneys results in slowly progressive renal failure. The patient frequently presents with osteodystrophy (p. 324) and hypertension is usually absent. By way of contrast a unilateral hypoplastic kidney frequently becomes the seat of chronic pyelone-phritis and it is a well-recognized cause of severe renal hypertension.

BLADDER NECK OBSTRUCTION

Severe degrees of bladder neck obstruction are seen almost solely in boys. The possibility of mild obstruction at the bladder neck causing recurrent urinary infection in girls has already been discussed (p. 319). The causes of severe bladder neck obstruction are (i) mucosal valves in the posterior urethra, (ii) fibro-elastosis of the tissues in the wall of the posterior urethra—Marion's disease (Bodian, 1957), (iii) neurogenic bladder dysfunction which may be congenital in spina bifida cystica, congenital absence of the sacrum and diastematomyelia, or acquired in spinal tumours or injuries. Neurogenic cases are often associated with incompetence of the anal sphincter. Very rarely bladder neck obstruc-tion is related to gross deficiency of the abdominal musculature and a few of these infants have also had a patent urachus which allows urine to drain from the umbilicus.

Clinical Features

The worst cases are due to urethral valves and they present from birth with dribbling overflow incontinence. The grossly distended bladder is readily palpable, as may be the kidneys. A micturating cysto-urethrogram may show the greatly distended posterior urethra and the valves; it will also reveal severe bilateral hydro-ureteronephrosis. Infection quickly supervenes and death occurs before long. Less severe degrees of bladder neck obstruction rarely produce symptoms until after the first year of life. These take the form of various difficulties in the act of micturition such as dribbling, hesitancy and frequency, or they are caused by urinary infection. A few children are not seen by a physician until they are in chronic irreversible renal failure. The diagnosis is con-firmed by intravenous pyelography, micturating cysto-urethrography and endoscopy.

Treatment

Various surgical measures are available for all but the most hopeless cases. These include periodic urethral dilatation, endoscopic resection of the bladder neck and plastic operations. When the blood urea is very high preliminary nephrostomy may be required to provide immediate drainage. In the severe neurogenic cases which are seen after operations on spina bifida it is sometimes necessary to perform bilateral cutaneous ureterostomy or to construct an ileal-loop bladder (Chapter XX).

THE MEGAURETER-MEGACYSTIS SYNDROME

In this condition bilateral dilatation of the ureters is associated with a greatly distended bladder which is apparently devoid of sensation, although there is no apparent organic obstruction at the bladder neck (Williams, 1959). The syndrome is more common in girls and presents with chronic or recurring pyuria. In the milder cases a trial should be given to chemotherapy and "triple voiding" but in the severe cases the treatment of choice is "Y-V" plastic operation on the bladder neck.

ECTOPIA VESICAE AND EPISPADIAS

These anomalies are associated with a defect in the lower abdominal wall so that in ectopia vesicae the bladder is open to the exterior and in epispadias the urethra lies open on the dorsum of the penis. In early infancy great care is necessary for the protection of the skin which should be treated with a buffered gel or aluminium paste. During the first year the first of a series of reparative operations may be possible. In the worst cases where urinary continence cannot be achieved it becomes necessary to construct an ileal loop bladder which drains urine on to the abdominal wall. The comfort of these unfortunate children can be greatly increased by suitably chosen "Chiron" urinals of the various types manufactured by Down Bros. of London.

HYPOSPADIAS

In this condition the external urethral meatus opens on to the ventral aspect of the penis (glandular and penile types) or in the perineum when the scrotum is bifid (perineo-scrotal type). Surgical repair, in several stages, should start in the second or third year of life. In some cases, however, meatotomy is required soon after birth for meatal stenosis. The mildest degrees of hypospadias can safely be left alone. *Surgical intervention should invariably be preceded by a buccal smear for sex determination because a few of these children are females virilized in utero by adrenal hyperplasia.* In them the correct treatment is cortisone and they should be reared as girls provided diagnosis is established before the age of 2 years (Chapter XVIII).

RENAL OSTEODYSTROPHY (Renal rickets.)

The term is used here to denote the bone changes which sometimes develop in cases of chronic glomerular failure with uraemia. It must be distinguished from the bone changes which may result from renal tubular disorders in which uraemia is not an inevitable accompaniment. The term "renal osteodystrophy" is preferred to "renal rickets" because the bone changes include more than rickets, and to "renal dwarfism" because dwarfism is not invariably present in older children. This condition is occasionally familial.

Aetiology

Osteodystrophy may develop in slowly progressive glomerular failure from any cause. The most common are bilateral renal hypoplasia, bilateral hydronephrosis, bilateral polycystic disease of the kidneys, and chronic pyelonephritis.

Clinical Features

In most cases the predominant symptoms are thirst and polyuria which may be extreme. These children are usually dwarfed, anaemic and thin. They often have a pale "renal" appearance, and the skin around the knees and lower thighs has a curiously mottled look. In some cases deformities are noted first. These are clinically typical of rickets, e.g. enlarged epiphyses and costo-chondral junctions, genu valgum or bowing of the femora and tibiae, pathological fractures. The urine is large in volume, of low specific gravity, it contains a trace of protein and may contain casts. Hypertension and retinal changes are usually conspicuous by their absence.

Biochemical Features

The blood urea is raised. The presence of metabolic acidosis is reflected in a lowered plasma CO_2 content (below 20 mEq/l.). In uncompensated cases the pH of the blood will fall below 7·38. This acidosis is due partly to the retention of acid metabolites by the kidney and partly to its inability to manufacture ammonium. Glomerular insufficiency also leads to the retention of phosphate and the serum level rises above 6·5 mg. per 100 ml. In some cases the serum calcium level is abnormally low (below 9 mg. per 100 ml.). A possible explanation of the hypocalcaemia is excess intestinal excretion of phosphate which combines with calcium in the gut to form calcium phosphate which interferes with the absorption of calcium. The tendency to hypocalcaemia is the cause of secondary hyperparathyroidism which is a characteristic feature of chronic renal failure and a cause of the bone changes (Fourman, 1960).

Radiological Changes

These are complex. First are the typical appearances of rickets such as cupping and fraying of the metaphyses, deepening of the epiphyseal plates and osteoporosis. There are also to be found in many cases the changes of osteitis fibrosa due to hyperparathyroidism. These include subperiosteal resorption best seen in the terminal phalanges, absence of the lamina dura, a ground glass or stippled appearance to the skull, and a characteristic irregularly distributed osteosclerosis, which is especially obvious at the base of the skull, in the clavicles and in the vertebral bodies which show transverse bands.

Treatment

The renal lesion is almost always irreversible and death from uraemia is the ultimate prognosis. In a few instances the renal lesion may be amenable to surgery, e.g. bladder neck obstruction. It is, however, always worthwhile treating the bone changes which in themselves can be a source of great disability. Healing of the rickets can be achieved with massive doses of calciferol 100,000–200,000 units daily. The serum calcium level must be monitored frequently, as it is easy and dangerous to produce hypercalcaemia from over-dosage. The metabolic acidosis can be relieved with sodium bicarbonate 15–45 gr. (1–3 gm.) four times daily or Albright's mixture:

> Sodium citrate   100 gm.
> Citric acid   60 gm.
> Water to   1 litre.
> *Label:* 15–45 ml. four times daily.

The aim of treatment is to maintain a normal blood pH (7·38–7·45) and plasma bicarbonate (20–24 mEq/1.).

RENAL TUBULAR DISORDERS

The renal tubules in health reabsorb various substances from the glomerular filtrate, e.g. glucose, aminoacids, sodium, potassium, bicarbonate, phosphate and calcium. Although absorption is their major function they also secrete creatinine, potassium and hydrogen ions. These functions are presumed to be dependent on intracellular enzyme reactions, failure of any leading to metabolic disorders of the type called "inborn errors of metabolism" (Chapter IX). It is, therefore, hardly surprising that a bewildering combination of tubular defects are sometimes encountered in individual subjects. The tendency in cystinuria for the formation of renal calculi has already been mentioned, also the invariable nephrocalcinosis of primary hyperoxaluria. One of the most common and benign of renal tubular defects gives rise to *renal glycosuria*, important only because it must be distinguished from the glycosuria of diabetes mellitus. We propose to discuss in this section only those relatively common tubular disorders which can result in grave ill-health.

IDIOPATHIC HYPERCHLORAEMIC RENAL ACIDOSIS OF INFANCY

First described in 1936 this disease was commonly reported in the United Kingdom during the period 1946–1954 (Hutchison and Mac-Donald, 1951; Lightwood *et al.*, 1953). Since then its incidence appears to have dropped greatly. Some have suggested, without supporting evidence, that this might be related to the withdrawal of mercury from the common "teething powders". The aetiology of the disease, however, is not known. As seen in infancy renal tubular acidosis does not cause bone changes. A similar disease of adults, on the other hand, causes osteomalacia (Albright *et al.*, 1946), but its relationship to the infantile condition is not clear.

Pathogenesis

The metabolic acidosis has been shown to be due to an inability of the proximal renal tubules to reabsorb bicarbonate from the glomerular filtrate so that the urine is usually alkaline, even in the presence of acidosis (Latner and Burnard, 1950). The hyperchloraemia is due to an increased tubular reabsorption of chloride (Pitts *et al.*, 1949).

Pathology

In fatal cases renal medullary calcinosis is a constant finding, although similar changes have been seen in young infants dying of unrelated causes. In contrast to renal tubular acidosis in adults the nephrocalcinosis of infancy is rarely radiologically visible during life.

Clinical Features

Some time between the ages of 6 weeks and 6 months the infant becomes ill with failure to thrive, anorexia, frequent vomiting and severe constipation. Over-breathing due to acidosis may be evident. The urine is usually alkaline to litmus. Mild urinary infection occurs in some cases. The blood biochemical changes are those of metabolic acidosis and hyperchloraemia (above 110 mEq/1.). Most affected infants recover completely with appropriate treatment.

Treatment

Marked clinical and biochemical improvement usually follows the administration of an alkali in the form of Albright's mixture (p. 326) 15–45 ml., or sodium bicarbonate 15–45 gr. (1–3 gm.) four times daily. It is important that sulphonamides are never prescribed for these infants because by inhibiting carbonic anhydrase they can limit the absorption of bicarbonate by the distal tubule.

RICKETS RESISTANT TO VITAMIN D.

(Phosphaturic Rickets: "Late Rickets")

In this disease rickets develops at a later age than is usual in infantile rickets (Chapter XXV) and it is resistant to vitamin D in ordinary doses. It appears to be causally related to a deficiency in the tubular reabsorption of phosphate. In a few cases renal glycosuria has also been reported but the other tubular functions seem to be unimpaired. The disease is presumed to be transmitted by a dominant gene on the X chromosome because affected males have only affected daughters, whereas affected females have equal numbers of affected and healthy children irrespective of sex. The condition is, therefore, more common in girls, but because they have one normal X chromosome it is more severe when it occurs in boys (Winters *et al.*, 1958; Stanbury, 1958).

Clinical Features

The child develops the classical features of rickets modified from the infantile variety only by the patient's age. They include enlargement of epiphyses, rachitic rosary, kyphoscoliosis and deformities of the limbs. Bilateral coxa vara frequently results in a characteristic waddling gait. The urinary excretion of calcium is small whereas the output of phosphate is excessive. This disease was in the past sometimes called "late rickets". The biochemical findings in the blood are the same as those usually found in infantile rickets, namely, a normal serum calcium (9–11·5 mg. per 100 ml.), reduced serum phosphate (less than 4·5 mg. per 100 ml.) and raised alkaline phosphatase. The radiological features also are those of uncomplicated rickets, e.g. cupped, frayed and broadened metaphyses, broadened epiphyses, osteoporosis, deformities and pathological fractures. In adults the picture is one of severe osteoporosis with pseudo-fractures (Looser's nodes), sometimes called Milkman's syndrome.

Differential Diagnosis

The age of the child combined with a history of an adequate dietary intake of vitamin D are sufficient to exclude infantile rickets. Coeliac rickets (Chapter XVI) must be excluded by tests of intestinal absorption, and renal failure by tests of glomerular function. The de Toni-Fanconi syndrome is most readily excluded by urinary aminoacid chromatography (see below).

Treatment

Large doses of calciferol (100,000–300,000 units daily) are required to heal the rickets. Unfortunately, in some cases treatment is rendered extremely difficult because of toxic effects. It is dangerous to permit the serum calcium to rise above 12 mg. per 100 ml., or the 24-hour urinary calcium output to exceed 400 mg.

THE DE TONI-FANCONI SYNDROME

(Cystinosis)

This disease is transmitted as an autosomal recessive trait. In the infantile cases with which we are concerned there is usually, but not invariably, evidence of *cystinosis*. Cystine crystals are found throughout the reticulo-endothelial system, but there is no gross excess of cystine in the urine as in cystinuria which is a quite separate inborn error of metabolism. The most prominent features of the disease are due to multiple deficiencies in the renal tubules so that there is impairment of the reabsorption of water, glucose, aminoacids, phosphate, potassium and uric acid. In some cases at least these tubular defects are probably related to the cystinosis. The metabolic acidosis, which is another feature of the disease, may be due to the defective formation of ammonium in the tubules. An excellent account of the disease in childhood has been given in a series of papers by Bickel and his colleagues (1952). The de Toni-Fanconi syndrome as seen in adults appears to be a separate entity which is never associated with cystinosis (Stowers and Dent, 1947).

Clinical Features

The symptoms usually appear in early infancy. They resemble those of hyperchloraemic acidosis. Thus failure to thrive, anorexia, vomiting and severe constipation are constantly present. Thirst and polyuria may also have been noted by the mother. A feature characteristic of cystinosis is photophobia. This is due to the presence of cystine crystals in the cornea and it is not always present. Rickets makes its appearance after some months of illness. Its appearance in a wasted infant is in contrast to infantile rickets, which affects only reasonably well-grown infants (Fig. 57). Severe deformities can develop in some patients. Simple urine testing in the ward sideroom usually reveals the presence of glycosuria and proteinuria, the former being of great diagnostic significance. During the course of a long illness life may be endangered at any time by severe attacks of dehydration, and by sudden renal losses of potassium which lead to prostration, muscle weakness and typical electrocardiographic changes. In the later stages of the disease hepatomegaly may develop. Ultimately glomerular failure with uraemia becomes superimposed. The radiological changes are typical of rickets.

Biochemical Features

In addition to glycosuria and proteinuria, chromatography reveals a generalized excess of aminoacids in the urine. The renal tubular origin of the aminoaciduria is reflected in normal blood aminoacid levels. The characteristic changes in the blood are hypophosphataemia, normal serum calcium, raised alkaline phosphatase, lowered plasma bicarbonate, and hypokalaemia. In the terminal stages of the disease the onset of glomerular failure may lead to a rise in serum phosphate and fall in serum calcium.

Diagnosis

This is based initially on the presence of glycosuria and aminoaciduria. The blood chemical changes also support the diagnosis. Cystinosis can be confirmed by the detection of cystine crystals in the cornea with a slit lamp, or by finding them in bone marrow or lymph node

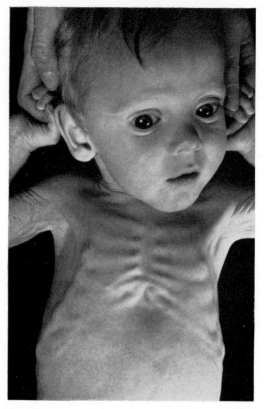

Fig. 57.—Rachitic rosary in 7-month infant suffering from de Toni-Fanconi syndrome; note generalized wasting.

biopsy material. As cystine crystals are soluble in formalin, tissues to be examined for their presence should always be fixed in alcohol.

Treatment

The rickets require large doses of calciferol for healing (50,000–300,000 units daily). The serum calcium level must be carefully monitored on this treatment and should not be permitted to rise above 12 mg. per 100 ml. The metabolic acidosis can be corrected with Albright's mixture (p. 326) 15–45 ml. four times daily or sodium bicarbonate 15–45 gr. (1–3 gm.) four times daily. If hypokalaemia is present some of the sodium salt should be replaced by potassium citrate or potassium bicarbonate. The daily intake of potassium salt may need to be as large as 5 gm. The prognosis is poor in spite of the considerable temporary improvement which treatment may bring. Encouraging results have recently been reported with D-penicillamine by Clayton and Patrick (1961). Confirmation in a larger number of cases is awaited.

NEPHROGENIC DIABETES INSIPIDUS

This is a very rare condition which must be differentiated from diabetes insipidus due to failure of production by the posterior pituitary of antidiuretic hormone (ADH). In nephrogenic cases the renal tubules fail to respond to vasopressin and to reabsorb water normally. The condition has been transmitted as a sex-linked trait in most of the reported families, only males being affected. In normal people ADH is thought to act by liberating hyaluronidase in the renal tubules. The resultant depolymerization of the ground substance and release of calcium increases permeability and allows water to be reabsorbed against the gradient of hypertonic urine (Ginetzinsky, 1958). This theory has been tested and found to be compatible with the facts in several families affected with nephrogenic diabetes insipidus (Dicker and Eggleton, 1963). Some cases have shown incompatible results, suggesting that there may be other types of case, e.g. that the ADH or administered vasopressin is destroyed before reaching the kidneys.

Clinical Features

The symptoms, excessive thirst and polyuria, start soon after birth. Failure to thrive, anorexia, constipation and vomiting are common. Infants frequently show hyperelectrolytaemia and azotaemia but these biochemical disturbances becomes less in those who survive infancy. Deprivation of fluids or a high environmental temperature leads to fever, prostration and dehydration because these patients cannot pass a urine of high specific gravity. This is a particular risk during infancy when the patient is unable to determine his own fluid intake. Some children with this disease show signs of organic brain damage which has been attributed to the hypernatraemia and dehydration which frequently exist during the period of infancy (Ruess and Rosenthal, 1963). Diagnosis can be confirmed by the failure of response to vasopressin and by the marked inability to concentrate the urine during water deprivation tests. These patients also show an absence of antidiuresis during the administration of hypertonic saline (Carter and Robbins, 1947).

Treatment

In infants it is important to offer water at frequent intervals to avoid the dangers of hyperelectrolytaemia and dehydration. A curious paradox is the useful effect which chlorothiazide and more recent derivatives of this group of diuretics have in reducing urinary output in this disease (Crawford et al., 1960). The mode of action is unknown, but patients on these drugs must at the same time be guarded from the risks of potassium depletion.

REFERENCES

ALBRIGHT, F., BURNETT, C. H., PARSONS, W., REIFENSTEIN, E. C., and ROOS, A. (1946). *Medicine (Baltimore)*, **25**, 399.

ARNEIL, G. C. (1961). *Lancet*, **2**, 1103.

BICKEL, H., SMALLWOOD, W. C., SMELLIE, J. M., BAAR, H. S., and HICKMANS, E. M. (1952). *Acta paediat. (Uppsala)*, **42**, Suppl. 90.

BLAINEY, J. D., BREWER, D. B., HARDWICKE, J., and SOOTHILL, J. F. (1960). *Quart. J. Med.*, **29**, 235.

BODIAN, M. (1957). *Brit. J. Urol.*, **29**, 393.

BODIAN, M., BLACK, J. A., KOBAYASKI, N., LAKE, B. D., and SCHULER, S. E. (1965). *Quart. J. Med.*, **34**, 359.

CARTER, A. C., and ROBBINS, J. (1947). *J. clin. Endocr.*, **7**, 753.

CLAYTON, B. E., and PATRICK, A. D. (1961). *Lancet*, **2**, 909.

CRAWFORD, J. D., KENNEDY, G. C., and HILL, L. E. (1960). *New Engl. J. Med.*, **262**, 737.

DAVSON, J., and PLATT, R. (1949). *Quart. J. Med.*, **18**, 149.

DICKER, S. E., and EGGLETON, M. G. (1963). *Clin. Sci.*, **24**, 81.

ELLIS, A. (1942). *Lancet*, **1**, 34 and 72.

FOURMAN, P. (1960). *Calcium Metabolism and the Bone.* Oxford: Blackwell Scientific Publication.

GINETZINSKY, A. G. (1958). *Nature (Lond.)*, **182**, 1218.

HEYMANN, W. (1961). *J. Pediat.*, **58**, 609.

HUTCH, J. A., MILLER, E. R., and HINMAN, F. (1963). *Amer. J. Med.*, **34**, 338.

HUTCHISON, J. H. (1965). *Practitioner*, **194**, 338.

HUTCHISON, J. H., and MACDONALD, A. M. (1951). *Acta paediat. (Uppsala)*, **40**, 371.

JOEKES, A. M., HEPTINSTALL, R. H., and PORTER, K. A. (1958). *Quart. J. Med.*, **27**, 495.

KOPELMAN, H., ASATOOR, A. M., and MILNE, M. D. (1964). *Lancet*, **2**, 1075.

LANGE, K., WASSERMAN, E., and SLOBODY, L. (1958). *J. Amer. med. Ass.*, **168**, 377.

LATNER, A. L., and BURNARD, E. D. (1950). *Quart. J. Med.*, **19**, 285.

LAWSON, D., MONCRIEFF, A., and PAYNE, W. W. (1960). *Arch. Dis. Childh.*, **35**, 115.

LEUTSCHER, J. A., and JOHNSON, A. B. (1954). *J. clin. Invest.*, **33**, 276.

LIGHTWOOD, R., PAYNE, W. W., and BLACK, J. A. (1953). *Pediatrics*, **12**, 628.

LORBER, J. (1962). *Arch. Dis. Childh.*, **31**, 452.

McGEACHIE, J., and KENNEDY, A. C. (1963). *J. clin. Path.*, **16**, 32.

METCOFF, J., and JANEWAY, C. A. (1961). *J. Pediat.*, **58**, 640.

MILNE, M. D. (1964). *Brit. med. J.*, **1**, 327.

MITCHELL, R. G. (1960). *Lancet*, **1**, 843.

NORMAND, I. C. S., and SMELLIE, J. M. (1965). *Brit. med. J.*, **1**, 1023.

PAYNE, W. W., and ILLINGWORTH, R. S. (1940). *Quart. J. Med.*, **9**, 37.

PITTS, R. F., AYER, J. L., and SCHEISS, W. A. (1949). *J. clin. Invest.*, **28**, 35.

POLITANO, V. A., and LEADBETTER, N. F. (1958). *J. Urol. (Baltimore)*, **79**, 932.

POTTER, E. L. (1946). *J. Pediat.*, **29**, 68.

ROSENHEIM, M. L. (1963). *Brit. med J.*, **1**, 1433.

RUESS, A. L., and ROSENTHAL, I. M. (1963). *Amer. J. Dis. Child.*, **105**, 358.

SCRIVER, C. R., EFRON, M. L., and SCHAFER, I. A. (1964). *J. clin. Invest.*, **43**, 374.

SHEARN, M. A. (1965). *New Engl. J. Med.*, **273**, 943.

SMELLIE, J. M., HODSON, C. J., EDWARDS, D., and NORMAND, I. C. S. (1964). *Brit. med J.*, **2**, 1222.

STANBURY, J. B., WYNGAARDEN, J. B., and FREDERICKSON, D. S. (1965). *The Metabolic Basis of Inherited Disease*, 2nd edit. New York: McGraw-Hill Book Co.

STANBURY, S. W. (1958). *Advanc. intern. Med.*, **9**, 231.

STOWERS, J. M., and DENT, C. E. (1947). *Quart. J. Med.*, **16**, 275.
VERNIER, R. L., WORTHEN, H. G., and GOOD, R. A. (1961). *J. Pediat.*, **58**, 620.
WILLIAMS, D. I. (1954). *Ann. roy. Coll. Surg. Engl.*, **14**, 107.
WILLIAMS, D. I., and STURDY, D. E. (1961). *Arch. Dis. Childh.*, **36**, 130.
WINTERS, R. W., GRAHAM, J. B., WILLIAMS, T. F., McFALLS, V. W., and BURNETT, C. H. (1958). *Medicine (Baltimore)*, **37**, 97.

CHAPTER XVIII

DISEASES OF THE ENDOCRINE SYSTEM

There have been enormous advances in the field of endocrinology in recent years and thousands of papers are published in the medical journals each year. The paediatrician must have sufficient knowledge in this vast subject to enable him to co-operate in practice with the bio-chemists, physicists and other experts to the advantage of his patients. He must not lose sight of the fact that the hormones exert their effects upon almost every tissue in the body, and conversely that the endocrine glands are secondarily affected in many forms of illness. The reader is referred for further details to the textbooks by Wilkins (1965) and Williams (1962).

THE PITUITARY GLAND

Disturbances of pituitary function are rare in children. Their diagnosis has frequently to be based upon a process of exclusion although the ability to measure human growth hormone in the serum by radio-immuno-assay has provided us with a valuable diagnostic tool. It is, as yet, available to the few who work in special centres.

HYPOPITUITARISM

Aetiology

At least half the cases in children are "idiopathic". The commonest demonstrable cause is the craniopharyngioma or suprasellar cyst which arises from Rathke's pouch (Chapter XI). A rare cause is xanthomatosis (Hand-Schüller-Christian disease) (Chapter XI).

Clinical Features

The usual presenting feature is dwarfism, but its pituitary origin can often only be proved beyond doubt when there is a demonstrable local lesion such as a craniopharyngioma with radiographic changes in the region of the sella turcica, visual field defects, "bursting" headaches, and other abnormal neurological signs such as those indicating increased intracranial pressure. In many instances the diagnosis rests upon the exclusion of other types of dwarfism, e.g. hypothyroid, primordial, and those due to bone diseases or severe renal, cardiac or intestinal disorders. The pituitary dwarf is usually of normal birth weight. In fact, slowing of growth only becomes apparent after a year or thereabouts, and it has been suggested that growth in early infancy does not depend upon growth hormone. The pituitary dwarf has normal body proportions but looks much younger than his years.

Bone-age is retarded and becomes more so in relation to height-age as age advances. Sexual development is indefinitely delayed (infantilism) and in adolescence there is an absence of sexual hair, the testes remain underdeveloped, and gonadotrophins are not detectable in the urine. For some reason pituitary dwarfism is much commoner in boys.

In a minority of cases there are signs of functional failure of the target glands such as the thyroid and adrenal (Martin and Wilkins, 1958). Gonadal hypofunction is not demonstrable before the normal age of puberty. Although overt signs of secondary hypothyroidism such as myxoedema or epiphyseal dysgenesis are rare, there is sometimes a lowered serum protein-bound iodine or raised serum cholestrol. A useful diagnostic test in some cases can be based upon the thyroid uptake of ^{131}I, 24 hours after a tracer dose. If this is low after the first dose but much higher when a second test is performed after the administration of thyrotrophin (TSH) 10 units intramuscularly twice daily for three days, there is strong presumptive evidence of hypopituitarism. Adrenocortical hypofunction can occasionally be inferred from an abnormally low urinary output of 17-ketosteroids and 17-hydroxycorticosteroids, and from an impaired ability to secrete a water load. There may be no increase of urinary 17-hydroxycorticosteroids in response to inhibition of 11-β-hydroxylase with metyrapone.

When facilities are present for the estimation of human growth hormone (HGH) a higher level of diagnostic precision is available than hitherto. Straight estimation of the serum level is not by itself of much value but a brisk rise in the HGH level in response to insulin-induced hypoglycaemia is of considerable diagnostic significance (Hunter and Greenwood, 1964), as is also the complete absence to such stimulation of a HGH response. Further diagnostic tests are possible if HGH can be obtained. Thus, estimations of the urinary nitrogen in the daily urines can be made for 5 to 9 day periods before the administration of the HGH, during HGH, and post-HGH. Hypopituitary children show a sharp fall in nitrogen excretion during HGH administration (10 mg. I.M. daily) reflecting an increased retention of between 30 and 45 per cent. This is apparently not found in non-hypopituitary dwarfs (Hubble, 1966). Furthermore, during the post-HGH period the pituitary dwarfs continue to retain an increased amount of nitrogen as compared with their pre-HGH or control period, a finding not recorded in other types of dwarfism.

Differential Diagnosis

In many types of dwarfism the diagnosis can be so firmly established that hypopituitarism is thereby excluded. These include metabolic disorders such as intestinal malabsorption, chronic renal failure, congenital heart disease, bronchiectasis, hypothyroidism, Turner's syndrome, and primary bone disorders such as rickets, achondroplasia and Morquio's disease. The main problem is to separate the pituitary dwarf from the primordial dwarf and the dwarfism arising from constitutional slow growth with delayed adolescence. The distinction may have to await the onset of puberty in some cases unless HGH tests of the type described above can be performed.

Treatment

It has been clearly shown that pituitary dwarfs, but not other types, show a rapid increase in growth rate on human growth hormone (HGH) in intramuscular doses as low as 5 mg. per day (Raben, 1962; Ziskind, 1962; Aarskog, 1963). Unfortunately, growth hormone prepared from human or primate pituitary glands is not available for routine use at the present time, and bovine preparations are of no value. At the time of puberty virilization should be encouraged in males with sublingual methyltestosterone 30 mg./day. This will not, of course, bring about normal maturation of the testes. Females require oestrogens (as stilboestrol 1–2 mg./day) given at first continuously and later cyclically. They may also be given methyltestosterone 10–20 mg./day to promote growth of pubic hair. Thyroxine is only indicated in the rare cases of pituitary hypothyroidism when epiphyseal dysgenesis has been demonstrated radiologically. If the urinary output of 17-hydroxycorticosteroids is reduced, cortisone in small doses (25 mg./day) may promote wellbeing. The place of the newer non-virilizing anabolic steroids is doubtful. Their tendency to bring about premature closure of the epiphyses probably limits their use to adolescence when they can be prescribed in an effort to promote skeletal and muscular development.

Constitutional Slow Growth with Delayed Adolescence

In this type of dwarfism there is often a family history of the same growth pattern in which both linear and skeletal growth lag behind in a parallel fashion. This contrasts with the increasingly delayed skeletal maturation in relation to height of hypopituitarism or hypothyroidism. Puberty is also delayed but normal sexual development ultimately takes place. Until this happens it may be impossible to differentiate this type of dwarfism from that due to lack of pituitary growth hormone. A buccal smear and the estimation of the urinary gonadotrophins in such cases will make it possible to exclude Klinefelter's syndrome.

Treatment

Androgens or gonadotrophins must not be prescribed in childhood because they may damage the testes. After the normal age of puberty (14–15 years) boys can be treated with intramuscular gonadotrophin 2,000–4,000 units twice weekly, or with a monthly dose of intramuscular testosterone enanthate in oil 200–400 mg. In girls treatment should be delayed until the age of 17 years when oestrogens and progestogens may be given cyclically to promote uterine bleeding.

PRIMORDIAL DWARFISM

This "label" undoubtedly includes several distinct entities which cannot yet be clearly distinguished. They all have in common a history of low birth-weight and dwarfism which dates from early infancy. The dwarfism may be of extreme degree but it is usually associated with a normal bone-age, normal sexual development and the capacity for procreation. In many cases radiographs show pseudo-epiphyses at the proximal ends of the metacarpals and there may be other minor bone abnormalities. The term Lorain-Lévi dwarfism, often given to such cases, is best avoided because the precise nature of the cases described by Lorain and Lévi is not certain. Some types of primordial dwarfism are undoubtedly genetic in origin; in others an environmental influence has seemed more probable. These patients do not respond to HGH.

Two principal types of primordial dwarfism can be recognized. In the *symmetrical* type, which may be inherited as a dominant or recessive trait, the characteristics are low birth-weight, normal sexual development and the ability to reproduce. In the *asymmetrical* type the characteristics are disproportionate growth and minor skeletal abnormalities. There may also be congenital heart disease or mental deficiency. One group is distinguished by slender bodies, small heads and old-looking features ("bird-headed dwarfs"); another by a stocky build and flattened nose ("snub-nosed dwarfs") (Black, 1961). Both these types are probably genetic in origin but some cases of primordial dwarfism seem to be related to disturbances in early or late pregnancy.

Treatment

None is available.

PROGERIA

Aetiology

This remarkable disease has sometimes been confused with Simmonds' disease which is due to total destruction of the anterior pituitary. In fact, progeria has few points in common with Simmonds' disease (which is unknown in childhood), and it should not be regarded as a pituitary disease.

Clinical Features

The child is normal in weight and appearance at birth. Growth almost ceases after the first birthday and the typical features of the condition are present after some three to five years (Fig. 58). The head is almost bald and the eyebrows are scanty. The eyes appear prominent and the nose is beak-shaped. There is a receding chin. The skin is atrophic with a texture like that seen in the aged. Similarly, there is paucity of subcutaneous fat over the face, trunk and limbs. Radiographs show osteoporosis. There is also delay in the primary dentition.

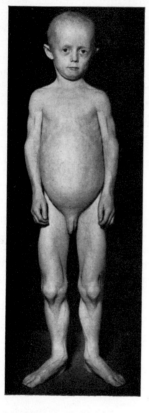

Fig. 58.—Typical case of progeria. Observe baldness, loss of subcutaneous fat, prominent eyes, scanty eyebrows, and aged appearance in boy aged 7 years.

The disease proves fatal during the second decade, usually from the effects of arteriosclerosis. Osteoarthritis may also be present in this process of premature senility.

Treatment

None is available.

HYPERPITUITARISM

Aetiology

Over-activity of the anterior pituitary is very rare in childhood. The commonest type involves over-production of growth hormone. This is often related to tumour or hyperplasia of the eosinophil cells although it has also been reported with a chromophobe adenoma. In childhood it results in gigantism, and after the epiphyses have united, in acromegaly. Cushing's syndrome was first related to tumour or hyperplasia of the pituitary basophil cells, but it is better regarded as a result of adrenocortical over-activity (see below). Some might regard thyrotoxicosis as due to hyperpituitarism and the over-production of thyrotrophin (thyroid stimulating hormone: T.S.H.), but this disease is discussed with the other thyroid disorders.

Clinical Features

In gigantism an excessive rate of growth starts in early childhood and continues for longer than normal due to a delayed puberty and epiphyseal closure. Hypogonadism is sometimes added to the picture in adult life. When the epiphyses begin to unite acromegalic features are frequently added, e.g. hypertrophy of the mandible (prognathism), coarse facial features due to nasal and maxillary overgrowth, thickening of the skin, huge spade-like hands and feet. Diabetes mellitus develops in some cases. A pituitary tumour may also produce local pressure effects on the optic chiasm and increased intracranial pressure.

Differential Diagnosis

Pituitary gigantism must be distinguished from hereditary tallness. In the latter the body proportions are normal, the bones show normal development, and there is a family history of large stature.

Treatment

Surgical removal of a pituitary tumour is indicated when there are obvious pressure effects. In other cases deep X-ray therapy to the pituitary fossa may be tried. Many cases end fatally in early adult life from intercurrent infection or progressive debility. In others the progress of the tumour results eventually in death from hypopituitarism.

DIABETES INSIPIDUS

Aetiology

This disease is due to deficient production of antidiuretic hormone (A.D.H.: Vasopressin) by the neurosecretory system, which includes the posterior lobe of the pituitary and also the supra-optic and paraventricular nuclei of the hypothalamus. This system also secretes oxytocin and, possibly, other hormones. The function of A.D.H. is to promote reabsorption of water by the renal tubules. It may also cause hypertension by its effects on smooth muscle. The output of A.D.H. is reduced by a fall in plasma osmolarity which explains the antidiuretic effect of intravenous hypertonic saline, and the diuresis which follows a water load.

Hypovolaemia, however, can overcome the effects of hypo-osmolarity and result in antidiuresis. It is necessary to distinguish pituitary diabetes insipidus from the nephrogenic variety (Chapter XVII) which does not respond to A.D.H.

The posterior pituitary may be damaged by tumour (craniopharyngioma), Hand-Schüller-Christian disease, fracture of the base of the skull, healing tuberculous meningitis and meningo-vascular syphilis. In some cases there is no discoverable cause. A hereditary form has been described, transmitted as a dominant trait.

Clinical Features

The characteristic picture is the sudden onset by day and night, of severe polyuria with resultant excessive thirst. Dehydration only develops if fluid intake is limited, voluntarily or during anaesthesia. In the child a common complaint is "enuresis". The urine is very dilute with a specific gravity of 1,005 or less. The water deprivation test reveals that the specific gravity does not rise. This must be carefully supervised so that the patient is not allowed to lose more than 5 per cent of his body weight (usually for a period of 6 to 8 hours). Another useful diagnostic test involves the use of hypertonic saline. The patient first drinks water, 20 ml. per Kg. body weight and the urine output thereafter is measured every 15 minutes until a diuresis occurs; he is then given 2·5 per cent sodium chloride solution intravenously, 0·25 ml./Kg./min. for 45 minutes. In true diabetes insipidus the normal marked antidiuresis does not occur. Finally, to distinguish nephrogenic diabetes insipidus 5 units of pitressin tannate in oil are given intramuscularly. In pituitary diabetes insipidus this causes immediate abolition of thirst and polyuria with a rise in the urinary specific gravity which should be checked every 15 minutes after the injection.

Differential Diagnosis

Compulsive water drinking is associated with other signs of psychological disturbance and there is a normal antidiuretic response to intravenous hypertonic saline. It is extremely rare in childhood. More common causes of thirst and polyuria are diabetes mellitus and chronic renal failure, both of which should be obvious after simple clinical examination and urine analysis.

Treatment

In most cases the diabetes insipidus of pituitary origin can be controlled by intramuscular pitressin tannate in oil, 5 units every 24–48 hours, or by the inhalation of pituitary snuff (Pitocin or Disipidin) 10–25 mg. every 2–6 hours. The long-term outlook depends principally upon the primary disease.

THE THYROID GLAND

Disorders of the thyroid gland are, with the exception of diabetes mellitus, the most common endocrine problems of childhood. The advent of radioisotope techniques has been followed by a vast increase in our knowledge of the physiology and disturbances of thyroid function. A detailed account of thyroid physiology can be found in the books by Pitt-Rivers and Tata (1959) and Pitt-Rivers and Trotter (1964), and in the published proceedings of a conference held in the Royal College

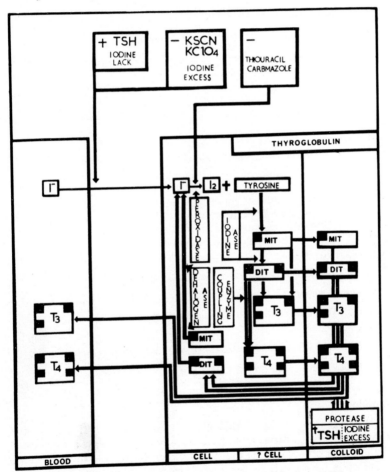

FIG. 59.—Biosynthesis of the thyroid hormones. T = tyrosine; MIT = mono-iodotyrosine; DIT = di-iodotyrosine; T_3 = tri-iodothyronine; T_4 = thyroxine (tetra-iodothyronine); TSH = thyroid stimulating hormone; + = reaction promoted; − = reaction inhibited.

of Physicians of London (Mason, 1963). A schematic representation of the biosynthesis of the thyroid hormones is shown in Fig. 59.

HYPOTHYROIDISM

A classification of the causes of hypothyroidism is shown in Table IV. It is designed upon an aetiological basis which will permit the clinician to approach diagnosis and treatment using modern methods.

TABLE IV

A CLASSIFICATION OF HYPOTHYROIDISM IN CHILDHOOD

I *DYSGENESIS OF THE THYROID GLAND* (Sporadic cretinism)

    (*a*) Congenital athyreosis   Congenital-Cretinism
    (*b*) Maldescent
    (*c*) Maldevelopment   Acquired-Juvenile
                                      Myxoedema

II *DEFICIENCY OF IODINE* (*Endemic Cretinism*)

III *INBORN ENZYME DEFECTS* (Familial cretinism).

    (*a*) Intrathyroid (Familial non-endemic goitrous cretinism)

        (i) Failure of thyroid trapping of iodine.
        (ii) Failure of organic binding of iodine.
        (iii) Failure of coupling of iodotyrosines.
        (iv) Failure of deiodination of iodotyrosines.
        (v) Production of abnormal thyroprotein.
        (vi) Other defects to be defined.

    (*b*) Extrathyroid

        ? Defect in peripheral utilization of thyroxine.

IV *INGESTION OF GOITROGENS* (*Accidental or therapeutic*)

    (*a*) Antenatal (iodine, thiouracil etc. in pregnancy)
    (*b*) Postnatal

V *PRIMARY THYROID DISEASE, e.g. Hashimoto, carcinoma etc.*

VI *PITUITARY HYPOTHYROIDISM*

Aetiology

(I) **Dysgenesis of the thyroid gland.**—The use of [132]I and ^{131}I has shown that non-goitrous hypothyroidism does not always arise because the infant is totally lacking in thyroid tissue. Indeed the sporadic cretin more often has an ectopic focus of thyroid activity situated somewhere between the root of the tongue and the normal site in the neck. Less often, thyroid tissue of inadequate amount is situated in the normal part of the neck (Hutchison, 1963). The amount of thyroid tissue may be so inadequate that hypothyroidism is present at birth (*cretinism*), or it may keep the child euthyroid until such time as he outgrows its capacity to meet his requirements when acquired hypothyroidism develops (*juvenile myxoedema*). In some totally athyroidic cases of cretinism Blizzard *et al.* (1959) have suggested that a process of thyroidal auto-immunization in the mother has resulted in thyroid antibodies crossing the placenta and destroying the foetal thyroid. In other cases a familial incidence has suggested a genetic influence (Ainger and Kelly, 1955). The author has seen several such cases in which either two siblings were cretinous or in which a cretinous mother has given birth to a cretinous child (Greig *et al.* 1966). It should be noted that the earlier belief that the maternal thyroid gland can vicariously substitute for that of the foetus is not tenable and that, in fact, thyroid hormone cannot cross the placenta in sufficient amount to prevent foetal hypothyroidism when the foetal thyroid is inadequate (Hageman and Villee, 1960).

(II) **Endemic cretinism.**—There can be no doubt that simple goitre and endemic cretinism can be produced by a deficiency of iodine-intake and that they can be prevented by the iodination of table-salt. There is some evidence, however, that sometimes the iodine-deficiency acts by unveiling an underlying inborn error of thyroid metabolism (Costa *et al.*, 1953) and early workers in this field frequently stressed the frequency of consanguinity in the parents of endemic cretins.

(III) **Inborn enzyme defects.**—This group which has been intensively studied in recent years (Hutchison, 1958; Joseph *et al.*, 1958; McGirr, 1960; McGirr, 1963) belongs to the inborn errors of metabolism (Chapter IX). The various enzyme defects which have been defined are genetically determined (Hutchison and McGirr, 1958; Fraser *et al.*, 1960). It is proposed in this chapter to give only a brief account of these complex thyroid disturbances and full details can be obtained in the references supplied.

(i) *Iodide trapping defect.*—This was recently described as a condition in which the thyroid gland is unable normally to trap and concentrate iodide from the blood stream (Stanbury and Chapman, 1960). The gland contains little iodide from which to manufacture hormone.

(ii) *Impaired organification of trapped iodine.*—In the normal thyroid, iodide trapped from blood is rapidly oxidized to free or elemental iodine. If the peroxidase which permits this step is deficient, the incorporation of iodine into a protein complex in combination with tyrosine cannot take place and hormone synthesis is reduced. Most of the patients with this defect have also had nerve deafness (Pendred's syndrome), and a few have had ichthyosis.

(iii) *Failure of coupling of iodotyrosines.*—Thyroxine is thought to be formed from the coupling of two molecules of diiodotyrosine; tri-iodothyronine from the coupling of one molecule of diiodotyrosine with one molecule of monoiodotyrosine. When the coupling process is blocked the thyroid gland is stuffed full of iodotyrosines but contains little or no fully fashioned hormone (thyroxine or triiodothyronine).

(iv) *Failure of deiodination of iodotyrosines.*—The thyroid hormones stored in the thyroglobulin are liberated into the blood stream by the action of thyroid protease. The iodotyrosines which are released from the thyroglobulin at the same time do not normally enter the blood stream because they are deoidinated by the enzyme dehalogenase, and the iodine so released re-enters the pathway of hormone synthesis. When dehalogenase activity is missing the iodotyrosines will enter the blood stream unchanged and will be lost in the urine. This will lead to constant loss of iodine from the body and ultimate hypothyroidism.

(v) *Production of an abnormal thyroprotein.*—In this group of patients an abnormal iodinated protein is found in the plasma. It precipitates with protein but unlike thyroxine it is not extractable with butanol. It has no hormonal activity although both iodotyrosines and iodo-thyronines can be liberated from it by hydrolysis (McGirr *et al.*, 1960). There is, in fact, a good deal of evidence that several different iodopro-teins have been involved in different cases, and it is probable that a number of distinct intrathyroid metabolic defects are still to be charac-terized (Murray *et al.*, 1965).

In each of these intrathyroid metabolic defects the production of hormones is diminished. This results in an increased output of pituitary TSH with consequent thyroid hyperplasia and goitre. These various types of "familial non-endemic goitrous cretinism" cannot be dis-tinguished from each other on clinical or histological evidence. Their elucidation is dependent upon detailed studies using ^{131}I. The interested reader is referred to the references already supplied. It is indicated in Table IV that there have been some goitrous cretins in whom evidence of other ill-defined intrathyroid defects exist.

The question of hypothyroidism arising from an extrathyroid failure in the peripheral utilization of circulating thyroxine remains in some doubt. We have described one non-goitrous cretin in whom there was no response to treatment with dry thyroid B.P., but who responded rapidly to triiodothyronine (Hutchison *et al.*, 1957). It is not possible to interpret the significance of these observations further than to suggest some failure in the utilization of thyroxine.

(IV) **Ingestion of goitrogens.**—Some drugs such as thiouracil, car-bimazole and potassium perchlorate are used in therapeutics for their thyroid blocking actions. Obviously in overdosage they will produce goitre and hypothyroidism. Certain drugs used for other purposes may, however, occasionally produce similar unwanted effects, e.g. sulphon-amides, para-aminosalicylic acid and phenylbutazone. It is an in-teresting fact that whereas a deficiency of iodide is a recognized cause of goitre, an excess can also cause goitre and hypothyroidism in a few susceptible individuals. The iodide is often ingested in the form of proprietary "asthma cures" and expectorants (Morgans and Trotter, 1959). Congenital goitrous hypothyroidism has also followed the ingestion of iodides and other goitrogenic drugs by the expectant mother during pregnancy (Petty and Di Benedetto, 1957). Soybean which is sometimes used as a substitute for milk in allergic infants has also produced goitre and hypothyroidism; the goitrogen has not been identified but its effect can be prevented with iodide (Shepard *et al.*, 1960).

(V) **Primary thyroid disease.**—Hashimoto's disease (auto-immune thyroiditis) has been diagnosed more frequently in children in recent years. It is probably less of a rarity than used to be thought and is described on page 351. Carcinoma of the thyroid gland is exceedingly uncommon before puberty in the United Kingdom. It is, apparently, not so rare in the U.S.A. where radiation for "thymic asthma", enlarged tonsils and acne vulgaris were once a common practice (Winship and Rosvoll, 1961).

(VI) **Pituitary hypothyroidism.**—Overt manifestations of secondary hypothyroidism are rare in childhood although in some cases of hypopituitarism there may a somewhat low level of serum protein-bound iodine. These cases show little response to thyroid treatment, in marked contrast to primary hypothyroidism.

Clinical Features

The diagnosis of severe cretinism should not be difficult (Van Wyk, 1956). Indeed, the manifestations are present within a few days of birth, in contrast to the statement in many textbooks. The presenting symptoms are feeding difficulties, noisy respiration or constipation. The undue prolongation of "physiological jaundice" should always arouse the suspicion of hypothyroidism (Åkerrén, 1954). The appearance of the infant is typical. The facial features are coarse and ugly with, often, a wrinkled forehead and low hairline. The hair may be dry and scanty. The large myxoedematous tongue protrudes from the mouth and interferes with feeding and breathing. The cry has a characteristic hoarseness. The neck appears short because of the presence of myxoedematous pads of fat above the clavicles. The skin, especially over the face and extremities feels dry, thick and cold. An umbilical hernia is common. The hands and fingers are broad and stumpy. The cretinous infant is frequently apathetic and uninterested in his surroundings. As time goes by, psychomotor retardation becomes obvious and partially irreversible. These features are depicted in Figs. 60 and 61. It should be noted that the common type of sporadic cretinism due to thyroid dysgenesis is much more common in girls. This is not true of the other types.

Milder degrees of cretinism and juvenile myxoedema (Fig. 62) produce much less striking features. None the less, the marked delay in diagnosis so commonly encountered is unnecessary and it results often in avoidable intellectual impairment. *The possibility of hypothyroidism should be considered in every infant or child in whom growth is retarded.* A normal linear growth completely excludes hypothyroidism. Most mild cases of hypothyroidism show sufficient characteristic manifestations to arouse the immediate suspicion of the alert physician. Thus the body proportions remain infantile with long trunk and short legs. A tendency to stand with exaggerated lumbar lordosis and slightly flexed hips and knees is common. The anterior fontanelle is late in closing. The deciduous teeth are slow in erupting and radiographs may show defects in the enamel. The face and hands are frequently mildly myxoedematous and the cerebral activities are slow and sluggish. The mandible is often underdeveloped and the naso-labial configuration may be obviously that of a much younger child. The deep reflexes are sometimes exaggerated with slow relaxation and there may be mild ataxia. In some

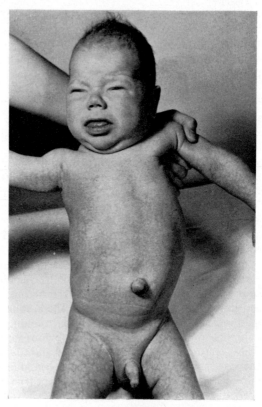

FIG. 60.—Sporadic cretin aged 4 months. Note coarse ugly features, large myxoedematous tongue, umbilical hernia.

cases of juvenile myxoedema, however, the only clinical indication of hypothyroidism is dwarfism with infantile proportions. In such cases sexual maturation is delayed (as in all hypothyroid children) so that the condition may be regarded as a "thyrogenic infantilism" (Zondek *et al.*, 1958).

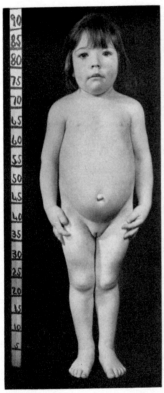 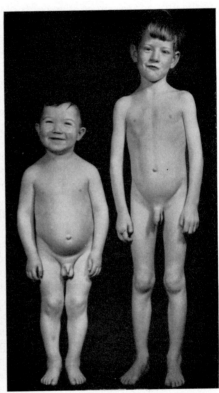

FIG. 61.—Untreated cretin aged 7 years. Observe infantile body proportions, coarse features and thick hands and feet.

FIG. 62.—Mild cretinism in boy aged 6½ years. Radioiodine tests showed thyroid activity in suprahyoid region. Note infantile body proportions

Diagnosis

The most important step in the diagnosis, without which the rest cannot follow, is the birth of suspicion in the mind of the clinician. A careful medical history and a thoughtful physical examination are often sufficient to confirm the diagnosis in themselves. Certainly they should rarely fail to put the physician on to the right track.

1. *Linear growth.*—Dwarfism is one of the only two invariable find-ings in hypothyroidism. This observation requires only a table or chart showing the mean heights of normal children of the community (Tanner and Whitehouse, 1959). The ratio of the upper to lower skeletal segment is also abnormal (infantile) in hypothyroid children. The lower segment is the distance from the top of the symphysis pubis to the ground; the upper segment is obtained by subtracting the lower segment from the total height. At birth the upper/lower ratio is 1·7/1; at 2 years it is 1·44/1; by 10–11 years the ratio is 1/1. Hypothyroid children have an unduly long upper segment because of their short legs.

2. *Skeletal maturation.*—Delayed ossification, to a more severe degree than the retardation in linear growth, is the other constant finding in hypothyroidism. The assessment of bone-age is based on radiographs of various epiphyseal areas, chosen according to the child's age, and their comparison with an ossification chart showing the normal ages at which the different centres should ossify (Wilkins, 1965; Mac-Kay, 1961). Thus foetal hypothyroidism can be presumed in the full-term baby if the upper tibial or lower femoral epiphyses, which normally ossify at 36 foetal weeks, are absent or if they show *epiphyseal dysgen-esis.* This appearance of dysgenesis of the epiphyses is pathognomonic of hypothyroidism. It may be florid at one area and absent at another, so that radiographs should always be taken of several areas of the skeleton. In some cases dysgenesis only appears after thyroid treatment has been started, but then only in those ossification centres which should have appeared in the normal child before that age. The presence of dysgenesis indicates that the hypothyroid state has existed before the affected centre would be normally due to ossify and it permits of an assessment of the age, foetal or postnatal, at which the hypothyroidism developed. The characteristic X-ray appearance (Wilkins, 1941) is of a misshapen epiphysis with irregular or fluffy margins and a fragmented or stippled substance (Fig. 63). *In the great majority of cases of hypothy-roidism measurements of the linear height, the upper and lower segments, and a few well-chosen radiographs will establish or exclude the diagnosis of hypothyroidism beyond doubt.* They will also determine the age of onset of the hypothyroid state.

3. *Biochemical tests.*—The *protein-bound iodine* (^{127}I) level in the serum is invariably lowered in non-goitrous hypothyroidism (normal range in childhood = 4–8 μg. per 100 ml.). This test is particularly useful in early infancy when assessment of bone-age may be less precise. The estimation is, however, technically difficult and only available in large centres. It has to be interpreted with great caution in goitrous cases in which normal values are not inconsistent with severe degrees of hypothyroidism. A raised *serum cholesterol* (above 300 mg. per 100 ml.) is highly significant, but normal values are not uncommon

in cretinism. The level rises briskly, however, some weeks after thyroid treatment is withdrawn in a case of hypothyroidism, and this observation can be useful confirmation when the initial diagnosis in a child having therapeutic doses of thyroxine is under suspicion. Other common findings in hypothyroid infants are a lowered alkaline phophatase and raised carotene (only after vegetables have been included in the diet). They are, however, of little diagnostic use.

4. *Radio-active iodine tests.*—These are never necessary to establish the diagnosis of hypothyroidism, but they can be used to provide a great deal of information about the pathogenesis. For the detection and

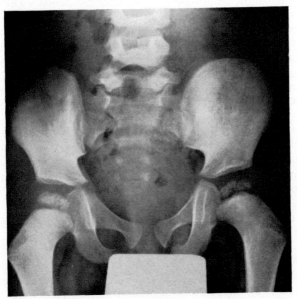

FIG. 63.—Epiphyseal dysgenesis in femoral heads. Note stippling and fragmented appearance.

location of thyroid activity in non-goitrous cretins ^{132}I (half-life 2·3 hr.) can be safely given followed by scanning of the neck for radio-activity two hours later. The wisdom of using ^{131}I (half-life 8 days) has been doubted by some because of its possible carcinogenic effects. It has provided a great deal of valuable information about the nature of goitrous cretinism and other thyroid disorders. Its use should be confined to workers with expert experience in the use of radioisotopes when the dangers are probably much less than those associated with many other commonly used diagnostic procedures. The reader will find references to technical details of the use of radio-active iodine methods in the books mentioned at the beginning of this section.

Treatment

The drug of choice for the treatment of hypothyroidism is sodium *l*-thyroxine. This iodinated aminoacid is stable whereas preparations of dry thyroid vary in activity from batch to batch and they deteriorate with the passage of time. A preparation containing both thyroxine and triiodothyronine in the proportions of 9 : 1 is now commercially available, but its advantage over thyroxine alone is doubtful. Cretins are very sensitive to the action of thyroid so that initial dosage should be small and increases rarely made more frequently than at intervals of two weeks. A safe initial dose is *l*-thyroxine 0·025 mg. per day. The dose can be doubled every two weeks until a satisfactory maintenance dose level has been reached. This varies between 0·1–0·3 mg. per day. In the early days of treatment the hypothyroid child frequently shows a disturbed mental performance, unaccustomed restlessness and temporary loss of weight. These manifestations do not indicate over-dosage. They are temporary and parents should be warned to expect them, coupled with an assurance that soon their child will be much better than ever before. The maintenance dose level is that which permits linear growth to proceed at a normal rate and does not leave the bone-age retarded. It is, however, undesirable to permit bone-age to advance too far (over two years) beyond chronological age or premature fusion of the epiphyses will result in dwarfism. The author regards these criteria as preferable to serial estimations of the serum PBI for the control of dosage. If the latter is to be used the serum PBI level should be maintained between 6–9 μg. per 100 ml. Treatment must, of course, be regularly continued for the duration of the patient's life.

Prognosis

The somatic response to adequate treatment is invariably good, but in many cases a disappointing retardation of intellect persists. The age at which treatment is started is obviously important; the sooner the better. None the less, the results may be poor in some cases. The demonstration by ourselves (Hutchison, 1963) and others that all cretins are not completely athyroidic makes it easier to understand these results in the light of the fact that the age of onset of the hypothyroid state and its severity varies from case to case. The amount of thyroid tissue available during foetal and early postnatal life will determine whether the infant is severely cretinous from birth, or only mildly cretinous, or precariously euthyroid for some years when juvenile myxoedema develops. These clinical categories are usually distinguishable by the physician and the mental prognosis in each has been discussed by Smith *et al.* (1957). When cretinism is severe from birth only 15 per cent of patients achieve an I.Q. above 90; in mild cretinism over 40 per cent reach an I.Q. of above 90; whereas in juvenile myxoedema an I.Q. over 90 may be expected in about 80 per cent of patients. It would seem that adequate hormone production during foetal and early postnatal life protects the brain against permanent damage from later hypothyroidism, whereas the absence of thyroid hormone during the period of most rapid brain growth results frequently in irreversible damage. Another factor which obviously influences the ultimate mental development of the individual child is the level of intelligence of the parents.

Auto-immune Thyroiditis (Hashimoto's Disease)

Aetiology

This is the only primary disease of the thyroid gland which causes hypothyroidism in childhood with any frequency. It is one of the best examples of a strictly organ-specific auto-immunity and the immunological phenomena are usually confined to the thyroid gland. Antibodies have been found to at least three thyroid autoantigens in this disease namely, thyroglobulin, a microsomal fraction and a soluble colloid fraction distinct from thyroglobulin. There is some evidence of a familial transmission of thyroid auto-immunity (Doniach *et al.*, 1965). None the less, the factor which initiates the disease is unknown.

Pathology

The outstanding feature is infiltration of the thyroid by lymphocytes, plasma cells and reticular cells. Hyperplasia of the epithelial cells is commonly seen. In more advanced cases the epithelial cells show degenerative changes and there may be extensive fibrosis with final destruction of the gland.

Clinical Features

In most children the only sign is a goitre (Nilsson and Doniach, 1964). It rarely has the firm rubbery consistency so typical of the adult form of the disease. In fact, almost any goitre in a child may be due to auto-immune thyroiditis and specific diagnostic tests for its confirmation or exclusion should be done much more frequently than heretofore. It may be smooth in consistency, feel granular and bosselated, or become lobulated. Only a minority of affected children go on to develop hypothyroidism but it is important to search for signs of this state in every case.

Diagnosis

The serum PBI level is usually within normal limits but in some children is in the high "thyrotoxic" range. This reflects not thyrotoxicosis but leakage of iodinated protein into the circulation from damaged acini. The serum PBI will be markedly reduced when the child is frankly hypothyroid. A characteristic finding is a much higher value for PBI than for butanol-extractable iodine (BEI), again reflecting the presence of an abnormal iodoprotein in the blood stream. Unfortunately, the estimation of the BEI in the serum is rarely available in this country. The same discrepancy is more easily shown between the PB^{131}I and the BE^{131}I after a tracer dose of radioiodine.

The most specific diagnostic tests have an immunological basis. They are the tanned red cell test, complement fixation test, cytoplasmic immunofluorescence and colloid immunofluorescence (Doniach et al., 1965). *Children with thyroiditis give lower titres than adults, but the more frequent performance of these tests in children with goitre and/or hypothyroidism would reveal that the disease is less rare than has been suspected on clinical grounds drawn from experience in adults.*

Thyroid biopsy, either by open operation or needle aspiration, is only indicated when the suspicion of carcinoma arises.

Treatment

Thyroxine should be prescribed, whether or not the child is hypothyroid, to suppress the excess secretion of pituitary TSH and diminish the size of the goitre. These children should be kept under prolonged medical supervision because some later develop other auto-immune diseases such as myasthenia gravis or pernicious anaemia.

HYPERTHYROIDISM

In contrast to hypothyroidism which is common, thyrotoxicosis is rare in childhood. It usually takes the form of Graves' disease with diffuse thyroid hyperplasia and exophthalmos. An uncommon type of hyperthyroidism is encountered in the newborn infant born to a previously thyrotoxic mother.

EXOPHTHALMIC GOITRE (GRAVES' DISEASE)

Aetiology

The serum of thyrotoxic patients contains a substance which has a TSH-like action but which has a much more prolonged thyroid stimulating effect. This substance has been called "long-acting thyroid stimulator" or LATS and it is the direct cause of Grave's disease (Adams, 1965; Carneiro et al., 1966). It does not originate in the pituitary gland and it is, indeed, believed to be an IgG (7S) gamma globulin and is probably to be regarded as a thyroid autoantibody. The antigen is presumably the site within the thyroid gland with which TSH interacts. The exophthalmos of Graves' disease does not correlate closely with the serum level of LATS. None the less, it is also probably derived from some form of thyroid auto-immunity.

Pathology

The thyroid follicles are hyperplastic and the gland is excessively vascular. Mitotic figures are common in the acinar cells and lymphocytic infiltration may be marked. The alveoli are almost devoid of colloid.

Clinical Features

The disease is more common in girls and rare before the age of 7 years. The parents may bring their child for medical advice with a variety of symptoms such as irritability, fidgetiness, deterioration in school performance, loss of weight in spite of good appetite, excessive sweating, palpitations or nervousness. The child looks thin, and often startled because of her stare and wide palpebral fissures. There may be obvious exophthalmos. Her skin will be flushed, warm and moist. A fine tremor of the outstretched hands is common. The abnormal cardiovascular signs in the child include sinus tachycardia, raised systolic blood pressure and a large pulse pressure. The thyroid gland is visibly enlarged and feels soft. A bruit may be audible over the gland. Emotional lability is frequently very obvious. The upper/lower segment ratio is usually low. Menstruation may be delayed in untreated girls.

Diagnosis

This is usually obvious on simple clinical observation. The most useful confirmation is a serum PBI above 8 μg. per 100 ml. A raised B.M.R. can only be reliable evidence in the older child. Bone-age is often advanced. Radioiodine tests are probably best avoided as they are never necessary to reach a diagnosis in the child.

Treatment

A trial of medical treatment should always be made. Suitable drugs and doses are carbimazole 10 mg. thrice daily or methylthiouracil 75 mg. thrice daily; after four weeks or thereabouts the doses can often be reduced to 10 mg. or 50 mg., respectively, daily. It is wise to give the maximal required dose to control the hyperthyroidism and to prevent myxoedema with thyroxine 0·1–0·15 mg. per day. In the author's experience the results of drug treatment are frequently disappointing.

In about 50 per cent of cases we advise partial thyroidectomy. The results in children have been gratifying and complications are uncommon. It must be remembered that all the anti-thyroid drugs can cause toxic effects, e.g. rashes, agranulocytosis, aplastic anaemia. On the other hand, post-operative hypothyroidism is rare and can, if necessary, be readily corrected with thyroxine. In childhood there is, of course, no justification for the use of radioiodine in treatment.

Neonatal Hyperthyroidism

There has been a considerable number of instances in which women who have or have had thyrotoxicosis have given birth to infants with the unmistakable signs of hyperthyroidism in the neonatal period. The infants have been restless, agitated, excessively hungry, and they have exhibited warm, moist flushed skin, tachycardia (190–220 min.), tachypnoea, exophthalmos and goitre. In the first infant to be reported, born to an untreated mother, the diagnosis was made antenatally because of foetal tachycardia (White, 1912). Some mothers have been previously treated by partial thyroidectomy (Lewis and Macgregor, 1957); others have received thyroid blocking drugs during pregnancy (Bongiovanni et al., 1956).

Neonatal thyrotoxicosis is a temporary state of about three months duration, but if it is not recognized and treated can prove fatal. Various theories of pathogenesis have been put forward but it now seems certain that the signs in the infant are due to the effects of LATS which has crossed the placenta from the mother (Sunshine et al., 1965). The transplacental passage of LATS accords with the known behaviour of IgG globulin which can cross the placental barrier freely, and the duration of the disease is compatible with the 20–30 day half-life of maternal antibodies in the foetal circulation. When the mother is frankly thyrotoxic up to the time of delivery of the baby the hyperthyroid state is present in the infant at birth, whereas if the mother has been rendered euthyroid by drugs or operation the neonatal thyrotoxicosis does not develop for three or more days.

The signs of thyrotoxicosis can be alarmingly severe and prompt treatment of the newborn infant is essential. This is with potassium iodide 2–5 mg. thrice daily. If the condition is not rapidly brought under control carbimazole should also be given, 2·5 mg. three or four times daily. The antithyroid medication should be continued for two to three months.

Simple and Sporadic Goitre

It is not uncommon to see children, usually girls, with simple goitres. The thyroids vary in size but they are usually diffuse and non-nodular. In adult life some become nodular, and thyrotoxicosis or malignant changes are not unknown.

Although these children are clinically euthyroid the serum PBI levels may be slightly subnormal indicating diminished hormone production which results in an increased output of TSH by the pituitary with resultant goitre.

The causes of sporadic goitre are many. In each case a careful history must be taken with special attention to diet, possible ingestion of drugs, and familial incidence of thyroid disorders or consanguinity in the parents. Most cases are probably due to iodine deficiency as shown by a low level of plasma inorganic iodine (Alexander *et al.*, 1962; Wilson, 1963). In some parts of the world other factors contribute. Thus, in Tasmania simple goitre has been attributed to a goitrogen in milk derived from weeds in the pastures on which the cows graze (Gibson *et al.*, 1960). Furthermore, certain foods such as swedes and turnips contain a goitrogen ("goitrin") which may be liberated by the action of enzymes in the intestine (Greer, 1962). Some cases of sporadic goitre, often familial, are due to partial deficiencies of the same intrathyroid enzymes already described under the causes of hypothyroidism, where the deficiency is of more severe degree. Others can be traced to the ingestion of goitrogenic drugs such as iodide, P.A.S., sulphonamides and cobalt.

Treatment

Simple goitre is best treated with thyroxine in doses just short of causing toxic effects. It may have to be continued for life. In cases which develop around the time of puberty, however, spontaneous recovery may occur. Goitrogenic drugs should obviously be withdrawn. The addition of potassium iodide to table-salt would prevent most simple goitres. It has frequently been advised in the United Kingdom but so far not implemented.

The Parathyroid Glands

Primary disorders of the parathyroid glands are exceedingly rare in paediatric practice. Indeed the most commonly seen disorder is the secondary hyperparathyroidism responsible in part for the bone changes which sometimes develop in chronic renal failure (Chapter XVII).

Hypoparathyroidism

Aetiology

Hypoparathyroidism is still sometimes seen after thyroidectomy, but the few cases reported in children have been of the "idiopathic" variety (Drake *et al.*, 1939; Steinbeg and Waldron, 1952; Bronsky *et al.*, 1958; Fourman, 1960). Rarely hypoparathyroidism in the infant has been associated with parathyroid disease in the mother (Benson and Parsons, 1964).

Clinical Features

The diagnosis is not difficult when a case presents with chronic tetany. The symptoms include paraesthesiae ("pins and needles"), muscle cramps and carpopedal spasm. Chvostek's and Trousseau's signs may be elicited. More often the outstanding feature is the presence of recurrent convulsions when an erroneous diagnosis of epilepsy may easily be made. Some affected children have also been mentally retarded and intracerebral calcification may occur. Useful diagnostic clues are delay in the second dentition and defective enamel, ectodermal dysplasia and deformed nails, loss of hair, and moniliasis in the mouth or nails. Cataract develops later in 50 per cent of cases. The characteristic biochemical changes are a low serum calcium (below 9 mg. per 100 ml.) and raised serum phosphate (above 7 mg. per 100 ml.).

"Pseudo-hypoparathyroidism" (Albright *et al.*, 1942) gives rise to a very similar clinical picture but it appears not to respond to parathyroid hormone, possibly because of a failure of the renal tubules to respond so that there is an abnormal reabsorption of phosphate. However, the hypocalcaemia responds to vitamin D or A.T. 10.

Treatment

The immediate treatment for tetany is an intravenous injection of 10 per cent calcium gluconate, 10–20 ml., repeated every few hours as necessary. Parathormone may also be given intravenously or intramuscularly, 30–200 units every 12 hours, to raise the serum calcium. For long-term treatment calciferol is as effective as A.T. 10, and cheaper. The daily dose is usually about 50,000 units but may need to be raised as high as 200,000 units. Its actions are to mobilize calcium from the bones and to increase its absorption from the intestine, also to increase the renal excretion of phosphate.

HYPERPARATHYROIDISM

Aetiology

Adenoma and hyperplasia of the parathyroid glands have both been found, the former being more common.

Clinical Features

In some cases bone pains and muscular weakness are the first symptoms. More often nephrocalcinosis and nephrolithiasis result in thirst and polyuria. Peptic ulceration is unduly frequent in these patients. Anorexia, vomiting and severe constipation are common and attributable to the hypercalcaemia. The bone changes of osteitis fibrosa generalisata are found. These include osteoporosis with patches of osteosclerosis. This produces a characteristic granular mottling or discrete rounded translucent areas in radiographs of the skull. Similar appearances are commonly found in the clavicles and iliac bones. Pathognomonic changes are frequently seen in the terminal phalanges of the hands where there is subperiosteal resorption of bone with a crenelated appearance, best seen with a hand lens. The lamina dura, a dense line of alveolar bone surrounding the roots of the teeth, disappears. A giant cell tumour (osteo-clastoma) may appear as a multilocular cyst on radiographs of the mandible or long bones. Occasionally the presenting sign is a pathological fracture at the site of such a tumour.

The most common biochemical features are a raised serum calcium level (over 11 mg. per 100 ml.) and lowered serum phosphate (below 3 mg. per 100 ml.). These values fluctuate and several estimations in the fasting patient at intervals may be required before the diagnosis is confirmed. The plasma alkaline phosphatase is frequently but not invariably raised. There is an increased urinary output of calcium (over 400 mg. per day on an ordinary diet). This observation should be followed by estimating the 24-hour calcium output on a low calcium diet (120 mg. per day); an output in excess of 180 mg. is abnormal. When the kidneys have been severely damaged by nephrocalcinosis a high serum phosphate level may simulate secondary hyperparathyroidism. In children, however, renal osteodystrophy includes the changes of rickets (Chapter XVII), which are not seen in primary hyperparathyroidism. Furthermore, hypocalcuria is the rule in renal failure, but hypercalcuria usually persists in primary hyperparathyroidism even when there is severe renal damage (Fourman, 1960).

Treatment

The parathyroid tumour or hyperplastic glands should be removed surgically. It is important to correct dehydration before operation by forcing fluids, if necessary by the intravenous route. Transient postoperative tetany is common and best treated with frequent intravenous doses of calcium gluconate. The results of operation are excellent provided the diagnosis has preceded irreversible damage to the kidneys.

THE ADRENAL GLANDS

The physiological chemistry of the adrenal cortex is exceedingly complicated. It follows that the disturbances which may arise in this system are also complicated, requiring highly sophisticated laboratory tests for their elucidation. Detailed descriptions have recently been provided by Visser (1966) and Cope (1966). The more important metabolic steps are shown in Fig. 64.

The function of the chromaffin cells of the adrenal medulla is to secrete the catecholamines dopamine, noradrenalin and adrenalin. Similar cells are present in the organ of Zuckerkandl and in other organs. They are the site of origin of phaeochromocytoma. There are also sympathetic ganglion cells in the adrenal medulla, and their precursors can be the site of origin of neuroblastoma. These cells can also produce dopamine and noradrenalin which may be found in excess in some cases of neuroblastoma (Chapter XI).

Congenital Virilizing Adrenal Hyperplasia

In this condition there is an over-production of adrenal androgens which results in virilization of the female (female pseudohermaphroditism) and in macrogenitosomia praecox in the male. The cause is a deficiency of one or other of the enzymes necessary for synthesis of the adrenocortical hormones. This defect is transmitted as an autosomal recessive trait, being manifest only in homozygotes. These conditions may be considered as inborn errors of metabolism (Chapter IX).

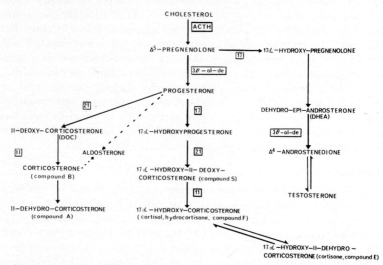

FIG. 64.—Pathways of steroid metabolism. 11 17 21 = hydroxylases. 3β—ol—de = 3β—ol— dehydrogenase.

Pathogenesis [See my notes from paper by Rati]

Deficiencies, variable in degree from case to case, of several adreno-cortical enzymes have now been defined (Wilkins, 1962). The most common involves 21-hydroxylase (Fig. 64). This results in a diminished production of cortisol and, by means of the familiar feed-back mechanism, in an increased output of pituitary corticotrophin (ACTH). The consequences are adrenocortical hyperplasia and increased production of 17α-hydroxyprogesterone. From this is manufactured an excess of 17-ketosteroids with androgenic properties which cause masculinization. The urine contains a marked excess of 17-ketosteroids and of pregnanetriol or pregnanetriolone which are derived from 17α-hydroxy-progesterone. If the deficiency of 21-hydroxylase is almost complete, acute adrenal insufficiency with excessive loss of salt in the urine will rapidly develop—"salt-losing syndrome". Less commonly there is a deficiency of 11-hydroxylase (Fig. 64). This results in the excessive production of compound S, of 17α-hydroxyprogesterone, and of 11-deoxy-corticosterone (DOC) which is a potent mineralocorticoid and cause of hypertension. In addition to an increased urinary excretion of

17-ketosteroids, large amounts of tetra-hydro-S (THS) derived from Compound S, and of pregnanetriol derived from 17α-hydroxyprogesterone are excreted. In a few of these patients the excess manufacture of etiocholanolone from 17α-hydroxyprogesterone causes periodic attacks of fever. The most recently defined enzyme defect involves 3β-ol-dehydrogenase (Fig. 64) (Bongiovanni, 1961; Hamilton and Brush, 1964). This results in deficient production of cortisol and other hormones with salt loss and functional adrenal failure. Pregnanetriol output in the urine is greatly decreased but there is an excessive excretion of 17-ketosteroids, Δ⁵-pregnenolone and dehydro-epiandrosterone. Affected females show virilization as in the other enzyme defects, but males show incomplete masculinization with bifid scrotum and undescended testes. This may be explained by the fact that 3β-ol-dehydrogenase is also necessary for the formation of Δ⁴-androstenedione (Fig. 64).

Clinical Features

Male infants with adrenal hyperplasia appear normal at birth with the exception of the rare cases due to 3β-ol-dehydrogenase deficiency (see above). After a short time virilization is revealed by enlargement of the penis, growth of pubic hair, excessive muscular development and advanced skeletal maturation (Fig. 65). These effects are due to the virilizing and protein-anabolic action of the excess androgens. The testes, however, remain small and atrophic. The increased stature ultimately gives way to dwarfism due to premature fusion of the epiphyses. In female infants the excessive androgenic effects upon the foetus produce more striking and unwelcome changes. In mild cases there is marked clitoral enlargement. At the other end of the scale there is a penile urethra and fused labia which simulate a scrotum so that the infant can readily be mistaken for a cryptorchid male (Chapter XVII). Pubic hair of male distribution may also appear soon after birth (Fig. 66). However, such female pseudohermaphrodites always possess a uterus, tubes, ovaries and a vagina which usually opens into the urethra. The buccal smear is, of course, chromatin positive (XX chromosomal constitution). The most common appearance is a large clitoris (phallus) with an opening in the perineum, the urogenital sinus, which is a common outlet for both urethra and vagina. Without treatment such a girl becomes progressively masculinized with excessive muscularity and advanced bone-age. In the past most of these girls were reared as "boys".

When a 21-hydroxylase defect is complete, an acute adrenal crisis occurs during the neonatal period with vomiting, diarrhoea, severe dehydration and oligaemic shock. The correct diagnosis is easy enough in the virilized female infant but in the male an erroneous diagnosis of pyloric stenosis, gastro-enteritis or septicaemia is easily made. *The clue to the correct diagnosis is the presence of abundant urinary chlorides in these "salt-losers", in contrast to the diminished urinary chlorides usually found in other types of dehydration.* The serum sodium and chloride levels are reduced, and the serum potassium level is high with corresponding E.C.G. changes. Salt-losing crises also occur in cases of 3β-ol-dehydrogenase deficiency. In 11-hydroxylase deficiency the

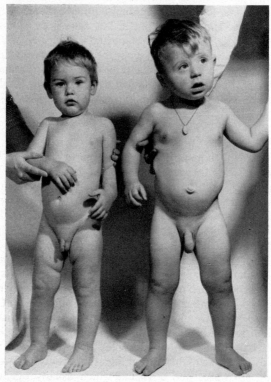

FIG. 65.—Macrogenitosomia praecox in boy aged $1\frac{3}{12}$ years due to congenital adrenal hyperplasia.

characteristic diagnostic feature is hypertension which disappears with treatment. In all types of adrenal hyperplasia excessive skin pigmentation is common.

Diagnosis

The most constant finding is a high urinary excretion of 17-ketosteroids (in relation to the patient's age), whereas the output of 17-hydroxycorticosteroids is not significantly abnormal. In cases of 21- and 11-hydroxylase deficiency the urinary pregnanetriol excretion is greatly raised, whereas the output of this metabolite is reduced in 3β-ol-dehydrogenase deficiency.

Differential Diagnosis

The severely virilized female can best be separated from the hypo-spadiac male by nuclear sexing methods. Macrogenitosomia praecox in boys with adrenal hyperplasia can be distinguished from true pubertas

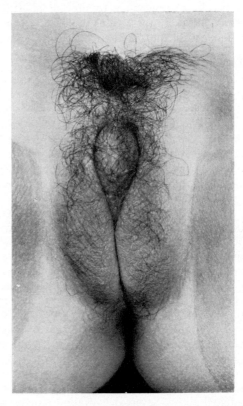

FIG. 66.—Masculinization of female genitalia due to congenital adrenal hyper-plasia.

praecox due to hypothalamic or "constitutional" causes by the fact that in the latter the testes show enlargement and biopsy will confirm spermatogenesis. The masculinizing ovarian arrhenoblastoma does not occur before puberty.

An important differentiation in the older child is between congenital adrenal hyperplasia and tumour, adenoma or carcinoma, of the adrenal cortex. Adrenal hyperplasia is pituitary-dependent which can be demonstrated by the dexamethasone suppression test (Liddle, 1960). Administration of this drug will markedly suppress the urinary output of 17-ketosteroids. Adrenal tumours remain unaffected in their hormonal activity by dexamethasone. Indeed, in these cases the output of 17-ketosteroids frequently reaches very high levels (above 30 mg./24 hr.). The tumour may be outlined by radiography and tomography after presacral insufflation of air or oxygen, or by intravenous pyelography.

The female foetus can be severely masculinized when various synthetic progestogens have been given to the pregnant woman in the first 12 weeks of pregnancy to prevent abortion (Suchowsky and Junkmann, 1961). In these cases the urinary output of 17-ketosteroids and pregnanetriol is not increased.

Treatment

This has been well described by Hubble (1960) and Wilkins (1962). Adrenocortical over-activity must be suppressed with cortisone or one of the newer synthetic steroids in physiological doses. Salt loss when present demands one of the salt-retaining steroids and an extra intake of salt. The treatment must be controlled by regular estimations of urinary steroid metabolites such as pregnanetriol, and by supervision of height increments and bone growth. In virilized girls the surgeon can often make future sexual life, and even pregnancy, possible by operation about the age of 4 years.

Initial rapid adrenocortical suppression should be obtained with intramuscular cortisone 25–100 mg./day according to the patient's age. This is followed by oral cortisone given in three or four daily doses in quantities sufficient to suppress the excessive output of 17-ketosteroids and pregnanetriol (15–75 mg. per day). Hamilton in the author's department obtains good results with prednisolone or prednisone (1 mg. = 4 mg. cortisone) while others have used dexamethasone (0·1 mg. = 5 mg. cortisone).

The "salt-loser" constitutes a grave neonatal emergency. Treatment can be difficult and it may be some weeks before the infant is out of danger. The first requirement is a mineralocorticoid such as deoxycorticosterone acetate, 1 mg. intramuscularly twice or thrice daily. This must be combined with intramuscular cortisone or hydrocortisone as advised above. Severe dehydration requires an intravenous infusion of 5 per cent dextrose in physiological saline (180 ml./Kg./day). Subsequently extra salt is given (2–5 gm./day) orally. In most cases it is necessary to give a salt-retaining preparation permanently. Suitable preparations are 9-alpha-fluorohydrocortisone 0·02–0·2 mg./day by mouth, or deoxycorticosterone trimethylacetate as a long-acting microcrystalline suspension 25 mg. intramuscularly every 4–6 weeks. A careful watch must be kept for oedema or hypertension.

With suppressive therapy children with adrenal hyperplasia usually do well. They should always carry a card stating the fact that they are on steroid therapy. Any infection, injury or surgical operation must be covered with intramuscular hydrocortisone hemisuccinate 100 mg. followed by reduced doses at six-hourly intervals for the next few days.

A difficult problem is posed by the girl who is so virilized that the surgeon cannot hope to reconstruct a vagina, and by the girl who has already been reared as a "boy" for more than three years. It is probably unwise to change the "boy's" sex in these circumstances and better to employ suppressive therapy combined with surgical removal of the uterus, tubes and ovaries. In most virilized females who have been treated with suppressive glucocorticoids from an early age it is both possible and important to correct the external genitalia, thus permitting a normal sexual life later on. Indeed, some such patients have now been successfully delivered of live babies in adult life. Most workers in this field agree that operation should be performed in the first 4 years of life, although not in early infancy. When only the clitoris is enlarged it often diminishes in size after some years of suppressive therapy. It may, however, require surgical treatment and an operation has been devised which preserves the glans which may be important for normal sexual experience in adult life.

CUSHING'S SYNDROME

This disease, in contrast to the adrenogenital syndrome, is very rare in childhood. A detailed discussion has been given by Wilkins (1962).

Aetiology

The clinical manifestations can be entirely attributed to hypersecretion of the adrenocortical hormones. In childhood the usual lesion is adrenal hyperplasia. Adenoma or carcinoma of the adrenal cortex is very rare. Only a few instances have been reported where the lesion was a pituitary basophil (or chromophobe) adenoma as originally described by Cushing. There is no known adrenocortical enzyme block, although cases showing features of both Cushing's and the adrenogenital syndrome have been described. The adrenal cortex in Cushing's syndrome is more sensitive than normal to ACTH stimulation. In cases due to adrenal hyperplasia there is an increased resistance to suppression of ACTH secretion by dexamethasone (Liddle, 1960); in cases due to tumour this resistance is complete.

Clinical Features

Those due to an increased production of glucocorticoids include buffalo-type obesity, moon-face, purple striae over abdomen, flanks and thighs, easy bruising, muscle wasting and weakness, osteoporosis, latent diabetes mellitus and polycythaemia (Fig. 67). Increased output of mineralocorticoids and aldosterone accounts for the hypertension and common hypokalaemic alkalosis. Excessive secretion of androgens may cause hirsutism, acne, baldness and clitorial enlargement. These patients are, in addition, highly susceptible to infection.

Diagnosis

The urinary output of 17-hydroxycorticosteroids is elevated, and there may be a raised output of 17-ketosteroids. The plasma 17-hydroxycorticoids are constantly high and they do not show the normal diurnal variation with a fall in the afternoon level. The dexamethasone suppression test (Liddle, 1960) is useful in differentiating adrenal hyperplasia from tumour. There may be a diabetic curve in the glucose tolerance test. Hypokalaemic alkalosis is not uncommon.

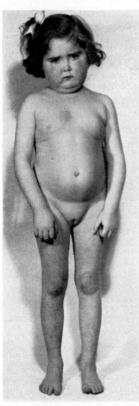

FIG. 67.—Cushing's syndrome in girl aged 3 years.

It should not be forgotten that all the features of Cushing's syndrome can be produced when ACTH or the corticosteroids are given in pharmacological doses in diseases such as nephrosis, rheumatoid arthritis and rheumatic fever.

Treatment

External irradiation of the pituitary gland can infrequently precipitate a remission. A tumour of the adrenal or pituitary should, of course, be excised when this is possible. In most cases of adrenal hyperplasia a satisfactory result can only be obtained by total bilateral adrenalectomy followed by replacement therapy (as in Addison's disease). Unfortunately, it appears that this treatment may be followed by the subsequent appearance of pituitary tumours and severe hyperpigmentation (Nelson et al., 1960). The prognosis of Cushing's syndrome is, therefore, an unhappy one.

ADDISON'S DISEASE

This is an exceedingly rare disease in paediatric practice but some cases are probably missed. Correct diagnosis is important because effective treatment is now available.

Aetiology

In most cases there is adrenocortical atrophy. It has recently been demonstrated that such patients show a high incidence of specific-type antibodies to adrenal, thyroid and stomach tissues and that there is an unduly high incidence among relatives of thyroid disorders and pernicious anaemia (Irvine, 1963). This condition may, therefore, be an "auto-immunity". Addison's disease is rarely due to tuberculosis of the adrenal glands in the United Kingdom nowadays. There is a familial form of acute adrenocortical failure which presents in the neo-natal period (Mitchell and Rhaney, 1959; Boyd and MacDonald, 1960). In these infants the adrenal glands are very small but they can be shown by histochemical studies to be very active. The term "hypoplasia" would be better replaced by "dysadrenocorticism". Familial types of Addison's disease have also been described in association with hypo-parathyroidism and moniliasis (Di George and Paschkis, 1957), and with spastic paraplegia (Harris-Jones and Nixon, 1955). The term "Addison's disease" does not include adrenal haemorrhage due to asphyxia neona-torum (Chapter III) or to meningococcal septicaemia (Chapter XX).

Clinical Features

In the older child the manifestations closely resemble those seen in the adult—extreme asthenia, cachexia, hypotension and microcardia. Pigmentation of skin and mucous membranes tends to be less marked in children. Dangerous adrenal crises may occur, often precipitated by infections. Hypoglycaemic convulsions are rare.

In the familial form of the disease acute adrenal failure develops with alarming rapidity during the neonatal period. Vomiting, diarrhoea and extreme dehydration can lead easily to an erroneous diagnosis such as pyloric stenosis, high intestinal obstruction or gastro-enteritis. *The pointer to adrenal insufficiency is the presence of abundant chlorides in the urine.*

Diagnosis

During a crisis characteristic blood chemical changes are found. These include low serum chloride and sodium, elevated serum potassium (with changes in the E.C.G.), and hypoglycaemia. The serum sodium/potassium ratio which is normally 30/1 falls below 20/1. In the absence of a crisis the blood chemistry may not be grossly abnormal and more refined tests are necessary. The simplest of these rests upon the inability of the kidneys in this disease to respond to a water-load with a normal diuresis. After an overnight fast the child is given water in a dose of 20 ml./Kg. to be drunk within 45 minutes. The urine is collected for the next five hours. If less than 80 per cent of the water-load is excreted there is impaired diuresis. The test can be repeated on the following day, the child having been given 100 mg. cortisone by mouth four hours before the start of the test. In Addison's disease a normal diuresis will then occur. Two more complicated tests may be employed;

Eight-hour I-V ACTH test.—A 24-hour urine collection is made. At its completion a second 24-hour collection is started and during the first eight hours of this collecting period 25 mg. ACTH in 500 ml. physiological saline is given by intravenous infusion. An eosinophil count is made just before and at the completion of the infusion. A drop in eosinophils of less than 50 per cent indicates adrenal insufficiency. So also does a rise in the 24-hour output of 17-hydroxycorticosteroids of less than 100 per cent.

I-V ACTH plasma corticoid test.—The plasma level of 17-hydroxycorticoids is estimated before and two hours after 10 mg. ACTH intravenously. A rise of less than 100 per cent signifies adrenocortical failure.

Treatment

The adrenal crisis should be treated along the lines described for "salt losers" in the adrenogenital syndrome. This includes intravenous 5 per cent dextrose in physiological saline; hydrocortisone hemisuccinate 100 mg. intramuscularly or intravenously followed by 50 mg. six-hourly; and deoxycorticosterone acetate 1 mg. intramuscularly twice or thrice daily.

Maintenance treatment must take into account the severity of the condition and the patient's age. It must aim at adequate growth, well-being and energy, a normal heart size, normal E.C.G., normal blood chemistry and blood pressure. Oral cortisone is given thrice daily in individual doses of 5–10 mg. Extra salt (2–5 gm./day) is included in the diet. In severe cases it is desirable to give a mineralocorticoid such as 9-alpha-fluorohydrocortisone 0·05–0·2 mg./day by mouth, or deoxycorticosterone trimethylacetate 25 mg. intramuscularly every four weeks.

The prognosis in older children should be good, although they are susceptible to periodic adrenal crises when they acquire intercurrent infections. Adrenal failure in the neonatal period, however, can prove a most difficult problem and death may occur in spite of the most energetic measures.

HYPERALDOSTERONISM (CONN'S SYNDROME)

This is an exceedingly rare condition. One type due to congenital adrenal hyperplasia, occurs mainly in boys. The other, due to adenoma, is a disease of adult females (Conn, 1955). The principal features are hypertension, oedema, polyuria, hypokalaemia, periodic paralysis, or tetany with positive Chvostek sign. The serum potassium may be below 3 mEq/l., and the plasma volume is increased by 30 per cent or more above the predicted normal. The serum potassium level can be raised to normal on spironolactone (Aldactone A) 50–75 mg. four times daily. The treatment of the congenital type is complete bilateral adrenalectomy followed by substitution therapy.

PHAEOCHROMOCYTOMA

This is very rare in childhood. The tumour may arise in the adrenal medulla (phaeochromocytoma) or from chromaffin cells elsewhere such as the organ of Zuckerkandl (paraganglioma). In children both adrenals may be simultaneously affected. In some cases the tumour is locally malignant.

Clinical Features

In some cases hypertension occurs in paroxysms which coincide with the liberation of the catecholamines by the tumour. These cause headaches, palpitations and epigastric pain. Sweating may be profuse and the child becomes prostrated. Frequently he has a characteristically "startled" expression with wide palpebral fissures and dilated pupils. More often, however, the hypertension becomes chronic and produces retinal changes (papilloedema and exudates), cardiomegaly and proteinuria. There may be hyperglycaemia and glycosuria. The intravenous pyelogram is usually normal unless the tumour itself is obstructing the ureter.

Diagnosis

A useful screening test involves the use of phentolamine (Rogitine). With the patient lying down an intravenous infusion of 5 per cent dextrose in water is set up. The blood pressure is recorded every minute until it is stable. Phentolamine 5 mg. is then injected into the tubing of the "giving set". A fall in blood pressure of over 35 mm. Hg systolic and 25 mm. Hg diastolic strongly supports the diagnosis. In every case it is essential to prove the diagnosis by demonstrating an excessive urinary excretion of catecholamines (over 200 mg./24 hr.) or of their breakdown product V.M.A. (3-methoxy-4-hydroxy-mandelic acid) (over 5 mg./24 hr.). The site of the tumour can often be defined by intravenous pyelography or presacral insufflation with oxygen.

Treatment

The tumour should be removed surgically whenever this is practicable. Chronic hypertension can be controlled while operation is being arranged, with phenoxybenzamine (Dibenyline) 10 mg. twice or thrice daily; it must be withdrawn 48 hours before operation. During the operation hypertension must be carefully controlled with intravenous phentolamine. After the tumour has been removed there is a danger of profound hypotension. This must be prevented by the continuous infusion of noradrenalin (Levophed), 8 mg. in 1,000 ml. 5 per cent dextrose in water, for 4–36 hours until the blood pressure remains spontaneously at a safe level. In bilateral adrenal tumours total adrenalectomy should be followed by substitution therapy.

THE GONADS

Disturbances of function of the sex glands are rarely evident before puberty. The paediatrician must, however, be familiar with these problems as his patients will reach adult life in good health only if he correctly diagnoses and treats the ailments of childhood. The most common problem in this field is the undescended testis (cryptorchidism), although this does not inevitably lead to hypogonadism. The problem has been a somewhat confused one, largely due to diagnostic misconceptions. It is considered separately on page 370 under the title "Absence of the Testes from the Scrotum".

HYPOGONADISM

Failure of the testicular function leads to the state of eunuchoidism. This may be due to such causes as testicular agenesis, mumps orchitis, bilateral cryptorchidism, prolonged malnutrition and castration. A specific variety of male hypogonadism is found in Klinefelter's syndrome in which the buccal smear is chromatin positive (as in the normal female). Chromosome analysis reveals a sex chromosome configuration such as XXY or XXXY. In some cases there has been mosaicism, e.g. XXY/XY. In the female, primary hypogonadism is much less common. The classical example is Turner's syndrome (gonadal dysgenesis) in which the buccal smear is chromatin negative and there is only one female sex chromosome (XO). Female hypogonadism will, of course, result from bilateral oophorectomy. Secondary hypogonadism can result in both sexes from failure in the production of pituitary gonadotrophins.

Clinical Features

With the exception of cryptorchidism the features of hypogonadism in the male only become manifest after the time of normal puberty. Growth continues for an abnormally long period because of delay in fusion of the epiphyses. Fat distribution is excessive and in the usual female sites, hips, thighs, breasts. The voice is high-pitched and "infantile". The penis is small and sexual hair is scanty. Gynaecomastia is especially common in *Klinefelter's syndrome* in which, also, the testes are small and devoid of normal sensation. The degree of eunuchoidism varies in cases of Klinefelter's syndrome according to the amount of androgen production but testicular biopsy always shows hyalinization in the cells of the seminiferous tubules and adenomatous clumping of the Leydig cells. Many of these people are mentally subnormal (Chapter XXII).

In *Turner's syndrome* the characteristic features are obvious from an early age. These include dwarfism, advanced epiphyseal fusion, webbing of the neck, excessive cubitus valgus, osteoporosis and other congenital abnormalities such as coarctation of the aorta, defects in the eyes, ears and bones, and mental subnormality. In some cases congenital lymph-oedema of the extremities is associated with severe cardiac or renal anomalies (Bonnevie-Ullrich syndrome). Menstruation does not occur and the uterus remains small and infantile. There is an excessive urinary output of gonadotrophins after the age at which puberty should have occurred.

One form of pituitary hypogonadism is *Fröhlich's syndrome* which can be caused by a tumour such as craniopharyngioma, encephalitis or trauma. This is, in fact, an excessively rare condition. The principal features are gross obesity combined with sexual infantilism. Ossification is delayed. It must not be confused with simple obesity (Chapter XII) which is very common. A variant of Fröhlich's syndrome, transmitted as an autosomal recessive trait, is the Laurence-Moon-Biedl syndrome which is characterized by obesity, genital hypoplasia, polydactyly or syndactyly, retinitis pigmentosa and severe mental retardation.

Another form of pituitary hypogonadism has been called "idiopathic eunuchoidism with low FSH." These patients present the classical picture of eunuchoidism and they may have cryptorchidism. However, unlike cases of primary hypogonadism they do not show an excessive urinary output of gonadotrophins.

Treatment

Primary hypogonadism in the male is treated with intramuscular testosterone or oral methyltestosterone. The diagnosis must first be proved by testicular biopsy and assay of urinary gonadotrophins, because these drugs can damage the healthy testis. Turner's syndrome is treated with oestrogens, possibly also progestogens, given cyclically. It is not, of course, possible to make these patients fertile. In cases with low urinary FSH the testes can be stimulated with chorionic gonado-trophin.

HYPERGONADISM

Aetiology

A very rare cause of pubertas praecox in boys is the interstitial (Leydig) cell tumour of the testis; it may be highly malignant. Germinal cell tumours such as seminoma or teratoma do not produce androgens. In girls isosexual precocity may be due to granulosa cell tumour of the ovary; it is usually benign.

Clinical Features

In both sexes the result of hyperactivity of the gonads is isosexual pubertas praecox. In boys the penis and testes enlarge and sexual hair appears at an unduly early age. In girls the genitalia enlarge, menstruation and ovulation occur and sexual hair develops. Bone-age is advanced. In boys there is an excess output of urinary 17-ketosteroids. In girls oestrogens reach and may surpass adult female levels.

Differential Diagnosis

Sexual precocity may have various causes such as hypothalamic lesions in both sexes, and adrenogenital syndrome in boys, although in the latter spermatogenesis does not take place and the testes remain small. It is important to appreciate, however, that the most common type of premature puberty is "constitutional", 90 per cent in girls, 50 per cent in boys. Here there is no discoverable lesion and future adult development is normal. Interstitial cell tumours of the testis and granulosa cell tumours of the ovary are invariably palpable.

ABSENCE OF THE TESTES FROM THE SCROTUM
("UNDESCENDED TESTES")

The terms used to describe the position of the testis in relation to the scrotum have been varied and confusing, e.g. undescended, imperfect descent, maldescent and so on. In this account only three major situations are recognized.

(i) The testis may be retractible. This is the situation in which the testis, which is normally in the scrotum, has been pulled out of it and upwards into the superficial inguinal pouch by the cremasteric reflex. This is *not* an undescended testis; but in at least 70 to 80 per cent of cases in which the testis is found to be absent from the scrotum it is, in fact, temporarily retractible. In such cases the testis can be coaxed back into the scrotum under suitable conditions as described below. This phenomenon is not seen after puberty.

(ii) The testis is undescended and lies either within the abdomen or in the inguinal canal. Scorer (1964) has produced good evidence that descent of the testis is usually complete before birth but may be delayed for about three months, especially in premature infants, and that, contrary to popular belief, does not take place spontaneously at any later age before or at puberty. Unilateral failure of descent is four times more common than bilateral.

(iii) The testis is ectopic. This means that it lies away from its line of natural descent and occupies a completely abnormal position in the perineum, femoral region or in front of the symphysis pubis. This is, in fact, an extremely rare anomaly.

Various figures have been quoted for the incidence of undescended testis. In some series the phenomenon of the retractile testis has resulted in a fallaciously high figure. From his observations in young infants Scorer (1964) found that in 2·7 per cent one or both testes had failed to reach the scrotum at birth. When the next three months had passed this incidence had fallen to the low figure of 0·8 per cent. Baumrucker (1946) found an identical incidence in a series of 10,000 recruits to the U.S. Army.

Clinical Features

The boy should always be examined in a warm room, in both the supine and standing positions, and the examiner's hands must be warm and gentle. The retractile testis can be found in the superficial inguinal pouch if the examiner's fingers are run downwards along the line of the inguinal canal. If the testis can then be manipulated into the scrotum it is not undescended to any degree requiring treatment. In true failure of descent the scrotum on the affected side is almost invariably smaller than on the other, and this is a useful diagnostic pointer. It is also important to palpate over the common sites for the ectopic testis— perineum, above the symphysis pubis, in the femoral area. Bilateral cryptorchidism should lead to a consideration of possible endocrine or chromosomal abnormalities such as Klinefelter's syndrome, hypopituitarism, and eunuchoidism with low gonadotrophin output. A buccal smear is indicated to confirm male sexing, and to exclude virilization of a female as the result of congenital adrenal hyperplasia (p. 357).

As the processus vaginalis only closes completely when the testis has reached its point of full descent it is common for failure of descent to be associated with an inguinal hernia. Occasionally after the surgeon has corrected a hernia the testis on that side is found to be situated somewhat higher than normal, and it may be smaller than the one on the other side. Scorer (1964) regards this as an example of incomplete descent although, in fact, the testis is in the scrotum. It is not, however, of great clinical significance.

Treatment

There will continue to be room for controversy until more is known of the natural history of the undescended testis; prospective studies from birth to adult life and fatherhood are lacking. The myth of spontaneous descent at or before puberty has been exposed. This arose because the retractile testis was wrongly regarded as undescended, and the pull of the cremasteric muscle disappears after puberty. It is almost certain that hormone treatment with gonadotrophins cannot cause the descent of the testis and large doses may damage the testis. This form of treatment should, therefore, be abandoned.

The problem of bilateral cryptorchidism is fairly clear. The untreated adult is almost invariably sterile and orchidopexy is obviously required, although spermatogenesis is likely to be acquired by only a few patients. The best age for operation is still undecided but many surgeons advise that it be performed before 9 years.

The unilateral undescended testis can be dealt with in a variety of ways. This type of patient with one scrotal testis is, of course, normally fertile so that orchidopexy on the affected side is justifiable more on cosmetic or psychological grounds than on the hope of achieving spermatogenesis. If the undescended testis is associated with an inguinal hernia it may be brought into the scrotum during operation for the hernia. Other surgeons, impressed by the increased incidence of neoplasia in the undescended testis, have advised that the unilateral case should be dealt with by abdominal orchidectomy.

THE PANCREAS

The only important endocrine disorders involving the pancreas in paediatric practice are found in diabetes mellitus (of two types), and in the babies of diabetic mothers.

Diabetes Mellitus

Aetiology

The precise cause of the common type of diabetes mellitus with ketosis is unknown, in spite of recent work on plasma insulin-like activity and insulin antagonists (Vallance-Owen and Lilley, 1961; Hales and Randle, 1963; Samaan and Fraser, 1963). In childhood the disease is invariably insulin-sensitive, but whether it is due primarily to diminished insulin production by the β-cells of the islets of Langerhans or to a raised level of insulin antagonists is uncertain. Diabetes can occur in acromegaly (increased production of growth hormone), in Cushing's syndrome (increased production of ACTH), and in thyrotoxicosis (production of LATS), but these types are of little relevance to the ordinary cases of the disease. Heredity is an important factor because a family history of the disease is obtainable in about 50 per cent of cases of juvenile diabetes. It has been suggested that transmission is as an autosomal recessive trait in which case, when both parents are diabetic, all their children should ultimately develop the disease. Others have suggested that the predisposition to diabetes mellitus is associated with an excess of albumin-bound insulin antagonist in the plasma, and that this characteristic is inherited as an autosomal dominant. All that can be stated with assurance is that inheritance is an important aetiological factor and there may, in fact, be different patterns in different families. The incidence of diabetes before puberty is about 1 in 2,000. The close relationship with obesity, which is well recognized in adults, does not apply during childhood.

Pathology

There has been great variation in the reported findings. Reduction in the islets or in the numbers of β-cells has been the most usual abnormality. Deficiency of insulin results in many metabolic upsets. The conversion of glucose to glycogen is diminished, hence the hyperglycaemia and glycosuria. The muscles are unable to utilize glucose as a source of energy. The glucose is excreted in the urine with water and sodium, hence the thirst and polyuria. Protein synthesis is impaired resulting in loss of weight, muscle weakness and slowing of growth. An important effect is a decrease in lipogenesis from carbohydrate and an increased breakdown of fat from which energy is derived. When the production of ketone bodies exceeds their utilization they accumulate in the blood and spill over into the urine; this leads to the state of ketoacidosis which results in coma.

Clinical Features

Diabetes mellitus is a much more acute disease in the child than in the adult. The onset is marked by excessive thirst, polyuria and rapid loss of weight. In the untreated case the urine is loaded with sugar and acetone. When the presence of diacetic acid is revealed by the ferric chloride test the child is in the stage of pre-coma. The plasma CO_2 will be reduced due to metabolic acidosis. At this stage there will develop anorexia, abdominal pain and frequent vomiting. Finally, in a state of profound dehydration with hypotension, sunken eyes, dry tongue, and scaphoid abdomen, the child lapses into the coma which precedes death. Respiration is rapid, sighing and pauseless. The blood pH is reduced. The serum sodium and chloride levels are also reduced. Haemoconcentration masks the severe losses of intracellular potassium in diabetic coma, but after the dehydration has been corrected there is marked hypokalaemia and the E.C.G. shows characteristic abnormalities.

Diagnosis

This is not difficult in the child because by the time medical advice is sought there is marked glycosuria and ketonuria. The blood sugar level is rarely below 200 mg. per 100 ml. and frequently much higher. A fasting blood sugar level over 120 mg. per 100 ml. is diagnostic of diabetes mellitus. It is rarely necessary to carry out a glucose tolerance test (after 1·5 gm. glucose per Kg. body weight); a blood sugar level of 130 mg. per 100 ml. two hours after the ingestion of glucose is diagnostic.

Differential Diagnosis

The author has seen a child in diabetic coma who had been treated for "enuresis" during the preceding six weeks. This can only happen when a physician commits the unforgivable sin of diagnosing "enuresis" without having tested the urine. Diabetes insipidus is extremely rare. The urine will not show the presence of glucose or acetone. Renal glycosuria is not associated with symptoms and the diagnosis is readily confirmed by a glucose tolerance test.

Course and Prognosis

Without treatment death in coma is inevitable within a few months or less. On the other hand, with adequate treatment and supervision the diabetic child is able to live a normal life, to attend an ordinary school, and to engage in all normal physical pursuits. The long-term prognosis must be guarded because at least 50 per cent of all diabetic children will develop serious complications in early middle age. These include diabetic retinopathy, cataract, renal glomerulosclerosis, coronary artery disease, peripheral vascular disease and various types of neuropathy. It seems that the risks of these complications are *not* related to the degree of control which is exercised over the blood sugar levels. None the less, poor control means repeated episodes of hyperglycaemic or hypoglycaemic coma, with risk of death or brain damage. The diabetic child with irresponsible or mentally impoverished parents is in a most unenviable position. He is not suitably placed in a residential school for physically handicapped children and there is a lack of schools suitable for this type of "socio-medical" case (Farquhar, 1962).

Treatment

Initially the diabetic child should be admitted to hospital for stabilization. Indeed, by the time of diagnosis he is only too often in a state of ketoacidosis requiring emergency treatment. When dehydration is severe there is also repeated vomiting. In these circumstances physiological saline should be given in large amounts by continuous intravenous infusion. After taking blood for sugar estimation, soluble insulin is urgently required and it needs to be repeated every 2 to 4 hours. The initial dose, depending upon the blood sugar level, varies between 40 and 80 units; about two-thirds should be given intramuscularly and one-third intravenously. The daily dosage during the state of ketoacidosis varies between 100 and 500 units. When the blood sugar level has fallen below 300 mg. per 100 ml. 5 per cent dextrose is added to the infusion fluid. Oral feeds are started when the plasma CO_2 has been restored to normal, when ketonuria has become slight or absent, and when vomiting has ceased. A careful watch should be kept on the serum potassium level, and E.C.G. monitoring is also advisable. Hypokalaemia is almost invariable after the dehydration has gone; it should be corrected with oral potassium chloride 1 gm. four times daily.

The diet of the diabetic child should give 40 per cent of the calories as carbohydrate, 20 per cent as protein and 40 per cent as fat. A convenient method is to use the Lawrence Line Diet (Lawrence, 1964) in which each Black line contains 10 gm. carbohydrate, and each Red line 7·5 gm. protein and 9 gm. fat. It is usual to give about twice as many Black as Red lines. The daily caloric requirement varies from 50 calories per lb. (110 per Kg.) at one year to 20 calories per lb. (45 per Kg.) at 14 years. Many physicians today prefer the "free" diet, in which the child is allowed the ordinary diet customary for his age and social environment. It is wise, however, to forbid certain articles such as sweets, chocolates, cakes and sweetened drinks. "Diabetic" sweets and chocolates may be used. The advantages of the free diet are ease of management, especially at school, and the lessened risks of hypoglycaemic attacks. It does result in somewhat higher blood sugar levels, frequently about 250 mg. per 100 ml. at some part of the day, but it is doubtful if this carries any real disadvantages.

While soluble insulin must always be used for the treatment of the child with ketoacidosis, it is an advantage to use a single daily injection of one of the long-acting insulins for permanent treatment. We have found the Lente insulins to be very satisfactory in most diabetic children. The most useful is Novo Lente (insulin zinc suspension), although in some children better control can be achieved with Semi Lente (amorphous insulin zinc suspension). Ultra Lente (crystalline insulin zinc suspension) is too long-acting. We have only rarely used protamine zinc insulin, alone or mixed with soluble insulin, in recent years. A few unstable or "brittle" diabetic children can only be safely controlled on soluble insulin given twice daily. For the insulin dosage customarily needed by children (10–60 units per day) the "double" strength insulin (40 units per ml.) is most convenient. Insulin should be injected subcutaneously into the thighs and upper arms in rotation.

Older children should be taught how to measure and administer their own insulin, and to test their own urine. The parents must also know this in addition to receiving instruction on the dietary regime prescribed for their child. This instruction must be thorough and complete before the child leaves hospital. The diabetic child must be allowed to live an entirely normal life of mental and physical activity. He is best supervised at a "diabetic clinic" where his parents learn from other parents and where he himself meets other diabetic children and hears of their accomplishments. The parents must be told that any intercurrent infection is an indication for an increase (never a decrease) in insulin dosage. The daily intake of carbohydrate can usually be maintained in the form of milk and glucose. Thus 7 fl. oz. (210 ml.) of milk plus 10 gm. glucose approximate to 2 Black and 1 Red Lawrence Line.

TEMPORARY NEONATAL DIABETES MELLITUS

This is a rare but easily missed condition which is present at birth or develops shortly thereafter (Hutchison *et al.*, 1962). The affected infants have almost invariably been of low birth weight in relation to the length of gestation, and have frequently shown the appearances commonly associated with dysmaturity or placental insufficiency, such as a long thin body and limbs, dry wrinkled and desquamating skin and meconium-stained nails. The onset of the diabetic state is sudden with rapid loss of weight (in spite of an adequate caloric intake) and severe dehydration (in spite of an adequate fluid intake). Thirst and polyuria are present but easily overlooked in the infant. These babies have a peculiar waxen pallor and liveliness of consciousness which are unusual in other states of severe dehydration (Fig. 68). The urine is loaded with sugar and there is severe hyperglycaemia. On the other hand, ketonuria and acidosis have been conspicuously absent in all the reported cases. *Diagnosis must depend on vigilance, which should ensure that the urine or blood is tested for sugar content in every newborn infant whose birth weight is disproportionately low in relation to the estimated maturity.*

The cause of this temporary diabetic state is not known. Repeated measurements of the plasma insulin by the immuno-assay technique in the author's department (Dr. I. C. Ferguson) have shown the levels to be at the higher level of the normal range.

Treatment and Prognosis

This type of diabetes is extremely responsive to insulin which should be given in soluble form, 2–4 units intramuscularly, before every feed. An intravenous infusion of half-strength physiological saline may be required when diagnosis has been delayed and dehydration is severe. After the acute stage has passed it may be possible to control the diabetic state with one daily subcutaneous injection of insulin zinc suspension. This type of neonatal diabetes mellitus is clearly a different condition from the common insulin-sensitive type of juvenile diabetes, because spontaneous recovery invariably takes place in a period of weeks or months. Several of the survivors, however, have suffered from some type of brain damage. This may have been due, at least in part, to hypoglycaemic episodes which should be avoided by careful attention to blood sugar levels and insulin dosage.

INFANTS OF DIABETIC MOTHERS

It has long been known that a high perinatal mortality is found in the offspring of diabetic mothers (but not of diabetic fathers). These babies have such a characteristic appearance that they might well be related (Gellis and Hsia, 1959). Indeed, the appearance of such an infant has frequently led to the diagnosis (later confirmed) of a pre-diabetic state in the mother. The infants of diabetic mothers have an unduly high weight and length for their gestational age (Farquhar, 1959). They are obese, covered with vernix caseosa, round-faced and plethoric. They lie on their backs with legs abducted and flexed and with their hands alongside their heads, a posture commonly adopted by the premature infant. They frequently tremble on being stimulated by noise. They show an undue susceptibility to develop the respiratory distress syndrome (Chapter II), also to have cyanotic attacks. They are frequently premature by dates, often because birth is by Caesarean section because of the known tendency toward intra-uterine death after the thirty-sixth week. Hypoglycaemia is

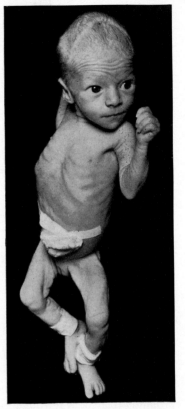

FIG. 68.—Neonatal diabetes mellitus. Observe lively expression in spite of dehydration with visible over-riding of sutures and marked wasting.

more consistently found 2–3 hours after birth than in normal infants, but it is corrected spontaneously in 4–6 hours. The most constant necropsy finding is hypertrophy of the islets of Langerhans, mainly due to hyperplasia of the β-cells. These facts correlate with the tendency to early postnatal hypoglycaemia. Baird and Farquhar (1962) have shown that diabetic mothers' babies have an abnormally high plasma insulin-like activity after a glucose load, and it seems likely that their characteristic obesity is due to their own excess production of endogenous insulin, stimulated by the maternal hyperglycaemia (Osler, 1960).

Treatment

These infants should be treated precisely as if they were small feeble prematures (Chapter II). The hypoglycaemia is transient and does not require correction. The respiratory distress syndrome may demand biochemical control of the treatment (Chapter II).

HYPOGLYCAEMIA

There is no critical level of blood glucose below which symptoms will occur. The normal blood glucose level varies between 80–120 mg. per 100 ml. Children can tolerate levels of 50 mg. per 100 ml. without symptoms, and newborn infants even lower levels. Hypoglycaemia may arise from an excessive amount of insulin in the circulation. This may result from an overdose of insulin in the diabetic child, in the infant of the diabetic mother (see above), and in an insulin-secreting adenoma of the pancreas which is exceedingly rare in childhood. Hypoglycaemia is also a feature of a variety of metabolic disorders, such as coeliac disease, galactosaemia, von Gierke's disease, hepatic disorders and adrenocortical failure where it only rarely causes characteristic clinical manifestations. Hypoglycaemia is a common occurrence in newborn babies. Predisposing factors seem to be placental insufficiency and pre-eclamptic toxaemia. This condition has received considerable attention in the past few years and is fully considered in Chapter II.

Clinical Features

In children the early symptoms are sweating, pallor, irritability or disobedience, and tachycardia. Later there are more severe neurological manifestations such as tremors, paralysis, convulsions and coma.

Treatment

Insulin-induced hypoglycaemic attacks in diabetic children should be promptly treated. A few lumps of sugar are sufficient to correct a mild attack. In severe episodes 10–20 ml. of 50 per cent glucose should be given intravenously and also 0·5 ml. of 1/1,000 solution of adrenalin hydrochloride subcutaneously.

REFERENCES

GENERAL

WILKINS, L. (1965). *The Diagnosis and Treatment of Endocrine Disorders in Childhood and Adolescence*, 3rd edit. Springfield, Ill.: Chas. C. Thomas.
WILLIAMS, R. H. (1962). *Textbook of Endocrinology*, 3rd edit. Philadelphia: W. B. Saunders Co.

PITUITARY

ÅARSKOG, D. (1963). *Amer. J. Dis. Child.*, **105**, 368.
BLACK, J. A. (1961). *Arch. Dis. Childh.*, **36**, 633.
HUBBLE, D. (1966). *Arch. Dis. Childh.*, **41**, 17.
HUNTER, W. M., and GREENWOOD, F. C. (1964). *Brit. med. J.*, **1**, 804.
MARTIN, M. M., and WILKINS, L. (1958). *J. clin. Endocr.*, **18**, 679.
RABEN, M. S. (1962). *New Engl. J. Med.*, **266**, 82.
ZISKIND, A. (1962). *Pediat. Clin. N. Amer.*, **9**, 395.

THYROID

Hypothyroidism

AINGER, L. E., and KELLY, V. C. (1955). *J. clin. Endocr.*, **15**, 469.
ÅKERRÉN, Y. (1954). *Acta. paediat. (Uppsala)*, **43**, 411.
BLIZZARD, R. M., CHANDLER, R. W., LANDING, B. H., SUTHERLAND, J. M., ESSEL-BORN, V. M., PETTIT, M., and GUEST, G. M. (1959). *Amer. J. Dis. Child.*, **98**, 565.
COSTA, A., COTTINO, F., FERRARIS, G. M., MARCHIS, E., MAROCCO, F., MORTARE, M., and PIETRA, R. (1953). *Medicina (Parma)*, **3**, 445.
DONIACH, D., NILSSON, L. R., and ROITT, I. M. (1965). *Acta paediat. (Uppsala)*, **54**, 260.
FRASER, G. R., MORGANS, M. E., and TROTTER, W. R. (1960). *Quart. J. Med.*, **29**, 279.
GREIG, W. R., HENDERSON, A. S., BOYLE, J. A., McGIRR, E. M., and HUTCHISON, J. H. (1966). *J. clin. Endocr.*, **26**, 1309.
HAGEMAN, D. D., and VILLEE, C. A. (1960). *Physiol. Rev.*, **40**, 313.
HUTCHISON, J. H. (1958). *Recent Advances in Paediatrics*, 2nd edit., Chap. 6. Edited by D. Gairdner. London: J. & A. Churchill.
HUTCHISON, J. H. (1963). In *The Thyroid and its Diseases*, p. 39, edited by A. S. Mason (Proc. Conf. R.C.P. Lond.). London: Pitman Medical.
HUTCHISON, J. H., and McGIRR, E. M. (1958). *Lancet*, **1**, 1035.
HUTCHISON, J. H., ARNEIL, G. C., and McGIRR, E. M. (1957). *Lancet*, **2**, 314.
JOSEPH, R., TUBIANA, M., and JOB, J. C. (1958). *Rev. franc. Étud. clin. biol.*, **3**, 167.
McGIRR, E. M. (1960). *Brit. med. Bull.*, **16**, 113.
McGIRR, E. M. (1963). In *The Thyroid and its Diseases*, p. 52, edited by A. S. Mason (Proc. Conf. R.C.P. Lond.). London: Pitman Medical.
McGIRR, E. M., HUTCHISON, J. H., CLEMENT, W. E., KENNEDY, J. S., and CURRIE, A. R. (1960). *Scot. med. J.*, **5**, 189.
MACKAY, R. H. (1961). In *Skeletal Maturation Chart*. Rochester, N.Y.: Kodak Medical Publications.
MASON, A. S., Ed. (1963). *The Thyroid and its Diseases* (Proc. Conf. R.C.P. Lond.). London: Pitman Medical.
MORGANS, M. E., and TROTTER, W. R. (1959). *Lancet*, **2**, 374.
MURRAY, I. P. C., McGIRR, E. M., THOMSON, J. A., and HUTCHISON, J. H. (1965). *Current Topics in Thyroid Research*, p. 813. New York: Academic Press.
NILSSON, L. R., and DONIACH, D. (1964). *Acta paediat. (Uppsala)*, **53**, 255.
PETTY, C. S., and DI BENEDETTO, R. L. (1957). *New Engl. J. Med.*, **256**, 1103.
PITT-RIVERS, R., and TATA, J. R. (1959). *The Thyroid Hormones*. Oxford: Pergamon Press.
PITT-RIVERS, R., and TROTTER, W. R. (1964). *The Thyroid Gland*, Vols. I and II. London: Butterworth & Co.
SHEPARD, T. H., PYNE, G. E., KIRSCHRINK, J. F., McLEAN, M. (1960). *New Engl. J. Med.*, **262**, 1099.
SMITH, D. W., BLIZZARD, R. M., and WILKINS, L. (1957). *Pediatrics*, **19**, 1011.
STANBURY, J. B., and CHAPMAN, E. M. (1960). *Lancet*, **1**, 1162.
TANNER, J. M., and WHITEHOUSE, R. H. (1959). *Lancet*, **2**, 1086.
VAN WYK, J. J. (1956). *Pediatrics*, **17**, 427.
WILKINS, L. (1941). *Amer. J. Dis. Child.*, **61**, 13.
WINSHIP, T., and ROSVOLL, R. V. (1961). *Cancer (Philad.)*, **14**, 734.
ZONDEK, H., KAATZ, A., LESZYNSKY, H. E., MARGOLIASH, E., and STEIN, J. A. (1958). *Brit. med. J.*, **1**, 546.

Hyperthyroidism

ADAMS, D. D. (1965). *Brit. med. J.*, **1**, 1015.
BONGIOVANNI, A. M., EBERLEIN, W. R., THOMAS, P. Z., and ANDERSON, W. B. (1956). *J. clin. Endocr.*, **16**, 146.

CARNEIRO, L., DORRINGTON, K. J., and MUNRO, D. S. (1966). *Lancet*, **2**, 878.
LEWIS, I. C., and MACGREGOR, A. G. (1957). *Lancet*, **1**, 14.
SUNSHINE, P., KUSUMOTO, H., and KRISS, J. P. (1965). *Pediatrics*, **36**, 869.
WHITE, C. (1912). *J. Obstet. Gynaec. Brit. Emp.*, **21**, 231.

Simple Goitre

ALEXANDER, W. D., KOUTRAS, D. A., CROOKS, J., BUCHANAN, W. W., MACDONALD
    E. M., RICHMOND, M. H., and WAYNE, E. J. (1962). *Quart. J. Med.*, **31**, 281.
GIBSON, J. B., HOWELER, J. F., and CLEMENTS, F. W. (1960). *Med. J. Aust.*, **1**, 875.
GREER, M. A. (1962). *Recent Progr. Hormone Res.*, **18**, 187.
WILSON, A. M. (1963). In *The Thyroid and its Diseases*, p. 64, edited by A. S. Mason
    (Proc. Conf. R.C.P. Lond.). London: Pitman Medical.

Parathyroids

ALBRIGHT, F., BURNETT, C. H., SMITH, P. H., and PARSON, W. (1942). *Endocrino-
    logy*, **30**, 922.
BENSON, P. F., and PARSONS, V. (1964). *Quart. J. Med.*, **33**, 197.
BRONSKY, D., KUSHNER, D. S., DUBIN, A., and SNAPPER, I. (1958). *Medicine (Balti-
    more)*, **37**, 317.
DRAKE, T. G., ALBRIGHT, F., BAUER, W., and CASTLEMAN, B. (1939). *Ann. intern.
    Med.*, **12**, 1751.
FOURMAN, P. (1960). *Calcium Metabolism and the Bone.* Oxford: Blackwell Scientific
    Publications.
STEINBERG, H., and WALDRON, B. R. (1952). *Medicine (Baltimore)*, **31**, 133.

ADRENALS

BONGIOVANNI, A. M. (1961). *J. clin. Endocr.*, **21**, 860.
BOYD, J. F., and MACDONALD, A. M. (1960). *Arch. Dis. Childh.*, **35**, 561.
CONN, J. W. (1955). *J. Lab. clin. Med.*, **45**, 3.
COPE, C. L. (1966). *Brit. med. J.*, **2**, 847, 914.
DI GEORGE, A. M., and PASCHKIS, K. (1957). *Amer. J. Dis. Child.*, **94**, 476.
HAMILTON, W., and BRUSH, M. G. (1964). *Arch. Dis. Childh.*, **39**, 66.
HARRIS-JONES, J. H., and NIXON, P. G. F. (1955). *J. clin. Endocr.*, **15**, 739.
HUBBLE, D. (1960). *Proc. roy. Soc. Med.*, **53**, 861.
IRVINE, W. J. (1963). In *The Thyroid and its Diseases*, p. 129, edited by A. S. Mason
    (Proc. Conf. R.C.P. Lond.). London: Pitman Medical.
LIDDLE, G. W. (1960). *J. clin. Endocr.*, **20**, 1539.
MITCHELL, R. G., and RHANEY, K. (1959). *Lancet*, **1**, 488.
NELSON, D. H., MEAKIN, J. W., and THORN, G. W. (1960). *Ann. intern. Med.*, **52**, 560.
SUCHOWSKY, G. K., and JUNKMANN, K. (1961). *J. clin. Endocr.*, **68**, 341.
VISSER, K. H. A. (1966). *Arch. Dis. Childh.*, **41**, 2, 113.
WILKINS, L. (1962). *Arch. Dis. Childh.*, **37**, 1, 231.
RAITI +NEWNS (1964). Arch. Dis. Childh. 39, 206, ---- (Aug. 64)

UNDESCENDED TESTES

BAUMRUCKER, G. O. (1946). *Bull. U.S. Army Med. Dep.*, **5**, 312.
SCORER, C. G. (1964). *Arch. Dis. Childh.*, **39**, 605.

PANCREAS

BAIRD, J. D., and FARQUHAR, J. W. (1962). *Lancet*, **1**, 71.
FARQUHAR, J. W. (1959). *Arch. Dis. Childh.*, **34**, 76.
FARQUHAR, J. W. (1962). *Scot. med. J.*, **7**, 119.
GELLIS, S. S., and HSIA, D. Y-Y. (1959). *Amer. J. Dis. Child.*, **97**, 1.

HALES, C. N., and RANDLE, P. J. (1963). *Lancet*, **1**, 790.
HUTCHISON, J. H., KEAY, A. J., and KERR, M. M. (1962). *Brit. med. J.*, **2**, 436.
LAWRENCE, R. D. (1964). *The Diabetic A.B.C.*, 13th edit. London: H. K. Lewis & Co.
OSLER, M. (1960). *Acta endocr. (Kbh.)*, **34**, 261.
SAMAAN, N., and FRASER, R. (1963). *Lancet*, **2**, 311.
VALLANCE-OWEN, J., and LILLEY, M. D. (1961). *Lancet*, **1**, 806.

CHAPTER XIX

DISEASES OF THE BLOOD

Modern haematology embraces many complicated techniques which must remain restricted to the full-time haematologist. They have added greatly to our understanding of the nature of some of the less common disorders, e.g. haemolytic anaemias, haemoglobinopathies, megalo-blastic anaemias etc. None the less, the blood disorders commonly encountered in paediatric practice can most often be dealt with by the use of the relatively simple standard techniques, which are within the competence of any physician who is prepared to devote a reasonable amount of effort to their performance. For certain important purposes such as the grouping and cross-matching of blood, and investigation of the blood clotting mechanisms, the paediatrician will be well advised to rely upon the expert haematologist.

The Normal Blood Picture in Infancy

Considerable variations in the normal values during the early days of life have been recorded by different workers. There are several reasons for this. Blood samples obtained by venepuncture in early infancy have lower values for haemoglobin and red cells than those obtained by heel-prick. Individual infants show a wide variation in levels. Different methods of haemoglobinometry may yield different results unless the apparatus has been accurately standardized. However, certain relatively flexible values can be stated and in routine clinical practice only fairly large departures from normal are likely to prove significant.

Haemoglobin

A level of 100 per cent will be regarded as equivalent to 14·8 gm. Hb. per 100 ml. The Hb. level of blood from the umbilical cord has a mean of 16·9 gm. per 100 ml. (114 per cent) with a range of 13·7–20·1 gm. per 100 ml. (Gairdner, 1958). A venous sample of the infant's blood some hours after birth will reveal a considerably higher Hb. level, mean 19·1 gm. per 100 ml. (129 per cent). This should be contrasted with the value for skin-prick blood at birth given by Mackay (1933) which was 143 per cent (21·2 gm. per 100 ml.). This rise in Hb. level just after birth is probably due to haemoconcentration following diminution in the plasma volume.

The haemoglobin levels during the first year of life have been given in terms of skin-prick blood by Mackay (1931). From about 140 per cent at birth the level falls to 75 per cent (11·1 gm. per 100 ml.) by the age of

8–12 weeks. Thereafter the Hb. level rises again to about 85 per cent (12·6 gm. per 100 ml.) at 6 months and remains there for the rest of the first year of life. Mackay's figures for the second half of the first year were obtained from babies receiving iron supplements and may be regarded as the optimum rather than the mean. Other workers take the normal Hb. level during this period to be more in the region of 75 per cent (Horan, 1950; Gairdner *et al.*, 1952). The explanation for the fall in Hb. level during the early weeks of life is that, although erythropoiesis continues at the high level found in the foetus for about three days after birth an abrupt decline in erythropoiesis then occurs and the marrow erythroid count falls from 40,000 per c.mm. to 6,000 (Gairdner, 1958). This is reflected in a fall in the reticulocyte count from 3–4 per cent just after birth to under 1 per cent one week later. These changes seem to be geared to the need to maintain the concentration of oxyhaemoglobin about 11 gm. per 100 ml. Thus, in the foetus with a Hb. level of 17 gm. per 100 ml. and an oxygen saturation of 65 per cent, the oxyhaemoglobin concentration is $17 \times 65 = 11$ gm. per 100 ml. after birth. When the lungs expand, the oxygen saturation rises to the adult level of 95 per cent; in this situation a Hb. level of just over 11 gm. per 100 ml. produces an oxyhaemoglobin concentration of 11 gm. per 100 ml. It must be realized that the postnatal fall in Hb. level is due to diminished activity of the erythroid elements in the bone marrow combined with the rapid increase in blood volume. It is *not* related significantly to increased red cell destruction. This fall is frequently exaggerated in the premature infant to result in the *early anaemia of prematurity* (Chapter II).

At birth 50–95 per cent of the haemoglobin is of the foetal type (Hb.-F) which resists denaturation with alkalis. It has a slightly different electrophoretic mobility and a quite different oxygen-dissociation curve from adult-type haemoglobin (Hb.-A). After birth Hb.-F is slowly replaced by Hb.-A so that after a year only small amounts of Hb.-F are still present. In certain diseases such as thalassaemia and sickle-cell anaemia Hb.-F contrives to be produced in excessive quantity. Its value to the foetus appears to be that it has a greater affinity for oxygen at low tensions than adult haemoglobin, and it releases carbon dioxide more readily.

Red cells.—The red cell count at birth varies between $6\frac{1}{2}$ and $7\frac{1}{2}$ millions per c.mm. The count falls to about $5–5\frac{1}{2}$ millions after two weeks and thereafter runs parallel to the Hb. level. Scanty eosinophilic normoblasts are found in the peripheral blood at birth. Erythrocytes at birth have a larger diameter (about 8·4 microns) than in the adult. The mean adult value of 7·2 microns is reached after one year.

White cells.—The total white cell count at birth is about 18,000 per c.mm. The adult level of 6,000–7,000 per c.mm. is not reached for 7–10 years. At birth about 60 per cent of the white cells are polymorphonuclears

(11,000 per c.mm.), and 15 per cent are lymphocytes (2,700 per c.mm.). During the ensuing two weeks the polymorphonuclears fall to within the normal adult range (3,500–4,500 per c.mm.) where they remain during the rest of childhood. On the other hand, the lymphocytes, predominantly of the large type in infancy, rise rapidly to about 9,500 per c.mm. at two weeks and only slowly fall during the next 12 years to the adult level of about 1,500–2,000 per c.mm. It is important to remember the comparatively high lymphocyte count in normal children if mistaken diagnoses such as glandular fever or leukaemia are to be avoided. The monocyte ratio in children tends to be somewhat higher than in adults. Eosinophils and basophils show no special characteristics.

IRON-DEFICIENCY OR NUTRITIONAL ANAEMIA OF INFANCY

This is the only deficiency disease seen commonly in the U.K. at the present time. There is no reason to believe that the high incidence noted during the second six months of life by Mackay (1933), Fullerton (1937) and the author (Hutchison, 1938) is significantly lower at the present time.

Aetiology

Several factors, singly or in combination, can result in this deficiency state. Unduly prolonged milk (human or cow's) feeding results in iron-deficiency. This is perhaps the most commonly found factor. Another important factor is the influence of birth weight. It is well known that premature infants and others of low birth weight (such as twins or triplets) are particularly likely to develop iron-deficiency anaemia. Infants, whatever their maturity, have a body iron content of about 75 mg. per Kg. fat-free body weight (Widdowson and Spray, 1951). However, the smaller infant grows more rapidly in proportion to his birth weight than the larger, with a correspondingly larger rise in his haemoglobin mass. As the absorption of iron is very low during the first four months of life the smaller infant more rapidly exhausts his storage iron (in liver and spleen) and develops overt signs of iron deficiency. Maternal anaemia has frequently been considered to lead to a lower level of storage iron in the foetus and so to an increased susceptibility to later iron-deficiency anaemia (Mackay, 1931; Strauss, 1933; Guest and Brown, 1957). This is unlikely to be a major factor in many cases. Finally, infections to which the iron-deficient infant is prone add to the condition and further aggravate the anaemia.

Clinical Features

Mild degrees of nutritional anaemia probably affect over 25 per cent of infants during their first year. The onset is rarely before the fifth month of life. When the anaemia is severe there is obvious pallor of skin and mucous membranes. Splenomegaly is common and there may be cardiomegaly and a haemic systolic murmur. The anaemia is microcytic and hypochromic. The serum iron is markedly reduced (normal mean = 100 μg. per 100 ml.), and the saturation of the iron-binding protein of the serum is reduced from 30 per cent to 10 per cent or less (Britton, 1963). The bone marrow shows normoblastic hyperplasia and an absence of stainable iron.

Prevention

In the full-term infant iron-deficiency is best prevented by the introduction of mixed feeding with foods rich in iron at the age of 4 months (Chapter I). In the premature infant iron should be given orally in the form of ferrous sulphate ½ gr. (30 mg.) thrice daily from the age of six weeks (Chapter II).

Treatment

In most cases the anaemia can be rapidly corrected at the rate of 1 per cent Hb. per day with oral iron. A suitable prescription is:

Ferrous sulphate 3 gr. (180 mg.)
Dilute hypophosphorous acid ½ ℳ (0·03 ml.)
Dextrose 15 gr. (1 gm.)
Chloroform water to 60 ℳ (4 ml.) thrice daily with food.

Alternative but more expensive preparations are:
Ferrous succinate (ferromyn elixir) 30 minims thrice daily; or Plesmet syrup (iron chelate) 60 minims thrice daily. Only rarely is it necessary to give iron-dextran complex (Imferon) intramuscularly. A suitable formula on which to calculate the dosage in milligrammes is:

$1·31 \times (19 -$ Hb. in gm. per 100 ml.$) \times$ weight in lbs.

It must be remembered that iron therapy will not work in the presence of a severe infection. When infection occurs in a severely anaemic child blood transfusion may have to be considered. This is a not uncommon occurrence.

MEGALOBLASTIC ANAEMIAS

True megaloblastic erythropoiesis is extremely rare in paediatric practice. The most common cause is malabsorption of folic acid in the older child with inadequately treated coeliac disease (Chapter XVI). A megaloblastic anaemia has been described in young infants in the U.S.A. There have usually been other signs of malnutrition in these infants such as scurvy, and infection also appears to be common. Other features have included leucopenia, thrombocytopenia, hepatosplenomegaly and achlorhydria. Permanent recovery follows treatment with folic acid. A factor in the malnutrition may have been the use of goat's milk (Zuelzer and Ogden, 1946). We have reported a case which may have had a similar aetiology, although leucopenia was not found and free hydrochloric acid was detected in the gastric juice after histamine (Hutchison and MacArthur, 1949). Recovery was brought about with folic acid.

Addisonian pernicious anaemia is exceedingly rare in childhood but it undoubtedly does occur as proved by the absence of intrinsic factor activity in some cases (Lambert et al., 1961). As seen in young children it differs radically from the adult form of the disease. Thus, gastric secretion of hydrochloric acid and pepsinogen is normal and the gastric mucosa appears healthy (McIntyre et al., 1965). There is a striking familial incidence and parental consanguinity is common. The anaemia responds rapidly to the administration of vitamin B_{12}, but during relapse there is, in addition to the blood findings, slowing of growth, retardation of bone-age and even delay in mental development. Minor neurological abnormalities are sometimes found such as absence of the deep reflexes and loss of vibration sense in the legs. This form of pernicious anaemia, probably due to a congenital metabolic error in the formation of intrinsic factor and seen in young children, can be distinguished from a form of the disease having its onset in adolescence. The latter is associated with atrophic changes in the gastric mucosa, as in the adult form of the disease and in some patients also with the presence of antibodies to intrinsic factor and gastric parietal cells. The adolescent pernicious anaemia, unlike the childhood form, resembles the adult disease further in often being associated with endocrine disturbances such as hypothyroidism. There is, clearly, strong evidence for separating the childhood and presumably congenital form of the disease as a distinct entity.

THE HAEMOLYTIC ANAEMIAS

The causes of haemolytic anaemia, which may be defined as one in which the life span of the red cells is shortened, have been summarized by Richmond (1962):

Defects within the red blood cell

Chemical with structural consequences
    Congenital spherocytosis
    Thalassaemia
    The haemoglobinopathies

Enzymatic
    G-6-P dehydrogenase deficiency

Undetermined
    Paroxysmal nocturnal haemoglobinuria (not seen in childhood).

Mechanisms extrinsic to the red blood cell

Infections

Chemical and physical agents

Red cell antibodies
Idiopathic
Symptomatic

Undetermined
—with and without systemic disease.

Further details can be obtained in the publications of Dacie (1960, 1962a, 1962b) and Prankerd (1959). Haemolytic anaemias due to blood group incompatibility between mother and child, and G-6-P dehydrogenase deficiency are considered in Chapter IV. Paroxysmal haemoglobinuria due to syphilis is described in Chapter X. It should also be pointed out that the common and classical manifestations of increased haemolysis such as acholuric jaundice, excess urobilinogenuria, reticulocytosis and hyperplasia of the bone marrow need not always be present. Indeed, even anaemia may be absent in mild cases because of the capability of the bone marrow to compensate for increased red cell destruction.

CONGENITAL SPHEROCYTOSIS (ACHOLURIC JAUNDICE)

Aetiology

This disease is transmitted as a Mendelian dominant trait, presumably resulting in the deficiency of a specific enzyme. The precise intra-erythrocytic abnormality is not known. Various enzyme defects have been suggested (Prankerd, 1959, 1960, 1961). A recent suggestion has been that the primary defect involves a block in the enzyme system responsible for the conversion of lysophosphatidyl ethanolamine to phosphatidyl ethanolamine, the spherocytosis and abnormal glycolytic mechanism in the red cells being secondary to the abnormal phosphatide mechanism (Kates *et al.*, 1961). It is certain that the major part of the haemolysis of the abnormal red cells takes place in the spleen (Dacie, 1962b).

Clinical Features

Congenital spherocytosis can cause haemolytic icterus in the neonatal period (Chapter IV). Even kernicterus has been described. It is, however, rare for the disease to appear in infancy. More commonly it presents during later childhood with pallor and lassitude; less often with jaundice and highly coloured urine. It may remain symptomless until adult life when biliary colic due to gall-stones is not uncommon.

Acute haemolytic crises with severe anaemia and icterus require emergency treatment but they are, in fact, uncommon. Splenomegaly is usually present whatever the degree of haemolysis in congenital spherocytosis. The blood shows an orthochromic anaemia. The red cells are unable to sustain a normal biconcave shape because of their metabolic defect. They are spheroidal with a smaller diameter than normal. It is usually easy to distinguish these microspherocytes in well-stained blood films. They appear unduly dark in colour and smaller in diameter than normal biconcave erythrocytes. Reticulocytosis is usually found. High figures may be reached during a crisis, but the absence of a reticulocytosis does not invalidate the diagnosis. The indirect bilirubin level in the serum is raised. This is also reflected in the presence of excess urobilinogen in the urine. Increased osmotic fragility of the red cells is an important diagnostic feature. The test is much more reliable when performed on a quantitative basis (Britton, 1963); it is not pathognomonic of congenital spherocytosis being sometimes abnormal in acquired haemolytic anaemia, and it may, infrequently, give normal results in the congenital cases. Coombs' test is negative. The marrow shows normoblastic hyperplasia. Rarely an aplastic crisis can occur with hypoplasia of the bone marrow resulting in anaemia, leucopenia and thrombocytopenia. A family history of the disease should always be sought.

Treatment

Splenectomy results in a return to normal health although it does not alter the metabolic defect in the red cells. It should always be advised in the child with congenital spherocytosis because even mild degrees of the disease interfere with growth and well-being. There has been a suggestion by some workers that splenectomy renders a child more susceptible to severe bacterial infections. Others have failed to substantiate this. There is, however, good evidence that the risk is greatest in infancy (King and Schumacker, 1952; Lowden et al., 1962), and the author has himself had good reason to regret advising splenectomy in infancy. In our opinion splenectomy should be postponed until after the first year of life. Control of the anaemia can meantime be achieved by blood transfusion provided that cross-matching is carefully performed by an expert. Rarely, in the neonatal period a rising serum bilirubin level may necessitate an exchange transfusion to eliminate the risk of kernicterus.

THALASSAEMIA (COOLEY'S ANAEMIA)

Aetiology

This is an uncommon disease in the U.K. being seen most often in children of Mediterranean stock, particularly from Italy, Sicily and Greece. It is inherited as an autosomal dominant characteristic. The

disease (thalassaemia major) is seen only in homozygotes, but heterozygotes frequently show minor haematological abnormalities (thalassaemia minor). There appears to be an intra-erythrocytic defect in the
formation of haemoglobin, and as haemoglobin is a constituent of the
surface of the red cell it is not surprising that this should result in the
presence of structurally abnormal cells.

Clinical Features

Subjects with *thalassaemia minor* have no symptoms but they show
the presence of mild anaemia, poikilocytosis, anisocytosis, some
bizarre-shaped cells and slight splenomegaly. The children of the mating
of two such heterozygotes have a 1 in 4 chance of suffering from
thalassaemia major. This condition is characterized by a chronic
haemolytic anaemia which becomes manifest early in infancy. Pallor
is constant and icterus not uncommon. Splenomegaly increases
throughout childhood. Hepatomegaly is also present, largely due to
extramedullary erythropoiesis. Pathognomonic skeletal changes can be
demonstrated radiographically. The membranous bones of the skull are
thickened and lateral views of the skull show the "hair on end" appearance. The facies has a mongoloid appearance due to thickening of the
facial bones. The hands may become broadened and thickened due to
changes in the metacarpals and phalanges (Caffey, 1951). These bone
changes are due to the long-continued hyperplasia of the bone marrow.
Blood examination shows a severe hypochromic anaemia with marked
anisocytosis and poikilocytosis. Many microcytic red cells lie side-by-
side with large (12–18μ.) bizarrely shaped cells. In some of the latter cells
an abnormal central mass of haemoglobin gives to them the appearance
of "target cells". Reticulocytosis is marked and Howell-Jolly bodies
may be numerous. The serum indirect bilirubin level is raised. There
is an increased serum iron level, while the iron-binding capacity is
fully saturated and lower than in normal children. The haemoglobin
in thalassaemia major consists of both Hb.-A and Hb.-F (Singer *et al.*,
1951). Apparently the continued formation of foetal type haemoglobin is an attempt to compensate for the impaired ability to produce
Hb.-A.

Treatment

Thalassaemia major can be treated only by repeated blood transfusions whenever the haemoglobin levels fall below 6 gm. per 100 ml.
In time this leads to haemosiderosis in which the increased content of
iron causes the skin to assume a muddy bronze colour, and there is an
increase in the size of the liver. Splenectomy may be indicated merely
to relieve the patient of the weight of an enormous spleen. Hypersplenism as reflected in leucopenia and thrombocytopenia is another
indication. It is doubtful if splenectomy can be justified solely in an

effort to increase the intervals between blood transfusions. The disease interferes seriously with growth and most affected children die before reaching adulthood.

SICKLE CELL DISEASE

Aetiology

This disease is almost confined to the Negro race. The homozygotes suffer from *sickle cell anaemia* in which all their haemoglobin is of the Hb.-S variety (Chapter IX). The heterozygotes reveal the *sickle cell trait* and their haemoglobin is composed of about 60 per cent Hb.-A and 40 per cent Hb.-S. Inheritance is by an autosomal dominant gene. The trait is found in about 7–9 per cent of American negroes, but it is much more prevalent in some African tribes. It provides increased resistance to malignant tertian malaria. Hb.-S has a distinctive electrophoretic pattern (Pauling *et al.*, 1949), which is due to its abnormal molecular structure (Ingram, 1956). This type of haemoglobin forms crescent-shaped crystals under reduced oxygen tension, and it is this property which is responsible for the sickled shape of the erythrocytes in people who possess the gene. Haemolysis in sickle cell anaemia appears to be due mainly to impaction of the sickled cells in the capillaries, especially in organs where the oxygen tension is low. Capillary obstruction leads to infarcts in various organs, e.g. spleen, intestine, bones, kidneys, heart, lungs and brain.

Clinical Features

The sickle cell trait is symptomless unless it is associated with another haemoglobinopathy or with thalassaemia (see below). Sickle cell anaemia often presents during the first year with pallor, listlessness and mild jaundice. In some cases there are recurrent haemolytic crises with acute symptoms such as severe abdominal pain and rigidity, pain in the loins, limb pains, localized paralyses, convulsions or meningism. Chronic haemolytic anaemia interferes with growth and nutrition so that the child is often stunted in later years. Splenomegaly may be marked, but sometimes disappears in later childhood. Cholelithiasis may develop as in other haemolytic anaemias. The blood shows a hypochromic anaemia, reticulocytosis, increased serum indirect bilirubin, decreased red cell osmotic fragility, and polymorphonuclear leucocytosis. In a crisis excess urobilinogenuria is marked. Sickled cells may be seen in ordinary blood films. They can always be produced by preparing a fresh drop of blood under a coverslip which is sealed off from oxygen with Vaseline. After 1–24 hours at room temperature sickled forms will be seen. The diagnosis can be confirmed by demonstrating the characteristic solubility of Hb.-S (Itano, 1953) or by paper electrophoresis (Smith and Conley, 1953; Chernoff, 1955). Children affected with sickle cell anaemia also have some Hb.-F in their circulation. There may also be striking bone changes in the X-rays such as demineralization, radial striations in the skull, and localized areas of aseptic necrosis.

Treatment

There is no specific treatment and blood transfusions are frequently required for anaemia. In crises, rest in bed and relief of pain are essential. With careful supervision and the use of blood transfusion only when it is necessary many children with sickle cell anaemia reach adult life. Splenectomy is indicated when there is evidence of hyper-splenism. Death can occur suddenly from cardiac failure, renal failure or cerebral infarction.

OTHER HAEMOGLOBINOPATHIES

Apart from Hb.-S a variety of other abnormal haemoglobins have been discovered in recent years. These have been designated C, D, E, G, H, and so forth, and some have been named according to places such as "Norfolk" and "Barts". These abnormal haemoglobins seem to result in increased haemolysis, at least in part, by their effects in distorting the shape of the red cells. They have a marked racial inci-dence. They are determined by alleles of the genes for normal Hb.-A. Their differentiation is dependent upon their different solubilities and electrophoretic mobilities (Ingram, 1961). In practice most abnormal haemoglobins can be identified by paper electrophoresis. Foetal type Hb.-F is, on the other hand, detected by tests for alkali denaturation (Singer, 1955).

The existence of these abnormal haemoglobins in both heterozygous and homozygous forms, as already described in sickle cell disease, has been demonstrated. In heterozygous form they result in slightly excess haemolysis of which the subject is frequently quite unaware. In homo-zygous form there may be features resembling those seen in thalassaemia and sickle cell anaemia such as hypochromic anaemia, target cells, reticulocytosis, hepatosplenomegaly, jaundice and shortened survival time of autogenous red cells (Hb.-C; Hb.-E; and Hb.-H). In most of the haemoglobinopathies, however, even the homozygous state produces only a very mild haemolytic condition. Haemoglobin M is distinct in its effects from the other abnormal haemoglobins in that it causes a rare type of methaemoglobinaemia which cannot be reversed by methylene blue or ascorbic acid (Chapter IX).

Some anaemic children have been found to have inherited the genes for two abnormal haemoglobins. They are, in fact, double heterozygotes. Thus there has been described *sickle cell disease with haemoglobin C (or D)*. In these cases the clinical features have resembled those of sickle cell anaemia in mild degree. *Sickle cell-thalassaemia* disease reflects the double heterozygous state for the genes of Hb.-S and thalassaemia. The clinical picture is that of chronic haemolytic anaemia with marked microcytosis, hypochromia, and with both sickle cells and target cells. Splenomegaly is usual. Differential diagnosis from sickle cell anaemia may require electrophoretic analysis, alkali denaturation tests, and careful investigation of both parents. Commonly one parent is heterozygous for Hb.-S (sickle cell trait) while the other shows the features of thalassaemia minor.

Treatment

In many patients in this group the relatively slow rate of haemolysis can be compensated by marrow hyperplasia. Blood transfusion should be used sparingly and only when anaemia is severe.

(IDIOPATHIC ACQUIRED HAEMOLYTIC ANAEMIA

Aetiology

This is not a common problem in paediatric practice but it can cause an acute emergency. This type of anaemia is one of the conditions in which the modern concept of "auto-immunity" finds convincing support. Indeed, the disease has been called "auto-immune haemolytic anaemia". The red cells are coated with auto-antibody which results in a positive direct Coombs' (antiglobulin) test. The common type of incomplete antibody results in a filtering off of the affected cells, principally by the spleen where they are destroyed (Dacie, 1962a, b). In more severe cases when the red cells are heavily coated with antibody, sufficient agglutination can occur in vivo to cause removal of the cells from the circulation by the liver as well as the spleen. In these cases splenectomy would probably prove to be an ineffective therapeutic measure. Rarely, haemolytic anaemia follows the use of drugs. Apart from the group related to deficiency of glucose-6-phosphate dehydrogenase (Chapter IV), the other cases are thought to be due to the formation of an antibody to the drug/red cell complex. Drugs which can act in this way include PAS and phenacetin. It may be, also, that haemolytic anaemias complicating viral or bacterial infections are due to antibodies formed against bacterial or viral products adsorbed by red cells.

Clinical Features

In some children the disease has an alarmingly acute onset (Lederer's anaemia) with fever, backache, limb pains, abdominal pain, vomiting and diarrhoea. Haemoglobinuria and oliguria may be present. Pallor develops rapidly and icterus is common. Frequently, the pallor, listlessness and mild icterus develop more insidiously. Splenomegaly is common. The urine may be dark in colour due to the presence of excess urobilinogen. The anaemia is usually orthochromic but it may be either normocytic or macrocytic. Reticulocytosis is often marked and there may be many erythroblasts in the peripheral blood. Spherocytosis with an increased fragility of the red cells may simulate congenital spherocytosis. However, in acquired haemolytic anaemia Coombs' test is positive. Auto-agglutination may be marked at room temperature. The serum indirect bilirubin level is raised. A polymorphonuclear leucocytosis is usual and myelocytes may be numerous. There is occasionally a thrombocytopenia, and purpura can also develop. Both haemolytic and aplastic crises may occur. A false positive serological test for syphilis is a well-known phenomenon.

Treatment

In some children with Lederer's anaemia complete recovery follows emergency blood transfusion. The donors must be most carefully selected to avoid mismatched transfusions, because the donor cells must be demonstrated to be incapable of adsorbing antibody. In the less acute cases the haemolytic process continues after transfusion. Corticosteroids are of great value in these circumstances and frequently abolish the need for further transfusions. The initial dosage should be prednisolone 15 mg. four times daily, continued until the haemolysis is brought under control. Thereafter the dosage is progressively reduced, the aim being the smallest maintenance dose compatible with a reasonable haemoglobin level (10–12 gm. per 100 ml.). When long-term steroid therapy proves necessary a careful watch must be kept for undesirable side-effects such as osteoporosis, diabetes mellitus etc. When haemolysis cannot be controlled with a reasonable dosage of steroid, possibly combined with intramuscular corticotrophin, 80 units of the gel daily, or when relapse follows withdrawal of these hormones, the question of splenectomy arises. Unfortunately, this operation is not always successful in relieving the anaemia. It is difficult, also, to decide at what stage to abandon the trial of conservative measures. In recent years it has proved possible to forecast the effect of splenectomy in individual patients by studying the fate of injected red cells which have been labelled with radioactive chromium (^{51} Cr.). The accumulations of radioactivity over the spleen, liver and praecordium are then compared. Splenectomy is only likely to be successful when excess counts are found over the spleen. A new approach has been the use of antimetabolites, such as mercaptopurine, to destroy the cells which produce the abnormal auto-antibodies (Schwartz and Dameshek, 1962). This is potentially dangerous and not recommended for routine use. A safer and more hopeful approach, which resulted in apparent complete recovery of two infants with auto-immune haemolytic anaemia, is thymectomy (Wilmers and Russell, 1963; Karaklis et al., 1964). This line of treatment is based upon recent knowledge that in the young animal the thymus plays an important immunological role, and on the theory that in the auto-immune diseases it may be the primary source of auto-antibody-producing cells. Whether thymectomy would prove as successful in auto-immune haemolytic anaemia in the older child or adult in whom the thymus has undergone involution is still to be determined.

THE HAEMOLYTIC-URAEMIC SYNDROME OF INFANCY

We have seen a considerable number of cases in which an acute "necrotizing" nephritis in infancy has presented clinically in the form of an acute haemolytic anaemia. The cause of the haemolysis is uncertain but the prognosis is often grave. There have been several reports in the literature (Gasser *et al.*, 1955; Lock and Dormandy, 1961; Griffiths and Irving, 1961). Although the present author's cases have all been due to a necrotizing form of glomerulonephritis the same clinical picture has been related to renal cortical necrosis, pyelonephritis and thrombotic microangiopathy.

Clinical Features

The infant presents with vomiting, diarrhoea, pallor and possibly jaundice. In some cases convulsive twitchings have been an early manifestation. Oliguria is constantly present but not always appreciated. Hypertension may be severe. The blood shows a severe anaemia, thrombocytopenia, reticulocytosis and raised serum indirect bilirubin. Some of the red cells are characteristically misshapen, a feature which should lead to the correct diagnosis. Two abnormal cell types are to be found. "Burr cells" have one or several sharp projections along their edges. "Triangular cells" and others with a "broken egg shell" shape are also common. The blood urea is frequently greatly elevated. The urine shows protein, red cells and granular casts. The protein level in the cerebrospinal fluid may be raised.

Treatment

The general lines have been described in Chapter XVII (for renal failure). Frequent blood transfusions may be necessary for the haemolytic anaemia. In progressive cases there is a place for the use of corticosteroids and peritoneal dialysis.

THE HYPOPLASTIC ANAEMIAS

This group of anaemias is poorly understood and clearly contains a considerable number of quite separate diseases which present clinically in somewhat similar ways. The defect in erythropoiesis may affect all elements of the marrow or only one, such as the erythropoietic tissue. There may be virtually no formation at all of the precursors of red cells, leucocytes or platelets. There may, on the other hand, be an abundance of primitive cells in the marrow which have suffered an arrest of maturation due to the deficiency of some unknown haemopoietic factor. It has also been suggested that in some cases in which the peripheral blood seems to reflect a hypoplastic marrow there is, in fact, normal marrow activity but a failure of its capacity to release mature cells into the circulation (Britton, 1963). These are, fortunately, not common conditions, but those to be considered here occur sufficiently frequently in paediatric practice to merit the attention of all who have to handle sick children.

CONGENITAL HYPOPLASTIC ANAEMIA (RBC's)

Aetiology

This disease presents in early infancy as an apparent hypoplasia of the erythron. Granulocytes and platelets are unaffected. It may, in fact, be more than a single disease process. In most cases the bone marrow shows a gross deficiency of erythroblasts. It has been suggested that this might be due to the absence of some essential chemical factor and there is, indeed, evidence of a metabolic block in tryptophane metabolism in some of these patients (Diamond et al., 1961). In other cases normoblasts in the peripheral blood and plentiful erythroblasts in the marrow have been taken to indicate a form of maturation arrest—erythrogenesis imperfecta (Cathie, 1950).

Clinical Features

The presenting feature is pallor, which becomes apparent in the early weeks or months of life. Irritability becomes obvious only when the anaemia is severe in degree. Physical examination is usually unrevealing. There are no haemorrhagic manifestations. Hepatic or splenic enlargement is unusual but may develop as a consequence of cardiac failure. Haemic systolic murmurs are common. The anaemia, often severe, is normocytic and normochromic. Reticulocytes are absent or scanty. The white blood cells and platelets show no abnormalities.

Course and Prognosis

This is greatly influenced by treatment. Repeated blood transfusions lead to haemosiderosis with the typical muddy bronze skin pigmentation. Cirrhosis of the liver ultimately develops with failure of sexual maturation. The long bones often show marked growth arrest lines. Osteoporosis and delayed bone-age are common. The children are frequently dwarfed, but mental development proceeds normally. The prognosis is, therefore, not good in the long term. On the other hand, spontaneous remissions have frequently been reported, even after puberty and several hundred transfusions.

Treatment

Repeated transfusions are required over periods of many years. Some cases have shown excellent response to corticosteroids (Allen and

Diamond, 1961). The dosage of prednisolone has varied between 30–60 mg. per day at the start of treatment. Evidence of success is first a rise in the reticulocyte count and then in the haemoglobin and red cells. The author has yet to see a satisfactory remission from steroid treatment in this disease and its failure in some cases but not in others argues in favour of a multiple aetiology. Splenectomy is not advised and some children so treated have subsequently died of severe infections to which they had not previously been susceptible. In an effort to delay the development of haemosiderosis in patients who require repeated transfusions the author has used the iron-chelating agent desferriox-amine. A dose of 500 to 1,000 mg. is given intravenously with each transfusion, and doses of 500 mg. are given intramuscularly thrice to seven times each week in the intervals between transfusions. A great increase in the urinary output of iron can be demonstrated with this treatment, and although it is unwelcome to the child it seems likely to achieve its objective.

FANCONI-TYPE FAMILIAL HYPOPLASTIC ANAEMIA

Aetiology

This disease affects all three elements of the bone marrow. It is genetically determined and a familial incidence is usual.

Clinical Features

Pallor may become obvious in the early days of infancy, but more often the onset is delayed until between the ages of 3 and 10 years. Purpura and ecchymoses are not uncommon and there may be bleeding from mucous membranes. Defects in the radius and/or thumb, or accessory thumbs are common. Other congenital abnormalities seen less frequently include microcephaly, hypogonadism, cleft palate, and anomalies of the heart or renal tract. In some cases mild hyperpigmentation of the skin, in others exaggerated tendon reflexes have been noted. The blood shows a normocytic, normochromic anaemia, leucopenia, granulocytopenia and thrombocytopenia. Reticulocytes are scanty or absent.

Treatment

Repeated blood transfusions can prolong life but death is usual during childhood. Transfusion haemosiderosis may complicate the picture. Corticosteroids alone are of no value. Some cases have shown a response to methyl testosterone or methandrostenolone in combination with corticosteroids (McKay, 1962).

ACQUIRED HYPOPLASTIC ANAEMIA

Aetiology

This is a rare disease in childhood and most cases are "idiopathic". The bone marrow is rarely completely aplastic in such patients. In some there is a reduction in all the blood-forming elements; in others (maturation arrest) there are plenty of precursors such as proerythroblasts and myeloblasts. Rarely, the marrow may be hyperplastic (in contrast to the hypoplastic peripheral blood) when an inability to release its mature cells has been postulated; this may be due to primary hypersplenism and this form of disease has been called "*splenic pancytopenia*" (Britton, 1963). Some cases of hypoplastic anaemia are secondary to the toxic effects of drugs such as chloramphenicol, benzene derivatives, and the arsphenamines. Chloramphenicol in particular has been misused in recent years. It is most dangerous when given in prolonged or repeated courses which should be completely avoided. This antibiotic should never be prescribed when the antibiotic sensitivities of the pathogen indicate that a safer alternative can be used.

Clinical Features

The onset may be acute or insidious with increasing pallor, listlessness, malaise, bruises, purpura and, sometimes, bleeding from mucous membranes. Death is due to haemorrhage into internal organs or to intercurrent infection. The blood shows a normocytic, normochromic anaemia, thrombocytopenia, leucopenia and granulocytopenia. The marrow must always be examined by needle biopsy or trephine. The appearances vary as outlined above. Marrow examination is, furthermore, the only way in which hypoplastic anaemia can be distinguished from aleukaemic leukaemia. The prognosis is hopeless when the marrow examination reveals gross hypoplasia of all the blood-forming elements, but in less severe cases there is always hope of a spontaneous or induced remission.

Treatment

Life can be prolonged, sometimes for long periods, by repeated blood transfusions. Packed red cells are preferable to whole blood, and fresh blood is a great advantage. In childhood some cases have shown striking remissions on treatment with methyltestosterone or methandrostenolone in combination with one of the corticosteroids (Shahidi and Diamond, 1961). Splenectomy is indicated only in cases of splenic pancytopenia when cure or amelioration can be predicted.

ALBERS-SCHÖNBERG DISEASE (OSTEOPETROSIS)

Aetiology

This is a genetic disorder of bone, usually autosomal recessive. The cortex and trabeculae of the bones are thickened and the marrow is crowded out. Extramedullary erythropoiesis in the liver and spleen may prevent anaemia for a variable period.

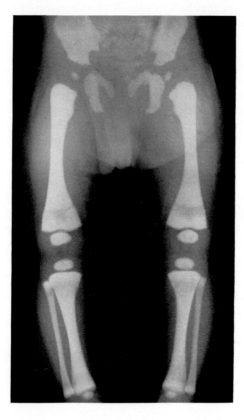

FIG. 69.—Osteopetrosis showing zones of decreased density at metaphyseal ends of long bones.

Clinical Features

The disease may present in infancy with progressive loss of vision due to optic atrophy, or with deafness. In later childhood the mode of presentation is a pathological fracture or increasing pallor. The anaemia is leuco-erythroblastic in type. There is progressive hepatosplenomegaly. The most characteristic diagnostic signs are to be found in radiographs of the skeleton (Figs. 69 and 70). The bones, including the base of the skull, ribs, vertebrae, scapulae and pelvis, show increased density.

Typical zones of decreased density can be seen at the metaphyses and running parallel to the borders of scapulae and ilia; these still contain marrow.

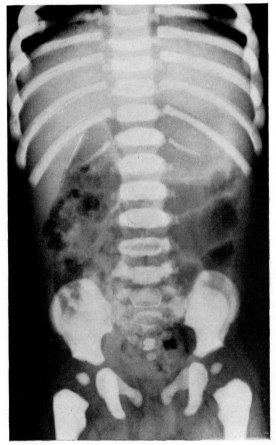

Fig. 70.—Osteopetrosis showing zones of decreased density in iliac bones.

Treatment

The only available measure is blood transfusion. Splenectomy is, of course, contra-indicated. The prognosis is hopeless.

THE PURPURAS

Purpura is an extremely common clinical phenomenon in childhood and has many causes. The principal pathogenic factors are capillary defects and thrombocytopenia, sometimes both being present. In most cases the purpura is symptomatic of another disease. It occurs due to decreased capillary resistance in acute infections such as meningococcal (and other) septicaemias, bacterial endocarditis, typhus and typhoid fever, scarlet fever etc. It may arise in scurvy, uraemia and snake-bite. Severe anoxia neonatorum sometimes causes petechiae, especially over the head, neck and shoulders. A similar mechanical effect is sometimes seen in the child who has had a severe and prolonged convulsion, and in whooping cough. Symptomatic thrombocytopenic purpura occurs in leukaemia, hypoplastic anaemia, and in states of hypersplenism such as Gaucher's disease (Chapter XII), Banti's disease (portal hypertension—Chapter XVI) and Felty's syndrome (rheumatoid arthritis—Chapter XXVI). Congenital defects in the capillaries are seen in such exceedingly rare conditions as hereditary haemorrhagic telangiectasia (Osler's disease) and cutis hyperelastica (Ehlers-Danlos syndrome). It will be clear, therefore, that purpura reflects a blood disorder in only a minority of cases. None the less, the more important primary diseases in which purpura is a prominent feature are conveniently discussed in this chapter.

HENOCH-SCHÖNLEIN (ANAPHYLACTOID) PURPURA

Aetiology

In most cases there is a history of a preceding sore throat or respiratory infection. In a few, evidence is obtainable from throat swab or ASO titre that the beta-haemolytic streptococcus is involved, but in the majority negative findings lend some support for the possibility that a virus antigen/antibody reaction is present (Bywaters *et al.*, 1957). Rarely, the disease can be related to an article of diet such as crab, chocolate etc. ("allergic purpura").

Clinical Features

A classical account has been given by Gairdner (1948). The disease has a wide variety of manifestations, but the diagnosis is rarely difficult and based essentially on *the rash of characteristic appearance and distribution*. The onset is ushered in by malaise, headache, anorexia and slight fever. The most prominent symptoms may arise from swollen, painful joints ("peliosis rheumatica"), or from areas of angioneurotic oedema elsewhere. In other children the onset is with severe abdominal pain with or without melaena. It is in such cases that a mistaken diagnosis of intussusception has sometimes led to an unnecessary laparotomy. There is nearly always some rash if it is adequately sought. In the majority of cases the rash is the most striking feature and the one which causes the parents to seek medical advice. It appears first as small separate urticarial lesions, both visible and palpable. These soon become dusky red or frankly purpuric and they no longer fade on pressure. As they resolve they may assume an ecchymotic appearance. In the typical case the rash is most profuse over the extensor surfaces of the knees, ankles and dorsum of the feet, arms, elbows and forearms; it is also marked over the buttocks (Fig. 71). The face is completely spared, but when the disease appears in an infant, which is quite rare, the face is often markedly involved (Fig. 72). In about 20 per cent of cases frank acute nephritis develops, but the Addis count is raised, indicating glomerular involvement, in over half the cases. There seems to be little doubt that glomerulonephritis complicating Henoch-Schönlein purpura has a less favourable prognosis than the classical post-streptococcal form of the disease. While most cases do, in fact, make a complete recovery, persistent or recurrent proteinuria and haematuria is an unfavourable feature of some, and renal biopsy frequently shows a progressive and irreversible lesion in the glomeruli. The bleeding time and platelet count are within normal limits.

Purpura fulminans.—This is probably an atypical form of anaphylactoid purpura, usually seen in young infants. It is, fortunately, rare. Large ecchymotic areas appear all over the trunk and extremities. Superficial gangrene is common. Anaemia may be present due to haemorrhage into the skin. Recovery is rare.

Treatment

There is no specific treatment for anaphylactoid purpura. Bed rest should be enforced until fresh lesions cease to appear. Penicillin is only indicated if beta-haemolytic streptococci are isolated from the throat. Glomerulonephritis should be managed along the usual lines (Chapter XVII). Severe abdominal pain may develop at any stage of the illness. It is best relieved with morphine in suitable dosage ($\frac{1}{8}$–$\frac{1}{6}$ gr. = 8–10 mg.). We have not found corticosteroids to be of value in this disease which rarely endangers life in childhood.

ESSENTIAL THROMBOCYTOPENIC PURPURA

Aetiology

Cases of the "idiopathic" type are now thought to be examples of auto-immunity with a similar pathogenesis to that described in acquired haemolytic anaemia (p. 392). Platelet antibodies have, however, proved much more difficult to demonstrate than those directed against red cells. Indeed, it is easier to demonstrate platelet antibodies in cases of thrombocytopenic purpura caused by drugs such as Sedormid and quinidine. The difficulties may be technical and the best technique at present seems to be a modification of Coombs' anti-globulin test called the anti-human-globulin consumption (A.H.G.C.) test (Dausset and Brecy, 1958; Van de Wiel et al., 1961). It should be pointed out, however, that bleeding does not arise from thrombocytopenia alone and there is probably concomitant capillary endothelial damage in this disease.

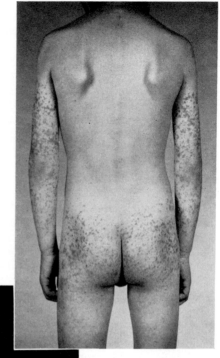

FIG. 71.—Anaphylactoid purpura showing typical distribution of rash over buttocks and extensor surfaces of arms and forearms.

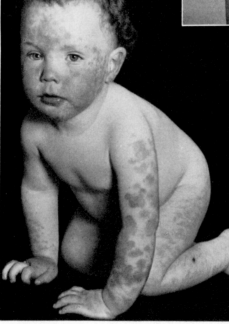

FIG. 72.—Anaphylactoid purpura in child aged 18 months showing involvement of skin of face.

Clinical Features

Most cases in childhood have an acute onset. There has frequently been a recently preceding upper respiratory infection or a zymotic disease such as measles, mumps or chickenpox. The first manifestation may be bleeding from mucous membranes such as epistaxis, bleeding gums or haematuria. Generalized purpura and/or ecchymoses are characteristic, often profuse. Life may be endangered in severe cases by blood loss or by subarachnoid haemorrhage.

Chronic or relapsing cases are also seen in which crops of purpura and ecchymoses appear over long periods. There may also be remissions and recurrences in the acute form. The spleen may be palpable but never becomes very large.

The blood shows a diminished platelet count. Bleeding occurs when the count falls below 40,000 per c.mm. The bleeding time is prolonged and clot retraction is defective, but the clotting time is normal. Hess's capillary resistance test is positive during the active phases. A post-haemorrhagic anaemia and leucocytosis may be present. The bone marrow may show paucity of megakaryocytes but more often these are abundant (? maturation arrest).

Treatment

In most children the acute attack of thrombocytopenic purpura under-goes spontaneous remission and does not again appear. This is a much happier prognosis than is usual in the adult and it should encourage the paediatrician to be patient. There is rarely any need for a quick decision about some form of specific treatment. When bleeding is severe and persistent, blood transfusion combined with steroid therapy is usually successful in precipitating a remission. This may be permanent or temporary, but in the last fifteen years the author has recommended splenectomy on very few patients. Unfortunately, splenectomy is fol-lowed by permanent return of the platelets to normal levels in only about 80 per cent of cases. For this reason we have been reluctant to recommend it unless the disease is persistent or there are repeated acute attacks.

Congenital Thrombocytopenic Purpura

It is well recognized that the infant of a mother who is suffering from thrombocytopenic purpura, or who has been so affected during the pregnancy may be born with severe thrombocytopenia. The infant usually exhibits generalized purpura and may die of severe visceral haemorrhages into organs such as the adrenals, brain and pericardium (Kaplan, 1959). The pathogenesis has been shown to be the passage of platelet antibodies across the placenta from mother to foetus (Jones et al., 1961). There have been recent reports of neonatal thrombocytopenia following the treatment of toxaemia of pregnancy with the thiazide group of drugs (Rodriguez *et al.*, 1964) and the author has seen two cases of purpura of this type where the mother had been given chlorothiazide. The affected infant should be treated from the time of diagnosis with a steroid such as prednisolone 5 mg. thrice daily for ten days, followed by progressive reduction in dosage until its discontinuance after 30–40 days.

FAMILIAL THROMBOCYTOPENIA, ECZEMA AND INFECTION

(Aldrich's Syndrome)

This is a very rare condition affecting only males and presumed to be inherited as a sex-linked recessive characteristic. It presents in infancy with typical infantile eczema. There is, in addition, a bleeding tendency in the form of oozing from mucous membranes and/or purpura. These children are highly susceptible to infections such as otitis media, pneumonia, meningitis and septicaemia, one of which is likely to prove fatal. The thrombocytopenia seems to respond poorly to ACTH or corticosteroids. There is a response to splenectomy but the wisdom of such a course in the light of probable further susceptibility to infections is open to doubt. As all three elements of this intriguing disease commonly occur quite separately the diagnosis could readily be overlooked unless the physician was aware of its existence (Aldrich *et al.*, 1954; Gordon, 1960). No quantitative deficiencies have been detected in any of the immunoglobulins in cases of this disease.

BLOOD CLOTTING DEFECTS

The mechanism of blood clotting is extremely complex, and the modern tests used to define the various congenital (and acquired) defects in this mechanism are only for the expert haematologist. The paediatrician must, however, have sufficient knowledge of the clinical types of clotting deficiency to use rationally the help which the haematologist has to offer.

Mechanism of blood clotting.—Only a brief description will be given. The basis of our present knowledge was laid down initially by Morawitz as follows:

$$\underset{\text{(Factor II)}}{\text{Prothrombin}} + \underset{\text{(Factor IV)}}{\text{calcium ions}} + \underset{\text{(Factor III)}}{\text{thromboplastin}} \rightarrow \text{Thrombin}$$

$$\text{Thrombin} + \underset{\text{(Factor I)}}{\text{fibrinogen (soluble)}} \rightarrow \text{Fibrin (insoluble)}$$

There are also anti-clotting factors normally present in blood. The most important is probably heparin which has an antithrombin activity.

Another is an enzyme (plasmin) which has a fibrinolytic activity; it exists in precursor form as plasminogen which is "activated" under certain circumstances, e.g. tissue damage.

However, many other factors are now known to be required in normal clotting. The formation of active thromboplastin in blood requires the presence of anti-haemophilic globulin (AHG: Factor VIII), Christmas factor (plasma thromboplastin component: PTC: Factor IX), and plasma thromboplastin antecedent (PTA: Factor XI), in addition to a platelet factor. The tissues also produce their own thromboplastin. The conversion of prothrombin to thrombin also requires additional factors, namely, proaccelerin (Factor V: labile factor), and proconvertin (Factor VII: stable factor). Two recently discovered factors necessary for the formation of thromboplastin are Stuart-Prower factor (Factor X) and Hageman factor (Factor XII).

It is clear that a congenital deficiency of any of these factors could result in deficiencies of haemostasis. A considerable number have been described but only haemophilia and Christmas disease bother the paediatrician frequently. The reader is referred to specialized texts for the rarer clotting deficiencies and for a detailed account of the tests required for their elucidation (Douglas, 1962; Britton, 1963).

HAEMOPHILIA (A)

Aetiology

The deficiency of anti-haemophilic globulin is inherited as a sex-linked recessive trait, only males being affected.

Clinical Features

It is rare for haemophilia to become manifest during the first year of life, presumably because the male infant acquires maternal AHG during foetal life. The outstanding feature is, of course, bleeding. This may take the form of prolonged oozing from a minor injury such as a cut lip or finger, from an erupting tooth, after the loss of a deciduous tooth or from the nose. There may be dangerous and persistent bleeding from circumcision, or tonsillectomy if the presence of haemophilia has not been discovered. A common event is severe haemarthrosis, especially in a knee-joint, after quite minor strain. A blow may result in a massive haematoma on any part of the body. A deeply situated haematoma may threaten life by pressure on vital structures such as the trachea or a large artery. In some children who are severely affected repeated haemarthroses may lead to fibrous ankylosis and crippling. Bleeding from the gastro-intestinal or renal tracts is not rare. Cases vary considerably in severity but run true to type within each individual family. There is a fairly high mutation rate and the absence of a family history of "bleeders" does not exclude the diagnosis.

Diagnosis

The classical blood finding in haemophilia is a prolonged clotting time. While this is certainly to be found in most cases it may become normal between attacks of bleeding, and in mild cases it may never be possible to demonstrate a delay in clotting. Furthermore, this simple and time-honoured test cannot distinguish true haemophilia from some of the other clotting factor deficiencies. It is, indeed, no longer acceptable as the sole basis of diagnosis which must rest upon more refined tests. The most valuable of these is *the thromboplastin generation test*. This test reveals the inefficient formation of thromboplastin, due in hae- mophilia to lack of AHG, which factor is found in normal plasma treated with aluminium hydroxide but which is absent from normal serum. There is, therefore, a demonstrable defect in clotting when the test is performed with the patient's alumina-plasma, normal serum, platelets and calcium chloride. Clotting proceeds normally, however, when normal alumina-plasma is used along with the patient's serum. The *one-stage "prothrombin time" test* gives a normal result in hae- mophilia. Indeed, it is possible by the expert use of these two tests to separate out the various deficiencies of clotting factors which have now been defined. In haemophilia the *prothrombin consumption test* is also abnormal in that almost no prothrombin is consumed.

Differential Diagnosis

Haemophilia may obviously be simulated clinically by a deficiency of any one of the clotting factors described above. None of these is as common as haemophilia, but the minor differences in clinical behaviour which they exhibit do not allow a firm diagnosis to be based upon any- thing less than a detailed laboratory investigation. The principal dis- tinguishing findings are presented below.

Treatment

The arrest of active bleeding requires that the concentration of AHG in the child's plasma be brought up to 30 per cent of normal. This re- quires the rapid transfusion of large volumes of *fresh blood* or of *freeze-dried fresh plasma*. Once bleeding has been stopped it is frequently necessary to continue or repeat the administration of freeze-dried plasma at a slower rate to maintain haemostasis. When major surgery is quite unavoidable it is now possible to obtain purified human, bovine or porcine AHG with which bleeding can be prevented during and after the operation. Their use requires that the plasma level of AHG be measured regularly throughout the period of administration. They are in short supply and extremely expensive. Bovine and porcine AHG are, unfortunately, antigenic so that they may each be used for one episode only. Local bleeding from minor wounds is an indication for removal of clot with hot water followed by the application of powdered thrombin (Thrombin Topical P. D. & Co.) under a pressure bandage. Stitches should not be inserted if possible. A haemarthrosis can best be surrounded by ice bags.

The *long-term management* involves the education of the child, and his parents, in a way of life which makes minor injuries less likely to be sustained. Attendance at an ordinary school is often possible through the co-operation of the teaching staff and the boy's friends. A useful adult life is usually attainable, especially in mildly affected cases, if the physician has advised and supervised his patient with understanding. One of the most difficult tasks is to convince the parents of the need for regular expert conservative dental care. The removal of a carious and neglected permanent tooth in an adult haemophiliac involves the medical staff in a major effort and the patient in a most unpleasant experience.

CHRISTMAS DISEASE (Haemophilia B)

Aetiology

The deficiency of Christmas factor is inherited as a sex-linked recessive trait. It accounts for about 15 per cent of all "bleeders", being much less common than true haemophilia A.

Clinical Features

The disease cannot be distinguished from haemophilia on clinical grounds. It can best be differentiated by means of the thromboplastin generation test. Defective clotting will be found when the test is performed with the patient's serum and normal alumina-plasma, whereas a normal response will be found with the patient's alumina-plasma and normal serum. The one-stage prothrombin time is normal, as in haemophilia A.

Treatment

Christmas factor is stable in whole blood, plasma or serum, so that any of these in sufficient quantity will stop bleeding. A concentrated factor IX preparation has been prepared from human plasma and can be used, when procurable, for unavoidable major surgery.

HAEMOPHILIA C

Aetiology

(P. T. A.)

The deficiency of factor XI is inherited as an incompletely recessive characteristic, affecting both males and females. Homozygotes bleed severely while heterozygotes bleed only mildly.

Clinical Features

The diagnosis of this rare disease can be shown in the thromboplastin generation test which will be abnormal only when it is performed with both the patient's alumina-plasma and the patient's serum. The one-stage prothrombin time is normal as in haemophilia A and B.

Treatment

As factor XI is stable, stored blood, plasma or serum in sufficient volumes will stop bleeding.

OTHER RARE CLOTTING DEFECTS

These have sometimes been referred to as "parahaemophilias". The bleeding tendency has been found in patients of both sexes but the various congenital defects, of factor V, factor VII, and factor X (Stuart-Prower) are probably very rare. In each of these deficiencies there is a prolongation of the one-stage "prothrombin time". If the test is performed with Russell's viper venom instead of brain extract the prothrombin time remains prolonged in factor X deficiency but is restored to normal in factor VII deficiency. These various clotting deficiencies can also be differentiated by specific qualitative tests which are based upon the different properties of the factors concerned.

The coumarin drugs, used frequently in adults for their anti-coagulant properties, depress the blood levels of prothrombin, factor VII, factor IX and factor X. The dosage is controlled so as to maintain the prothrombin time about 20–30 per cent of normal. Salicylates may have a similar effect when given in large doses.

Another very rare congenital clotting deficiency involves factor XII (Hageman). The one-stage prothrombin time is normal but there is abnormal thromboplastin generation and diminished prothrombin consumption. This deficiency is apparently not associated with excessive bleeding after surgery.

The cause of haemorrhagic disease of the newborn, which simulates temporarily the effects of the coumarins, has been discussed in Chapter V. The commonly accepted explanation of this neonatal emergency is that it is due to prothrombin deficiency, but it is likely that the principal deficiency is of factor VII. This probably explains the uncertain thera-peutic effects of vitamin K analogue. On the other hand, vitamin K deficiency may occur in fat-absorption defects such as coeliac disease, and a failure in the synthesis of prothrombin occurs in some cases of severe damage to the liver parenchyma.

Treatment

The congenital defects in this group are best combated with trans-fusions of fresh blood. Overdosage with coumarins can be corrected rapidly with fresh blood or with vitamin K_1, 10–30 mg. intravenously or orally.

CONGENITAL AFIBRINOGENAEMIA

Aetiology

This severe and rare disease is transmitted as an autosomal recessive characteristic, both sexes being equally affected. It has been suggested that some milder cases of fibrinogenopenia represent the heterozygous state.

Clinical Features

Severe haemorrhagic episodes may first appear in the neonatal period, e.g. in the form of haemorrhage from the umbilical cord. In other respects the clinical picture simulates that of haemophilia although haemarthrosis is rarely seen. The blood is completely incoagulable and a useful test is the complete absence of fibrin deposition in the plasma when it is heated to 56° C. The plasma fibrinogen level (normal 220–360 mg. per 100 ml.) is nil or grossly reduced.

The congenital condition has to be distinguished from the acute fibrinogenopenia which may occur when thromboplastic substances are liberated into the blood. This disaster is liable to occur in pregnancy as amniotic fluid has high thromboplastic activity, and in operations upon the lungs.

Treatment

Bleeding in congenital cases can be temporarily controlled by blood transfusion or by the transfusion of concentrated fibrinogen. In acquired cases the excess fibrinolysis can be controlled with epsilon-amino-caproic acid, 5–10 gm. in 25 per cent solution intravenously over one hour and followed by 2 gm. per hour for some hours (McNicol *et al.*, 1962).

THE LEUKAEMIAS
(see Chapter XI)

AGRANULOCYTOSIS

Aetiology

This is, fortunately, extremely uncommon in children. It may, of course, be part of other blood diseases such as hypoplastic anaemia. It may also complicate a severe or fulminating bacterial or virus infection. A few cases are "idiopathic". The majority, however, are due to an idiosyncrasy towards drugs of which a vast number are capable of causing agranulocytosis. In some cases the presence of antibodies towards a drug-leucocyte antigen (e.g. amidopyrine, sulphonamides) has been demonstrated. Other commonly used drugs include thiouracils, troxidone, phenytoin, potassium perchlorate, carbimazole, phenylbutazone, chloramphenicol and carbutamide.

Clinical Features

The onset is usually sudden with fever, severe toxaemia, limb pains, anorexia and vomiting, and sore throat. Severe necrotic and membranous lesions may affect the mouth and throat, less commonly the vulva or rectum. Jaundice and purpura are uncommon but do occur. The characteristic haematological finding is severe leucopenia with gross neutropenia. The red cells or platelets are also affected in some cases.

A chronic cyclical neutropenia has been described in a few children who suffered from recurrent attacks of mild infection and malaise.

In *primary splenic neutropenia* the marrow shows myeloid hyperplasia in spite of peripheral neutropenia, and there is usually splenomegaly (Wiseman and Doan, 1942).

Prognosis

Acute "idiopathic" or drug-induced cases carry a grave prognosis. The type associated with splenomegaly and maturation arrest in the marrow does better.

Treatment

The first essential is careful enquiry about possible drugs and their immediate withdrawal. Bacterial infection should be prevented with intramuscular penicillin; if already present a suitable antibiotic should be given in full doses. Chloramphenicol is completely contra-indicated. Drugs such as pentose nucleotide and folic acid are valueless. Pyridoxine (500 mg. per day intravenously) and corticosteroids in full doses may be of value. Blood transfusion is indicated only if there is anaemia. Splenectomy is only likely to be curative in cases with splenomegaly and myeloid marrow hyperplasia.

REFERENCES

ALDRICH, R. A., STEINBERG, A. G., and CAMPBELL, D. C. (1954). *Pediatrics*, **13**, 133.
ALLEN, D. M., and DIAMOND, L. K. (1961). *Amer. J. Dis. Child.*, **102**, 416.
BRITTON, C. J. C. (1963). *Disorders of the Blood*, 9th edit. London: J. & A. Churchill.
BYWATERS, E. G. L., ISDALE, I., and KEMPTON, J. J. (1957). *Quart. J. Med.*, **26**, 161.
CAFFEY, J. (1951). *Amer. J. Roentgenol.*, **65**, 547.
CATHIE, I. A. B. (1950). *Arch. Dis. Childh.*, **25**, 313.
CHERNOFF, A. (1955). *New Engl. J. Med.*, **253**, 322.
DACIE, J. V. (1960). *The Haemolytic Anaemias*, Part I, 2nd edit. London: J. & A. Churchill.
DACIE, J. V. (1962a). *The Haemolytic Anaemias*, Part II. London: J. & A. Churchill.
DACIE, J. V. (1962b). *Brit. med. J.*, **2**, 429.
DAUSSET, J., and BRECY, H. (1958). *Vox sang. (Basel)*, **3**, 197.
DIAMOND, L. K., ALLEN D. M., and MAGILL, F. B. (1961). *Amer. J. Dis. Child.*, **102**, 403.
DOUGLAS, A. S. (1962). *Anticoagulant Therapy*. Oxford: Blackwell Scientific Publications.
FULLERTON, H. W. (1937). *Arch. Dis. Childh.*, **12**, 91.

GAIRDNER, D. (1948). *Quart. J. Med.*, **17**, 95.
GAIRDNER, D. (1958). *Recent Advances in Paediatrics*, 2nd edit. London: J. & A. Churchill.
GAIRDNER, D., MARKS, J., and ROSCOE, J. D. (1952). *Arch. Dis. Childh.*, **27**, 128 & 214.
GASSER, C., GAUTIER, E., STECK, A., SIEBENMANN, R. E., and OECHSLIN, R. (1955). *Schweiz. med. Wschr.*, **85**, 905.
GORDON, R. R. (1960). *Arch. Dis. Childh.*, **35**, 259.
GRIFFITHS, J., and IRVING, K. G. (1961). *Arch. Dis. Childh.*, **36**, 500.
GUEST, G. M., and BROWN, E. W. (1957). *Amer. J. Dis. Child.*, **93**, 486.
HORAN, M. (1950). *Arch. Dis. Childh.*, **25**, 110.
HUTCHISON, J. H. (1938). *Arch. Dis. Childh.*, **13**, 355.
HUTCHISON, J. H., and MACARTHUR, P. (1949). *Lancet*, **1**, 916.
INGRAM, V. M. (1956). *Nature (Lond.)*, **178**, 792.
INGRAM, V. M. (1961). *Haemoglobin and its Abnormalities*. Springfield. Ill.: C. C. Thomas.
ITANO, H. A. (1953). *Arch. Biochem.*, **47**, 148.
JONES, T. G., GOLDSMITH, K. L. G., and ANDERSON, I. M. (1961). *Lancet*, **2**, 1008.
KAPLAN, E. (1959). *J. Pediat.*, **54**, 644.
KARAKLIS, A., VALAES, T., PANTELAKIS, S. N., and DOXIADIS, S. A. (1964). *Lancet*, **2**, 778.
KATES, M., ALLISON, A. C., and JAMES, A. T. (1961). *Biochim. biophys. Acta (Amst.)*, **48**, 571.
KING, H., and SCHUMACKER, A. B., Jr. (1952). *Ann. Surg.*, **136**, 239.
LAMBERT, H. P., PRANKERD, T. A. J., and SMELLIE, J. M. (1961). *Quart. J. Med.*, **30**, 71.
LOCK, S. P., and DORMANDY, K. M. (1961). *Lancet*, **1**, 1020.
LOWDON, A. G. R., WALKER, J. H., and WALKER, W. (1962). *Lancet*, **1**, 499.
McINTYRE, O. R., SULLIVAN, L. W., JEFFRIES, G. H., and SILVER, R. H. (1965). *New Engl. J. Med.*, **272**, 981.
MACKAY, H. M. M. (1931). *Spec. Rep. Ser. med. Res. Coun. (Lond.)*, No. 157.
MACKAY, H. M. M. (1933). *Arch. Dis. Childh.*, **8**, 221.
McKAY, E. (1962). *Arch. Dis. Childh.*, **37**, 663.
McNICHOL, G. P., FLETCHER, A. P., ALKJAERSIG, N., and SHERRY, S. (1962). *J. Lab. clin. Med.*, **59**, 15.
PAULING, L., ITANO, H. A., SINGER, S. J., and WELLS, I. C. (1949). *Science*, **110**, 543.
PRANKERD, T. A. J. (1959). *Brit. med. Bull.*, **15**, 54.
PRANKERD, T. A. J. (1960). *Quart. J. Med.*, **29**, 199.
PRANKERD, T. A. J. (1961). *The Red Cell: An Account of its Chemical Physiology and Pathology*. Oxford: Blackwell Scientific Publications.
RICHMOND, J. (1962). *Scot. med. J.*, **7**, 381.
RODRIGUEZ, S. U., LEIKEN, S. L., and HILLER, M. C., (1964). *New Engl. J. Med.*, **270**, 881.
SCHWARTZ, R., and DAMESHEK, W. (1962). *Blood*, **19**, 483.
SHAHIDI, N. T., and DIAMOND, L. A. (1961). *New Engl. J. Med.*, **264**, 953.
SINGER, K., CHERNOFF, A. I., and SINGER, I. (1951). *Blood*, **6**, 413.
SINGER, K. (1955). *Amer. J. Med.*, **18**, 631.
SMITH, E. W., and CONLEY, C. L. (1953). *Bull. Johns Hopk. Hosp.*, **93**, 94.
STRAUSS, M. B. (1933). *J. clin. Invest.*, **12**, 345.
VAN DE WIEL, T. W. M., VAN DE WIEL-DORFMEYER, H., and VAN LOGHEM, J. (1961). *Vox sang. (Basel)*, **6**, 641.
WIDDOWSON, E. M., and SPRAY, C. M. (1951). *Arch. Dis. Childh.*, **26**, 205.
WILMERS, M., and RUSSELL, P. (1963). *Lancet*, **2**, 915.
WISEMAN, B. K., and DOAN, C. A. (1942). *Ann. intern. Med.*, **16**, 1097.
ZUELZER, W. W., and OGDEN, F. N. (1946). *Amer. J. Dis. Child.*, **71**, 221.

CHAPTER XX

DISEASES OF THE NERVOUS SYSTEM

Many of the diseases with obvious neurological signs remain some-what of a mystery from the aetiological point of view. The necropsy findings are not always helpful in determining the primary disturbance which may have occurred months or years previously. Not surprisingly the treatment of such conditions is usually totally unsatisfactory. It is, therefore, proposed to deal with them rather briefly. On the other hand, some diseases of infective origin can now be cured provided diagnosis and treatment are established early, and these merit more detailed consideration. One of the most dramatic changes in medicine in the past 25 years has been our ability to cure diseases which used to strike terror into the hearts of parents (e.g. pyogenic and tuberculous meningitis) because of their frightful mortality rates. None the less, deaths and permanent brain damage still occur too frequently due to unnecessary delays in diagnosis or to inadequate treatment. Finally, some of the common diseases of the past, such as otogenic brain abscess, are now rarely encountered in children because of the efficient antibiotic treatment of otitis media and they hardly deserve attention in a book of this nature. A useful textbook for reference has been written by Ford (1960).

ACUTE INFECTIONS OF THE NERVOUS SYSTEM

ACUTE MENINGITIS

The common types of meningitis are pyogenic, aseptic and tuber-culous. Rare forms (not further considered here) are mycotic (torulosis, nocardiosis, histoplasmosis,) syphilitic, malarial and protozoal (toxo-plasmosis).

PYOGENIC MENINGITIS

Aetiology

Almost every bacterium is capable of infecting the meninges but only a few are common causes of pyogenic meningitis. Excluding the neonatal period (Chapter VI) the most common is the meningococcus. In infants and children a sporadic incidence is usual, but epidemics have frequently occurred in adults in army camps and the like. The disease is seen most commonly in the late winter and early spring. Next in frequency are cases due to *Haemophilus influenzae*; the disease is usually preceded by an upper respiratory infection. The common remaining meningeal infection is due to the pneumococcus; this may be secondary to pneumonia or upper respiratory infection but "primary" meningeal infections are not uncommon. In infants both staphylococcal and streptococcal meningitis are occasionally seen, most often secondary to infection elsewhere, e.g. bone, umbilicus, skin or middle ear. A meningomyelocele may also act as a portal of entry, especially after surgical treatment. Infections of the meninges due to Gram-negative bacteria are peculiar to the neonatal period (Chapter VI).

Clinical Features

The general symptomatology is common to all types of pyogenic meningitis and the causal organism is most often determined by examination of the cerebrospinal fluid. There are a few somewhat characteristic signs peculiar to meningococcal infections. The important one from the diagnostic point of view is a generalized purpuric rash ("spotted fever") although this is seen only in a minority of cases (Fig. 73). It is never seen in other types of meningitis. It may occur in fulminating cases of meningococcal septicaemia without meningitis or before it develops. It is also characteristic of meningococcal meningitis to develop suddenly and unheralded, whereas there is usually a preceding history of respiratory infection of some degree in cases due to the haemophilus or pneumococcus.

The onset of pyogenic meningitis itself is usually sudden with high fever, irritability, headache in older children, vomiting and general malaise. Convulsions are common. Young infants show tenseness and bulging of the anterior fontanelle, a most valuable sign of increased intracranial pressure, and head retraction is not uncommon. The older the child the more likely is there to be nuchal rigidity, but its absence in the baby by no means excludes the diagnosis. Kernig's sign is useful in older children and rarely observed in infants. We have found no value in Brudzinski's sign. Likewise *tâche cérébrale*, a linear wheal formed by drawing a finger nail or pencil across the skin, is of little real diagnostic significance. Blurring of consciousness of varying degree is the rule and increases in severity as the disease progresses. Focal neurological abnormalities such as paralytic squints, facial palsy or hemiplegia sometimes develop. Extreme restlessness and mental confusion are more common in older children and partly caused by the intense headache. Deafness due to damage to the auditory nerve is greatly to be feared because it is usually permanent. Papilloedema is infrequently found.

In infants the disease sometimes has a more insidious onset, especially in meningococcal cases, with diarrhoea and vomiting, irritability and "bogginess" of the anterior fontanelle. The diagnosis is easily missed, sometimes with grave consequences. The state of the anterior fontanelle is the vital clue to most cases in which other characteristic signs are absent.

Diagnosis

Lumbar puncture is indicated whenever the possibility of meningitis has crossed the physician's mind. In pyogenic cases the cerebrospinal fluid will be turbid or frankly purulent. The cell count varies from 1,000–10,000 per c. mm. The vast majority of cells are polymorphonuclears. Films of the centrifuged deposit may reveal Gram-negative intra- and extra-cellular diplococci in meningococcal cases, Gram-positive diplococci, often very numerous, in pneumococcal cases, and Gram-negative pleomorphic coccobacilli in cases due to haemophilus. The final cause is determined by culture. The protein content of the fluid is raised (above 40 mg. per 100 ml.), the sugar is greatly reduced (below 45 mg. per 100 ml.) and the chloride is reduced (below 650 mg. per 100 ml.).

Complications and sequelae

In the acute stage hydrocephalus may first develop, and thereafter progress or become arrested. Permanent brain damage with mental deficiency or spastic palsies are more common in the youngest infants, in part due to the greater difficulties and hence delay in diagnosis. Symptomatic epilepsy is less common. It may be assumed, however, that after the period of early infancy the persistence of a neurological deficit reflects either a delayed diagnosis or inadequate treatment. The possible exception to this is nerve deafness which can develop early in the illness and unpredictably.

Treatment

Pyogenic meningitis ought rarely to be fatal today. In meningococcal and pneumococcal cases both penicillin and sulphadiazine should be administered in full doses. Benzylpenicillin should be given intramuscularly every six hours in doses of 250,000–2,500,000 units according to age. Sulphadiazine should be given every four hours (100–150 mg./Kg./day), orally if the child can swallow, intramuscularly if vomiting is severe. When dehydration or severe vomiting necessitate intravenous fluid therapy with 5 per cent dextrose in half-strength physiological saline, the early doses of the drugs may be injected into the tubing. At the time of the first lumbar puncture it is our practice to inject 5,000–10,000 units of benzylpenicillin intrathecally. If the case turns out to be meningococcal further intrathecal therapy is unnecessary and undesirable. In pneumococcal cases daily intrathecal penicillin is given for 5–7 days, and thereafter at lengthening intervals until the cell count in the cerebrospinal fluid has fallen below 100 per c. mm. Some physicians dislike the use of intrathecal penicillin and rely upon a sufficient concentration crossing the blood-brain barrier by giving really massive doses intramuscularly. Provided the lumbar punctures are performed with full aseptic precautions, using proper needles with well-fitting stilettes, we prefer to give the antibiotic both intrathecally and intramuscularly. The antibacterial treatment must be continued for at least 10 days. In pneumococcal cases we frequently withdraw the sulphadiazine after 7–10 days and continue penicillin until the cerebrospinal fluid is almost normal; we then give a second course of sulphadiazine to obviate relapse which is not unknown in these cases.

When the causal organism is the haemophilus the therapeutic approach must be different. The most effective drug combination is chloramphenicol (150 mg./Kg./day) and sulphadiazine, each given six-hourly by mouth or intramuscular injection according to the state of the patient. In very severe cases it may be an advantage also to give streptomycin sulphate, 50 mg./Kg./day in two intramuscular doses, and 25–50 mg. daily by the intrathecal route.

When treatment is adequate a prompt improvement can usually be expected with subsidence of fever within 48–96 hours. If fever persists with continuing irritability and bulging of the fontanelle the presence of a subdural collection of fluid should be suspected. This is most commonly encountered in cases due to the haemophilus. This should be sought by subdural taps through the coronal suture on both sides. Evacuation of fluid may be required on several occasions before the accumulation of the xanthochromic protein-rich fluid stops. This complication of pyogenic meningitis was never seen by us in the pre-antibiotic era.

The child with meningitis requires a high standard of professional nursing and cannot be treated at home or in small ill-equipped hospitals. Anaemia may have to be corrected by blood transfusions. Convulsions are best controlled with intramuscular paraldehyde (0·15 ml./Kg.). It is our usual practice to perform lumbar punctures in older children under the influence of rectal thiopentone.

THE WATERHOUSE-FRIDERICHSEN SYNDROME

Acute bilateral adrenal apoplexy is most commonly seen in fulminating cases of meningococcal septicaemia. Death is usual before meningitis has had time to develop, and may, in fact, take place after an illness of only a few hours duration. The characteristic clinical picture (Arneil, 1946) is seen in an infant who suddenly becomes ill with irritability, vomiting and diarrhoea, and tachypnoea or Cheyne-Stokes breathing. The heart rate is very rapid. The infant becomes rapidly semi-comatose. Peripheral cyanosis is associated frequently with a patchy, purple mottling of the skin which resembles postmortem lividity. The child may die at this stage, about 6–8 hours from the onset of the illness. In less fulminating cases a diffuse purpuric and ecchymotic eruption appears which is very characteristic of meningococcal septicaemia (Fig. 73). The blood pressure may be so low as to be unrecordable. In the toddler the course of the illness tends on the whole to be less rapid than in the infant. The meningococcus is not always successfully isolated in blood cultures but can sometimes be cultured from the fluid contents of purpuric blebs on the skin. Indeed, the author has seen Gram-negative intracellular diplococci in ordinary blood films in a few cases, so overwhelming is the septicaemia.

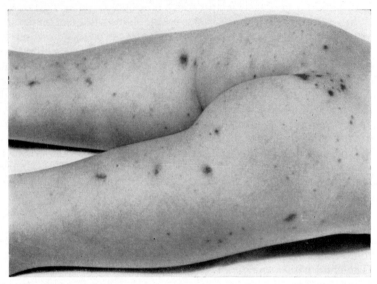

Fig. 73.—The typical purpuric and ecchymotic rash of meningococcal septicaemia. Some of the lesions may become necrotic with the formation of slowly healing ulcers.

Treatment

In cases where the adrenal cortex has been destroyed by haemorrhage recovery is impossible. In some cases of fulminating meningococcal septicaemia, however, there is intense congestion of the adrenal glands without much haemorrhage. It is in these cases, which are clinically indistinguishable from the fully-developed Waterhouse-Friderichsen syndrome, that energetic treatment can save life and lead to complete recovery. A continuous intravenous infusion of 5 per cent dextrose in half-strength physiological saline should be set up. The penicillin and sulphadiazine should be given by direct injection into the tubing as described above. Hydrocortisone hemi-succinate 100 mg. should be injected intravenously via the tubing at the start of treatment, to be followed by 50 mg. six-hourly for 24–48 hours; thereafter decreasing doses of cortisone are given orally for another few days.

ASEPTIC MENINGITIS (including Acute Poliomyelitis)

This disease presents a perennial problem. Sporadic cases occur throughout the year with annual outbreaks in summer and autumn.

From time to time sizable epidemics occur. Poliomyelitis is included under this heading because its precise diagnosis requires expert virological investigations, and other viruses can cause a clinically identical illness with meningitis and paralysis.

Aetiology

Many viruses can cause aseptic meningitis. These include poliomyelitis virus (Types 1, 2 and 3), Coxsackie virus, ECHO virus, the mouse virus of lymphocytic choriomeningitis, arbor viruses such as that of louping ill, and the viruses of mumps, herpes simplex, herpes zoster, measles, varicella, infective hepatitis and glandular fever. Mumps virus frequently causes meningitis without any of the other manifestations of this disease. Coxsackie virus can cause meningitis and paralysis which is indistinguishable clinically from classical poliomyelitis, and this can occur, of course, in persons who have been immunized against polio virus types 1–3. Non-viral agents which can cause aseptic meningitis include *leptospira* (*icterohaemorrhagiae* and *canicola*), *treponema pallidum, toxoplasma gondii* and *trichinella spiralis*.

Clinical Features

The onset is usually sudden with headache, muscle pains, anorexia, vomiting, malaise and diarrhoea or constipation. Fever is frequently above 102° F. In some cases, especially of poliomyelitis, there is a preceding illness about one week earlier with fever, headache, malaise, sore throat and abdominal pain. The temperature chart in such cases shows two "humps", sometimes called "the dromedary chart". The child may be drowsy, apathetic and irritable when disturbed, but blurring of consciousness is uncommon. Slight nuchal rigidity is usually found. Spinal stiffness is common, especially in poliomyelitis. This may result in the child being unable to kiss his knees when sitting up. Furthermore, he may have to support himself when sitting by placing his hands on the bed behind him, "the tripod sign". Kernig's sign is commonly present. In the infant the anterior fontanelle may be tense and full. In the older child a transient urinary incontinence is sometimes noted. Papilloedema is distinctly uncommon.

Lower motor neurone paralysis with loss of power, flaccidity and diminution or loss of deep reflexes may effect any of the voluntary muscle groups, being followed by a variable degree of recovery, or by muscle atrophy and ultimate shortening of the affected extremity. Deformities such as pes cavus, talipes or scoliosis may later become a problem of management. Life is endangered in cases of bulbar paralysis with inability to swallow and obstruction of the airway, and when the muscles of respiration are involved. When encephalitis is also present there may be serious disturbances of cerebration and focal signs such as spasticity, ataxia, intention tremor and sensory disturbances. Paralysis is only likely to develop in cases due to the poliomyelitis or Coxsackie viruses.

Diagnosis

The cerebrospinal fluid is clear or only slightly hazy. The cell count varies from 50–500 per c. mm. and the predominant cell is the lymphocyte. The total protein content is normal (20–40 mg. per 100 ml.) in the early stages although increased globulin is revealed by a positive Pandy test. Subsequently there is often a rise in total protein to 200–300 mg. per 100 ml. while the cell count falls, a dissociation between protein and cells which is particularly frequent in poliomyelitis. The sugar and chloride levels are normal and cultures remain sterile. The viral aetiology can often be determined by culture of the stools in monkey kidney, human amnion, or human thyroid or by injection into suckling mice. The serum (at least two specimens taken with a ten-day interval) may be tested for neutralizing antibody or complement fixation in rising titre.

Treatment

In non-paralytic cases, the great majority, spontaneous recovery rapidly follows the diagnostic lumbar puncture. Symptomatic measures to relieve fever, headache or muscle pain are required but there is no specific treatment. The child should be isolated from other patients. A careful watch for paralysis must be maintained.

When there is paralysis the first requirement is to prevent stretching of the muscles by keeping the limb in a neutral position with suitable splinting and padding. Passive movements under expert physiotherapists are helpful, followed soon by carefully graded active movements. In the case with severe muscle spasm, warm compresses and hot packs bring relief. The orthopaedist should be brought into the management at an early stage. When there is bulbar palsy the patient is best placed in the prone position with head lower than feet. Pharyngeal suction should be performed at frequent intervals. In the worst cases tracheostomy followed by intermittent positive pressure respiration is required. This should be undertaken in centres experienced and fully equipped for such an arduous but life-saving method of treatment. This regime is also preferred by many to the tank type of respirator (iron-lung) for cases of pure respiratory paralysis. In such cases a broad spectrum antibiotic is also necessary to combat the risks of secondary bacterial infection in the poorly ventilated lungs. The prognosis in bulbar and respiratory cases has been enormously improved in recent years but their management demands a high standard of medical and nursing care, the full details of which can only be learned in a special centre.

TUBERCULOUS MENINGITIS
(see Chapter X)

ACUTE ENCEPHALITIS

The term "encephalitis" is often used to include organic disturbances of the brain which are poorly understood, in addition to its correct use in describing infections affecting the brain substance. The difficulty of nomenclature can partly be resolved by the use of the term "encephalopathy", but it will remain until further knowledge is acquired as to the varied noxious influences which can damage the nervous system.

Aetiology

All of the viruses mentioned in connection with aseptic meningitis can cause acute encephalitis. Others include influenza virus, cytomegalic inclusion disease in infancy (Chapter IV), and the viruses of rabies, encephalitis lethargica, and the zymotic diseases such as measles and varicella. In addition to the viral encephalitis which may occur early in the infectious fevers such as measles, rubella, chickenpox and smallpox, an encephalitic illness of later onset may occur during the period of recovery. This is characterized histologically by extensive demyelination in the brain substance and the pathogenesis has been postulated to be an antigen-antibody reaction of some type, the damaged brain tissue having acquired antigenic properties. There remains further an ill-defined condition which simulates viral encephalitis clinically but in which the cerebrospinal fluid does not show an increase in cells or protein and which has been called "acute toxic encephalopathy". It is frequently fatal and significant histological findings are remarkably inconspicuous (Lyon et al., 1961). It may complicate upper respiratory infections, the infectious fevers, and has followed the use of pertussis vaccine.

Clinical Features

These are extremely protean. The disturbances of cerebration vary from the gradual onset of stupor or coma to the sudden onset of violent convulsions. Headache, irritability, mental confusion or abnormal behaviour may be marked. Focal neurological signs of many kinds are encountered such as cranial nerve palsies, speech disturbances, spastic palsies, cerebellar disturbances and abnormalities in the various reflexes. Spastic paraplegia with urinary incontinence or retention indicates spinal cord involvement. In most cases the cerebrospinal fluid shows a mild pleocytosis and increase in protein. Virological studies are often successful in determining the causal agent.

The outcome is always doubtful. Death is not uncommon, but many cases end in complete recovery. Others are left with permanent disability such as mental deterioration, hemiplegia or paraplegia, and epilepsy. In some children an apparently good recovery is followed later by learning difficulties or behaviour problems.

Treatment

Apart from general nursing measures it is open to doubt whether any treatment significantly influences the outcome. Convulsions must be controlled with intramuscular paraldehyde and the oral use of anti-convulsant drugs (p. 443). A clear airway must be ensured in the coma-tose patient by nursing him head lower than feet in the semi-prone position, and by frequent pharyngeal suction. Rarely a tracheostomy is required. Frequently tube-feeding or intravenous fluids are indicated. The electrolyte balance must be maintained. In post-infectious cases corticosteroids such as prednisolone or dexamethasone are worth a trial on the assumption that this is an allergic form of encephalitis. Their value is, however, difficult to assess in individual patients.

ACUTE INFECTIVE POLYNEURITIS

(Guillain-Barré Syndrome)

Aetiology

This condition must be distinguished from the polyneuritis of diphtheria and from the rare polyneuritis due to lead poisoning or drug intoxications. The disease has been assumed to have a viral origin although no specific virus has been identified. A similar condition in-frequently complicates glandular fever (Chapter X). A preceding upper respiratory infection is common. The pathological changes are poorly defined but the disease may, in fact, be more accurately regarded as a polyradiculitis affecting both the anterior and posterior spinal roots.

Clinical Features

After an upper respiratory febrile illness the child develops increasing muscular weakness and tenderness with loss of the deep reflexes. The proximal muscles of the limbs and those of the trunk are more severely affected than the distal musculature. Muscle atrophy is often remarkably slight. Sensory changes tend to be minimal. Their distribution seems to correspond more to the dermatomes than to the peripheral nerves. Intercostal and diaphragmatic paralysis may endanger life. Bilateral facial paralysis is common but bulbar palsy is rare. Tachycardia and cardiomegaly may be present. In the typical Guillain-Barré syndrome the cerebrospinal fluid shows a high protein content with little or no pleocytosis, but these changes are inconstant and may be late in ap-pearing. If death from respiratory paralysis or intercurrent respiratory infection can be avoided the child usually makes a slow but complete recovery over a period of months. _Landry's acute ascending paralysis_ is sometimes a variant of this disease, although other cases are due to acute poliomyelitis.

Treatment

The influence of ACTH or corticosteroids is difficult to assess. These hormones should only be used in advancing cases with a poor prognosis. Respiratory paralysis may require the use of a tank type of respirator. Physiotherapy is useful during convalescence.

ACUTE CEREBELLAR ATAXIA

Aetiology

Cerebellar ataxia is a common phenomenon in young children. There are many clearly defined causes, e.g. infratentorial tumours, post-infective encephalitis, otogenic cerebellar abscess (now very rare), and the various leucodystrophies and hereditary types of cerebellar ataxia. These are not included under the term "acute cerebellar ataxia" which refers to cases of sudden onset and unknown causation (Shanks, 1950). A virus has been suggested but never proved. The same applies to the idea of an allergic response to a virus infection.

Clinical Features

In the typical case the onset of cerebellar signs in a child aged 2–5 years is sudden. There may have been a preceding upper respiratory infection but its significance is difficult to assess. The principal feature is the typical reeling ataxia. There may be a tremor or wobble of the head. Hypotonia is common and the deep reflexes may be diminished. The child may be irritable or abnormal in personality but there is no blurring of consciousness. Other cerebellar signs may be elicited, e.g. nystagmus, intention tremor, dysmetria or disturbance of speech. The ocular fundi are normal. Vomiting may occur but there are no other indications of an increase in intracranial pressure. The cerebrospinal fluid is usually normal.

The differential diagnosis from the other causes of cerebellar ataxia (see above) is essential and usually possible on careful assessment of the history and physical findings. Air-ventriculography should be performed by a neurosurgeon if there is still suspicion of a tumour.

In most instances complete recovery can be expected within a period of weeks. A few cases, often those with an insidious onset, progress steadily but it is likely that they are of different aetiology, possibly in the spino-cerebellar ataxia group.

Treatment

Symptomatic measures only are possible

ACUTE INFANTILE HEMIPLEGIA

Aetiology

This is a characteristic clinical syndrome seen in both infants and children and perhaps better called "acute hemiplegia in childhood". Most cases are associated with a preceding pyrexial illness such as tonsillitis, cervical adenitis, tooth infection or sometimes tonsillectomy. As the disease is rarely fatal the aetiology has remained uncertain. It has most often been attributed to cortical thrombophlebitis although the affected children have not shown the spreading bilateral involvement and papilloedema to be expected with this pathology. Internal carotid arteriography after the acute illness has subsided has usually shown no abnormality. However, Bickerstaff (1964) has clearly demonstrated in cases investigated within a few days of the onset the presence of abnormalities in the internal carotid and first part of the middle cerebral arteries. These have ranged from complete occlusion to very marked narrowing of the lumen of the carotid and its branches, and in other cases there have been irregularities of the lumen. A good case is made out that this arterial obstruction is the consequence of an inflammatory arteritis of the carotid following throat or neck gland infection.

This syndrome does not, of course, include cases of congenital hemiplegia, brain tumour, otogenic encephalitis (now rarely seen), encephalitis following the infectious fevers or the results of trauma.

Clinical Features

The disease may present in one of two ways. In the more common, the child suddenly goes into status epilepticus with high fever and deep coma. The convulsions may be generalized or unilateral. After some hours or days of critical illness the fits cease and consciousness slowly returns. Hemiplegia is then found to be present, with dysphasia in right-sided cases. The upper motor neurone weakness and spasticity affect principally the face and arm, and recovery in the leg precedes and exceeds that of the arm.

In the second mode of presentation the child, after a recent febrile illness, suddenly develops a hemiplegia, with or without dysphasia; convulsions do not occur and if there is loss of consciousness it is of short duration.

In either type of case signs of recovery are obvious after a week or two although the hemiplegia rarely completely disappears. Intelligence may be unimpaired although in some cases serious mental retardation or epilepsy persist permanently. If the hemiplegia remains severe defective growth and shortening of the arm and leg result.

The cerebrospinal fluid shows no abnormality at the inception of the illness but some days later a slight rise in cells and protein may develop.

Later on air encephalography shows enlargement of the ventricle on the affected side of the brain with displacement of the ventricular system to that side and enlargement of the sulci. This atrophic change is, in fact, most marked in the territory supplied by the middle cerebral artery, but sometimes it is also seen in the territory of the anterior cerebral artery. The posterior part of the hemisphere is rarely affected.

Treatment

Other causes of convulsions such as meningitis and encephalitis should be excluded by early lumbar puncture. Status epilepticus is best treated with intramuscular paraldehyde (0·15 ml./Kg. = 1 ml. per stone) repeated as necessary. Persisting tonsillar or dental sepsis should be treated with intramuscular benzylpenicillin. The consequences of the disease can be so disastrous that careful consideration should be given to the use of anticoagulants although their value in carotid artery disease is very much open to doubt. Unfortunately, the clinical syndrome develops so quickly in most cases that maximal damage has already occurred before anticoagulants can be administered. Bickerstaff (1964) has suggested that the damage might be limited by the use of hypothermia, and where carotid angiography shows marked oedema of the hemisphere by intravenous hypertonic urea. During the stage of recovery physiotherapy is valuable.

THE PROGRESSIVE DEGENERATIVE DISEASES

This is a "mixed bag" of diseases most of which are not amenable to treatment. They are uncommon in everyday practice and they will receive only short discussion.

SCHILDER'S DISEASE

(Encephalitis periaxialis diffusa)

The cause of this extensive cerebral demyelinating process is unknown. The onset is usually between the ages of 5 and 13 years and the disease results in progressive dementia and decerebrate rigidity. If the occipital lobes are first affected, visual field defects and later cortical blindness are the initial features. Equally often the onset is with spastic palsies of various distribution but ultimately affecting the whole body and all four limbs. Aphasia, convulsive seizures, dementia, pseudo-bulbar palsy, emotional lability may all develop in varying degree. Increased intracranial pressure with bilateral sixth nerve palsies, papilloedema, and cerebral vomiting are seen in some cases. In others there is a true optic neuritis. The cerebrospinal fluid may be normal or show a mild pleocytosis and increase of protein. Remissions rarely occur and death takes place within a year or two. There is no effective treatment.

THE LEUCODYSTROPHIES *(Cerebral sclerosis)*

This group of diseases, some of which are familial, is poorly understood. Some have regarded them as allied to Schilder's disease, others
as allied to the lipoidoses (Chapter XII). The most common is the
familial *cerebral sclerosis of Krabbe* in which there is extensive degeneration of the white matter. Symptoms start between the ages of 4
and 6 months with incessant crying followed by apathy. Generalized
muscular rigidity is marked and seizures occur with head retraction and
extension of the arms and legs. There may also be generalized clonic
convulsions. Feeding must soon be carried out by tube. Blindness may
develop with or without optic atrophy. The blood lipids may be elevated.
Death occurs within a year.

In the *cerebral sclerosis of Greenfield* the brain shows, in addition to
extensive demyelination, numerous deposits of galacto-lipids which
stain metachromatically with toluidine blue. The onset is during the
second or third years of life with weakness of the arms and legs, either
spastic or flaccid, ataxia, squints, ptosis, nystagmus and ultimate
mental deterioration. Convulsions may occur. In a few cases the
diagnosis has been confirmed during life by demonstrating granules in
the urine which show metachromatic staining with toluidine or methylene blue (Austin, 1957).

Another strongly familial type is the *cerebral sclerosis of Pelizaeus-
Merzbacher* in which degeneration of the white substance is progressive.
The symptoms start in infancy with rotary nystagmus and later spasticity of the legs followed by the arms. Ataxia, intention tremor, and
scanning speech then make their appearance. After some years there is
gross mental deterioration. There may later be choreo-athetosis or
Parkinsonism. Remissions are common and death may be delayed
until middle age. In all of these degenerative disorders specific diagnosis
usually must await postmortem examination.

FRIEDREICH'S ATAXIA

This disease may be inherited either as a recessive or a dominant
trait. It makes its appearance in childhood and before puberty with pes
cavus, kyphoscoliosis and some degree of ataxia. There is evidence of
damage to the spino-cerebellar tracts (e.g. ataxia, nystagmus, intention
tremor) and the dorsal columns (e.g. absent deep reflexes and loss of
vibration and postural sensation). Degeneration of the pyramidal tracts
results in extensor plantar responses. Optic atrophy and dysarthria
may appear late in the course of the disease, and occasionally there is
mental deterioration. Cardiac manifestations also occur due to an
interstitial myocarditis, e.g. tachycardia, systolic murmurs and S-T
changes in the ECG. Death may be delayed for 10–15 years, but it may
occur earlier from cardiac failure. There is no specific treatment, but

orthopaedic measures may be helpful. Several other rare types of hereditary cerebellar ataxia have also been described.

HEREDITARY SPASTIC PARAPLEGIA

This condition may be inherited as a dominant, recessive or sex-linked recessive disease. It is characterized by the onset during childhood of progressive uncomplicated spastic paraplegia. Severe flexion deformities may develop. The diagnosis rests upon the family history.

WERDNIG-HOFFMANN PROGRESSIVE SPINAL PARALYSIS

This is a relatively common disease of infancy inherited as a recessive trait and showing a marked familial incidence. The principal pathological feature is progressive loss of the motor neurones in the anterior horns of the spinal cord. The disease may be present at birth or appear within a few weeks. There is flaccidity and weakness of the muscles of the trunk and limbs. The proximal muscles tend to be more severely paralysed than the distal. The deep reflexes are absent or soon disappear. When the intercostal and other accessory muscles of respiration become affected dyspnoea and inspiratory intercostal recession develop. In due course involvement of the diaphragm renders the infant extremely prone to respiratory infections, one of which ultimately proves fatal. The loss of power to suck further aggravates the terminal stages of the illness. Life is rarely prolonged beyond the age of 5 years. There is no specific treatment.

The term *amyotonia congenita* is best abandoned. It implies only a "floppy infant" for which there are many causes in addition to Werdnig-Hoffmann disease. These include Tay-Sachs disease (Chapter XII), flaccid diplegia (Chapter XXI), infantile myasthenia gravis (Chapter XXIV), and idiopathic hypercalcaemia (Chapter XXV). None of these conditions should be difficult to distinguish from Werdnig-Hoffmann disease.

The principal difficulty is to differentiate Werdnig-Hoffmann disease from *benign infantile hypotonia* (Walton, 1957). Here too, extreme hypotonia dates from or soon after birth. The deep reflexes although very sluggish can usually be elicited and muscle fibrillations, commonly seen in Werdnig-Hoffmann disease, do not occur. The true diagnosis in benign infantile hypotonia becomes clear with the passage of time (5–9 years), when slow but not always complete recovery takes place. Muscle biopsy reveals the atrophy of denervation in Werdnig-Hoffmann disease, but the appearances remain normal in benign infantile hypotonia.

CHARCOT-MARIE-TOOTH PERONEAL MUSCULAR ATROPHY

This rare disease may be transmitted as a dominant, recessive or sex-linked recessive characteristic. It starts with progressive weakness and lower motor neurone type of flaccid atrophy of the peroneal and tibial muscles and of the small muscles of the feet. The result is paralytic talipes equino-varus. Later wasting of the calf muscles gives the legs an odd inverted wine bottle appearance. At a late stage weakness and wasting affect the hands and forearms. The disease rarely extends above the knees. The ankle-jerks are lost but the knee-jerks remain brisk. Some loss of vibration and positional sensation is common. Optic atrophy has been described in adult life.

KINNEAR WILSON'S DISEASE
(Hepatolenticular Cirrhosis)
Aetiology

This disease, inherited as an autosomal recessive is an inborn error of metabolism (Chapter IX), in which there is an excessive accumulation of copper in the brain, liver, cornea and other tissues. There is also an increased absorption of copper from the intestine and a lowered level of caeruloplasmin (the copper-binding protein of the serum). The pathogenesis has been reviewed by Walshe (1959), Stanbury et al. (1965) and Walshe and Cumings (1961).

Clinical Features

These develop in childhood or adolescence. In many cases they are predominantly neurological, e.g. coarse and sometimes bizarre tremors which may simulate severe chorea, extreme emotional instability with bouts of laughing and weeping, dysarthria, difficulty in swallowing and dementia. A characteristic finding is the Kayser-Fleischer ring, a golden-brown discoloration due to deposition of copper at the corneal limbus. In recent years it has been increasingly recognized that Wilson's disease may present with solely or predominantly hepatic manifestations, e.g. jaundice, hepatomegaly, ascites or haematemesis due to portal hypertension. Indeed, Wilson's disease should be considered in all children with prolonged jaundice or obscure hepatomegaly (Walshe, 1962).

Diagnosis

The most characteristic findings are a greatly excessive urinary output of copper and a reduced serum level of caeruloplasmin. Other common findings are disordered liver functions tests, amino-aciduria and portal cirrhosis in a liver biopsy.

Treatment

Marked improvement can be achieved by the mobilization of copper from the tissues with various chelating agents. The first to be used was dimercaprol (BAL) which has to be given parenterally. The most useful is penicillamine which is active when given by mouth in doses of 0·9–1·2 gm./day in three equal amounts. It should be given in the form of D-penicillamine. A low-copper diet (excluding cocoa, nuts, liver, shell-fish, mushrooms and spinach) is also advised. Copper absorption may further be reduced with potassium sulphide, 20 mg. thrice daily, which forms insoluble copper sulphide in the gut.

ATAXIA-TELANGIECTASIA (LOUIS-BAR SYNDROME)

This condition has now been defined as a specific entity (Boder and Sedgwick, 1963), probably transmitted as an autosomal recessive characteristic. The clinical features are diagnostic when fully developed. The first to appear is a progressive cerebellar ataxia in the course of the second or third year of life, occasionally even earlier. There may be, in addition, choreo-athetotic movements and a tendency to turn the eyes upwards when focusing (Smeby, 1966). Telangiectases make their appearance between the ages of 3 and 7 years. They are found on the bulbar conjunctiva, malar eminences, ears, antecubital fossae and elsewhere. Patches of poorly pigmented skin are often present over the face and neck but the hair is not affected. These children suffer severely from infections of the sinuses and lungs; indeed, bronchiectasis is a frequent cause of death. In other cases death has been due to malignant disease (e.g. lymphosarcoma). A constant feature of all the investigated cases, and one which explains the extreme susceptibility to severe sino-pulmonary infection, is absence or gross reduction in the serum IgA (B2A) globulin. Occasionally there has been a total gamma globulin deficiency (Peterson et al., 1964). Post-mortem examination has usually revealed absence of the thymus, or one of extremely small size and abnormal cellular content which resembles that of the foetal thymus before lymphoid induction. There is no specific treatment yet available. Infection should be controlled with suitable antibiotics. Malignant change might be temporarily altered with corticosteroids.

THE PHAKOMATOSES

TUBEROUS SCLEROSIS (Epiloia)

This is a hereditary disease transmitted as a dominant trait. It is characterized in its fully developed form by mental deficiency, epileptic seizures and a rash of butterfly distribution and papular character on the face and nose (adenoma sebaceum). Other skin lesions include "shagreen" patches and café-au-lait spots. In some cases there are teratomata or hamartomata of the kidneys, liver and lung. The heart may be the seat of a rhabdomyoma. Radiologically visible intracranial calcification may be found and is due to the presence of nodular masses in the brain (phakomata). This disease is probably akin to neuro-fibromatosis described below.

NEUROFIBROMATOSIS (von Recklinghausen's Disease)

This hereditary disease is also transmitted as a dominant characteristic. In childhood a progressive and severe kyphoscoliosis in association with multiple *café-au-lait* spots on the skin is a common mode of presentation. In some cases palpable neurofibromata are to be detected along the course of subcutaneous nerves. Osteitis fibrosa cystica (without hyperparathyroidism) may show as the presence of multiple cystic areas in radiographs of bones. The brain may be the site of formation of nodules similar to those found in tuberous sclerosis.

THE STURGE-WEBER SYNDROME

In this disease there is an association between an extensive cutaneous port-wine haemangioma of the upper face and scalp, which is strictly limited by the mid-line, and a similar vascular anomaly of the underlying meninges on the same side. The infant usually starts to have convulsions confined to the contralateral side of the body. The cause is obvious from the distribution of the facial haemangioma (Fig. 74). In time a spastic hemiparesis develops on the contralateral side. Later in childhood, but rarely in infancy, radiographs of the skull show a characteristic double contour or "tram-line" type of calcification (Fig. 75). Mental deterioration ultimately appears and progresses. Glaucoma may also develop and require surgical intervention. The mode of inheritance of this disease is not clear, but the author has seen an affected child whose father suffered from typical neurofibromatosis.

VON HIPPEL-LINDAU DISEASE

This is a rare genetically determined combination of haemangiomatous cystic changes in the retina and cerebellum, sometimes also in kidney, liver and pancreas. It may present with the signs of a cerebellar tumour or with loss of vision due to retinal detachment. Surgical intervention on both the cerebellum and retina is sometimes successful.

HYDROCEPHALUS

Aetiology

Hydrocephalus is due to an excessive volume of cerebrospinal fluid and it is associated with increased intracranial pressure. It may be due to congenital causes such as the Arnold-Chiari malformation in spina

FIG. 74 (*see opposite*).—Capillary haemangioma in trigeminal area of face and scalp. Associated with convulsions and mental retardation due to haemangioma of meninges—Sturge-Weber syndrome.

FIG. 75 (*see opposite*).—Radiograph of skull of child shown in Fig. 74. Note intracranial calcification in occipital area—Sturge-Weber syndrome.

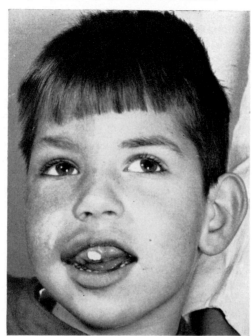

FIG. 74.

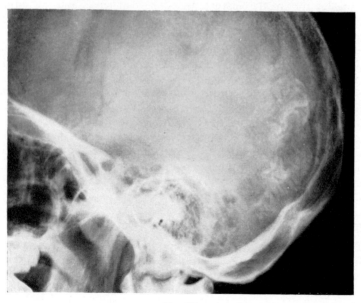

FIG. 75.

bifida cystica (see below), stenosis or forking of the aqueduct of Sylvius, atresia of the foramina of Magendie and Luschka, failure of development of the basal subarachnoid cisterns, and congenital toxoplasmosis. Rarely the disease is inherited as a recessive sex-linked condition (Edwards *et al.*, 1961). Acquired causes of hydrocephalus include the reactions of the meninges to pyogenic or tuberculous meningitis, intracranial tumours, intracranial haemorrhage at birth, metastatic tumours and brain abscess. In non-communicating hydrocephalus a dye such as phenolsulphonphthalein, when injected into one of the greatly dilated ventricles, fails to reach the subarachnoid space. When communication exists between the fourth ventricle and the subarachnoid space the hydrocephalus is of the communicating type. The distinction is important in relation to surgical treatment. The reader is referred for fuller details to Dorothy Russell's (1949) work on this condition.

Clinical Features

The appearance and size of the head are related more to the age of onset of the hydrocephalus than to its cause. Thus, hydrocephalus can obstruct the course of labour. In most cases the hydrocephalus only appears after birth. In infancy it causes a progressive enlargement of the head which assumes a globular shape with over-hanging forehead and disproportionately small face. The increasing enlargement should be assessed by regular measurements of the skull circumference. The fontanelles are greatly enlarged and somewhat tense, and the sutures may gape widely. Dilated veins are often prominent over the scalp. The eyeballs tend to be pushed downwards so that a rim of sclera is visible between the iris and upper eyelid. Neurological manifestations include squints, optic atrophy, and spastic paraplegia or quadriplegia. The degree of mental retardation is variable and not closely related to the thickness of the cerebral cortex. In severe cases failure to thrive and marasmus are common.

When the obstruction to the cerebrospinal fluid pathway occurs later in childhood there may be little or no enlargement of the head, but there will then be such signs of increased intracranial pressure as headache, cerebral vomiting, a cracked pot sound on percussion of the skull, papilloedema, and radiographic changes in the bones of the vault (Fig. 36).

Differential Diagnosis

This is rarely difficult. The most important differentiation in infancy is from chronic subdural haematoma (Chapter III), because the latter condition is eminently curable. Subdural taps should always be performed in doubtful cases. In the rare disorder called *macrocephaly* there is generalized enlargement of the brain although the child is mentally defective. It can be differentiated from hydrocephalus by pneumo-encephalography.

Treatment

It is essential to realize that about 40 per cent of all cases of hydro-cephalus in infancy undergo spontaneous arrest (Laurence and Coates, 1962). Surgical treatment should probably be confined to cases in which serial measurements of head circumference show progressive and rapid enlargement. Hydrocephalus develops in about 80 per cent of cases of meningomyelocele (Lorber, 1961), especially when the site is dorso-lumbar. It can be diagnosed by ventriculography in the early weeks of life and before the head enlarges. It is probably not influenced by repair of the meningomyelocele. Operation is indicated in all but the mildest cases of this nature. Operation must always be preceded by detailed investigations to confirm the diagnosis beyond doubt and to demonstrate the type of hydrocephalus. These include air-encephalography or air-ventriculography, and the intraventricular injection of phenol-sulphonphthalein. Many surgical manoeuvres have been devised for this disease (Scarff, 1963). The most popular are perhaps ventriculo-peritoneal drainage, and the use of the Spitz-Holter valve to drain cerebrospinal fluid from the lateral ventricle into the superior vena cava or atrium. Torkildsen's operation drains cerebrospinal fluid from the ventricle to the cisterna magna, but it is only practicable in carefully chosen cases. In all operations involving plastic tubes or silicone valves there is a likelihood of later obstruction to the flow of fluid. There is also a risk of chronic bacteraemia from colonization of the valve or tube. It is notoriously difficult to assess the long-term results of operations for hydrocephalus. Undoubtedly they should be undertaken only by ex-perienced surgeons working in large centres (Macnab, 1958).

CONGENITAL ANOMALIES OF THE C.N.S. AND ADJACENT STRUCTURES

This group includes defects of the cephalic end of the neural tube with failure of development of the cerebrum—*anencephaly*—and of the caudal end with deficiencies in the spine and spinal cord. Many of the more gross abnormalities are incompatible with life and will not receive further discussion here. A good account has been given by Morison (1963). We will discuss only those anomalies in which surgical correction or amelioration is frequently possible.

DEFECTS IN THE SKULL

These are *meningocele* in which meninges only protrude through a bony defect, *encephalocele* in which both meninges and brain tissue protrude, and *hydroencephalocele* in which the hernial sac also contains part of the ventricular system. These defects associated with cranium bifidum are almost always in the mid-line somewhere between the bridge of the nose and the foramen magnum. Some such herniations can occur into the orbit or into the pharynx. Those situated most posteriorly in the suboccipital region are most likely to be amenable to surgery. Only a minority of these defects offers much hope of surgical cure (Ingraham, 1944).

SPINAL DEFECTS

A simple defect in the neural arches of one or more vertebrae is relatively common and in itself of no importance—*spina bifida occulta*. When a bony defect is associated with an abnormality of the meninges or spinal cord a much more serious situation arises—*spina bifida cystica*. Indeed this is one of the important causes of perinatal mortality. In its most benign form only the mesoderm which forms the vertebral column is defective and a portion of dura and arachnoid protrude through the defect—*meningocele*. The spinal cord is usually in its normal position. The meningocele appears as a fluctuant swelling, variable in size, covered by intact true skin, and situated anywhere between the cervical and sacral area. Simple meningoceles are not associated with any neurological deficits. When the defect of the mesoderm is accompanied by an ectodermal defect as well, the neural tube (of ectodermal origin) has remained in contact at some area with the surface ectoderm and it is adherent to the wall of the hernial sac; this is a *myelomeningocele*. The nerve roots from the involved section of the spinal cord are present in the meningeal sac which in myelomeningocele is nearly always in the lumbo-dorsal region. This means that the terminal portion of the spinal cord and the roots of the cauda equina are involved. Clinically the sac shows ulceration because it is covered by neuroepithelium instead of true skin. This covering is thin, transparent and very liable to break down with consequent leakage of cerebrospinal fluid and bacterial sepsis. Until very recent years over 90 per cent of babies born with myelomeningocele died of meningitis, progressive hydrocephalus or the complications of flaccid paraplegia. Only one infant in a hundred grew to live a normal life. However, development of methods to control the hydrocephalus by ventriculocardiac drainage has completely altered this grim picture, *provided that closure of the spina bifida cystica is performed as an emergency procedure within 12–24 hours of birth*. Nowadays in the best centres 70 per cent of affected infants survive. Of these, about one third have normal or only mildly paralysed legs; one third have a coincidental myelodysplasia with flaccid paralysis, but of a degree compatible with the ability to walk after corrective orthopaedic measures; and in the remaining third severe flaccid or mixed paraplegia demands either splintage or a wheelchair. Most of these children have a measure of bladder paralysis. This should be suspected in the newborn if there is continuous dribbling of urine when the infant is picked up by the armpits. Unless this condition is treated early the neurogenic bladder leads soon to back pressure, bilateral hydroureteronephrosis and urinary infection. Nearly all children with myelomeningocele also have some degree of bowel paralysis, and its presence would be suggested by a patulous toneless anus. An even more severe lesion is called a *myelocele* where the spinal cord lies exposed on the surface as a ribbon of disorganized neural tissue. This is, in fact, very rare and it is incompatible with life. *Always do IVP as ?, associated renal anomaly*

The Arnold-Chiari malformation.—This is found only in association with myelomeningocele and it is invariably complicated by hydrocephalus which may be obvious at birth or develop after some months. It is frequently the ultimate cause of death in these infants after apparently successful surgical treatment of the spina bifida unless early measures are taken to arrest its progress. The actual malformation consists of two prolongations of the cerebellum down over a greatly elongated medulla oblongata. Indeed a large portion of the medulla lies below the foramen magnum through which also pass the tongue-like cerebellar projections.

Treatment

The results of operation in the pure meningocele are excellent. In this type of spina bifida cystica, which is relatively uncommon, the sac is completely covered by normal skin and there is no neurological deficit. Surgical operation is not urgent and may be left for eight months or thereabouts.

In myelomeningocele, the most common variety of spina bifida cystica, the position is very different. Here the sac is covered with papery thin neuroepithelium which readily ulcerates with leakage of cerebrospinal fluid. Not only is there a grave risk of pyogenic meningitis, but there is good evidence that any neurological deficit can rapidly worsen as the contents of the sac are exposed to the air after the infant's birth (Sharrard *et al.*, 1963). The outlook for these unfortunate infants has been transformed by emergency operation to close the defect in skin and meninges within 24 hours of birth (Eckstein and Macnab, 1966). *"decapping"* About 80 per cent of infants with myelomeningocele have a significant degree of hydrocephalus. About a half of these will require ventriculo-cardiac drainage, using the Spitz-Holter valve, during the neonatal period (first month); many of the others will require this operation during the next six months. A few will require a second operation for the insertion of a new valve, but control of the hydrocephalus now ensures that most of the surviving children are of normal intelligence.

Every infant operated upon for myelomeningocele should have the urinary tract examined by intravenous pyelography during the first month of life. The major threat to life lies in the risk of pyelonephritis so that the urine should be examined regularly for significant pyuria and bacteriuria. It is frequently possible in infants of both sexes to avoid serious back pressure effects by instructing the parents in the technique of manual bladder expression. Ultimately all the girls and some of the boys will require urinary diversion operations such as uretero-ileostomy. In other boys resection of the bladder neck followed by the fitting of a suitable urinal is preferred. The best surgical procedures for urinary incontinence due to neurogenic bladder are still being investigated, but surgery of this sort is usually delayed until the child is over two years of age. During this period intravenous pyelography and cystography may be necessary on several occasions. Control of the bowel is usually easier, with the help of laxatives and occasional bowel washouts. Minor surgery may be required for rectal prolapse.

Another major long-term concern is the management of lower limb deformity and paralysis. When closure of the spinal lesion is carried out as an emergency procedure a few hours after birth about 30 per cent of the survivors will have only minimal or no lower limb paralysis. The remainder, however, have some paralysis, and this may be complete or severe. In the last group there may be, in addition, lower limb deformity caused by intra-uterine pressure on the paralysed extremities. It follows that many orthopaedic measures may be required in the individual child. These vary from the fitting of suitable splints and braces, instruction in walking, and physiotherapy, to major operations such as iliopsoas transplant, femoral osteotomy and tendon transplants in the feet. In a few children over the age of eight years major bony operations become necessary for spinal curvature.

The modern management of spina bifida cystica has been described in some detail to indicate how complicated a business it can be and involving paediatric or neuro-surgeons, orthopaedic surgeons and urologists. In addition, these children are prone to illness requiring the services of the paediatrician, such as pyelonephritis, meningitis and pneumonia. There are also problems of educational and social management which involve the educationists and medical social workers. It is also pertinent to observe that the decision to treat these unfortunate infants soon after birth, in the knowledge that many will survive to require prolonged and sometimes unpleasant therapeutic measures, involves for many a preliminary ethical question. It is easy to understand the viewpoint of those who doubt the wisdom or humanity of active treatment. On the other hand, a conservative approach still permits a proportion of these babies to live, but much more severely crippled by progressive hydrocephalus and paralysis than if prompt closure of the spinal defect had been undertaken. The majority of medical men now believe that on medical grounds alone everything that is practicable should be done, and the climate of public opinion would, in any event, no longer permit the paediatrician, whatever his personal beliefs, to withhold emergency surgical treatment. It is not within the compass of this book to discuss the economic implications of the modern treatment of spina bifida cystica but they are obviously far-reaching.

INTRACRANIAL TUMOURS
(see Chapter XI).

SPINAL TUMOURS

Spinal tumours such as glioma are very rare in children but the cord may be compressed by tumours arising from adjacent tissues, e.g. eosinophilic granuloma of bone, neurofibroma, secondary deposits from neuroblastoma or lymphosarcoma etc. The symptoms are variable but root pains are common, there may be signs of lower motor neurone weakness in the muscles supplied by the involved spinal segments and possibly spastic weakness or changes in the reflexes below the level of the tumour. Sensory changes are not common in the early stages and often difficult to demonstrate in the young child. Bladder or bowel control may be disturbed. A very common physical sign is a stiff back.

Stiffness of the lumbar spine is a constant feature of an intraspinal dermoid tumour. These have been seen in children who have suffered earlier from tuberculous meningitis and who have had frequent lumbar punctures. The dermoid tumour arises from implanted skin fragments and will not occur if only needles with well-fitting stilettes are used. In some of the affected children there has also been weakness and wasting in the thigh muscles and absent knee and ankle jerks (Blockey and Schorstein, 1961).

Treatment

Only the intraspinal dermoid is usually completely removable. In some cases such as eosinophilic granuloma excellent results can be obtained with irradiation. In most spinal tumours palliation is all that is available. However, the correct diagnosis must always be reached by myelography, laminectomy and biopsy.

THE AUTONOMIC NERVOUS SYSTEM

PINK DISEASE (INFANTILE ACRODYNIA)

This once common and distressing disease of infancy has become quite rare in Britain since mercury (in the form of grey powder or calomel) was removed from the proprietary "teething" or "soothing" powders, so beloved of British mothers and so completely lacking any rational justification.

Aetiology

There is strong evidence that the ingestion of mercury in small amounts is closely connected with pink disease (Warkany and Hubbard, 1948). None the less only a minority of the many infants given mercury developed pink disease, and the disease can occur in babies who have apparently never ingested mercury and in whose urine no traces of the metal can be found. It may be that factors or causes other than an unusual sensitivity to mercury explain some cases.

Clinical Features

The onset is most often during the early "teething" period with increasing irritability and sleeplessness, severe anorexia, failure to gain weight, and excessive sweating especially over the head and neck. There is often a severe hypotonia although the deep reflexes are retained. Photophobia is striking and the infant often adopts a characteristic knee-elbow position with his face buried in the pillow. The hands and feet look swollen and grossly hyperaemic although they feel cold to the touch. The palms and soles may desquamate. The nose and cheeks may also be unduly red. Generalized but fleeting erythematous rashes may be seen. The invariable tachycardia is marked and its absence excludes the diagnosis completely. The teeth may become loose and the gums swollen and hyperaemic. Hypertension is common. These children are highly susceptible to respiratory infections which can be dangeous to life or produce permanent bronchiectasis. In their absence complete recovery can be predicted, but only after 3–6 months of a miserable and trying illness. Every effort should be made to treat the child outside the hospital where ward infection and even sudden death can occur.

Treatment

There is no effective specific treatment. A chelating agent such as dimercaprol (BAL) has proved to be disappointing. Symptomatic measures include encouraging the infant to take milk, ensuring an adequate intake of vitamins, relieving sleeplessness with chloral hydrate or barbiturates and treating intercurrent infections. The mother will require steady support from her physician.

Prevention

It should be accepted by all medical practitioners that there is no place in the paediatric pharmacopoeia for mercurial preparations of any kind.

FAMILIAL DYSAUTONOMIA

This is a rare familial, probably autosomal recessive disease, seen more commonly in Jewish children (Riley, 1957).

Aetiology

The clinical features led the author to suggest the presence of an overproduction of acetylcholine at the nerve endings of the parasympathetic nervous system (Hutchison and Hamilton, 1962). On the other hand, on the basis of an abnormal excretion of the metabolites of catecholamines Smith *et al.* (1963) postulated a defect in the function of the sympathetic nervous system.

Clinical Features

In severe cases the diagnosis is usually made in infancy but milder cases can remain undetected for years. The striking features are severe hypotonia and muscle weakness with absence of the deep reflexes, excessive salivation, continual sweating and an inability to produce tears. The corneal reflex is usually absent. Difficulty in swallowing is common. There may be markedly delayed psychomotor development. Recurrent pyrexial attacks unassociated with signs of infection may cause anxiety. Periodic erythematous blotching of the skin may occur. Transient episodes of arterial hypertension have been reported, whereas in some cases there has been postural hypotension. In the older child attacks of cyclical vomiting are not infrequent. Another feature is an apparent indifference to pain. Urinary frequency has also been a symptom in some patients. In others motor incoordination can be demonstrated. Smith and Dancis (1963) have reported an abnormal response to an intradermal injection of histamine which can be used as a diagnostic test.

Treatment

No specific treatment is available. Behaviour disturbances in some affected children require expert psychiatric attention. The most severely affected children may die in infancy of severe pulmonary complications related to the excessive production of mucus and saliva. In these episodes antibiotics may prove to be life-saving.

CONVULSIONS IN INFANCY AND CHILDHOOD

We have considered convulsions of all sorts and from many causes together in this chapter. This is because not only is epilepsy common in children, but also because the nature of other types of infantile convulsions and the extent to which they are fundamentally epileptic are inseparable problems. Some would regard all convulsions as denoting "epilepsy". Most paediatricians would prefer to reserve the term "epilepsy" for the child who is subject to recurring seizures or lapses of consciousness, and to exclude from this group those convulsions which are not repeated over a prolonged period of time and for which a substantial localized or generalized "provoking" cause can be determined.

Aetiology

Although there was a tendency in the past to regard almost any preceding event as a cause of convulsions, and although today no one would accept such minor peripheral irritations as threadworms, constipation or teething as causative, the majority of convulsions in infancy can be related to a specific provocation. These include birth injury (Chapter III), neonatal tetany, the tetany of rickets (Chapter XXV), intracranial infections, tumours and injuries, and developmental anomalies of the brain. In the pre-school child the most common provoking cause for a generalized seizure is the brisk fever of an acute infection. The speed and height of the temperature rise are more important than the precise nature of the infection which may be otitis media, tonsillitis, pyelonephritis, pneumonia, bacillary dysentery or any of the common infectious fevers. Indeed, the high incidence of convulsions in childhood is largely due to the high incidence of infections.

On the other hand, none of the factors cited above invariably provoke a convulsion in every infant or child. We must, therefore, postulate a convulsive tendency, variable in degree, in some subjects. It is tempting to suggest that in its highest degree it results in idiopathic epilepsy, whereas in those who possess the tendency in lesser degree a convulsion will occur only when provoked by some specific stimulus and that further convulsions will probably not occur in the absence of the stimulus. The neurologist has always tended to insist upon the unity of all convulsions but the paediatrician has baulked at the use of the label "epilepsy", with all its sinister implications, in the case of the child who has had a solitary febrile fit. It is probably best to restrict the term "epilepsy" to spontaneously occurring losses of consciousness which are entirely dependent upon inherited or inborn convulsive tendencies, and to prefer the word "convulsion", suitably prefixed, for the provoked attacks. But the close inter-relationship between the two groups, which overlap each other, must never be forgotten. It should be stressed further that in a high proportion of epileptic children and in a smaller proportion with provoked convulsions, a family history of epileptic seizures or of infantile convulsions is obtainable.

There remains to mention a few causes of convulsions in infancy and childhood which the wise physician always keeps in mind when faced with the problem of the convulsing child, especially when the circumstances seem in any way unusual or when treatment seems disappointing. In some young infants repeated seizures are due to an inborn error of brain metabolism, whereby the daily requirements of pyridoxine greatly exceed that in a normal diet. This state is known as *pyridoxine dependency* and it is rapidly amenable to treatment (Scriver and Hutchison, 1963). Various other metabolic disturbances, in addition to hypocalcaemia already mentioned, can cause convulsions; these include hypoglycaemia, hyponatraemia from water intoxication or from retention of water in acute infections of the brain tissues, hypernatraemia from disease of the hypothalamus or frontal lobes or from severe hypertonic dehydration, and lead poisoning. Finally, hypertensive encephalopathy as a cause of convulsions in childhood is not excessively rare.

Clinical Types

Various clinical types of epileptic seizure are well recognized. The electroencephalographic changes are frequently characteristic in the different clinical types, but this correlation is by no means firm and a good deal of overlap and mixing of types exist. In any event, the interpretation of electroencephalographs is a task for the expert.

Grand mal.—This is the commonest clinical manifestation of epilepsy and the only form which provoked seizures take. Its features are too well known to require detailed description—sudden loss of consciousness, possible injury from falling, tonic followed by clonic spasms, tongue biting, possibly urinary or faecal incontinence, frothing at the mouth. It is followed by postictal sleep, or a period of confusion or automatism. A careful examination is essential to exclude a provoking cause which requires specific treatment. In febrile attacks the convulsion is short, solitary, and occurs at the onset of the illness. A prolonged or recurrent convulsion in a febrile child may well herald idiopathic epilepsy and the physician should be guarded in his prognosis in these circumstances. In grand mal epilepsy the EEG shows most often frequent high voltage spikes, but there may instead or in addition be spike and wave or slow wave patterns.

Hypocalcaemic convulsions should always be suspected when a newborn infant develops generalized twitchings during the first week of life and after an uncomplicated birth. *Neonatal tetany* is much more common in the artificially fed infant, possibly because of the high phosphate content of cow's milk. The diagnosis is confirmed by finding a low serum calcium (below 8 mg. per 100 ml.) and a raised serum phosphate (above 7 mg. per 100 ml.). The possible effects of hypoglycaemia in the newborn have been considered in Chapter II and are much more difficult to evaluate. When grand mal seizures occur in early infancy due to *pyridoxine dependency* there are usually some additional and characteristic clinical features which should alert the physician to the underlying cause. These are an immense irritability and a sensitivity to small noises that indicates true hyperacusis; a remarkable fluttering of the eyelids and upward rolling of the eyes; and extreme repetitive convulsive twitchings. Both the clinical and electroen-cephalographic abnormalities can be abolished completely with one intramuscular injection of pyridoxine hydrochloride 10 mg., although continued oral medication will be required to keep the infant well and to prevent permanent mental deficiency.

Myoclonic attacks.—These may occur as the sole manifestation of epilepsy or in children who also have grand mal seizures. The attacks are quite transient and consist of a sudden convulsive jerk of the head and neck, or of a limb, without loss of consciousness.

A characteristic type of myoclonus occurs in a rare childhood disorder called *subacute inclusion-body encephalitis* or *subacute sclerosing pan-encephalitis*. This disease appears to be mid-way between the progressive degenerations of the nervous system and the acute encephalitides. Its clinical characteristics are easily recognizable. A child of school age makes repetitive stereotyped involuntary movements with rhythmic regularity (2–6 per minute). Each begins with shocklike abruptness typical of the myoclonic jerk, but then the elevated limb remains "frozen" for a second or two before, and unlike the myoclonic jerk, it gradually melts away (Metz *et al.*, 1964). The EEG shows high-amplitude slow wave complexes having the same rhythmicality as the myoclonic jerks and superimposed on an otherwise normal record. As the disease progresses there is progressive mental deterioration, focal paralysis and, finally, decerebrate rigidity. Death is the usual outcome. The cerebrospinal fluid shows a raised globulin level and a "paretic" type of colloidal gold reaction.

Akinetic seizures.—In these attacks the child suddenly drops to the floor with transient unconsciousness. There may also be other types of epileptic episode and akinetic seizures are commonly seen in mentally retarded children.

Infantile spasms.—These have been variously called "salaam fits", and "lightning fits". The onset is before the age of 12 months. The infant may have appeared to develop normally before the onset of the attacks or to have been brain damaged from birth. Mental deficiency is an almost invariable and irreversible accompaniment of infantile spasms once they have developed. The condition responds poorly to anticonvulsant drugs. The attacks, which are often extremely numerous each day, consist of sudden transient jerks of the whole body, head and limbs. Most often the head and trunk flex suddenly forward while the hands jump up alongside the head (salaam fits), but the spasm may also be opisthotonic in nature. The fits often become less frequent with the passage of time, and may cease spontaneously. The EEG shows gross abnormalities; the most severe and characteristic has been termed "hypsarrhythmia". This amounts to total chaos with asynchrony, high amplitude irregular spike-and-wave activity, no organized discharges, and no normal background activity (Gibbs *et al.*, 1954;

Jeavons and Bower, 1961). There is evidence of perinatal brain damage or of postnatal neurological disease in some of these infants, but in many the cause of the disorder is unidentifiable.

Petit mal.—This diagnosis should be reserved for those children who show, brief, often frequent, lapses of consciousness unassociated with twitching or loss of balance and in whom the EEG shows a characteristic 3 per second spike-and-wave pattern. Petit mal must not be confused with abortive grand mal seizures. These may be very brief but there is usually loss of balance or posture, and frequently the eyelids twitch or there are other muscle movements never seen in true petit mal. The distinction is important in treatment. Petit mal attacks may be very frequent in childhood and show a tendency to disappear towards puberty (pyknolepsy). Unfortunately, they are not infrequently replaced by grand mal.

Psychomotor seizures (temporal lobe epilepsy).—This type of epilepsy is relatively uncommon in childhood. It may take various forms, each rather bizarre, and their epileptic basis should be indicated by their continued recurrence without obvious cause. There is an aura in psychomotor attacks more often than other types of epilepsy in childhood. It may take many forms, e.g. sudden fear, unpleasant smells or tastes, abdominal pain or tinnitus. The attack itself frequently consists of abnormal repetitive movements, e.g. jaw movements, eye fluttering or blinking, or staring, clasping or fumbling with the hands. Sudden difficulty in speaking or incoherence is common. The most distressing features involve mental disturbances, e.g. violent tantrums, dream-like states, or the *déjà vu* phenomenon. Various types of visual, auditory or olfactory hallucinations may occur. There may be postictal confusion or sleepiness. The EEG typically shows a focal discharge from the temporal lobe, slow wave or spike-and-wave (Chao *et al.*, 1962). Not all cases of psychomotor epilepsy have a temporal lobe discharge and not every case with a temporal lobe focus is associated with psychomotor attacks.

Jacksonian seizures.—In the typical case a grand mal seizure starts in one area, face, arm or limb, and spreads in an orderly fashion until one half or the whole body is affected. The site of the organic lesion may thus be localized. Conjugate deviation of the head and eyes to one side may indicate a lesion in the opposite frontal lobe. Tingling in a foot incriminates the opposite parietal lobe. A visual aura points to the temporal or occipital lobe. However, in children it is not uncommon to have Jacksonian attacks in the absence of a focal lesion in the brain. When one half of the body is affected the attack may be followed by a transient hemiparesis—*Todd's paralysis*.

Status epilepticus.—This dangerous state has been described as the Sword of Damocles which hangs over every epileptic head. It may develop suddenly, but is a particular danger if anticonvulsant treatment is suddenly withdrawn and against which parents must be carefully warned.

Diagnosis

The first task of the physician must be to exclude an organic cause for the convulsions, by careful history taking and complete clinical examination. When convulsions recur, radiography of the skull and electroencephalography are essential. Lumbar puncture should only be performed when there is a reasonable suspicion of an organic basis, because this minor operation is unpleasant for the child and not wholly devoid of risk. In exceptional cases the neurosurgeon may be required to carry out cerebral angiography or pneumoventriculography. The author prefers not to label a child "epilepsy" before the age of 2 years.

Prognosis

"Idiopathic" convulsions in infancy frequently herald mental retardation. Poorly controlled epilepsy is often associated with a slow mental deterioration through the years. Severe EEG abnormalities, frequent akinetic or myoclonic seizures, and infantile spasms all augur a gloomy prognosis. On the other hand, solitary "febrile" convulsions, hypocalcaemic tetany, and epileptic seizures which can be well controlled by drugs are most often associated with normal psychomotor development, and they are not incompatible with a high intellectual performance.

Treatment

(i) *General.*—In the case of provoked convulsions it is obvious that early diagnosis followed by specific treatment is essential. The treatment appropriate to many causes such as meningitis, hypertensive encephalopathy, intracranial tumour etc. is discussed in the appropriate chapters. The common "febrile" convulsion is best treated by tepid sponging to lower the temperature and the infection itself may be amenable to specific therapy. The time-honoured hot mustard bath is completely contra-indicated as it can only increase the patient's body temperature. The best treatment for a prolonged convulsion (over 15 minutes) or for status epilepticus is intramuscular paraldehyde 0·15 ml./Kg. body weight (1 ml. per stone). This must always be taken from a sealed ampoule because paraldehyde in a bottle can undergo dangerous decomposition. It is also essential to ensure that paraldehyde is never administered from a disposable plastic syringe. A 5 ml. glass syringe should be used. The dose can be repeated in 30 minutes if the convulsion continues. Alternative drugs are intramuscular sodium phenobarbitone 5 mg./Kg., or phenytoin sodium 100 mg. per dose. We have found paraldehyde to be as effective as any and it has a wide safety margin. The deeply comatose child should be nursed in the prone position and the pharynx kept clear by frequent suction. Cyanosis should be relieved in an oxygen tent.

Neonatal tetany can be quickly relieved with oral calcium chloride in solution, 5 gr. (0·3 gm.) four-hourly for three days; the calcium is not absorbed but the chloride ion enters the blood to produce a metabolic acidosis. Alternatively, the serum calcium level may be raised with 10 per cent calcium gluconate, 3 ml. intramuscularly. Convulsions related to a relative deficiency of pyridoxine will stop after 10 mg. pyridoxine by any route. Thereafter the continuous maintenance dose must be worked out in hospital on the basis of biochemical tests (Scriver and Hutchison, 1963). A test dose of pyridoxine is worth a trial in every case of "idiopathic" convulsions in infancy which does not respond to anticonvulsants.

(ii) *Anticonvulsants.*—It is important to control or prevent if possible the recurring seizures of the epileptic. This may require frequent initial consultations with the physician until the optimum dose and drug or combination of drugs have been determined. The best drug with which to start treatment is phenobarbitone. In infants it can be given in powder form, ⅛ gr. (8 mg.) four or five times daily. In older children a suitable initial dose is ½ gr. (30 mg.) twice daily. It is rarely fruitful to increase the dose in children above 1 gr. (60 mg.) thrice daily. Phenobarbitone is cheap, effective and safe. Only rarely does a drug rash or fever necessitate its discontinuance. When fits are not adequately controlled with phenobarbitone in the maximum dose short of causing excessive drowsiness, phenytoin sodium, in the form of tablets, capsules or the oral suspension, should be added or substituted. A suitable initial dose is 50 mg. twice daily, increasing gradually if necessary to 100 mg. thrice daily. Phenytoin is an extremely effective drug but frequently produces an unwelcome although reversible hypertrophy of the gums. Rarely the appearance of a rash is an imperative indication for its withdrawal because of the danger of agranulocytosis. The presence of ataxia is an indication of overdosage. We have recently found another hydantoin, ethotoin (Peganone), to be very free of side-effects; the initial dose is 250 mg. twice daily, increasing to 500 mg. or more thrice daily. A powerful drug for grand mal has been developed in primidone (Mysoline). Unfortunately, its usefulness is limited by the frequency with which it causes severe ataxia. Megaloblastic anaemia is a side-effect seen in adults but this is rare in children. The initial dose should be 125 mg. (as ¼ tablet or 30 min. of the oral suspension) twice daily, increasing slowly to a maximum of 250 mg. thrice daily. The latest addition to the anticonvulsants, and claimed to be of especial value in temporal lobe epilepsy, is sulthiame (Ospolot). We have occasionally found it to be of value also in poorly controlled cases of grand mal in doses varying from 50 to 200 mg. thrice daily.

These drugs are of great value in grand mal and to a much less extent in myoclonic, akinetic and psychomotor attacks. In true petit mal they are of little value. Fortunately, effective drugs for petit mal exist, but it is important to realize that they may actually aggravate the tendency to grand mal. The most useful and safe is ethosuximide (Zarontin) 125–250 mg. twice or thrice daily. Other effective drugs are troxidone (Tridione) and paramethadione (Paradione) 150–300 mg. twice or thrice daily; unfortunately, these drugs often produce an intolerance to light ("the glare phenomenon"), and drug rashes and agranulocytosis are by no means negligible risks. Some children require a combination of drugs for mixed grand mal and petit mal attacks. Brain-damaged epileptic children respond much less well than cases of "idiopathic" epilepsy.

Infantile spasms are remarkably unresponsive to any of the anticonvulsant drugs although they sometimes cease spontaneously with time. In many cases the fits can be stopped or markedly reduced in frequency with ACTH (corticotrophin) given intramuscularly in doses of 40 mg. per day, or with prednisolone given orally in doses of 20 mg. per day. We frequently find that a 21-day course of treatment is sufficient, although in some cases prolonged but reduced dosage is necessary. Unfortunately control of the fits is rarely accompanied by significant intellectual improvement.

(iii) *Social management.*—The epileptic child whose convulsions can be prevented or rendered infrequent should attend an ordinary school and live as normal a life as possible. The physician must by explanation and advice bring the parents to accept the need for an unrestricted existence and even to accept a few risks. Certain restrictions such as riding a bicycle in the city streets or mountain climbing are clearly unavoidable, but they should be reduced to the minimum. Psychological difficulties can often be prevented by wise counsel and psychiatric treatment is only rarely required. Special schooling may be necessary for the mentally handicapped epileptic. On the other hand, the epileptic who comes from an unstable home and in whom seizures are poorly controlled can often derive enormous benefit, therapeutic, educational and psychological, from admission to an institution or colony for epileptics. There are also voluntary societies devoted to the problems in society of the epileptic, and their assistance should be sought if later difficulties of social adjustment or employment arise. It is an unfortunate fact that the epileptic adult often proves "difficult" with his fellows in Industrial Rehabilitation Units, sheltered workshops and vocational training centres so that he derives less benefit than he might. It is also sad to relate that members of the general public, including non-medical professional people, are often ill-informed about epilepsy so that they are less helpful towards the epileptic than they would be towards other handicapped persons. None the less, the majority of epileptics who are of normal intelligence are today enabled to live useful and almost normal lives in a wide variety of professions and trades.

BREATH-HOLDING ATTACKS

These occur not infrequently in infants or toddlers and they are usually precipitated by pain, indignation or frustration. Shortly after the onset of a fit of loud crying the infant suddenly stops breathing in expiration and becomes cyanosed. If inspiration does not quickly follow the infant loses consciousness and goes rigid with back arched and extended limbs. He may have a few convulsive twitches. Respiration always starts again with rapid recovery and there is no danger to life. The susceptibility to breath-holding attacks is usually short-lived and they cease spontaneously as the child matures. The EEG shows no abnormality between or during attacks (Gauk *et al.*, 1963). These attacks are not epileptic and they do not require any treatment. Their differentiation from epileptic seizures, in the absence of personal observation, rests upon a good history from an observant mother. When there is doubt an EEG should be advised.

REFERENCES

ARNEIL, G. C. (1946). *Arch. Dis. Childh.*, **21**, 171.

AUSTIN, J. H. (1957). *Neurology (Minneap.)*, 7, 415.

BICKERSTAFF, E. R. (1964). *Brit. med. J.*, **2**, 82.

BLOCKEY, N. J., and SCHORSTEIN, J. (1961). *J. Bone Jt. Surg.*, **43B**, 556.

BODER, E., and SEDGWICK, R. P. (1963). *Clinics develop. med.*, **8**, 110

CHAO, D., SEXTON, J. A., and PARDO, L. S. S. (1962). *J. Pediat.*, **60**, 686.

ECKSTEIN, H. B., and MACNAB, G. H. (1966). *Lancet*, **1**, 842.

EDWARDS, J. H., NORMAN, R. M. and ROBERTS, J. M. (1961). *Arch. Dis. Childh.*, **36**, 481.

FORD, F. R. (1960). *Diseases of the Nervous System in Infancy, Childhood and Adolescence*, 4th edit. Oxford: Blackwell Scientific Publications.

GAUK, E. W., KIDD, L., and PRICHARD, J. S. N. (1963). *New Engl. J. Med.*, **268**, 1436.

GIBBS, E. L., FLEMING, M. M., and GIBBS, F. A. (1954). *Pediatrics*, **13**, 66.

HUTCHISON, J. H., and HAMILTON, W. (1962). *Lancet*, **1**, 1216.

INGRAHAM, F. D. (1944). *Spina Bifida and Cranium Bifidum*. Cambridge, Mass.: Harvard Univ. Press.

JEAVONS, P. M., and BOWER, B. D. (1961). *Arch. Dis. Childh.*, **36**, 17.

LAURENCE, K. M., and COATES, S. (1962). *Arch. Dis. Childh.*, **37**, 345.

LORBER, J. (1961). *Arch. Dis. Childh.*, **36**, 381.

LYON, G., DODGE, P. R., and ADAMS, R. D. (1961). *Brain*, **84**, 680.

METZ, H., GREGORIOU, M., and SANDIFER, P. (1964). *Arch. Dis. Childh.*, **39**, 554.

MORISON, J. E. (1963). *Foetal and Neonatal Pathology*, 2nd edit. London: Butterworth & Co.

PETERSON, R. D., KELLY, W. D., and GOOD, R. A. (1964). *Lancet*, **1**, 1189.

RILEY, C. M. (1957). *Advanc. Pediat.*, **9**, 157.

RUSSELL, D. S. (1949). Observations on the Pathology of Hydrocephalus. *Spec. Rep. Ser. med. Res. Coun. (Lond.)*, (No. 265). London: H.M. Staty. Office.

SCARFF, J. E. (1963). *J. Neurol. Neurosurg. Psychiat.*, **26**, 1.

SCRIVER, C. R., and HUTCHISON, J. H. (1963). *Pediatrics*, **31**, 240.

SHANKS, R. A. (1950). *Arch. Dis. Childh.*, **25**, 389.

SHARRARD, W. J. W., ZACHARY, R. B., LORBER, J., and BRUCE, A. M. (1963). *Arch. Dis. Childh.*, **38**, 18.

SMEBY, B. (1966). *Acta paediat. (Uppsala)*, **55**, 239.

SMITH, A. A., and DANCIS, J. (1963). *J. Pediat.*, **63**, 889.

SMITH, A. A., TAYLOR, T., and WORTIS, S. B. (1963). *New Engl. J. Med.*, **268**, 705.

STANBURY, J. B., WYNGAARDEN, J. B., and FREDRICKSON, D. S. (1965). *The Metabolic Basis of Inherited Disease*, 2nd edit. New York: McGraw-Hill Book Co.

WALSHE, J. M. (1959). *Ann. intern. Med.*, **51**, 1110.

WALSHE, J. M. (1962). *Arch. Dis. Childh.*, **37**, 253.

WALSHE, J. M., and CUMINGS, J. N. (1961). *Wilson's Disease: Some Current Concepts.* Oxford: Blackwell Scientific Publications.

WALTON, J. N. (1957). *J. Neurol. Psychiat.*, **20**, 144.

WARKANY, J., and HUBBARD, D. M. (1948). *Lancet*, **1**, 829.

CHAPTER XXI

(0.2%) # CEREBRAL PALSY 2 : 1000 (U.K.)

The term "cerebral palsy" is used here to denote "a disorder of movement and posture resulting from a permanent, non-progressive defect or lesion of the immature brain" (Mitchell, 1961). More detailed accounts can be found in the books by Woods (1957), Illingworth (1958), Henderson (1961) and Ingram (1964). An enormous amount of interest in the problems of cerebral palsy has been generated in the past twenty-five years. Some of this has been so emotionally charged that it has at times been misdirected. Some workers in the field have been led to make unrealistic claims for various therapeutic and educational methods. Even now we are a long way from understanding the problem sufficiently to plan a completely rational and reasonably economic system of diagnostic, therapeutic and educational help for affected children. The incidence of cerebral palsy in the U.K. is in the region of 2 per 1000 in childhood. The problem is, therefore, a large one. It is essential to stress, also, that children who suffer from cerebral palsy frequently have other severe handicaps in addition. Approximately 50 per cent of cerebral palsied children have an Intelligence Quotient (I.Q.) below 70, as compared with 3 per cent of the general population. Furthermore, while 75 per cent of the general population have I.Q.'s above 90 this applies to only 25 per cent of the cerebral palsy group. Epileptic seizures are common in cerebral palsied children. Henderson (1961) reported an incidence of 25 per cent. Squints occur in almost one half of all affected children. Refractive errors are common, especially degenerative myopia in children of low birth weight. Blindness is not uncommon, especially in the severely spastic group. Other ophthalmological abnormalities include defects of the choroid, retina and optic nerves. Visual field defects are especially common in hemiplegics. Deafness, frequently unsuspected, is common, especially in athetoid cases when it is of high tone distribution. It should be looked for in every affected child. Even dental problems are common, such as gingivitis due to defective chewing, tooth grinding in the mentally defective, and malocclusion. Enough has been said to justify the author's view that the results of treatment in the cerebral palsied group should be stated with reserve. Some of the highly optimistic claims in this field can apply only to a very small minority of children.

Aetiology

It is frequently impossible to determine the precise cause of cerebral palsy in individual patients. None the less, a good deal is known about the various causative factors and their varying influence in the different clinical types of cerebral palsy. In some cases there are *prenatal* influences as in cerebral agenesis due to clear genetic factors or unknown origins, rubella in the first trimester of pregnancy, toxoplasmosis transmitted across the placenta, and X-irradiation. Some cases of severe spastic tetraplegia with mental deficiency belong to this group. On the other hand, milder cases of spastic tetraplegia and of paraplegia, a group sometimes called "diplegics", show a remarkably high incidence of premature birth and low birth weight. The precise nature of this relationship is not clear although anoxia may be an important factor. Certainly anoxia is the most important *natal* aetiological factor. It is commonly found in athetoid children. Another common cause of athetosis is kernicterus due to blood group incompatibility or to the hyperbilirubinaemia of prematurity, although the widespread use of replacement transfusion has greatly reduced the incidence of these cases. Other *postnatal* causes include acute infantile hemiplegia (Chapter XX), meningitis, subdural haematoma and virus encephalitis. Birth trauma, apart from anoxia, has become relatively uncommon in modern obstetric practice.

Classification of Cerebral Palsy

There have been several different types of classification but the problem is difficult due to the frequent occurrence of "mixed" neurological abnormalities in individual patients, and because of our inability to determine the aetiology in many cases. The classification used here is a modification of that approved by the American Academy for Cerebral Palsy and described by Mitchell (1961). This divides cases according to the functional disorder present, its anatomical distribution, and its severity:

Type of Motor Disorder.
  A. Spasticity
  B. Athetosis
  C. Rigidity
  D. Ataxia
  E. Tremor
  F. Hypotonia
  G. Mixed.

Anatomical Distribution.
  Tetraplegia
  Paraplegia
  Triplegia
  Double Hemiplegia
  Hemiplegia
  Monoplegia.

Degree of Severity.
 Mild
 Moderate
 Severe.

A. **Spasticity.**—The spastic group shows the features of lesions of the pyramidal tracts such as muscle spasm which may be of the "claspknife" variety, spastic postures of the limbs, exaggerated deep reflexes, ankle clonus, and after the age of 2–3 years an extensor plantar response. The most common type is *spastic tetraplegia* in which all four limbs are involved. Mitchell (1961) subdivides this into Types I and II. In the common type I spastic tetraplegia the legs are more severely involved than the arms. Variants of this group are *spastic paraplegia* in which the arms are apparently unaffected by ordinary clinical standards, and *spastic triplegia* (which is rare) in which one arm appears to be normal. This group is traditionally called "cerebral diplegia". It is often associated with premature birth; cyanotic attacks or convulsive twitching are common soon after birth and the intelligence is usually only moderately reduced. The degree of motor dysfunction is frequently symmetrical. In the much less common type II spastic tetraplegia the spasticity is extremely severe in all four limbs, so that contractures develop early and disuse muscle atrophy may be marked. Epileptic fits are common. Pregnancy and birth have usually appeared to be normal which, when considered alongside the not infrequent presence of microcephaly and of other major or minor physical abnormalities, suggests a prenatal failure of development. These children are invariably severely mentally retarded. They have frequently shown abnormal neonatal behaviour such as lethargy, reluctance to feed or convulsions in spite of an uneventful birth, and it is difficult to decide whether these abnormalities occur in the individual baby from birth trauma or because of an abnormally formed brain. The term *double hemiplegia* is reserved for a few children with spastic tetraplegia in which the arms are manifestly more severely affected than the legs. A prenatal defect is often suggested by a family history of mental abnormality or of epilepsy. *Spastic hemiplegia* is a remarkably "pure" type of cerebral palsy which may be prenatal in origin but is frequently postnatal and due to causes such as acute infantile hemiplegia, meningitis, cerebral thrombophlebitis and subdural haematoma. In some cases the birth details strongly suggest intracranial haemorrhage or other cerebral damage. The right side is more often affected than the left, and the arm more severely than the leg. Sensory loss is common, e.g. diminished sensation to touch and pain or astereognosis. Hemianopia is not infrequent. Convulsions are common and only sometimes confined to the affected side. Some of these children are of normal or even high intelligence but many are retarded in varying degree. Finally, *spastic monoplegia* implies involvement of one limb only. This is probably a group of mixed aetiology. Thus brachial monoplegia is likely to represent a partial hemiplegia, whereas crural monoplegia may represent a partial paraplegia and fall into the "cerebral diplegia" category.

B. **Athetosis.**—Various clinical sub-types of athetosis have been described although their neuro-anatomical basis cannot be differentiated. The most common type involves the limbs, trunk and face in irregular, slow, writhing or rotating movements which are, of course, involuntary. The term "choreo-athetosis" has been used for cases in which the writhing athetotic movements have a quick jerkiness which somewhat simulates the movements of Sydenham's chorea. In very young children who are later destined to be athetoids there may be a hypotonic phase during which involuntary movements of writhing type are slight and easily overlooked. In others, hypertonicity with opisthotonic spasms or writhing movements of the trunk occur, sometimes called "dystonic athetosis". In some athetoid children there is a marked degree of muscle tension which inhibits the involuntary movements to some degree although the disability is severe. This type is sometimes referred to as "tension athetosis". When athetosis has been caused by kernicterus there is often a high-tone deafness and unless this fact is recognized the degree of mental retardation may be seriously over-estimated. A more common cause of athetosis in the U.K. today is birth trauma, either anoxic or less often due to intracranial haemorrhage. It is important to remember that in the athetoid group the degree of mental retardation may be quite unrelated to the severity of the athetosis, in contrast to the close relationship which is usual between the mental defect and motor disability in the spastic group.

C. **Rigidity.**—It is unfortunate that the word "rigidity" has been used with different meanings by different workers. As used here it is *not* intended to include the contracted muscles of the spastic child nor the tension sometimes accompanying athetosis. The term is used to describe the "lead pipe" or "cogwheel" muscle stiffness seen typically in lesions of the extrapyramidal system. This amounts to an uneven resistance experienced by the physician when he flexes or extends the patient's limbs. It is, in practice, a distinctly uncommon variety of cerebral palsy and always accompanied by mental deficiency.

D. **Ataxia.**—In some children, a small proportion of cerebral palsies, the clinical manifestations indicate a cerebellar defect, e.g. ataxic reeling gait, intention tremor and past pointing, nystagmus, hypotonia and diminished deep reflexes.

E. **Tremor.**—This type of cerebral palsy is rare and characterized by a constant, severe coarse tremor. Spasticity and athetosis are rare but true extrapyramidal rigidity is not infrequently also present.

F. **Hypotonia.**—In a few children cerebral palsy takes the form of a hypotonic tetraplegia without any spasticity or over-activity of the deep reflexes. This group has sometimes been called "flaccid diplegia". Many infants destined to develop typical spastic tetraplegia pass through a flaccid or hypotonic phase. The true situation is usually revealed by adductor muscle spasm but in some cases differentiation from flaccid diplegia depends upon continued observation. In benign infantile hypotonia (Chapter XX) there has usually been a normal birth and later mental development, whereas flaccid diplegics have often had asphyxia neonatorum and are invariably mentally retarded.

The Early Diagnosis of Cerebral Palsy

In very severe cases the diagnosis is easy from the early weeks of life, e.g. in type II spastic tetraplegia with severe generalized spasticity and gross mental retardation. In cases of typical kernicterus which survive the acute stage of hyperbilirubinaemia the certainty of brain damage makes subsequent interpretation of the neurological signs easy (Chapter IV). In many cases, however, early diagnosis is extremely difficult and, on occasions, impossible. It can be beyond the skill of the most experienced to decide just when adductor muscle tone is outside normal limits or when the knee jerks are pathologically brisk. The author will freely admit to having been confused rather than assisted by attempts to elicit and interpret most of the primitive reflexes described in the literature, although persistence of the Moro reflex beyond the age of eight to ten weeks is good cause for suspicion of cerebral palsy. The Landau reflex is also of some value, It is seen normally in infants between the age of three months and 1½ years. When the baby is held in the air in the prone position with the examiner's hand under the lower part of the anterior wall of the chest there is extension of the head, arching (to a variable degree) of the spine, and some extension of the hip joints. The Landau reflex is absent in most cases of cerebral palsy, lower motor neurone disease and severe mental deficiency. Valuable indications of spastic cerebral palsy in the young infant are poverty of movement and facial expression, extended or crossed legs when the infant is suspended by the armpits, marked adductor spasm, exaggerated deep reflexes, and in the upper limbs a persistently clenched hand with thumb adducted after the first three months (Illingworth, 1966). At a later age the child may walk on his toes with a typical spastic gait and the plantar responses will by then be extensor. There may be a dissociation in his various developmental stages when mental progress may run ahead of motor skills.

In cases of hemiplegia the contrast between the spastic and normal sides of the body is obvious at an early age to the careful and unhurried observer. Athetosis may only become obvious after the age of two years. The features of kernicterus have already been described in Chapter IV. The child who is later to develop athetotic movements shows delayed motor development in infancy. Opisthotonic spasms with intervening periods of generalized hypotonia and "floppiness" have frequently been reported in infants who later developed frank athetosis. Illingworth has stressed the ease with which the early manifestations of athetosis, such as ataxia in carrying out voluntary movements, can be mistaken for those of cerebellar ataxia. In early infancy it may be impossible to distinguish between the mentally retarded child and the spastic child who is also mentally retarded, but the true situation will become clear as time passes. It is always important to keep in mind that delay in speech in cerebral palsied children may be due to spasticity or athetosis of the tongue, or to high tone deafness. Such delay when associated with athetotic grimacing of the face may lead to an erroneous diagnosis of mental retardation. This can only be avoided by taking a careful history from the time of conception and when doubt remains by formal intelligence testing which must be performed by an experienced psychologist.

Management

For a balanced account of this complex medical, social and educational problem the reader is referred to Kershaw (1966). The problem has many facets such as physiotherapy, orthopaedic surgery, speech therapy, hearing aids, and education. It is the responsibility of the paediatrician to co-ordinate the whole management as far as possible. The earlier in the child's life treatment can be begun the better will be the result. In many cases of cerebral palsy the general facilities long available from the Local Authorities in this country are quite adequate. Thus the spastic child who is mildly retarded mentally and with only slight physical disability can be quite well educated at an ordinary school, although he may receive some physiotherapy at a local clinic or hospital. The more severely retarded child with slight physical disability can be managed well enough in a special school for the mentally handicapped. On the other hand, the spastic or athetotic child who is severely crippled but of normal intelligence is best educated in a special school (day or residential) for cerebral palsied children. Such schools are extremely expensive because they must carry a big and highly-trained staff of physiotherapists, speech therapists, educational psychologists, and specially trained teachers. They must also be visited regularly by paediatrician, otorhinolaryngologist, orthopaedic surgeon, audiometrician, and other specialists. There is no doubt that these special schools for spastics achieve some impressive results in the fields of both general and physical education. The residential type of school can also serve a most useful function in difficult cases by admitting children for a short period of weeks during which a much more accurate assessment of the mental and physical disabilities can be made. In the individual child this may then allow his future management at home or at a day school to be more usefully planned. It should be realized that the child who is severely damaged both mentally and physically can never be taught to live an independent and useful existence within the general community. He can be considerably helped in a special school for spastics provided his mental retardation is not too severe. In adult life he will require hostel or institutional care. If his mental defect is severe and he cannot be adequately cared for at home admission to an institution for mental defectives is the only reasonable course to advise.

Perhaps the most difficult problem of all, although it is not a common one, is the spastic child of high intelligence who is severely handicapped physically. Although he has the ability to learn, his physical defects, e.g. of speech and motor functions, frequently make a real higher education impossible. None the less, if he can be found a place in one of the few highly specialized schools for spastics, where he can receive expert physical treatment as well as an advanced education, even a University course may be within his grasp. In the few exceptional successes of this sort which the author has personally encountered, he has been impressed by the vital element for success in the form of quite outstanding, almost obsessional, parents who had made the most remarkable efforts and self sacrifices on behalf of their child.

It is obvious that for a physical disability such as cerebral palsy physiotherapy has an important part to play, along with general education, speech training, and the amelioration of other physical defects of hearing, vision etc. The physiotherapy must be conducted by workers who have a special interest in the cerebral palsied, and supervised by paediatricians, orthopaedists or neurologists similarly motivated. The results are difficult to assess objectively. They appear to be best in the moderately severe spastics and poorest in the athetotics. They must be accepted as of very limited value, but when added to other measures such as special education the results are in some instances highly gratifying. Even more difficult to assess is the place of orthopaedic surgery in cerebral palsy. Ill-conceived operations have frequently done the patient more harm than good. Increasing realization of this fact has greatly reduced the number of spastic children submitted to open surgery, although the orthopaedic surgeon can frequently assist by fitting special leg-irons, boots and the like. The need for the correction of deformities, such as flexion contractures of the thighs and knees, would be diminished if all spastic children had their tight muscles stretched by parents or physiotherapists at frequent intervals each day. None the less, all severely palsied children should have the benefit of expert orthopaedic opinion at regular intervals.

A word must be said of the vital part to be played by the parents, especially the mothers, of cerebral palsied children, and of the guidance which they should receive from their physician. Simple inexpensive equipment for use in the home is available or can be cheaply constructed.

Thus a special chair which will allow the spastic child to sit upright can be made for him by a suitable manufacturer. These are available in the U.K., made to order, at the local Limbfitting and Appliance Centre. Walking aids of various types can be obtained on the advice of the orthopaedic surgeon. Special handles for feeding utensils, wide based cups, and suction discs to hold plates in position can be extremely useful. The mother will have to spend much time helping her child to feed himself with a spoon because in this simple way muscle control and co-ordination are encouraged. Some of the difficulties of the cerebral palsied child are probably due to a defective "body image", so that his sense of position in space is faulty and incomplete. This makes dressing and undressing difficult and here again much patience and encouragement are required. The problems can be simplified somewhat by the use of zip fasteners, slip-on shoes and simple forms of clothing which do not involve the use of buttons. Various forms of help for parents are available from the Local Authority and various voluntary bodies in the community.

Finally, it should be stated that there is a very limited place for drugs in cerebral palsy. Muscle relaxants such as Myanesin have been tried but the results are disappointing. Anticonvulsant drugs are indicated in epilepsy (Chapter XX) but their effects are frequently disappointing in brain-damaged children. In a few older children or adolescents with congenital hemiplegia complicated by frequent and uncontrollable epileptic seizures, the operation of hemispherectomy has abolished the seizures. The hemiplegia is apparently not much worsened and cerebration may be improved.

REFERENCES

HENDERSON, J. L. (1961). *Cerebral Palsy in Childhood and Adolescence*. Edinburgh: E. & S. Livingstone.

ILLINGWORTH, R. S. (1958). *Recent Advances in Cerebral Palsy*. London: J. & A. Churchill.

ILLINGWORTH, R. S. (1966). *The Development of the Infant and Young Child: Normal and Abnormal*, 3rd edit. Edinburgh: E. & S. Livingstone.

INGRAM, T. T. S. (1964). *Paediatric Aspects of Cerebral Palsy*. Edinburgh: E. & S. Livingstone.

KERSHAW, J. D. (1966). *Handicapped Children*, 2nd edit. London: Wm. Heinemann (Medical Books).

MITCHELL, R. G. (1961). *Cerebral Palsy in Childhood and Adolescence*, Chapt. IV, Edited by J. L. Henderson. Edinburgh: E. & S. Livingstone.

WOODS, G. E. (1957). *Cerebral Palsy in Childhood*. Bristol: John Wright & Sons.

CHAPTER XXII

MENTAL DEFICIENCY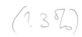

The literature on this subject is vast in its extent and in some measure reflects the magnitude of the problem. Indeed, this increases numerically year by year as modern therapeutics keeps alive mental defectives who would in the past have died in childhood of intercurrent infections; and also relatively, as our increasingly complex society makes it more and more difficult to find a niche for the intellectually or socially incompetent. For further reading the interested are referred to the text-books by Clarke and Clarke (1958) and by Tredgold and Soddy (1963). Within recent years there has occurred a change of outlook in enlightened members of the community towards the handling of the mentally subnormal. Instead of a tendency to hide them away from sight at home or in institutions, and an attitude of hopelessness, there is a growing realization that the mentally handicapped child is as entitled to education and the opportunity to develop his capabilities as the normal child. The Local Authorities and Education Authorities have steadily improved their services. Various voluntary bodies, such as the Society for Mentally Handicapped Children, have done excellent work in initiating services which have not so far been supplied from public funds. They have also done good work in an educative capacity to enlighten public opinion. One of the biggest problems, as yet unsolved, is how to make it possible in a complex society for the mentally subnormal adult to be accorded the right to work. It is obvious that this problem cannot be solved within the rigid framework of economics and "profit and loss" accounting. There are no reliable figures of the prevalence within the British community of mental deficiency. It is probable that as much as 3 per cent of the population have an Intelligence Quotient (I.Q.) of 70 or less.

Definitions

The terms mental deficiency, mental subnormality, mental retardation, mental handicap or amentia are taken to mean a failure of development of the mind. This is in contrast to dementia which means a disintegration of the fully developed mind.

There are, of course, varying degrees of severity of mental retardation. These may be conveniently classified as follows, although the terms used are no longer employed in official documents in the United Kingdom: Idiot = I.Q. 0–25; Imbecile = I.Q. 25–50; Feeble-minded (moron) = I.Q. 50–70. Those with an I.Q. below 50 are likely always to need care and attention and unlikely to be educable in any formal sense. Those with an I.Q. between 70 and 90 are not included within the group of mentally retarded children, but they are likely to be educationally backward and to be placed in the lower educational stream of a normal school. Some, in fact, require the facilities and specially trained staff of a special school.

Aetiology

The vast majority of cases of mental retardation can be placed in one of two broad aetiological groups, (a) *primary amentia* which is due to inheritance or defects in the child's genetic material; (b) *secondary amentia* in which the brain, derived from a normal germ plasm, has been damaged by environmental influences which may be operative prenatally, natally, or postnatally. In a few cases both genetic and environmental factors combine to result in brain damage. It must be stressed, however, that in individual patients it is quite often impossible to determine the precise cause of the mental deficiency. For example, in the case of a severely retarded child apnoeic and cyanotic attacks in the first week of life could indicate brain damage resulting from anoxia *or* respiratory difficulties due to malfunctioning of an abnormally formed brain.

Inheritance.—An increasing number of single gene defects are being uncovered as causes of mental deficiency. These fall into the category of inborn errors of metabolism (Chapter IX). They are now numerous and include phenylketonuria, maple syrup urine disease, argininosuccinic aciduria, Hartnup disease, galactosaemia (Chapter IX), pyridoxine dependency (Chapter XX), Niemann-Pick disease, Gaucher's disease, Tay-Sachs disease, gargoylism (Chapter XII), and others such as Sturge-Weber syndrome, tuberous sclerosis and neurofibromatosis (Chapter XX). It is likely that further metabolic errors associated with mental deficiency will be defined in future and it is to be hoped that effective methods of treatment may be developed, as in the case of phenylketonuria. Some cases of sporadic cretinism and all cases of non-endemic familial goitrous cretinism are also due to single gene defects (Chapter XVIII). Another rare example is familial dysautonomia (Chapter XX).

In recent years some types of mental retardation have been clearly related to gross chromosomal abnormalities. The most severe degrees are produced by non-disjunction during gametogenesis in the mother, leading to trisomy for one of the small acrocentric autosomes. In these conditions the long recognized correlation with advancing maternal age has been explained on the assumption that the ageing ovum is more prone to favour non-disjunction. *Mongolism* is the most common of the trisomies and in these children the cells contain 47 chromosomes (instead of the normal 46); this is due to the presence of three autosomes

No. 21 in the Denver system, often called "trisomy 21" (Harnden, 1961; Baikie, 1962). The common type of mongolism due to trisomy 21, and related to advancing maternal age (over 35 years), is sporadic in its occurrence and the mother of such a child is no more likely than any other woman of the same age to give birth to another mongol in a future pregnancy. It has long been known, however, that in some families, usually when the mother is under the age of 25 years, mongolism appears in more than one child. Chromosome studies in these cases have shown that the affected children have 46 chromosomes in most of their cells; there may be, for example, 4 chromosomes in the 21–22 group as in the normal person, but 5 instead of 6 chromosomes in the 13–15 group, and an extra submetacentric chromosome in the 6–12 group. This is likely to be due to a translocation having arisen between chromosomes 21 and 15 to give the additional chromosome in the 6–12 group. This type of *"translocation mongol"* has, in fact, the genetic material of chromosome 21 in triplicate. In the mother of such a child, however, there may be only 45 chromosomes in each cell; 3 instead of 4 in the 21–22 group, 5 instead of 6 in the 13–15 group, and an additional chromosome of the type seen in the mongol child in the 6–12 group. The translocation between chromosomes 21 and 15 "carried" by this mother (which results in mongolism in her child) is due to translocation arising during gametogenesis in the maternal grandmother or her parents (Carter *et al.*, 1960). There have been other variants of translocations involving chromosome 21, e.g. where the mother had only 45 chromosomes due to an apparent 21/21 or 21/22 translocation; or where the mongol child and his father are both chromosome mosaics (Hamerton *et al.*, 1961). When chromosome analysis of the parents of an affected child shows an abnormality they should be warned that there is a risk of the order of 2 in 3 of a second affected child.

There are two other types of trisomy which are much less common than mongolism (Smith *et al.*, 1961). Each causes such severe and multiple abnormalities, including mental retardation, that death is inevitable in early infancy. In D_1 *trisomy* there are 3 chromosomes instead of 2 in one of the 13–15 group. This results in convulsions, deafness, microphthalmia, colobomata, cleft lip and palate, haemangiomata, cardiac defects, flexion deformities of fingers, and polydactyly of feet. In *No. 18 trisomy* there is an additional chromosome 18 which results in failure to thrive, hypertonicity, flexion of fingers with the index finger overlapping the third, low set ears, micrognathia, dorsiflexion of big toes, Meckel's diverticulum, cardiac defects, inguinal and umbilical herniae, prominent occiput, and renal abnormalities. Other cases have shown some of the abnormalities noted above but they have had 46 chromosomes (not 47 as in trisomy) and have been interpreted as partial trisomies.

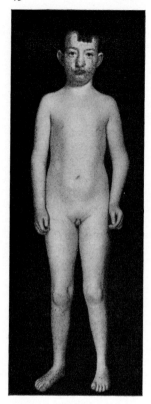

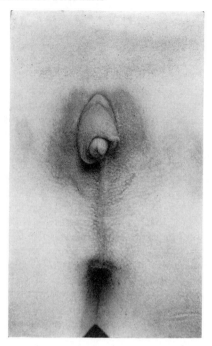

FIG. 77.—Genitalia of boy shown in Fig. 76. Bilateral cryptorchidism.

FIG. 76.—Klinefelter's syndrome in 10-year-old boy. I.Q. 30. Chromosome type XXXXY.

Abnormalities of the sex chromosomes also cause mental retardation but of much less severe degree than that usually seen in mongolism, D_1 trisomy, or 18 trisomy when autosomes are involved. The common sex chromosomal abnormalities are Klinefelter's syndrome with a chromosome status of XXY, XXXY or even XXXXY (Figs. 76 and 77) (Chapter XVIII) and Turner's syndrome XO (Chapter XVIII). Other female mental defectives have had a sex chromosome configuration of XXX called the "triple-X state" or (inaccurately) the "super-female" (Fraser et al., 1960).

Most of the genetically determined types of mental deficiency discussed so far have been of severe degree. On the other hand, rather more than 75 per cent of all mental defectives fall into the feeble-minded category (I.Q. 50–70) and cannot be attributed to single gene or gross chromosomal abnormalities. None the less, it is accepted that genetic influences play the major part in determining the child's intelligence (Penrose, 1956). It is commonplace that persons of high intelligence marry others of high intelligence and that their children are mostly of superior intelligence. Similarly the children born into families of lower than average intelligence tend also to be of somewhat poor intellectual calibre. The dullest of these children will have I.Q.'s between 50 and 70. This type of feeble-mindedness has sometimes been called "*simple primary amentia*" and it is due to multifactorial inheritance. There is good evidence that environmental influences also affect intelligence and, of course, the children of highly intelligent parents normally enjoy a much better environment than the children of dull or backward parents. None the less, although a good environment can improve a child's intellectual performance while a bad influence such as emotional deprivation or insecurity in early life can retard him, his potential ability is almost wholly derived from his inheritance.

Environment.—In some cases mental deficiency has resulted from damage to a normally developing brain by some noxious environmental influence. This may operate at various periods in the stage of development. *(Similar to causes of C.P.)*

Prenatal.—Rubella during the first 12 weeks of pregnancy can certainly damage the foetal brain. Toxoplasmosis may also be associated with mental defect. Maternal irradiation has been shown to result in mental deficiency with microcephaly, and sometimes microphthalmia, as in the survivors of the Hiroshima and Nagasaki atomic attacks. Congenital syphilis is very rare in the United Kingdom today. The effect upon a child's intelligence of adverse environmental factors during the mother's pregnancy, such as poverty, malnutrition, excessive smoking and emotional stress are difficult to assess. They can increase the risk of mental retardation by their association with a raised incidence of premature birth, and it is well recognized that premature babies are more frequently retarded than controls (Drillien, 1963).

Natal.—There is a well documented association between some of the complications of pregnancy and abnormalities of the brain including mental deficiency. These complications such as antepartum haemorrhage, toxaemia, breech presentation and complicated or instrumental delivery are frequently associated with intrapartum foetal anoxia. It is, however, extremely difficult to assess the importance of intrapartum or neonatal anoxia as a cause of later neurological disability (Chapter I). The problem has been well reviewed by Illingworth (1966).

Postnatal.—The association of kernicterus with mental retardation has been discussed in Chapters IV and XXI. Other postnatal causes of mental defect include meningitis, encephalitis, subdural haematoma, head injury and lead poisoning.

Diagnosis

In most cases the diagnosis of mental retardation can be made in the first year of life provided the physician is familiar with the stages of development in the normal baby, and that he realizes the variations which may occur in perfectly normal babies (Illingworth, 1966). It is essential that a thoughtful history be obtained from the parents, to be followed by a detailed physical examination of the child. Frequently the child must be seen on several occasions before a final conclusion is possible. There may be factors which indicate that the child is "at risk" and more likely to be retarded than others. These include prematurity, complications of pregnancy or labour, a history of asphyxia neonatorum, deep jaundice in the newborn period, convulsions or cyanotic attacks, maternal rubella or a family history of mental deficiency. The basis of the diagnosis of mental retardation may be conveniently discussed under four headings.

Physical abnormalities.—Certain physical features are undoubted evidence of associated mental defect. These include the characteristic signs of mongolism, microcephaly, cretinism (Chapter XVIII), and gargoylism (Chapter XII). Other physical abnormalities are often, although not invariably, associated with mental handicap. In this group are cerebral palsy, the bilateral macular choroido-retinitis of toxoplasmosis (Chapter X), Turner's syndrome (Chapter XVIII) and hydrocephalus. Certain other physical "stigmata" are seen more commonly in mental defectives than in normal people, but in themselves they can do no more than direct the physician's attention towards a more careful assessment of the child's intellectual development. Such peculiarities are a high narrow (saddle-shaped) palate, abnormally simple ears, hypertelorism, marked epicanthic folds, and short curved fifth fingers.

Delayed psychomotor development.—It is characteristic of the mentally retarded child that his development is delayed in all its parameters. He is slow in showing an interest in his surroundings, slow in attempting to handle or play with objects, slow to sit or stand unsupported and to walk on his own, late in speaking, late in acquiring bladder and bowel control. A lack of concentration or sustained interest is also obvious. Thus, after handling a new toy or object for a minute or two he loses interest and throws it down. His lack of interest in things around him may raise the suspicion of defective vision, just as his lack of response to sounds is apt to lead to a mistaken impression of deafness. Infantile practices tend to persist beyond the normal period, e.g. putting objects into his mouth, excessive and prolonged posturing of his hands and fingers before his eyes, drooling and slobbering. The physician must obviously be familiar with the various developmental stages of normal infants and children before he is in a position to make a judicious assessment of an individual patient. Sheridan (1960) and Illingworth (1966)

Table V
Developmental Steps in the Normal Child

4 *weeks*	Head flops back when lifted from supine to sitting position. Sits with rounded back while supported. Grasp reflex elicited by placing object in palm. Responds to sudden noise. Sucks vigorously.
8 *weeks*	Almost no head lag when pulled into sitting position. Sits with almost straight back and head only nods occasionally. Grasp reflex slight or absent. Smiles readily: vocalizes when talked to. Follows objects with head and eyes.
12 *weeks*	No head lag when pulled into sitting position. Sits supported with straight back: head almost steady. No grasp reflex: holds objects in hand for short time. Watches own hand movements. Turns head towards sounds. Recognizes feeding bottle placed before eyes.
6 *months*	Lifts head from pillow. Sits unsupported when placed in position. Rolls from supine to prone position. Holds feeding bottle. Grasps objects when offered. Drinks from cup. Transfers objects from one hand to the other. Responds to name. Held standing can bear weight on legs and bounces up and down. No more hand regard: finds feet interesting.
12 *months*	Understands simple sentences and commands. Can rise to sitting from supine position. Pulls to standing position by holding on to cot side. Walks holding hand or furniture. Speaks a few recognizable words. Points to objects which are desired. Throws objects out of pram in play.
15 *months*	Walks unsteadily with feet wide apart: falls at corners. Can get into standing position alone. Tries untidily to feed himself with spoon. Plays with cubes: places one on top of another. Indicates wet pants. Now seldom puts toys in mouth. Shows curiosity and requires protection from dangers.

18 *months*	Can walk upstairs holding on to hand or rail. Can carry or pull toy when walking. Can throw ball without falling. Points to three or four parts of body on request. Indicates need for toilet. Lifts and controls drinking cup. Feeds himself with spoon: only slight spilling. Points to three to five objects or animals in picture book.
2 *years*	Runs safely on whole foot: can avoid obstacles. Can kick a ball without losing balance. Can walk upstairs: holds rail coming downstairs. Turns door handles. Forms short sentences: vocabulary of 50 words. Spoon-feeds without spilling. Can put on hat, shoes and pants. Demands constant adult attention. Dry most nights if "lifted" at 11 p.m.
3 *years*	Walks upstairs with alternating feet. Washes and dries hands with supervision. Rides tricycle. Draws a man on request—head, trunk and one or two other parts. Can count up to 10. Discusses a picture. Asks frequent questions. Listens to and demands stories. Likes to help mother in house, father in garden. Eats with fork and spoon.
4 *years*	Can dress and undress. Asks incessant questions. Climbs ladders and trees. Engages in imitative play, e.g. doctor or nurse. Uses proper sentences to describe recent experiences. Can give name, age and address. Draws man with features and extremities. Matches four primary colours correctly. Plays with other children. Alternately co-operative and aggressive with adults or other children.
5 *years*	Runs quickly on toes: skips on alternate feet. Can tie shoe-laces. Can name common coins. Draws recognizable complete man. Names four primary colours: matches 10–12 colours. Uses knife and fork. Co-operates more with friends: accepts rules in games. Protective towards younger children and pets. May know letters of alphabet and read simple words.

have supplied excellent accounts of the development of the normal child. A brief outline of the more positive developmental steps is shown in Table V. The best assessment is to be expected from the man who has had long and intimate contact with normal children in the Child Welfare Clinic or in his own family practice, provided he has in his undergraduate period developed the capacity to observe and to appreciate the significance of his observations.

Abnormal behaviour and gestures.—Mentally retarded children frequently engage in types of behaviour and mannerisms which are obviously abnormal for their age. Thus, in early infancy the retarded baby may be excessively "good" in that he will lie in his pram for long periods without crying or showing restlessness, interest in surroundings, or boredom. In other cases there is constant or prolonged and apparently purposeless crying. Teeth grinding when awake is a common and distressing habit of many low-grade defectives. The older defective may exhaust his mother by his aimless over-activity which may at times endanger his life. Certain rhythmic movements although by no means confined to mentally retarded children are more commonly indulged in by them and for more prolonged periods. These include head-banging, body-rocking to-and-fro, and head-rolling. Low-grade defectives frequently lack the normal capacity for affection, they may be prone to sudden rages, and they may assault other younger children.

Convulsions.—Most epileptics are of normal intelligence. None the less, epileptic seizures occur more frequently among mentally retarded children than those who are normal. They are particularly common in defectives who find their way into institutions. It is also a fact that frequently repeated generalized seizures lead to slowly progressive intellectual deterioration.

Differential Diagnosis

The diagnosis of mental deficiency is obviously one in which the physician must not be wrong or he will cause the parents unjustifiable and unnecessary grief and anxiety. Some infants have a "slow start" but catch up later, and in the absence of manifest physical signs, such as microcephaly or mongolism, a firm diagnosis of mental retardation should only be made after a period of observation during which *the rate of development* is assessed. It is easy to confuse mental deficiency with cerebral palsy. Indeed the two frequently co-exist. Careful neurological examination, repeated on several occasions, will reveal the motor handicaps of cerebral palsy. The deaf child has frequently been diagnosed as mentally defective, sometimes with tragic results. This mistake should not occur when the physician takes a detailed history and follows it with a careful physical examination. The deaf child will, of course, show a lively visual interest and his motor skills will develop normally. A difficult if not very common problem is the aphasic child who fails to develop speech. He is readily confused with the mental defective, although here too a careful history and period of observation will reveal that in other respects his psychomotor development is proceeding normally. Particular caution is required in the intellectual assessment of the child who has been emotionally deprived by the break-up of his home, death of his mother, or who has been otherwise bereft of normal security. It may require a long period outside an institution before he can be assessed.

Infantile autism is probably a schizophrenic illness in the young child. Until recently many autistic children were wrongly labelled mentally defective. In a sense such children are defective because they cannot be normally educated and the prognosis is not good. None the less, the autistic child has often a revealingly intelligent expression, and in his reactions to objects and various test materials shows considerable innate ability to the careful observer. The most characteristic features of infantile autism are a complete lack of interest in personal relationships which contrasts with an interest in inanimate objects; frequently a preoccupation with parts of objects but not in their real functions; abnormal posturings, as with the hands and fingers, or abnormal interest in parts of the body; a tendency to react violently and unhappily to changes in environment; loss of speech or failure to acquire it, or the meaningless use of words or phrases; grossly abnormal mannerisms such as rocking, spinning or immobility (catatonia). The most outstanding feature of the autistic child is the way he rejects social contacts. None the less, although he is aloof, does not respond to a greeting with a smile, does not wave goodbye and so forth, he is yet aware of social contact. Thus, he may engage furiously in one of his more irritating mannerisms when someone enters his presence and cease whenever he is left alone. There is an odd high incidence of professional and educated people among the parents of autistic children. Such children, of course, are wrongly placed in institutions for the mentally defective. Some have responded considerably to psychotherapy as out-patients or in-patients in departments of child psychiatry. None probably become normal children.

INTELLIGENCE TESTS

Psychometric tests are of considerable although limited value in providing an estimate of a child's probable potential ability. They cannot, naturally, take into account the influence of such variables as zeal, ambition, interest, encouragement or the lack of it, good or bad teaching, and so forth. There are many aspects of intelligence and personality and the various tests assess these in different degrees. It is not proposed here to describe these tests in detail; they are reliable only in the hands of the expert. The most commonly used are: the Gesell tests for infants (1947) and the modifications of Cattell (1947) and Griffiths (1954); for older children the Stanford-Binet scale and the revised test of Terman and Merrill, also the Wechsler Intelligence Scale for Children; for adolescents and adults the Wechsler Adult Intelligence Scale and Raven's Progressive Matrices (Clarke and Clarke, 1958). There are also several useful personality tests of which the best for the mentally retarded are the Rorschach test and the Goodenough "Draw-a-Man" test. In the case of the school child it is also important to enquire as to his educational progress. An evaluation of the results of various tests competently performed is of great value in planning suitable education or training for the mentally handicapped child.

SPECIFIC TYPES OF MENTAL DEFECT

Some types of mental deficiency have already been described in previous chapters. Phenylketonuria (Chapter IX) and cretinism (Chapter XVIII) are especially important in that timely diagnosis and treatment can often prevent or ameliorate the mental subnormality.

MONGOLISM (DOWN'S SYNDROME)

Mongolism is the most common type of low-grade defect (idiot or imbecile). Only a rare case falls into the feeble-minded category. The physical features are so characteristic that the diagnosis is almost always possible at birth. The eyes are almond-shaped and slant upwards and outwards. There are marked epicanthic folds which are confined to the inner angles in contrast to those seen in Asiatics which include most of the upper eyelid. The nose tends to be small with a flat bridge. The skull is brachycephalic with a flat occiput and the neck is usually slender. The tongue, which is normally shaped and pointed, frequently protrudes from the unduly small mouth; this is quite different from the large, fleshy myxoedematous tongue of the cretin. As the years go by the mongol's tongue becomes deeply fissured transversely due to constant sucking between the lips. The ears are often abnormally simple or shell-shaped. The hands tend to be broad with short fingers and, in particular, the little finger is excessively short due to hypoplasia of the second phalanx and it is curved towards the ring finger. The palm frequently shows only a single palmar crease. There is an excessively wide gap between the large and second toes and on the soles there is a skin crease at this point. The hair is usually straight and rather sparse. A common characteristic is marked muscular hypotonia and laxity of ligaments. Radiographs reveal a typical mongoloid pelvis (Caffey and Ross, 1956). The eyes may show cataract, squint or a speckled iris. Blepharoconjunctivitis is common.

Mongols frequently show other major developmental anomalies, e.g. oesophageal atresia or imperforate anus. The most common involve the heart, e.g. Fallot's tetralogy, ventricular septal defects or ostium primum defects. Death may also occur in childhood from respiratory infections to which mongols are highly susceptible. Development of the genitalia and secondary sex characteristics is delayed. The mongol is usually an affectionate happy child, often fond of music, and amenable in the home. The antibiotics have made survival to adult life possible for most mongols who do not also suffer from other severe defects, but few survive beyond early middle age.

MICROCEPHALIC IDIOCY

This type of mental defect is recognizable in the neonatal period. It is genetically determined and may be familial. Apart from its smallness the head has a characteristic shape with narrow forehead, slanting frontoparietal areas, pointed vertex and flat occiput. The neck is short and the sudden movements of the head give the child a bird-like appearance. The ears are often large and abnormally formed. There may be a receding chin. Generalized muscular hypertonicity is a common feature. Convulsions frequently develop. These children are invariably low-grade defectives, devoid of the capacity for affection and sometimes dangerous to younger children.

This genetic condition can be distinguished from microcephaly which is secondary to severe brain damage such as toxoplasmosis, encephalitis and maternal irradiation during pregnancy.

MANAGEMENT OF MENTALLY SUBNORMAL CHILDREN

It must first be stated that with the exception of cretinism, phenylketonuria and galactosaemia there is at the present time no specific treatment for the mentally handicapped. The only drugs of value are anticonvulsants for children who also have epileptic seizures, and sedatives for restless hyperkinetic children.

Secondly, the author would state his opinion that once the physician has reached a definite diagnosis of mental retardation in a child, but not before, he must impart this information to the parents. This distasteful task requires time, tact, abundant sympathy and understanding, but it must be discharged in simple unambiguous phrases. In the case of the very young child the doctor would be wise not to commit himself too firmly or too soon to an assessment of degree or to a forecast as to educability. These matters can be resolved with time, and it is the physician's duty to see the child and his parents regularly, and to be prepared to give of his time to answer their many questions. In particular, the irrational feelings of guilt which many parents have on hearing that their child is mentally retarded must be assuaged by quiet discussion and explanation. Some parents will refuse to accept the situation at first. They may "go the rounds" of the specialists seeking a happier diagnosis. This is completely understandable. At the end of the day they will still require and merit all the help which their personal physician can offer. This is often particularly necessary when a mentally retarded child is at home with normal brothers and sisters where many different stresses and strains can arise.

The child with an I.Q. between 50 and 70 is usually educable at a special school (day or boarding). His progress there will depend not only upon his innate ability but on the support and training he receives, and has earlier received, from his parents. The child who proves unable to benefit from formal education in the three "R's" at a special school, can be placed in an occupation or training centre. Here he is taught social behaviour and simple manual skills. While the child whose I.Q. is around 50 is never likely to be educable to the extent that he can be self-supporting, it is a considerable advantage to him to become socially acceptable. Some Local Authorities have instituted special "Child Assessment and Advisory Clinics" to which family doctors or medical officers of the Child Welfare Service can refer pre-school children suspected of delayed development. These centres are staffed by specially trained medical officers of the Child Welfare Service, and they are visited regularly by consultant paediatricians and psychiatrists, as well as by educational psychologists. They serve a most useful purpose, not only in advising doctors and the parents of retarded children, but in arranging suitable placement of the children in schools when they reach the age of five years. It is undesirable that a mentally retarded child should be sent to an ordinary school if he is intellectually quite unable to benefit from such education. Suitable placement at the beginning will frequently avoid the behaviour problems and frustrations from which the retarded child must suffer if he is kept for long in an ordinary school competing with children of normal intelligence. The ability of a child to benefit from education at a special school or his suitability only for a training centre is not solely dependent on his I.Q. Some children who do well at special schools have lower I.Q.'s than others who have to be transferred to training centres. Important factors are the child's personality and behaviour patterns, his home environment, and his willingness to learn.

Low-grade defectives, the idiots and imbeciles of the traditional classification, nearly always require to be placed in special long-stay institutions for the mentally defective. As a general rule the earlier this category of child is placed in an institution (Health Service or private) the better, because a prolonged stay at home may cause the parents to neglect their other normal children, or the parents of a first-born defective child to deny themselves further children. However, each case must be assessed on its merits with due regard for the parents' wishes, the home and financial circumstances, the ages and reactions of the other children in the family, and the behaviour and general condition of the retarded child. Some of the voluntary societies run short-stay homes in which the retarded child can stay while the parents have a holiday on their own, or during illness or pregnancy in the mother. The mongol child is more often kept at home because he is happy and good-natured. The defective with aggressive or destructive tendencies is likely to be placed in an institution at an earlier age. Some retarded children find their way into institutions because they break the law and prove to be out of control, although they may be less severely retarded than other children who remain happily at home. There is, furthermore, a shortage of accommodation in suitable institutions in the U.K. and severely retarded children too frequently have to spend several years on a waiting list before a place can be found for them. This can result in great distress in some homes and it is in such circumstances that voluntary bodies can often help the parents and the child. Paediatricians in the hospitals of the National Health Service can also help in emergency situations by admitting the retarded child for a limited period to the ordinary paediatric ward or to an associated convalescent home.

The paediatrician is frequently asked about the employment prospects of retarded children, although it is not strictly a paediatric problem. Provided the child is physically fit he will be capable in many instances of simple manual work. Many jobs in modern industry are repetitive and not requiring a great deal of intelligence. It must be realized, however, that the feeble-minded adult is incapable of forethought, of planning his future financial or marital arrangements, even although he may be capable of efficiently performing a repetitive type of skill. This fact makes his future prospects unpredictable and not a matter for optimism. There has recently grown up the idea that hostels for the mentally handicapped could allow them to become economically self-supporting, while still having available constant advice and a measure of supervision. In practice, it will be a long time before suitable hostels can be built and before there is a sufficiency of trained staff and social workers. It may take even longer to educate the general public to see the desirability of such provisions.

REFERENCES

BAIKIE, A. G. (1962). Symposium: *Genetics in Medicine*. Edinburgh: Royal College of Physicians.

CAFFEY, J., and ROSS, S. (1956). *Pediatrics*, **17**, 642.

CARTER, C. O., HAMERTON, J. L., POLANI, P. E., GUNALP, A., and WELLER, S. D. V. (1960). *Lancet*, **2**, 678.

CATTELL, P. (1947). *The Measurement of Intelligence of Infants and Young Children*. New York: The Psychological Corporation.

CLARKE, A. M., and CLARKE, A. D. B. (1958). *Mental Deficiency: the Changing Outlook*. London: Methuen & Co.

DRILLIEN, C. M. (1963). *The Growth of Development of the Prematurely Born Infant.* Edinburgh: E. & S. Livingstone.

FRASER, J. H., CAMPBELL, J., MacGILLIVRAY, R. C., BOYD, E., and LENNOX, B. (1960). *Lancet*, **2**, 626.

GESELL, A. L., and ARMATRUDA, C. S. (1947). *Developmental Diagnosis.* New York: Paul B. Hoeber Inc.

GRIFFITHS, R. (1954). *The Abilities of Babies.* London: Univ. of London Press.

HAMERTON, J. L., BRIGGS, S. M., GIANELLI, F., and CARTER, C. O. (1961). *Lancet*, **2**, 788.

HARNDEN, D. G. (1961). *Tools of Biological Research*, Third Series. Edited by H. J. B. Atkins. Oxford: Blackwell Scientific Publications.

ILLINGWORTH, R. S. (1966). *The Development of the Infant and Young Child: Normal and Abnormal*, 3rd edit. Edinburgh: E. & S. Livingstone.

PENROSE, L. S. (1956). *The Biology of Mental Defect.* London: Sidgwick & Jackson.

SHERIDAN, M. D. (1960). *The Developmental Progress of Infants and Young Children.* (Min. of Hlth.) London: H.M. Staty. Office.

SMITH, D. W., PATAU, K., and THERMAN, E. (1961). *Lancet*, **2**, 211.

TREDGOLD, R. F., and SODDY, K. (1963). *Tredgold's Textbook of Mental Deficiency (Subnormality)*, 10th edit. London: Baillière, Tindall & Cox.

CHAPTER XXIII

BONES AND JOINTS

There are many diseases of the skeleton. Most are not amenable to curative treatment. Some can be treated successfully by the orthopaedic surgeon, e.g. club-foot, congenital dislocation of the hip and Perthe's disease. It has seemed to the author that a useful dissertation upon these many problems would require a book in itself. The interested reader is referred to one of the textbooks devoted to skeletal disorders. In this chapter consideration has been confined to a few diseases which frequently enter into the differential diagnosis of other acute medical disorders and which are, therefore, commonly encountered by the paediatric physician.

ACUTE OSTEITIS (OSTEOMYELITIS)

The incidence of this disease in childhood, which is mainly between the ages of 4 and 12 years, has not altered significantly in the author's experience during the past 30 years. On the other hand, the advent of penicillin brought about a dramatic fall in the mortality rate from something in the region of 30 per cent before 1941 to less than 2 per cent at the present time. Osteitis in the neonatal period has, indeed, become more common in recent years. It has special bacteriological and clinical features which have been discussed in Chapter VI.

Aetiology

The vast majority of cases (95 per cent) are due to a coagulase-positive *Staph. aureus.* In children over 50 per cent are penicillin-sensitive, in contrast to neonatal osteitis where the causal staphylococci are almost invariably penicillin-resistant. In many cases there is a recent history of minor trauma to the affected bone as well as evidence of some small septic focus such as a boil or an infected abrasion. The theory is that the child with a symptomless bacteraemia develops osteitis when the well vascularized metaphysis is injured by a kick or knock. In a very small minority of cases other causal organisms are found such as haemolytic streptococci and pneumococci. In the newborn a few cases are due to *E. coli* and other Gram-negative bacteria.

Osteitis is distinctly more common in children from the lower income, poorly housed sections of the community where personal cleanliness is not of a high standard. It is also more common in boys than girls in the proportion of 4:3 (White and Dennison, 1952).

Pathology (see lecture notes on Pathology)

Although the disease may affect any part of the skeleton, the bones most commonly affected in order of frequency are femur, tibia, humerus and radius. The condition starts as an inflammatory hyperaemia and congestion at the metaphysis. This leads to greatly increased intraosseous pressure which explains the intense unremitting pain in the untreated case. By the time pus forms there is a severe septicaemia. Pus may also burst through the cortex and form a subperiosteal abscess. The stripping of the periosteum from the bone, together with vascular thrombosis, leads to necrosis of bone and the formation of a sequestrum. The periosteum lays down new bone which may almost completely envelop the dead part of the shaft. This enveloping bone is called the involucrum. The cartilaginous epiphyseal plate limits the spread of the infection, although if it is damaged bone growth becomes distorted subsequently. In the pre-antibiotic era the whole medullary cavity became filled with pus. Septic emboli often led to pyaemia with pyopericardium, pyothorax and acute suppurative nephritis. As the periosteum is closely attached to the bone around the region of the epiphyseal plate spread of the infection into the joint is a late development. The exception is the hip-joint where the metaphysis is itself intraarticular.

Clinical Features

In most cases the onset is acute with high fever, rigors, severe malaise and anorexia, and constant intense pain localized to the site of infection. Tenderness is confined to the infected area of bone but it is exquisite. When the infection reaches the subperiosteal space there is visible swelling and redness and the skin feels warm. These superficial signs, however, are late in appearing when osteitis affects the neck of the femur or the bones of the pelvis. The child is bright eyed with a flushed face. Tachycardia is marked. In severe cases he may be delirious and confused, even semi-conscious. The signs can be considerably modified by the casual use of antibiotics before the diagnosis has been established. Indeed, this use of antibiotics is only too likely to lead to delay in diagnosis, during which time severe bone destruction may take place. A polymorphonuclear leucocytosis is an almost invariable finding. On the other hand, radiography is of no diagnostic value in the early days of the illness, the characteristic bone changes (Fig. 78) only appearing after about two weeks. These take the form of irregular areas of rarefaction, most marked in the metaphysis; and later of sequestrum formation. In antibiotic-treated cases the dense involucrum formation, which was once so striking a radiographic appearance, is not a marked feature. In fact, decalcification in the metaphysis may become so severe that a pathological fracture can occur if the child is allowed to bear weight on the affected limb too soon (Dennison, 1948). Finally, it should be mentioned that in cases in which diagnosis and treatment are late, the presence of chronic hyperaemia and sequestrum formation can lead to considerable lengthening of the affected limb.

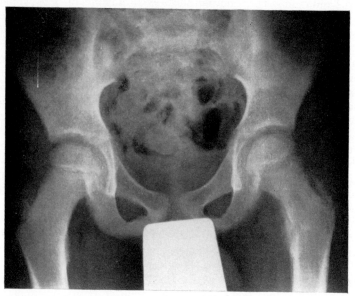

Fig. 78.—Radiograph showing acute osteitis of neck of left femur: note areas of rarefaction and loss of definition of bone outlines.

Differential Diagnosis

In most untreated cases the diagnosis of acute osteitis presents no serious problem. The unremitting well-localized severe pain and tenderness are not seen in cellulitis in the superficial tissues. On the other hand, when antibiotics have been given empirically before accurate diagnosis the problem can become most difficult, and blood cultures are then frequently sterile in the presence of active bone sepsis. We have stressed in earlier sections of this book the undesirability of prescribing antibiotics for the fevered child before a precise diagnosis has been made. Only too often this practice is to the patient's ultimate disadvantage because of the diagnostic, bacteriological and therapeutic problems which almost inevitably result. When the neck of the femur is the site of osteitis it is sometimes difficult to be sure that the child does not have rheumatic fever with acute monoarthritis of the hip-joint. A marked leucocytosis (over 20,000 per c. mm.) favours osteitis. Abnormal cardiac signs would point clearly to rheumatic fever. Salicylate would rapidly relieve rheumatic arthritis while having little effect on osteitis. In any event, the use of antibiotics should be withheld until a diligent examination, blood count and blood culture have been carried out. We have more than once seen an erroneous diagnosis of acute poliomyelitis made in the toddler who was suffering from acute osteitis of the upper end of one tibia. This can cause fever, pseudoparesis of the affected leg and diminution or absence of the knee-jerk. In osteitis the well-localized bone tenderness, brisk leucocytosis and normal cerebrospinal fluid should serve to resolve any doubts.

Acute leukaemia may also present with bone pain and fever. The pain is, however, rarely localized to one site and the peripheral blood will almost invariably show some significant abnormality. Finally, a fracture can occur in the young child when he is not under direct observation, presenting later as localized pain and tenderness. In this circumstance there will, of course, be no fever or toxaemia.

Treatment

The child suspected of acute osteitis should be admitted to hospital without delay. It is a regrettable fact that most cases of this disease still take longer than 72 hours to reach hospital. Before any specific treatment is started a blood culture, total white cell count and differential count should be performed. If there is severe dehydration or toxaemia an intravenous infusion of 5 per cent dextrose in half-strength physiological saline should be set up. The affected limb should be immobilized in a suitable splint but it must never be hidden inside a plaster cast.

There is room for controversy over the choice of antibiotic and the place for surgical intervention in acute osteitis. These problems have been discussed by Mann (1963). The views expressed here are based upon the author's personal experience and modified to some extent by many discussions of the problem with surgical colleagues. Before stating them it is well to stress that the principal causes of chronic osteitis and other complications are late diagnosis and treatment, or inadequate treatment with an ill-chosen antibiotic; especially if it has been given by the oral route. In such circumstances neither antibiotic nor surgical operation can prevent bone necrosis.

Resolution of early acute osteitis requires the prompt use of an antibiotic to which the causal organism is sensitive. It must be given in full doses, by the parenteral route, and it should preferably be bactericidal rather than bacteriostatic. The acute nature of the disease demands the start of treatment before the causal organism and its antibiotic-sensitivities can be known, although the importance of taking steps to acquire this information and of modifying the treatment in its light cannot be over-emphasized. These facts would seem to us to indicate that the drug of initial choice should be methicillin 100 mg./Kg./day or cloxacillin 50 mg./Kg./day, each to be given in four six-hourly intramuscular doses.

This choice will ensure the defeat of the penicillin-resistant staphylococcus. If the organism is successfully cultured and shown to be penicillin-sensitive a change should be made to benzylpenicillin 500,000 units intramuscularly every six hours. Infections by Gram-negative organisms are rare. They can be best treated with intramuscular streptomycin 50 mg./Kg./day or ampicillin 50 mg./Kg./day. The duration of antibiotic therapy is a difficult problem. Some have tried to solve it by repeated bone-marrow biopsy and culture from the affected metaphysis. This requires general anaesthesia and is probably better avoided. Others advise the continuance of the drug until the E.S.R. falls to normal, but this certainly leads to unnecessarily prolonged treatment. In most cases three weeks is probably an adequate period.

The proponents of early operation and bone drilling claim that it permits isolation of the causal organism in a higher percentage of cases, reduces the extent of bone necrosis and relieves pain (Harris, 1962). Others deny that operation is ever required (Neligan and Elderkin, 1965). It seems to us to be unlikely that operation, whenever performed, can significantly alter the fate of the bone. The drainage of a subperiosteal abscess when this has formed would, however, seem to conform to well-established surgical principles. The timing of such interference requires good clinical judgment. Clear indications are the spread of tenderness well beyond the metaphysis, visible swelling, warmth and redness of the skin, and fluctuation. Subsequent management, and particularly the decision to allow the child to resume weight-bearing, is best undertaken by the orthopaedic specialist. Osteitis of a vertebral body is peculiarly "benign". It responds to antibiotics and operation is hardly ever required.

Chronic Osteitis

This may follow the late or inadequate treatment of acute osteitis. There is often extensive sequestration and formation of involucrum. Chronic bone pain is common and particularly distressing during the night. Necrotic pieces of bone may finally discharge through the skin and lead to the formation of a fistula. Pyaemic foci may develop elsewhere in the body.

Primary chronic osteitis and the formation of a Brodie's abscess is uncommon in children. The condition is characterized by a dull boring pain, usually in the area of a long-bone metaphysis. The diagnosis is confirmed by X-ray.

Treatment

After some days on a suitable antibiotic by the parenteral route open operation is undertaken to remove sequestra and infected granulation tissue. The cavity in the bone is widely opened. An appropriate antibiotic is instilled, the wound is sutured, and the limb is immobilized.

Systemic antibiotic-therapy is continued for a week or two after operation.

ACUTE PYOGENIC ARTHRITIS

Acute suppurative arthritis arising directly from the blood-stream is only seen commonly in the young infant. It is then usually secondary to an infection elsewhere in the body and is, in fact, part of a pyaemic process. The most common organism is a penicillin-resistant staphylococcus but the condition can be caused by Gram-negative bacilli, haemolytic streptococci, meningococci, gonococci, typhoid bacilli and pneumococci. In older children suppurative arthritis is almost invariably a sequel to acute osteitis which has escaped early diagnosis or has been inadequately treated, possibly with the wrong antibiotic. The causal organism is, therefore, the *Staph. aureus* which is penicillin-sensitive in at least 50 per cent of cases. The hip-joint is most commonly affected.

Clinical Features

General signs of pyogenic infection are to be expected unless antibiotics have previously been empirically used. These include fever, anorexia, pain, irritability, toxaemia and polymorphonuclear leucocytosis. The affected joint will be swollen, extremely tender on palpation and its movements will be severely limited by pain and muscle spasm. In osteitis uncomplicated by suppurative arthritis, on the other hand, gentle handling usually allows the physician to demonstrate a normal range of joint movements. Visible swelling, and redness and warmth of the overlying skin are naturally more readily seen in the case of superficial joints such as the knee, shoulder or ankle, whereas arthritis of the hip-joint is readily overlooked in the infant until dislocation has occurred.

Treatment

Diagnostic aspiration of fluid allows identification of the causal organism and its antibiotic sensitivities. An appropriate antibiotic should be given intramuscularly in full doses, and should also be instilled repeatedly into the joint cavity. Open operation and drainage is only necessary when the pus is too thick to come through a needle.

INFANTILE CORTICAL HYPEROSTOSIS (Caffey's disease)

This is a somewhat mysterious but not very uncommon disease of the bones which is peculiar to young infants. It has many of the features of an infection and a virus aetiology has been suggested although no direct evidence to this effect has been obtained. It was first clearly described by Caffey (1946).

Clinical Features

The patient is usually an infant in the first six months of life. The onset is with fever, irritability and obvious tenderness on handling.

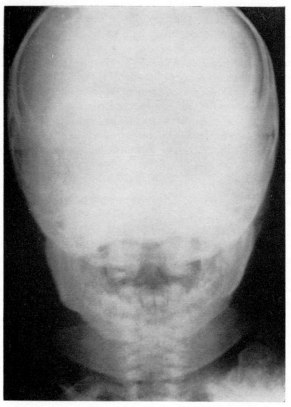

FIG. 79.—Radiograph showing cortical hyperostosis of severe degree in the mandible of an infant.

Always affects mandible (NX A9 now does).

The underlying lesion is a periosteitis with new bone formation and cortical thickening. The bones most commonly affected are the mandible, clavicles, ribs, scapulae and long bones of the limbs. Before there are radiological abnormalities in the bones there is swelling and oedema of the overlying soft tissues. Swelling over the mandible may simulate mumps. The soft tissue swellings over the limbs have a hardness and tenderness which is characteristic. The overlying skin may be shiny but discoloration and warmth of the type seen in bacterial osteitis or cellulitis does not occur. The E.S.R. is always raised. The plasma

c̄ ·Ill → soft tissue swelling ·— → periostitis č new bone formation · Recurrent.
High ESR + A·Phos.

alkaline phosphatase level is usually elevated. The disease is one of re-missions and relapses. Painful swellings may subside only to reappear later at different or even the same sites. The characteristic radiographic changes (Figs. 79 and 80) may take twelve months to disappear. Complete recovery is the rule.

Differential Diagnosis

The condition has been mistaken for multiple osteitis of infancy but the widespread distribution of the bone lesions, the absence of pus formation and of polymorphonuclear leucocytosis should make this mistake unlikely. Overdosage with vitamin A for a long period can produce similar clini-cal and radiological features but the mandible is not affected and the infant is usually nearing the age of one year; hyper-vitaminosis A is rarely seen in the United Kingdom.

Treatment

None of the available anti-bacterial drugs has any effect upon the disease which after months of remissions and relapses recovers spontaneously.

Also responds to steroids if severe & symptoms

"THE BATTERED BABY" SYNDROME

(MULTIPLE EPIPHYSEAL INJURIES)

This is not a rare syndrome but its true aetiology is frequently not appreci-ated because medical men are reluctant to believe that criminal assaults by parents on their babies are common, and also because the guilty parents not unnaturally withhold the relevant medical history (Caffey, 1957; Griffiths and Moynihan, 1963). It is usually from squalid homes that the battered baby syndrome is encountered, and the

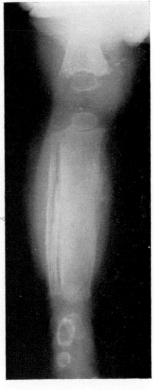

FIG. 80.—Hyperostosis affecting tibia and fibula of same infant as in Fig. 79.

parents are usually of subnormal intelligence. There are, however, exceptions to this generality and it is sometimes difficult to understand how one child of a family may be cruelly mishandled while other siblings receive care and kindness. In some instances, however, the explanation

NO.

for this behaviour lies in the fact that the mishandled child is mentally retarded and, therefore, rejected. The basic lesions of this syndrome are the separation of fragments from the metaphyses, and the separation of periosteum from the shafts of the bones with subperiosteal bleeding. The osteoblasts of the stripped periosteum continue to lay down new bone, so that external hyperostoses form along the shafts of the injured bones. The nature of the trauma is shaking, twisting or pulling of the infant's limbs. It is common also in these unfortunate infants to find fractures, especially of the ribs and clavicles, which can be due only to direct violence. In some of the reported cases death has been due to concomitant head injuries with subdural haematoma.

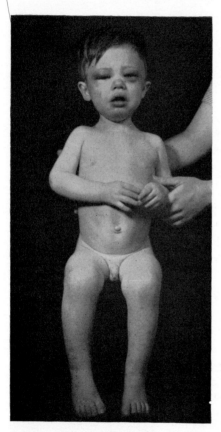

FIG. 81.—"Battered baby". Note extensive ecchymoses of face and temporal regions and swollen right elbow.

Clinical Features

The child is usually brought to the doctor with painful swellings, limitation of movement and possibly bruising in the region of the ends of the long bones. If a history of trauma were to be spontaneously forthcoming there would be no diagnostic problem. The true diagnosis is also easy when the child shows obvious "black eyes" and bruises of the face or sides of the head (Fig. 81). Such signs are, however, uncommon and in their absence the doctor is sometimes misled into an irrelevant differential diagnosis, including scurvy, osteitis, infantile cortical hyperostosis (although the mandible is not affected) and leukaemia. As the presence of fever and leucocytosis are common after haemorrhage several unnecessary and expensive investigations may be initiated.

The fact that traumatic lesions are not infrequently inflicted on babies by their parents must be more widely appreciated by medical men, and direct enquiry of the parents should be made. Even when violence is not admitted, or untruthfully ascribed to other children, the radiological appearances are so typical that they can be correctly interpreted without regard to the parent's clinical history. Soon after the injury the X-ray shows a tell-tale detachment of small bone fragments from the metaphyses and soft-tissue swelling. After several days there is visible hyperostosis due to the depositions of new bone in and beneath the

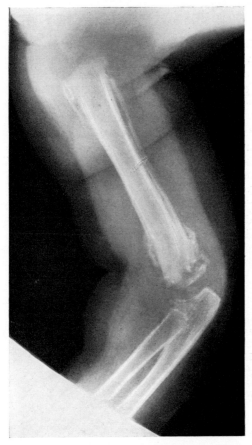

FIG. 82.—Fragmentation of lower metaphysis of humerus and deposition of new bone under periosteum along the shaft in the "battered baby" syndrome. These appearances are diagnostic of mishandling.

stripped periosteum (Fig. 82). Many of these cortical thickenings are lumpy with rough edges. Occasionally, direct injury to the epiphyseal cartilage can result in shortening of the shaft with splaying and cupping

of the shortened end. Whenever the battered baby syndrome is suspected radiographs of the skull and ribs, in addition to the ends of long
bones, should be taken. Linear fractures of the skull are common, and
it is somewhat characteristic to find several unsuspected fractures of the
ribs, often of different duration.

Treatment

It is characteristic that the infant makes a good and spontaneous
recovery in hospital, but if the true situation is not appreciated he may
be sent home to further mishandling, and even to the danger of a violent
death. It is the doctor's duty to reach the correct diagnosis, to confront
the parents with the situation, and to take such relevant steps as he
thinks necessary to guard against a recurrence. In some cases valuable
information concerning the family background can be obtained from
the family doctor, the Health Visitor or the Medical Officer of Health,
which can assist the doctor in determining his future action. In any case
this will be partly dependent on local circumstances. In most instances
the doctor in hospital should inform either the Children's Officer of
the local authority or the local Inspector of the National Society for the
Prevention of Cruelty to Children. The decision to inform the police is
ethically difficult but doctors have duties as citizens as well as medical
advisers. If the parents insist on removing the injured child from the
hospital the doctor may decide to inform the police, letting the parents
know of his intention. The British Paediatric Association (1966) have
published a useful memorandum on the subject of "the battered baby".

REFERENCES

BRITISH PAEDIATRIC ASSOCIATION (1966). *Brit. med. J.*, **1**, 601.
CAFFEY, J. (1946). *J. Pediat.*, **29**, 541.
CAFFEY, J. (1957). *Brit. J. Radiol.*, **30**, 225.
DENNISON, W. M. (1948). *J. Bone Jt. Surg.*, **30B**, 110.
GRIFFITHS, D. LL., and MOYNIHAN, F. J. (1963). *Brit. med. J.*, **2**, 1558.
HARRIS, N. H. (1962). *Brit. med. J.*, **1**, 1440.
MANN, T. S. (1963). *Brit. med. J.*, **2**, 1561.
NELIGAN, G. A., and ELDERKIN, F. M. (1965). *Brit. med. J.*, **1**, 1349.
WHITE, M., and DENNISON, W. M. (1952). *J. Bone Jt. Surg.*, **34B**, 608.

CHAPTER XXIV

DISEASES OF MUSCLES

Disorders which primarily affect muscle fibres, their membranes or the myoneural junctions are mercifully rare. Only the least rare will be discussed in this chapter. In particular, those disorders which usually first become manifest in early adult life, such as dystrophia myotonica (Walton and Nattrass, 1954) and polymyalgia rheumatica (Gordon, 1960), have been excluded from detailed consideration. Glycogen storage disease affecting skeletal muscles may simulate some of the other varieties of muscular weakness. Two types (limit dextrinosis and cardiomegalia glycogenica) are described in Chapter IX. Other extremely rare types have been discussed by Thomson *et al.* (1963).

MYOTONIA CONGENITA (Thomsen's Disease)

This is an extremely rare hereditary disease of the muscles, of unknown aetiology. It usually appears during childhood in the form of a delayed relaxation after voluntary contracture. The disability becomes less as the muscles continue to be used, and is worst following upon a period of rest. The legs are most severely involved so that the start of walking is often stiff and halting. The patient may also be unable to let go his grasp on an object after he has clasped it in his hand. The muscles may be somewhat hypertrophied. Stimulation of a muscle group by percussion results in an abnormally prolonged contraction with a visible concavity at the site of stimulation. Faradic or galvanic stimulation results in contraction for as long as the current is applied followed by a prolonged relaxation phase—the myotonic reaction. Life is not shortened.

Differential Diagnosis

In adult life myotonia congenita must be distinguished from *dystrophia myotonica*, in which the delayed relaxation following voluntary contraction is associated with atrophy, and where in contrast to myotonia congenita the muscles of mastication and of the face and neck are affected at an early stage. In dystrophia myotonica there may be other severe disabilities such as baldness, cataract and testicular atrophy.

Treatment

Considerable symptomatic relief can be obtained with oral quinine sulphate or hydrochloride 5 grains (0·3 gm.) twice or thrice daily.

PROGRESSIVE MUSCULAR DYSTROPHY

If the very rare distal and ocular varieties are excluded and also some atypical cases and those associated with thyrotoxicosis, cases of this disease fall into three groups which are clinically distinguishable and genetically separate—namely the pseudohypertrophic (Duchenne) type, the facioscapulohumeral (Landouzy-Déjérine) type and the limb-girdle (Erb) type (Walton, 1964).

The pathological features common to them all are cellular degeneration, the muscle fibres appearing small or swollen with accumulation of nuclei along the sarcolemmal sheaths, and replacement of muscle by connective tissue so that individual fibres are widely separated by intervening fibrous and areolar tissue. In the pseudohypertrophic variety much fatty infiltration gives the muscles a characteristic yellow colour on cross-section. Affected adults show an excessive urinary output of creatine and a diminished excretion of creatinine, but these parameters are of little or no value in childhood.

DUCHENNE TYPE (PSEUDOHYPERTROPHIC) MUSCULAR DYSTROPHY

Aetiology

Over 90 per cent of cases are transmitted as a sex-linked recessive trait so that only males are affected, while the disease is transmitted by females. There is also a sub-variety of pseudohypertrophic muscular dystrophy which, while also inherited in sex-linked recessive fashion, is clinically less severe than the classical form of the disease. The minority of cases, also exhibiting a milder form of the disease, are transmitted in an autosomal recessive manner so that very occasionally girls can be affected by the disease.

Clinical Features

The onset is usually before the third or fourth years of life, although the significance of the early symptoms is not infrequently overlooked. There may be a history of delay in walking, or of a failure of the gait ever to become steady. The child may fall unduly often, or his great difficulty in climbing stairs may be the parent's principal anxiety. Ultimately the gait assumes a characteristic waddle so that the feet are placed too widely apart and there is an exaggerated lumbar lordosis. Weakness of the shoulder muscles may render the child unable to raise his hands above his head. When he is lifted by his armpits he is apt to slide through the examiner's hands because of the weakness of his shoulder girdle muscles. A quite characteristic phenomenon is seen when the child, lying on his back on the floor, is asked to stand up. He will roll to one side, flex his knees and hips so that he is "on all fours" with both knees and both hands on the ground; he then extends his knees and reaches the erect posture by "climbing up his own legs", using his hands to get higher up each leg in alternate steps.

The muscles which first show weakness are those around the shoulders and hips and thighs. Pseudohypertrophy tends to be best seen in the supra- and infra-spinati, deltoids, triceps, quadriceps and the muscles of the calves. Atrophy is usually first obvious in the pectoralis major, biceps and gluteal muscles. Winging of the scapulae is often prominent due to weakness of the serratus magnus muscles. Tendon reflexes become progressively diminished and finally cannot be elicited as muscle weakness increases. By the age of 10 years the child is usually confined to a wheelchair, although he remains remarkably cheerful. Skeletal and postural deformities may later become severe. The skin of the legs may become blue or mottled due to poor peripheral circulation. Death is usual during adolescence from intercurrent respiratory infection, or the heart may fail from involvement of the myocardium.

Diagnosis

In the fully developed case the clinical picture is quite characteristic. The diagnosis can be confirmed in early cases by muscle biopsy. In recent years it has been discovered that several enzymes are consistently found to be present in excess in the serum of sufferers from progressive muscular dystrophy. Indeed, it is now possible to identify shortly after birth, those males who will later manifest the disease (Walton, 1964). The serum aldolase level is normally below 10 Bruns units per ml., whereas in muscular dystrophy of the Duchenne type levels of 20–170 are found (Clayton et al., 1963). Even more revealing are the serum levels of creatine phosphokinase (Hughes, 1962). These show a rise in the apparently healthy female carriers of the disease (Walton, 1964), and this correlates with the fact that minor dystrophic changes can be detected in muscle biopsy specimens from known female carriers. The upper normal level of serum creatine phosphokinase is 3·5 units per ml., but values of up to several hundred units have been recorded in cases not yet showing clinical signs.

Treatment

There is as yet no satisfactory treatment for muscular dystrophy although many substances such as vitamins, hormones and aminoacids have been tested. Initial claims for success with a proprietary mixture of nucleotides and nucleosides (Thomson and Guest, 1963) were discounted when a control trial failed to show that any improvement in the serum creatine phosphokinase levels or muscle power followed their use (Pearce, et al., 1964). Physiotherapy is frequently prescribed with beneficial psychological effects upon the child and his parents.

FACIOSCAPULOHUMERAL MUSCULAR DYSTROPHY

Aetiology

This form of dystrophy is transmitted as an autosomal dominant trait and can affect both sexes.

Clinical Features

The onset may be in early childhood or early adult life, most often with weakness and lack of expression in the facial muscles (Fig. 83). In

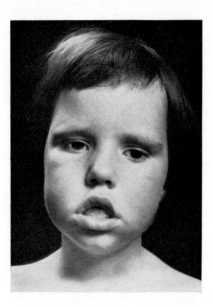

FIG. 83.—Facioscapulohumeral dystrophy: note typical lack of expression and inability to smile.

time the child cannot close his eyes, wrinkle his forehead or purse his mouth. The lips project forwards due to weakness of the orbicularis oris to give the appearance of "tapir mouth". Weakness of the shoulder girdle muscles, especially the pectoralis major, serratus magnus, trapezius, spinati, deltoid, triceps and biceps results in winging of the scapulae, inability to raise the arms above the head and looseness of the shoulders. Then the pelvic girdle becomes affected, glutei, quadriceps, hamstrings and iliopsoas, so that there is lumbar lordosis and a broad-based gait. This form of muscular dystrophy usually runs a prolonged and relatively benign course well into adult life. Indeed, the face only may be affected during most of childhood and severe crippling may be long delayed. The diagnosis can be confirmed by muscle biopsy or by finding elevated serum levels of aldolase or creatine kinase.

Treatment

None is available at the present time.

LIMB-GIRDLE MUSCULAR DYSTROPHY

Aetiology

This form of dystrophy in which pseudohypertrophy is uncommon is probably inherited as an autosomal recessive characteristic. Males and females are equally affected.

Clinical Features

These rarely appear during the first decade. Weakness first becomes obvious in the muscles of the shoulder girdle with winging of the scapulae and difficulty in raising the arms. Later the muscles of the pelvic girdle become affected. The facial muscles are never affected. The disease runs a slow course but usually leads to death before the normal age.

This type of muscular dystrophy is extremely rare in paediatric practice.

MYASTHENIA GRAVIS

Aetiology

There seems to be a defect of conduction at the myoneural junction compatible with a decreased acetylcholine effect in the motor end-plate. Simpson (1960) has suggested that myasthenia gravis may be an autoimmune disorder; the thymus may produce an antibody to muscle end-plate protein which acts as an acetylcholine competitive-blocking substance. Others (van der Geld et al., 1963) have added to the evidence in favour of this concept by demonstrating antibodies against skeletal muscle, thymus and thyroid tissue in the sera of myasthenic patients. The relationship of myasthenia gravis to hyperplasia of the thymus gland is now well established; in myasthenic patients who have a thymoma there is an even higher incidence of antibodies and their clinical condition tends to be more severe. A further feature of the myasthenic patient is his resistance to depolarizing agents such as succinylcholine and decamethonium. It is interesting that the healthy newborn infant shows a similar tolerance of depolarizing agents (Churchill-Davidson and Wise, 1963), although its relevance to the aetiology of myasthenia gravis is still obscure.

Clinical Features

Cases of myasthenia gravis have been reported as early in life as the first year, but the onset is rarely before the age of ten years. The ocular muscles are usually first affected; the child presents with ptosis (Fig. 84) or complains of diplopia; the muscle weakness tends to be more severe as the day goes on so that there may be marked ptosis or strabismus,

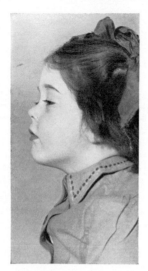

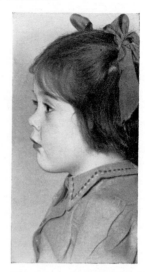

Fig. 84.—Bilateral ptosis in 4-year-old girl suffering from myasthenia gravis.

Fig. 85.—Same girl as in Fig. 84 a few minutes after a subcutaneous injection of neostigmine.

usually bilateral. The bulbar muscles are often next affected although this may not occur for some years. The voice is then weak, swallowing and chewing become difficult, and there may be asphyxial episodes due to the aspiration of upper respiratory secretions and saliva. When the facial muscles are affected a lack of expression is a striking feature. In the worst cases the muscles of the limbs and those responsible for respiration are affected. These features are always less obvious, and may totally disappear, after a night's rest. Muscle atrophy or fibrillary twitchings do not occur. The deep reflexes are usually present and may even be exaggerated. Although the thymus gland is hyperplastic this is not radiologically obvious unless there is an actual thymoma, when a large opacity may be visible in the superior mediastinum.

An interesting and highly dangerous form of myasthenia gravis is that which can affect the newborn infant of a myasthenic mother. The manifestations include a weak cry, generalized severe hypotonia, feeble sucking reflex and attacks of choking and cyanosis. They are temporary and recover within a few weeks, but are not infrequently fatal unless treatment is promptly instituted. Ptosis and paralysis of the extra-ocular muscles are apparently uncommon in neonatal myasthenia (Teng and Osserman, 1956).

As in the adult, the myasthenic child may run a prolonged course of remissions and relapses, but there is a tendency for the disease to reach a static phase some five years from the onset (Simpson, 1960; Walton,

1964). There is always a risk of death from aspiration of food into the respiratory passages, from respiratory failure if the diaphragm and intercostal muscles are affected, or from intercurrent respiratory infection.

Diagnosis

This should be suspected in the presence of ptosis, strabismus, bulbar palsy or severe muscular hypotonia during infancy or childhood. The manifestations can be immediately relieved by the hypodermic injection of neostigmine salicylate 0·25–1·0 mg. along with atropine sulphate 1/200–1/100 gr. (0·3–0·6 mg.) (Fig. 85). In infancy the heart-rate should be watched after this test, as occasionally a dangerous degree of bradycardia may require further doses of atropine. A drug of similar action to neostigmine but transient in its effects is to be found in edrophonium (Tensilon). It can be given intravenously in an initial dose of 2 mg. If there is no untoward response and no dramatic relief a further dose of 4–8 mg., according to age, should be given after a minute or so. The use of one of these drugs will always settle any doubts about the diagnosis.

Treatment

This should always be medical in the first instance and many patients can be adequately treated in this fashion. It must be recognized that different muscles show variable sensitivity towards the action of the anticholinesterase drugs. If an overdose is prescribed because certain muscles remain weak on a particular dosage, prolonged depolarization of muscle end-plates develops and causes transmission failure and paralysis (cholinergic crisis). The short-acting edrophonium may be used to determine whether the dose is optimal. If an intravenous injection fails to increase the efficiency of the respiratory muscles, when given after the drug which is being used for maintenance therapy, or if weakness is increased, the child is already having too much of the anticholinesterase drug. This test should only be performed after preparations have been made for assisted respiration.

The most useful drug for continuous treatment is pyridostigmine bromide (Mestinon) given orally in a dosage of 10–60 mg. every 3–8 hours according to the child's age and clinical response. Pyridostigmine gives fewer parasympathomimetic effects and smoother control than neostigmine bromide given orally in a dosage of 5–15 mg. every 6–8 hours. On the other hand, a more rapid relief of muscular weakness is obtained with neostigmine, and side-effects such as colic, sweating or bradycardia can be relieved with atropine sulphate 1/100 gr. (0·6 mg.) given orally. In some patients pyridostigmine and neostigmine can with advantage be used in combination. In the few resistant cases the effects of anticholinesterase drugs may be enhanced by potassium chloride 1 gm. twice or thrice daily.

The position of thymectomy in the treatment of myasthenia gravis in childhood is not yet clearly defined because of the relative rarity of the disease, and the reasonably satisfactory results usually obtained from medical treatment. Good results follow thymectomy in 70 per cent of young adults (Henson *et al.*, 1965). The indications for operation are a duration of the disease of under two years, and inadequate control of the muscular weakness with drugs. Improvement after thymectomy is gradual, and the operation should not be performed as an emergency procedure in a myasthenic crisis. In cases of malignant thymoma the best results follow deep X-ray therapy before surgical removal of the tumour and thymus gland.

FAMILY PERIODIC PARALYSIS (Teenage boys)

The classical form of this disease has its onset during the second decade. It is more common in males. Attacks of extreme muscular weakness, each lasting for several hours, occur in the early morning, or after a period of rest following brisk exertion, or soon after a heavy carbohydrate meal. The muscles of speech, swallowing and respiration are spared. During the attacks the serum potassium level is markedly reduced (below 3 mEq. per litre), but as there is a positive balance of potassium it seems that there must be a movement of the retained potassium into the muscle cells. The finding of a normal resting membrane potential during an attack, even when potassium has moved into the cell, is probably due to an associated inward movement of water (Shy *et al.*, 1961; Walton, 1964). Between attacks there are no symptoms and, indeed, some of these patients have shown a particularly robust physique. Other significant findings during an attack are a rise in the serum sodium concentration, and the typical electrocardiographic changes of hypokalaemia (flattened T waves, depression of the ST segment and prolongation of the QT interval with large U waves). Attacks can be induced in these patients with glucose or insulin, or with a combination of both (Stanbury *et al.*, 1965). In most instances the disease is transmitted as an autosomal dominant trait but apparently sporadic cases also arise, usually in males. Families in which periodic paralysis occurs have frequently shown an increased incidence of migraine, epilepsy and progressive muscular atrophy.

While the above description applies to the classical disease, more or less identical symptoms have been found in patients in whom the serum potassium does *not* fall during attacks (Tyler *et al.*, 1951). The name *adynamia episodica hereditaria* was suggested by Gamstorp (1956). In this form of periodic paralysis the attacks usually last for 30–40 minutes. The serum potassium is either normal or elevated during an attack (McArdle, 1962). Indeed, attacks can be induced by potassium chloride. This condition seems also to be inherited in autosomal dominant fashion.

In a third type of periodic paralysis (Poskanzer and Kerr, 1961) the attacks may last for weeks. Here too the serum potassium level is normal and attacks can be precipitated with potassium.

Treatment

In the common hypokalaemic variety of periodic paralysis the obvious treatment is the administration of potassium. This must not be done without first having established the existence of a lowered serum potassium level, because in the types of periodic paralysis associated with a normal or raised serum level the administration of potassium could be very dangerous.

In the hypokalaemic attacks the oral administration of potassium chloride 3–10 gm. is effective. Its value in preventing attacks is less but the use of 3–5 gm. at night is probably worthwhile. A diet low in carbohydrate is indicated, especially in the later part of the day, and excessive exertion should be avoided.

In *adynamia episodica hereditaria* attacks are said to be prevented by acetazolamide or hydrochlorothiazide. In the third type described above acetazolamide combined with 9 alpha-fluorohydrocortisone (0·1 mg./day) may prevent attacks.

ARTHROGRYPOSIS MULTIPLEX (AMYOPLASIA CONGENITA)

This is a rare disease of unknown aetiology. It is characterized by congenital stiffness of several joints. The hips and elbows are usually flexed, the knees often extended. The surrounding muscles can be shown radiologically to be grossly hypoplastic. The spinal movements, however, are not limited. Fibrous ankylosis of some joints may occur, in others spontaneous dislocation. There may be other deformities such as club feet, cleft palate, absence of sacrum or club hand. There is no specific treatment.

MYOSITIS OSSIFICANS PROGRESSIVA

In this disease of unknown cause calcium is deposited in the inter-muscular septa, fascial sheaths and tendons. The condition might be better called "myositis calcificans" as the calcium deposition is not always in the form of true bone.

Clinical Features

The onset is in early childhood. The first sign is a swelling in the muscles of any part of the body, often over the back. It is initially tender and may be surrounded by oedema. After it subsides a hardness can be felt in the muscles and calcification can be demonstrated radiologically (Fig. 86). This story is repeated in widespread parts of the skeletal musculature. In some cases calcified masses ulcerate through the skin. Some of these masses become very large; they may even become attached to bone and severe crippling can result. There is no abnormality in the blood chemistry. Children affected with this disease frequently

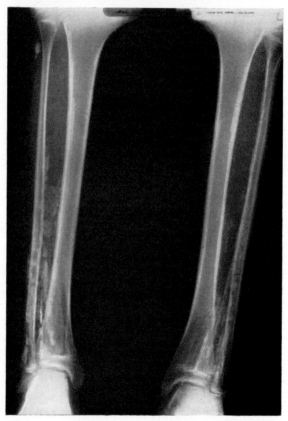

Fig. 86.—Radiograph of legs in myositis ossificans progressiva showing extensive metastatic calcification.

show hypoplasia of the thumbs and great toes, or other minor developmental anomalies. This disease must be distinguished from myositis fibrosa (see below) and dermatomyositis (Chapter XXVI).

Treatment

No specific therapy is available. In a case seen by the author (Fig. 86) a trial of corticosteroids failed to produce any benefit. E.D.T.A. has also been tried without improvement in the ossification.

MYOSITIS FIBROSA

There is a gradual degeneration of skeletal muscle and its replacement by fibrous tissue, but calcification does not occur. The aetiology is obscure.

Clinical Features

The disease first appears in the muscles of the calves and thighs which become progressively stiffened, hardened and contracted as fibrous tissue replaces muscle. There is, however, no pain. Slowly the process advances into the muscles of the back, shoulders, neck, abdomen, hips and chest. Flexion deformities ultimately lead to the child becoming bed-ridden. There may be a terminal state of cachexia.

Treatment

Physiotherapy is the only measure likely to slow down the development of deformities and immobilization.

REFERENCES

CHURCHILL-DAVIDSON, H. C., and WISE, R. P. (1963). *Anesthesiology*, **24**, 271.
CLAYTON, B. E., WILSON, K. M., and CARTER, C. O. (1963). *Arch. Dis. Childh.*, **38**, 208.
GAMSTORP, I. (1956). *Acta paediat.* (*Uppsala*), **45**, Suppl. 108, 1.
GORDON, I. (1960). *Quart. J. Med.*, **116**, 473.
HENSON, R. A., STERN, G. M., and THOMPSON, V. C. (1965). *Brain*, **88**, 11.
HUGHES, B. P. (1962). *Brit. med. J.*, **2**, 963.
MCARDLE, B. (1962). *Brain*, **85**, 121.
PEARCE, J. M. S., GUBBAY, S. S., HARDY, J., PENNINGTON, R. J. T., NEWELL, D. J., and WALTON, J. N. (1964). *Brit. med. J.*, **2**, 915.
POSKANZER, D. C., and KERR, D. N. S. (1961). *Amer. J. Med.*, **31**, 328.
SHY, G. M., WANKO, T., ROMLEY, P. T., and ENGEL, A. G. (1961). *Exp. Neurol.*, **3**, 53.
SIMPSON, J. A. (1960). *Scot. med. J.*, **5**, 419.
STANBURY, J. B., WYNGAARDEN, J. B., and FREDRICKSON, D. S. (1965). *The Metabolic Basis of Inherited Disease*, 2nd edit. New York: McGraw-Hill Book Co.
TENG, P., and OSSERMAN, K. (1956). *J. Mt. Sinai Hosp.*, **23**, 711.
THOMSON, W. H. S., and GUEST, K. E. (1963). *J. Neurol. Neurosurg. Psychiat.*, **26**, 111.
THOMSON, W. H. S., MACLAURIN, J. C., and PRINEAS, J. W. (1963). *J. Neurol. Neurosurg. Psychiat.*, **26**, 60.
TYLER, F. H., STEPHENS, F. E., GUNN, F. D., and PERKOFF, G. T. (1951). *J. clin. Invest.*, **30**, 492.
VAN DER GELD, H., FELTKAMP, T. E. W., VAN LOGHEM, J. J., OOSTERHUIS, H. J. H., and BIEMOND, H. (1963). *Lancet*, **2**, 373.
WALTON, J. N. (1964). *Lancet*, **1**, 447.
WALTON, J. N., and NATTRASS, F. J. (1954). *Brain*, **77**, 169.

CHAPTER XXV

DISTURBANCES OF NUTRITION

Nutritional deficiencies, other than those which are secondary to inborn errors of metabolism and malabsorption, and with the exception of iron-deficiency anaemia, are rare in the United Kingdom today. Some, such as kwashiorkor and vitamin B-complex deficiencies, have never been seen in this country so that the author cannot write of them from personal experience. In this chapter attention is given to deficiency of vitamins A, C and D which are commonly lacking in the basic diet of the human infant. Chronic vitamin A poisoning and idiopathic hypercalcaemia are also discussed; they are, in a sense, the results of our highly effective efforts to abolish vitamin A and D deficiency.

INFANTILE RICKETS

Rickets is a metabolic disturbance of growth which affects bone, skeletal muscles, and sometimes the nervous system. The type under consideration is due primarily to an insufficiency of vitamin D. The naturally occurring animal vitamin is D_3 (cholecalciferol). It can be formed in the human by irradiation of 7-dehydrocholesterol in the skin with ultra-violet light; or it can be ingested in the form of fish-liver oils, eggs, butter or margarine. The ultra-violet irradiation of ergosterol produces vitamin D_2 (ergocalciferol) which, in humans, is equally antirachitic with vitamin D_3. It is, however, not a natural animal vitamin. There is no vitamin D_1.

Aetiology

The deficiency of vitamin D which once resulted in so much infantile rickets, with its toll of permanent deformities, and deaths during childbirth, arose principally because of the limited amount of sunshine and skyshine in our Northern hemisphere. Furthermore, in our large industrial cities the skyshine contained very little ultra-violet light after filtering through the dust, smoke and fog. The need in a cold climate for heat-retaining clothing and the tendency to remain indoors in inclement weather further deprived the infants of ultra-violet irradiation. The natural diet of the human infant contains little vitamin D, especially if he is artificially fed on cow's milk. Indeed, cereals which are commonly used have a somewhat rachitogenic effect because the phosphorus in cereals is in an unavailable form, phytic acid (inositol-hexaphosphoric acid) which combines with calcium and magnesium in the gut to form the complex compound, phytin. It is obviously essential to fortify the infant's diet with vitamin D if he is to avoid rickets, although this would not be necessary in the wholly breast-fed infant living in the countryside of a sunny land. In recent years we have seen a good deal of rickets in the children of coloured races in the United Kingdom because of the combination of skin pigmentation, deficient ultra-violet light, and a diet which, while possibly adequate in their country of origin, is lacking in sufficient vitamin D (Dunnigan *et al.*, 1962).

Another important causative factor, necessary for the development of rickets, is growth. The marasmic infant does not develop rickets when he is vitamin D deficient unless he starts to grow. On the other hand, the premature infant of low birth-weight, who grows rapidly, is especially prone to develop rickets.

Pathogenesis

Remarkably little is known about the physiological actions of vitamin D. It is essential for the intestinal absorption of calcium. It also increases the absorption of phosphorus but this is probably related to its primary effect on the absorption of calcium. It appears also to have a direct effect on bone by increasing resorption of calcium from fully calcified bone and making it available for the formation of new bone. The effects of vitamin D on the kidney when given in large doses is to increase the excretion of calcium and phosphorus, but in the presence of rickets the urinary output of phosphorus is decreased. In rickets the serum citrate level is reduced (normal 2–3·5 mg. per 100 ml.) and the citrate content of bone, intestine and kidney is also low. Citrate ions bind calcium in a soluble unionized complex and it has been suggested that the actions of vitamin D depend on an increase in the citrate concentrations in the tissues (Fourman, 1960).

The first effect of vitamin D-deficiency is thought to be a fall in the concentration of calcium in the extracellular fluid. This results in parathyroid stimulation which usually maintains the serum calcium level at or near the normal. On the other hand, the phosphaturic effect of increased parathyroid hormone results in a lowered serum phosphorus level. This produces the low (Ca) × (P) product which is such a characteristic feature of active rickets. This stage is quickly followed by a rise in the plasma alkaline phosphatase, and then by the radiological and clinical features of rickets.

Pathology

In the normal infant there is a zone of cartilage between the diaphysis and the epiphysis—the epiphyseal plate. At the epiphyseal end this cartilage is actively growing (proliferative zone); whereas at the diaphyseal end, where mature cartilage cells are arranged in orderly columns, osteoblasts lay down calcium phosphate to form new bone.

In rickets the cartilage near the diaphysis (resting zone) shows a disordered arrangement of capillaries and although osteoblasts are numerous normal calcification does not take place. This is called osteoid
tissue. In the meantime active growth of the proliferative zone continues
so that the epiphyseal plate is enlarged and swollen. Osteoid tissue instead of normal bone is also formed under the periosteum. There is also,
in severe cases, a general decalcification of the skeleton so that curvatures and deformities readily develop.

Clinical Features

The diagnosis of infantile rickets is not difficult but its rarity in the
United Kingdom has resulted in its being unfamiliar to many of the
younger physicians. It is, however, still seen in a few of the more "unsatisfactory" families living in the slums of large cities (Arneil and
Crosbie, 1963), and in some instances these cases have been well advanced before diagnosis and treatment. A careful dietary history with
especial reference to the ingestion of vitamin D-fortified milks and
cereals, and of vitamin supplements, should reveal the child who is at
risk. In the era before the second World War rickets usually had its
onset about the age of six months, and even earlier in premature infants.
In recent years the cases of rickets have had a later onset because most
infants in the United Kingdom are fed on calciferol-fortified dried
milks during the early months of life. However, if liquid cow's milk
is needlessly substituted when mixed feeding is started, and if the
calciferol-fortified pre-cooked cereals and vitamin D supplements are
not given, rickets is likely to develop between the age of a year and
eighteen months.

There are few subjective symptoms of rickets. Head sweating is probably one. General muscular hypotonia encourages abdominal pro-
tuberance; this can be increased by flaring out of the rib margins, and
by fermentation of the excess carbohydrate so commonly included in
the diets of ignorant people. The rachitic child commonly suffers from a
concomitant iron-deficiency anaemia (Chapter XIX). His frequent
susceptibility to respiratory infections is related more to his squalid
environment and to over-crowding than to the rickets. The same
applies to the unhappy irritable behaviour which rachitic children sometimes exhibit.

The objective signs of rickets are found in the skeleton. The earliest
physical sign in the baby is craniotabes. This is due to softening of the
occipital bones where the head rubs on the pillow. When the examiner's
fingers press upon the occipital area the bone can be depressed in-and-
out like a piece of old parchment. Another common early sign is the
"rachitic rosary" or "beading of the ribs" due to swelling of the
costochondral junctions. The appearance is of a row of swellings, both
visible and palpable, passing downwards and backwards on both sides

of the thorax in the situations of the rib ends (Figs. 57 and 87). Swelling of the epiphyses is also seen at an early stage, especially at the wrists, knees and ankles (Fig. 87).

In severe cases the shafts of the long bones may develop various curvatures leading to genu varum, genu valgum and coxa vara. A particularly common deformity, shown in Fig. 87, is curvature at the

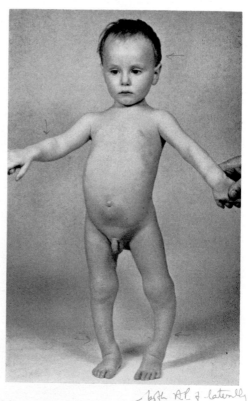

Fig. 87.—Child aged 1 10/12 years with rickets. Note swollen radial epiphyses, enlarged costochondral junctions, bowing of tibiae, and lumbar lordosis.

q protuberant abdomen
+ frontal bossing

both AP & laterally

junction of the middle and lower thirds of the tibiae. This is often due to the child, who may "have gone off his feet", being sat on a chair with his feet projecting over the edge in such a fashion that their weight bends the softened tibial shafts. Bossing over the frontal and parietal bones, due to the subperiosteal deposition of osteoid, gives the child a broad square forehead, or the "hot-cross-bun head". The anterior fontanelle may not close until well past the age of eighteen months, although this delay can also occur in hypothyroidism, hydrocephalus, and even in some healthy children. Another deformity affecting the bony thorax results in Harrison's grooves. These are seen as depressions or sulci on each side of the chest running parallel to but above the diaphragmatic attachment. This sign, however, may also develop in cases of congenital heart disease, asthma and chronic respiratory infection. Laxity of the spinal ligaments can allow the development of various spinal deformities such as dorso-lumbar kyphoscoliosis. In children who have learned to stand there may be an exaggerated lumbar lordosis. The severely rachitic child will also be considerably dwarfed. Pelvic deformities are not readily appreciated in young children but in the case of girls can lead to severe difficulty during childbirth in later years. The pelvic inlet may be narrowed by forward displacement of the sacral promontory, or the outlet may be narrowed by forward movement of the lower parts of the sacrum and of the coccyx.

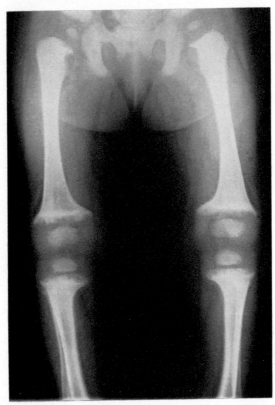

Fig. 88.—Florid rickets showing splaying and fraying of ends of the long bones. Early healing is indicated by the thin white lines of calcification near the diaphyses.

Radiological Features— *best seen at lower ends of radius + ulna.*

The normally smooth and slightly convex ends of the long bones become splayed out with the appearance of fraying or "cupping" of the edges. The distance between the diaphysis and the epiphysis is increased because the metaphysis consists largely of non-radio-opaque osteoid tissue. The periosteum may be raised because of the laying down of osteoid tissue, and the shafts may appear decalcified and curved. In the worst cases green-stick fractures with poor callus for-

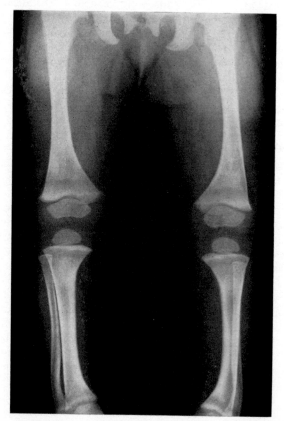

FIG. 89.—Radiographs from same case as in Fig. 88. Rickets has healed.

mation may occur. The earliest sign of healing is a thin line of preparatory calcification near the diaphysis (Fig. 88) followed by calcification in the osteoid just distal to the frayed end of the diaphysis. In time both the ends and shafts of the bones usually return to normal (Fig. 89).

Biochemical Features

The typical findings are a normal serum calcium level (9–11 mg. per 100 ml.) whereas the serum phosphate level (normally 5–7 mg. per 100 ml. in childhood) is markedly reduced to between 2 and 3 mg. per 100 ml. The normal serum calcium in the presence of diminished intestinal absorption of calcium is explained on the basis of increased parathyroid activity which mobilizes calcium from the bones. The serum phosphate falls due to the phosphaturia which results from the effect of parathyroid hormone on the renal tubules. A serum calcium $\times$ phosphorus product above 40 excludes rickets, while a figure below 30 indicates active rickets. This well-known formula is useful in clinical practice but it has no real meaning in terms of physical chemistry. The plasma alkaline phosphatase level (normal 15–20 King-Armstrong units) is markedly raised in rickets and only returns to normal with effective treatment. It is, in fact, a very sensitive and early reflection of rachitic activity but it can, of course, be raised in a variety of unrelated disease states such as hyperparathyroidism, obstructive jaundice, fractures, malignant disease of bone and the "battered baby" syndrome (Chapter XXIII).

Differential Diagnosis

Few diseases can simulate infantile rickets. In hypophosphatasia (Chapter IX) some of the clinical and radiological features resemble those seen in rickets, but their presence in the early weeks of life excludes vitamin D-deficiency. Other features such as defective calcification of the membranous bones of the skull, low plasma alkaline phosphatase and hypercalcaemia are never found in rickets. At one time *achondroplasia* was ascribed, wrongly, to foetal rickets. In fact the two diseases have nothing in common save dwarfism. The characteristic features of achondroplasia—short upper limb segments, large head with relatively small face and retroussé nose, trident arrangement of the fingers, lordosis, waddling gait, and X-ray evidence of defective endochondral ossification—are unmistakably different from anything seen in rickets. The globular enlargement of the hydrocephalic skull (Chapter XX) is quite distinct from the square bossed head of severe rickets. The bone lesions of congenital syphilis (Chapter X) are present in the early months of life and associated with other characteristic clinical signs such as rashes, bloody snuffles, hepatosplenomegaly and lymphadenopathy. In later childhood the sabre-blade tibia of syphilis shows anterior bowing and thickening different from rachitic bowing and in the absence of skeletal deformities elsewhere. Some healthy toddlers show an apparent bowing of the legs due to the normal deposition of fat over the outer aspects; this is unimportant and temporary, and there are no other signs of skeletal abnormality. Other normal young children have a mild, and physiological, degree of genu valgum due to a mild valgus position of the feet; in rachitic genu valgum there will be other rickety deformities. Other types of rickets due to coeliac disease (Chapter XVI) and renal diseases (Chapter XVII) must be excluded by appropriate investigations. Their existence is, however, almost always indicated in a carefully taken clinical history.

Prevention

700units/day. (double in winter.)

The normal vitamin D requirements of the healthy British infant have been discussed in Chapter VII. Rickets is seen today only in British families of low intelligence who fail to avail themselves of the medical advice so freely available from the Child Welfare Services of the Local Authorities. It is necessary for Health Visitors to seek out the types of family known to them to be at risk, but too often they find a lack of co-operation from the parents. The advantages of using a vitamin D-fortified milk preparation throughout the first year of an infant's life, and of calciferol-fortified cereals where mixed feeding has started, might be more widely advertised through the various mass media of communication such as radio and television.

Treatment

Although rickets can be healed by exposure to ultra-violet light it is cheaper and more reliable to administer vitamin D in adequate dosage by mouth. A suitable daily dose is 1,600–2,000 International Units (I.U.) orally. This can be achieved with one of the official B.P. or proprietary concentrated preparations such as Adexolin (Glaxo) 40–50 drops per day. Although a low intake of calcium does not by itself cause rickets there should be an adequate amount of calcium in the infant's diet (approx. 1 gm./day). This is contained in 1–1½ pints (600–900 ml.) of milk per day. An alternative method of treatment, especially useful where it is suspected that the parents are unreliable and unlikely to administer a daily dose of vitamin D, is the oral or intramuscular administration of one massive dose of vitamin D ("Stoss therapy"). High potency Radiostol (B.D.H.) 6 ml. orally contains approximately 600,000 I.U. Sterogyl-15 (Roche) 1·5 ml. intramuscularly also contains 600,000 I.U. It is, however, uncertain how much of such a large dose the body can utilize although rapid healing of the rickets can be confidently expected.

Even major deformities will disappear with adequate treatment, and surgical correction is rarely required. The child should be kept from weight-bearing until the X-rays show advanced healing to prevent aggravation of the deformities.

The parents of the rachitic child obviously require education in nutrition and child care. They should be urged to take the child, after treatment, for regular supervision by their family physician or at the local Child Welfare Clinic.

INFANTILE TETANY (SPASMOPHILIA)

Aetiology

Tetany can occur in a variety of situations such as hypoparathyroidism, respiratory alkalosis due to hysterical overbreathing, metabolic alkalosis due to pyloric stenosis, high intestinal obstruction or the excess administration of sodium bicarbonate, and in hypokalaemic alkalosis. In infancy, however, the common types of tetany are seen in the neonatal period in some infants fed on cow's milk preparations (Chapter XX), and in older babies or children suffering from rickets. We are here concerned only with rachitic tetany which is most likely to develop in the early spring. It is by no means confined to severe cases of rickets and seems often to be precipitated by a mild febrile illness.

Pathogenesis

The appearance of tetany depends upon a fall in the ionizable fraction of the serum calcium. Provided the non-ionizable protein-bound calcium is normal, tetany is likely to appear when the total serum calcium level falls below 8 mg. per 100 ml. (There is no method of estimating the level of ionized calcium which is suitable for the routine laboratory.) It is not known what brings about the marked fall in the serum calcium in some cases of rickets. In a few cases the administration of vitamin D has this effect, possibly by increasing the un-ionized calcium at the expense of the ionized fraction. Alkalotic tetany, on the other hand, may exist with a normal serum calcium level because the ionized calcium fraction alone is lowered. Conversely, a low total serum calcium level is not necessarily associated with tetany. In the nephrotic syndrome, for instance, the low protein-bound calcium level is accompanied by a normal amount of ionized and diffusible calcium.

Clinical Features

The increased neuromuscular irritability of hypocalcaemia may produce overt clinical manifestations (*active tetany*), or it may be detected only by means of certain specific tests (*latent tetany*).

Active tetany most often presents in infancy in the form of generalized epileptiform seizures (Chapter XX). The possibility of hypocalcaemia is usually suggested by the history which reveals an inadequate intake of vitamin D, and by such signs of rickets as craniotabes or a "rachitic rosary". In the period when infantile rickets was common in Glasgow, convulsions during the first two years of life were more commonly due to hypocalcaemia than to any other cause (Shanks, 1949), and estimation of the serum calcium was a routine investigation in every convulsing child. While this situation has disappeared from the United Kingdom it must still pertain in several parts of the world where rickets is common. In other infants tetany may reveal itself in the form of laryngismus stridulus in which laryngeal spasm causes attacks of apnoea and cyanosis, each followed by a deep inspiration and crowing noise. A fatal outcome can result from such an attack. A third manifestation of active tetany is carpo-pedal spasm; the hands and metacarpo-phalangeal joints are strongly flexed, the fingers are extended and the thumbs are adducted across the palms (*main d'accoucheur*), while the feet are inverted and the toes flexed.

Latent tetany should be looked for in every child with rickets. The most useful test is the facial phenomenon (Chvostek's sign) in which a twitch of the facial muscles on one side can be elicited by tapping over the facial nerve where it crosses the ramus of the mandible. Trousseau's sign is elicited by compressing the arm with the hand or sphygmomano-meter cuff when overt carpal spasm is produced within 1–3 minutes. Erb's sign which rests upon the demonstration of an undue excita-bility of the motor nerves to galvanic stimulation is rarely employed. The ECG may also show such abnormalities as a prolonged Q-T interval in hypocalcaemia.

Treatment

Active tetany complicating infantile rickets may be effectively treated in any one of three ways. The serum calcium level can be rapidly raised by the intravenous or intramuscular injection of 10–20 ml. of 10 per cent calcium gluconate, repeated every eight hours as required. Alternatively, the convulsions can be controlled with chloral hydrate 5–7½ gr. (0·3–0·5 gm.) four-hourly by mouth while the serum calcium level responds to intramuscular calciferol 600,000 units. The author prefers the third method which depends on raising the serum ionized calcium by the production of a metabolic acidosis. This can be achieved quickly with oral calcium or ammonium chloride, 15–30 gr. (1–2 gm.) four-hourly for three days; at the same time treatment with vitamin D should be started. The course of events should, in any event, be fol-lowed in the biochemical laboratory.

INFANTILE SCURVY

This disease was once common in the United Kingdom, but has now virtually disappeared. The author has seen two cases in low-grade mental defectives within the past ten years. The disease is still encountered in some of the less prosperous countries of the world.

Aetiology

The primary cause is an inadequate intake of vitamin C (ascorbic acid), a vitamin which the human is unable to synthesize within his body. It is rare in the breast-fed infant unless the mother suffers from sub-clinical avitaminosis C. Cow's milk contains only about a quarter of the vitamin C content of human milk and this is further reduced by boiling, drying or evaporating. Scurvy seemed to be especially common in infants who received a high carbohydrate diet.

Pathology

Vitamin C deficiency results in faulty collagen tissues including those of bone, cartilage and teeth, and the intercellular substance of the capillaries is also rendered defective. This results in spontaneous hae-morrhages and defective ossification affecting both the shafts and the metaphyseo-epiphyseal junctions. The periosteum becomes detached from the cortex and extensive subperiosteal haemorrhages occur; these explain the intense pain and tenderness, especially of the lower ex-tremities, which these unfortunate infants suffer.

Clinical Features

The first symptoms, increasing irritability, anorexia, malaise and low-grade fever, develop between the ages of seven and fifteen months. The most striking feature is the obvious pain and tenderness which the infant exhibits when he is handled, e.g. during napkin changing or if he is lifted. The legs are most severely affected and they characteristically assume a position ("frog position") in which the hips and knees are flexed and the feet are rotated outwards. We have seen the mother carry the infant into the physician's consulting room lying on a pillow in an effort to avoid hurting him further. The gums become swollen and discoloured and may bleed; this is seen only after teeth have erupted, and the teeth may become loose in the jaws. Periorbital ecchymosis ("black eye") or proptosis due to retro-orbital haemor-rhage is common, but haemorrhages into the skin, epistaxis or gastro-intestinal haemorrhages are not commonly seen in infantile scurvy. The anterior ends of the ribs frequently become visibly and palpably swollen but this does not affect the costal cartilages as in rickets; the sternum has the appearance of having been displaced backwards. Microscopic haematuria is frequently present. A mild orthochromic anaemia is characteristic.

Scorbutic rosary.

Also pseudo-paralysis.

Radiological Features

The diagnosis is most reliably confirmed by X-rays. The shafts of the long bones have a "ground-glass" appearance due to loss of the normal trabeculations. A dense white line of calcification (Fraenkel's line) forms proximal to the epiphyseal plate, and there is often a zone of translucency due to an incomplete transverse fracture immediately proximal to Fraenkel's line. A small spur of bone may project from the end of the shaft at this point ("the corner sign"). The epiphyses, especially at the knees, have the appearance of being "ringed" by white ink. Subperiosteal haemorrhages only become visible when they are undergoing calcification but a striking X-ray appearance is then seen (Fig. 90).

"Soap-bubble" appearance

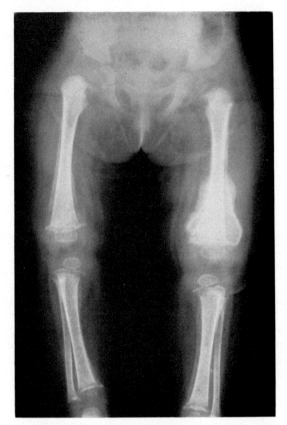

FIG. 90.—Radiograph from a case of infantile scurvy in the healing stage with calcified subperiosteal haematomata. Note also "ringing" of the epiphyses, Fraenkel's white line and proximal zone of translucency.

Differential Diagnosis

The clinical picture of scurvy rarely presents difficulties in interpretation. Pseudo-paresis of a limb due to the pain of subperiosteal haemorrhage might be confused with poliomyelitis but the other features of scurvy should quickly define the position. Similarly, the generalized nature of the bone changes in scurvy should abolish any early suspicion of osteitis. The pseudo-paresis of congenital syphilis occurs at a very much earlier age. Blood diseases which can cause pain in the bones, such as leukaemia, can be excluded by examination of the peripheral blood. The easiest mistake is to overlook the existence of mild scurvy in the child suffering from florid rickets; the radiological appearances of both diseases will be present.

Treatment

The most rapid recovery can be obtained with oral ascorbic acid, 200 mg. per day. There is no advantage in parenteral administration. Excess vitamin C is excreted in the urine and there is no such thing as vitamin C poisoning. The vitamin C requirements of the normal infant are discussed in Chapter VII; they must obviously be ensured after the scurvy has been cured.

(→ 25 mg./day in infants.)
(→ 50 mg./day if older.)

AVITAMINOSIS A

This has never been a common disease in the United Kingdom but cases were reported before the second World War (Spence, 1931; Harris and Abbasy, 1939). Since 1945 the author has seen one case from a particularly squalid home in Glasgow. In many of the under-developed areas of the world vitamin A deficiency is a common cause of blindness and it is not uncommonly associated with marasmus or kwashiorkor. The age-group most affected is from 6 months to 4 years.

Requirements — 1500 u. (< 1 yr) → 4,000 u.

Aetiology

The human intestinal epithelium can synthesize vitamin A from carotene. Both human and cow's milks contain satisfactory amounts of vitamin A whereas vegetables are rich in carotene. Lack of vitamin A is, therefore, only going to arise when a child is fed for long periods on a grossly sub-standard diet, e.g. of cereals, skimmed milk and flour.

Pathology

Avitaminosis A leads to defective regeneration of the visual purple of the retina, to arrest of growth and to increased susceptibility to infection because various types of epithelium undergo atrophy or change to stratified squamous epithelium, e.g. skin, bronchial tree, urinary tract.

Clinical Features

The first objective sign is night blindness. This is followed by xerosis; *xerophthalmia*— the conjunctiva and later the cornea become dry and injected. Bitot's spots may be seen on the bulbar conjunctiva as small yellowish-white triangular patches. Photophobia is marked. In advanced cases the cornea may become opaque and necrotic (keratomalacia) leading to blindness. The skin may become dry and roughened—follicular hyperkeratosis. Intercurrent infections such as pneumonia and pyelonephritis may prove fatal. The serum carotene level is early reduced. In severe cases the serum vitamin A level is also very low.

& mental & physical retardation.

Treatment

Oral vitamin A, 20,000 units daily for seven days followed by 2,500 units daily. The eye lesion is completely reversible at the stage of conjunctival and corneal xerosis but once keratomalacia develops, and this can proceed unsuspected behind the photophobic child's closed eyelids, blindness is inevitable.

CHRONIC VITAMIN A POISONING

Several reports of this disease have come from the more prosperous countries, especially the U.S.A. (Caffey, 1950). It is related to the mother who makes her infant's vitamin requirements somewhat of an obsession so that greatly excessive doses (over 15,000 units daily) are given. Only some infants seem susceptible to these effects. They include malaise, failure to thrive, anorexia and pruritus. The most characteristic change is found radiologically to be a hyperostosis, particularly of the middle portion of the shafts of the long bones. This is associated with tender swelling of the limbs. The jaw is not affected as it is in infantile cortical hyperostosis (Chapter XXIII). The liver may be enlarged. Skin manifestations are alopecia, seborrhoeic-type dermatitis and angular stomatitis.

IDIOPATHIC HYPERCALCAEMIA OF INFANCY

This disease was first reported in the United Kingdom by Lightwood in 1952. Although it has been seen in other countries it seemed to occur with a greater frequency in the U.K. until in recent years it has again showed a diminished incidence.

Aetiology

The resemblance of the features of idiopathic hypercalcaemia to those of vitamin D poisoning was quickly recognized. All the affected infants had been wholly or partially fed on cow's milk preparations, and some had received from various sources (dried milk, vitamin supplements, fortified cereals) unnecessarily large doses of calciferol, e.g. 4,000 units per day. On the other hand, none had received really massive doses of vitamin D and some only quite small amounts. None the less, there was a natural suspicion that the development of this apparently new disease might be related to calciferol (Bonham Carter et al., 1955). Forfar et al. (1956) noted the correlation in these cases between the hypercalcaemia and hypercholesterolaemia; they suggested that there might be a disorder of sterol metabolism in which cholesterol derivatives with toxic effects as well as a vitamin D-like effect were produced in excess. Fellers and Schwartz (1958) found in three severe cases of idiopathic hypercalcaemia that the serum contained much higher levels of vitamin D-like activity than would be expected from their previous intake of this vitamin, also that these levels persisted for many months after the cessation of vitamin D ingestion. They suggested that the anti-rachitic substance in the serum of their patients was not naturally occurring vitamin D_3 but some toxic sterol. In fact, the hypothesis could be that infants who develop this disease on calciferol have a pre-existing inborn error in the metabolism of vitamin D and other sterols. Certainly, the incidence of idiopathic hypercalcaemia in the U.K. has been reduced since the calciferol content of Cod Liver Oil Compound, Dried Milks and Fortified Cereals was reduced in 1958 (Report of Joint Sub-Committee on Welfare Foods, 1957).

Pathology

The only constant finding is medullary nephrocalcinosis. Occasionally metastatic calcification is found in other tissues such as the mitral valve ring.

Clinical Features

The form of the disease first described by Lightwood usually recovers completely and has been referred to as the "benign" type. Shortly after Lightwood's description a "severe" type with a much less happy prognosis was described (Fanconi *et al.*, 1952). Intermediate forms may also occur (Joseph and Parrott, 1958).

Benign type.—The onset is some time between the age of six weeks and eight months with anorexia, frequent vomiting, failure to thrive and severe constipation. The infant becomes marasmic and exhibits severe generalized hypotonia. Numerous hard faecal masses are palpable in the abdomen. Thirst and polyuria may have been noted by an observant parent. The urine is acid and contains some protein. There may be a low-grade pyuria. The diagnostic finding is a raised serum calcium (above 12 mg. per 100 ml.). In many cases the blood urea and serum cholesterol levels are also raised. The electrocardiograph shows characteristic changes of considerable diagnostic value in this type of hypercalcaemia. These are a broad T wave, usually of high voltage, and a short S-T interval (Coleman, 1959). The clinical picture resembles that seen in hyperchloraemic renal acidosis (Chapter XVII) and the differentiation rests upon the blood chemistry.

Severe type.—In addition to the features described above several more serious manifestations occur. The most serious and irreversible is mental retardation. Many of these infants have a characteristically "elf-like" face with low-set ears, long thick upper lip and prominent epicanthic folds (Fig. 91). Hypertension and a loud precordial systolic murmur are commonly present. Hyperostosis of marked degree is constantly found on X-rays, affecting especially the base of the skull, orbits, vertebrae and epiphyses. Marked azotaemia and hypercholesterolaemia are found in addition to hypercalcaemia. Death may occur from renal failure. The survivors are stunted physically and retarded mentally.

Treatment

Vitamin D-containing foods and preparations must be completely withdrawn. The infant should be fed on a specially prepared low-calcium milk such as Locasol (Trufood), or Cow and Gate Low Calcium milk, until the serum calcium level has returned to normal and weight

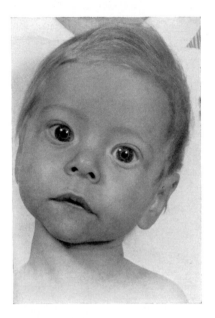

FIG. 91.—Typical facial appearance in severe type of idiopathic hyper-calcaemia.

gain has again started. In severe cases with marked hypercalcaemia, cortisone can be used for a few weeks to achieve a more marked res-ponse. A suitable dosage is 25 mg. four times daily for 7–10 days followed by gradual reduction. The serum potassium level must then be monitored.

REFERENCES

ARNEIL, G. C., and CROSBIE, J. C. (1963). *Lancet*, **2**, 423.
BONHAM CARTER, R. E., DENT, C. E., FOWLER, D. I., and HARPER, C. M. (1955). *Arch. Dis. Childh.*, **30**, 399.
CAFFEY, J. (1950). *Pediatrics*, **5**, 672.
COLEMAN, E. N. (1959). *Brit. med. J.*, **2**, 467.
DUNNIGAN, M. G., PATON, J. P. J., HAASE, S., McNICOL, G. W., GARDNER, M. D., and SMITH, C. M. (1962). *Scot. med. J.*, **7**, 159.
FANCONI, G., GIRARDET, P., SCHLESINGER, B. E., BUTLER, N. R., and BLACK, J. A, (1952). *Helv. paediat. Acta*, I, 314.

FELLERS, F. X., and SCHWARTZ, R. (1958). *New Engl. J. Med.*, **259**, 1050.
FORFAR, J. O., BALF, C. L., MAXWELL, G. M., and TOMPSETT, S. L. (1956). *Lancet*, **1**, 981.
FOURMAN, P. (1960). *Calcium Metabolism and the Bone*. Oxford: Blackwell Scientific Publications.
HARRIS, L. J., and ABBASY, M. A. (1939). *Lancet*, **2**, 1299 and 1355.
JOSEPH, M. C., and PARROTT, D. (1958). *Arch. Dis. Childh.*, **33**, 385.
LIGHTWOOD, R. (1952). *Proc. roy. Soc. Med.*, **45**, 401.
REPORT OF JOINT SUB-COMMITTEE ON WELFARE FOODS (1957). London: H.M. Staty. Office.
SHANKS, R. A. (1949). *Arch. Dis. Childh.*, **24**, 208.
SPENCE, J. C. (1931). *Arch. Dis. Childh.*, **6**, 17.

CHAPTER XXVI

CONNECTIVE TISSUE DISEASES

In this chapter we are concerned with a group of diseases which have been called the connective tissue or collagen diseases. They are less common in childhood than during adult life and their aetiology is not well understood. In each condition inflammatory changes are found to involve tissues of mesenchymal origin. In recent years the concept of "auto-immunity" has been developed, largely arising out of the brilliant thinking of Burnet (1959), and this has been related to the pathogenesis of a large number of disease-states including those to be described. Auto-immunity may be thought of as a breakdown in the normal immunological functions of an individual so that his immunity-producing mechanisms fail to discriminate between "self" and foreign substances and produce antibodies against his own tissues. The subject is complex and in an active stage of exploration by many workers (Miller, 1963; Burnet, 1963; Anderson, 1963). It is proposed to give here only an outline of the present concept of auto-immunity. It should first be pointed out, however, that even when auto-immune responses can be demonstrated in diseases which affect connective tissues in many parts of the body, this fact does not in itself constitute sufficient evidence of cause and effect.

"AUTO-IMMUNITY"

In the normal subject the response to invasion by a foreign substance (antigen) is the production of antibody by lymphoid cells of the reticulo-endothelial system. According to Burnet's clonal selection theory these antibodies are manufactured by large families or "clones" of genetically distinct lymphoid cells, each clone being capable of reacting with only one or two antigens and of producing one or two specific antibodies. In auto-immune states, however, some "forbidden clones" of lymphoid cells, possibly developed as a consequence of spontaneous mutation, fail to recognize their host's own tissues as "self" and react with them as if they were foreign antigens. Burnet has suggested that in the normal subject clones capable of making antibodies against "self" have been destroyed during foetal life. Their existence or appearance in post-natal life is seriously abnormal and detrimental to the individual, who may develop the manifestations of one of the auto-immune diseases. It is, furthermore, important to recognize that there are other aspects to immunity than the classical antibody-mediated reactions. There is also an important type of *in vivo* reaction which is dependent upon cellular immunity or delayed hypersensitivity. This is seen in the tuberculin reaction and also in the rejection of homografts. Little is known of the mechanism of cellular immunity but it may be extremely important in the auto-immune states.

There are two distinct groups of auto-immune disease. In one the antibodies found in the serum are organ specific, e.g. Hashimoto's thyroiditis, pernicious anaemia, Addison's disease and myasthenia gravis. There are tissue specific antibodies also in acquired haemolytic anaemia and idiopathic thrombocytopenic purpura, but in contrast to the diseases just mentioned they cannot be reproduced in experimental animals by the injection of tissue cells along with Freund's adjuvant. In the connective tissue diseases, however, the serum antibodies are not active against one specific organ. Indeed, there are several detectable antibodies; some react with the genetic material (DNA) of the cell nuclei, some with nuclear histones, and others with cytoplasmic fractions. The hypothesis that the cause of the connective tissue diseases lies in the phenomenon of auto-immunity is attractive but it has yet to be shown that any of these antibodies are, in fact, the cause of the widespread tissue damage.

Finally, it may be pointed out that all the diseases of the group under discussion share certain common features, viz: hypergammaglobulinaemia; circulating auto-antibodies; tissue infiltration with lymphoid cells; favourable response to corticosteroids.

RHEUMATOID ARTHRITIS (STILL'S DISEASE)

This is not a rare disease in childhood. It runs a more acute course than is usual in adults but its pathological features are the same. It is important to realize that many tissues can be involved and, in fact, that arthritis may never develop in some patients.

Pathology

The synovial membranes of joints, the pericardium, lymph nodes and other tissues show lymphoid infiltration, oedema and degenerative changes in the connective tissue. The articular cartilages may be ulcerated so that true bony ankylosis sometimes follows.

Clinical Features

These have been well described by Schlesinger *et al.* (1961). The onset is most often between the age of 1½ and 5 years, a younger group than that affected by rheumatic fever. In the older child the first symptoms are often those with which we are familiar in the adult, such as the insidious development of pain and swelling affecting the small joints. In the young child, however, rheumatoid arthritis is to be regarded as a generalized disease of acute onset and rapid progress. The most common features are high remittent fever, generalized lymphadeno-pathy (including the epitrochlears), splenomegaly, polymorphonuclear leucocytosis, and a rash. The rash has an irregular outline, is erythematous and blotchy, and changes its shape and distribution continuously; it somewhat resembles the erythema marginatum of rheumatic fever. In some cases there are also subcutaneous nodules, as in rheumatic fever. Acute pericarditis commonly occurs in rheumatoid arthritis in children (Chapter XIV) but endocardial lesions are quite rare. Joint manifestations are usually present at an early stage although they may initially amount only to arthralgia without visible swelling. It must be stressed, however, that it is not uncommon for the joints to remain symptom-free for many months, and in such cases many fruitless investigations and courses of antibiotics may have been tried. The author has found the typical rash to be a most useful diagnostic pointer.

When the joints are involved they are frequently large ones, e.g. knees, hips, ankles, elbows and wrists. The cervical spine is another commonly affected site, presenting with pain, limitation of movement and torticollis. The affected joints may swell with fluid or show more of a periarticular thickening. The surrounding muscles atrophy, sometimes with startling rapidity. Increasing limitation of movement and muscle weakness can lead to severe crippling. Hypochromic anaemia is often present and it does not respond to haematinics. The disease frequently runs a course of remissions and relapses. In most instances it "burns itself out" after some years, but by then the child may be moderately or severely crippled. Death may occur from intercurrent infection or from amyloid disease.

A few less common clinical manifestations must be mentioned. Involvement of the temporomandibular joints can cause great discomfort and difficulties in eating. Rarely the sternoclavicular joints and chondrocostal junctions can become swollen and very painful. Iridocyclitis can result in much photophobia, lacrimation and pain; cataract and blindness are not unknown. In a few children stridor and hoarseness can reach alarming proportions due to involvement of the crico-arytenoid joints.

In the early stages of arthritis radiographs may show no abnormality or soft tissue swelling may be obvious around the affected joints. Muscle atrophy may be visualized. As the articular cartilage is eroded there is progressive narrowing of the joint space; ultimately true bony union may take place between the opposing bones. Osteoporosis is frequently marked in the bones near the affected joints. Small foci of bone destruction may be seen in the juxta-articular ends of the bones.

Diagnosis

There are few useful laboratory tests in Still's disease. The ASO titre is usually normal. The E.S.R. is always raised when the disease is active. Tests for the rheumatoid factor in the serum (Latex fixation test, Rose-Waaler Test), which are usually positive in adult sufferers, are rarely positive in even severely affected young children. Many of the children have raised serum gamma globulin levels but this is of limited value. The diagnosis must, in most cases, rest upon the typical clinical features and course of the disease.   WBc·f

Prognosis

In general there are three possible end-results. The disease may resolve leaving the child physically fit or only mildly handicapped; it may leave the child severely crippled, perhaps chair-ridden; or inter-current infection to which these children are prone may cause death during the active stage of the disease. In any event the clinical course is always a long one of relapses and remissions.

or → Amyloid.

Treatment

The general care amounts to complete rest in bed and local rest to the joints during the acute stage with constitutional symptoms. Every effort must be made to prevent permanent deformities. When fever and malaise have settled, graded activity should be encouraged. Physiotherapy with active and passive joint movements is of rather limited value. The orthopaedic surgeon may have to perform synovectomy in some badly disorganized joints. The ophthalmologist's aid may be required in the management of iridocyclitis.

The author has lived through a period when a wide variety of toxic drugs have been tried in rheumatoid arthritis. These include gold salts, massive doses of calciferol, nitrogen mustard, phenylbutazone, anti-malarials such as chloroquine, and protein-shock. It is our opinion that in children only salicylates and corticosteroids have any significant effect, and their toxic effects are more than outweighed by their beneficial effects. We have the impression that better results are obtained by using both together than either singly. None the less, in mild early cases aspirin alone can sometimes control the disease and abolish pain, fever and malaise. In most cases corticosteroids must also be used. The effects are usually dramatic with rapid subsidence of arthritis, fever, rash, malaise, lymphadenopathy and splenomegaly. When the corticosteroid is withdrawn there is often a "rebound phenomenon" with a flare up in the symptoms. This may be capable of control with aspirin but in some cases a maintenance dosage of corticosteroid must be continued for years. The doses of aspirin and prednisolone which we generally employ are the same as those given for rheumatic fever (Chapter X). The most likely side-effect of steroid to be looked for in rheumatoid arthritis is osteoporosis which may result in compression-collapse of a vertebral body. The arrest of linear growth in children on long-term steroid therapy is also unwelcome, but may have to be accepted in a serious systemic disease which can endanger life. Blood transfusion is occasionally necessary to correct the anaemia. An open air hospital school is valuable for the child from poor home conditions. The paper by Schlesinger *et al.* (1961) indicates that much better results can be expected with salicylates and steroids than used to be the case. The author, likewise, now feels that there is justification for guarded optimism in most early cases. Long-standing cases with severely damaged joints still do very badly and corticosteroids should be used in severe cases as soon as the diagnosis is certain. In a very rare case the features of one of the other connective tissue diseases may appear in the course of the years.

DISSEMINATED LUPUS ERYTHEMATOSUS

This generalized disease of connective tissue runs a long course of relapses and remissions but it is always lethal in the course of time. These patients show a remarkable capacity for manufacturing antibodies against their own tissues (Holborow, 1963).

Pathology

There is widespread involvement of tissues. The primary lesion of connective tissue appears to be fibrinoid necrosis. Characteristic histological lesions are found especially in the kidneys (thickening of the basement membrane of the glomeruli to produce the appearance of "wire loops"), and spleen (perivascular fibrosis to form concentric rings). Another histological feature of lupus lesions, often found within the fibrinoid areas, are haematoxylin-staining irregular bodies which are thought to contain altered nuclear material.

Clinical Features

The onset is most often with irregular fever, arthralgia with or without obvious swelling of joints, anorexia, general malaise and generalized lymphadenopathy. Hepatomegaly and splenomegaly are common although not always present in the early stages of the illness. Periodic thrombocytopenic purpura is common. The classical rash of "butterfly" distribution over the bridge of the nose, cheeks and lower eyelids makes the diagnosis easy. It is by no means invariably present at the onset of the disease and may never appear. It is essentially an erythematous eruption, it often forms adherent scales, and it may be markedly photosensitive (Fig. 92). The rash may spread over the scalp, neck, upper chest, arms and to the buttocks or legs. In some cases involvement of small blood vessels leads to purpuric or erythematous patches over the palms, soles and fingertips; they may even become necrotic and ulcerate. In other cases there is a somewhat characteristic dusky bluish erythema on the palms and palmar aspects of the fingers.

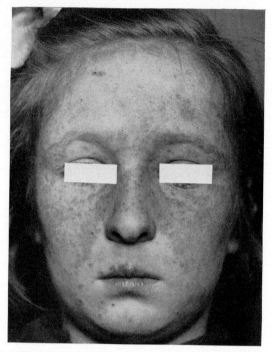

Fig. 92.—Typical "butterfly" rash of disseminated lupus erythematosus.

There may be pericarditis with friction, myocarditis with abnormalities in the ECG, and a verrucose endocarditis (Libman-Sacks syndrome) with murmurs. The most lethal lesions occur in the kidneys in most cases. These are associated with the nephrotic syndrome, hypertension and azotaemia. The urine contains an excess of protein and red cells, and there may be many casts. The nephrotic picture may disappear with treatment but renal hypertension with glomerular failure is inexorable. Other less common features are acquired haemolytic anaemia and leucopenia.

Diagnosis

The E.S.R. is invariably raised. Hypergammaglobulinaemia is usually marked. A false positive serological test for syphilis is common. Serum auto-antibodies may create great difficulties in the cross-matching of blood.

Confirmation of the diagnosis is, however, usually found in the presence of one or more of the multiple auto-antibodies which are found in this disease. These include antinuclear antibodies, antibodies to separate nuclear constituents, cytoplasmic antibodies, antibodies against various blood cells, and in some cases rheumatoid factors (Rose-Waaler test). The test most commonly performed is to search for the so-called L.E. cell. In smears made from incubated bone-marrow or blood from these patients, polymorphonuclear leucocytes with inclusion bodies in their cytoplasm can be found. The inclusion bodies are composed of altered nuclei from other leucocytes. A number of different antibodies to nuclear constituents can also be demonstrated when any unfixed tissue or blood smear is exposed to lupus serum by Coon's immunofluorescent method. For further details the reader is referred to the book by Gell and Coombs (1963). The most prominent immunological disorder in systemic lupus erythematosus is an overproduction of gammaglobulin associated with multiple auto-antibodies with specificities for many tissues. There may also be abnormalities of cellular hypersensitivity or immunity. A similar dysfunction is sometimes seen in other connective tissue disorders, and a familial link between DLE, rheumatoid arthritis, polyarteritis and the other disorders described below is known to exist.

Treatment

In children it is probable that only the corticosteroids offer any hope of amelioration. In adults chloroquine has sometimes proved useful but this applies principally to chronic discoid lupus erythematosus. The progress of the systemic disease can undoubtedly be slowed down with steroid therapy, and the child enabled to live an ambulant existence, often for some years. Once started the steroid drug must usually be continued, in the smallest dose capable of suppressing the clinical manifestations, for the rest of the patient's life. Withdrawal of steroids is rapidly followed by a severe relapse. We have preferred (from familiarity) to prescribe prednisolone. The initial dosage should be in the region of 60–80 mg./day, reducing by stages every 10–14 days. The maintenance dose in this disease can rarely be reduced below 5 mg./day and is more often 10–15 mg./day. The side-effects of steroids become marked but can be accepted in such a serious and lethal disease.

DERMATOMYOSITIS

The muscles and skin bear the brunt of the attack in this type of connective tissue disorder but many other tissues may be involved in the course of the disease. It is less lethal than DLE but in patients who have recovered, considerable physical disability may ensue.

Pathology

The small arterioles show perivascular "cuffing" with lymphoid cells and there is medial proliferation. The striated muscle fibres show loss of striation. The cells of the sarcolemma may be enlarged and multi-

nucleated. The myelin sheaths of the peripheral nerves may show degeneration. In the skin fibrinoid necrosis of connective tissue may be a
marked feature.

Clinical Features

The onset is sometimes with periorbital oedema. There is then a very
characteristic violet dusky rash mainly involving the upper eyelids,
although it may spread over the forehead, bridge of the nose and malar
regions. At times a rash occurs over the elbows, buttocks and thighs.
The rash is rarely as red or scaly as in systemic lupus erythematosus. In
some cases characteristic dusky erythematous patches appear over the
dorsal aspects of the interphalangeal joints of the hands. More often
the first symptoms are aching in the legs or shoulders with increasing
muscle weakness. Indeed weakness is striking whereas wasting is slight.
On the other hand, the affected muscles are tender to palpation and
abnormally firm in consistency. The skin overlying the affected muscles
often feels indurated and may show a rash. Fever is slight or absent.
The E.S.R. may or may not be raised. Rarely signs of visceral involvement appear, e.g. hepatosplenomegaly, abnormal ECG or proteinuria. In the stage of resolution diffuse calcification may become radiologically visible in the fascial planes and subcutaneous tissues (*calcinosis
universalis*). If the muscles of respiration are severely involved death
may occur from intercurrent infection. In other cases the disease tends
to burn itself out after a few years. Crippling deformities may remain
but some children are able to return to normal activities.

Diagnosis

The clinical picture is usually characteristic although it may take
months to become so. The serum transaminase levels are often high
due to destruction of muscle. Coon's immunofluorescent antinuclear
factor test is positive in some cases. There may be hypergammaglobulinaemia.

Treatment

The child should be kept as ambulant as possible and physiotherapy
is helpful in preventing contractures. Corticosteroids undoubtedly
reduce the severity of the symptoms and the patient feels much less ill.
The dosage is as for lupus erythematosus, but it is frequently possible to
contain the disease on smaller maintenance doses. Gastro-intestinal
haemorrhage is a distinct risk in dermatomyositis treated with steroids.

PROGRESSIVE SYSTEMIC SCLEROSIS (SCLERODERMA)

This generalized disease is extremely rare in childhood. It must be
distinguished from the less rare and relatively benign type of localized

scleroderma (morphoea). Indeed, for the disease under discussion the word "scleroderma" is unsuitable and the term "progressive systemic sclerosis" is much to be preferred.

Pathology

In the skin and other tissues (e.g. of the alimentary system) there is a great increase in the size of the collagen bundles due apparently to some chemical change in the ground substance rather than to any increase in the size of the individual fibrils. In some cases a pathognomonic histological change is found in the renal arterioles in the form of mucoid degeneration. This leads to narrowing of the lumen, ischaemia, hypertension, and so to further renal damage.

Clinical Features

The onset is usually with tightness and atrophy of the skin over the hands and fingers, leading to progressive limitation of movement. There may have been a preceding period during which the child suffered from Raynaud's phenomena. The skin over the affected areas, (and these can include the face, limbs and trunk), becomes progressively tight, shiny and often pigmented. It cannot be lifted off the underlying tissues in the usual folds. The face may be rendered immobile and mask-like, the mouth puckered and the nose beaked and pointed. The fingers become thin and tapered; the tips may ulcerate and extrude small granules of calcium. Involvement of the oesophagus or bowel may in time cause dysphagia, constipation or diarrhoea, and abnormal appearances may be found in a barium series. Renal involvement may lead to death from uraemia. Recent reports indicate that antinuclear antibodies can be demonstrated in a high proportion of cases of progressive systemic sclerosis.

Treatment

The disease runs a prolonged course of many years duration. It may sometimes recover leaving little disability but this is unusual. There is no evidence that any form of treatment alters the outcome although in the face of inexorable progression a trial of steroid therapy would probably be justifiable.

POLYARTERITIS (PERIARTERITIS) NODOSA

In this disease there is widespread angiitis affecting the arterioles and smaller arteries. It contrasts with Henoch-Schönlein purpura in which only capillaries are damaged and with the adult disease affecting the large arteries sometimes called Takayasu's or "pulseless" disease. It may also have some affinity with the temporal arteritis seen in adults. In some cases the antigen has been a drug such as sulphonamide or horse serum (e.g. ATS). In most the evidence favours an auto-immune response.

Pathology

The principal lesion is a fibrinoid necrosis of the subintima and inner media of small arteries. There is also a perivascular infiltration with polymorphonuclear and eosinophil leucocytes. Almost any part of the body may be so affected with arterial occlusions that the symptomatology is extremely varied.

Clinical Features

There may be a defined onset with fever, malaise, loss of weight and excessive tachycardia. In other cases the onset is vague and depends on the system first involved. Polyneuritis with muscle pains and tenderness, weakness and wasting, and diminished deep reflexes is common. Renal involvement leads to hypertension, azotaemia, proteinuria and cylindruria. Involvement of the coronary vessels may result in cardiac pain with characteristic ECG changes. The signs of cerebral or mesenteric thrombosis are likely to indicate an emergency situation. In a few instances aneurysmal dilatations of superficial vessels produce small palpable lumps. Eosinophilia occurs in about 20 per cent of cases. Anaemia, leucocytosis and wasting may each be a marked feature in some cases. Bizarre rashes may occur. The diagnosis, *once thought of by the physician*, should be sought in a muscle biopsy or preferably by biopsy of a nodule when such are palpable.

Treatment

The author has seen several impressive remissions of the disease induced by steroid therapy but the ultimate prognosis is very poor. It is doubtful if any form of treatment affects the duration of the disease.

REFERENCES

ANDERSON, J. R. (1963). *Brit. med. Bull.*, **19**, 251.
BURNET, F. M. (1959). *The Clonal Selection Theory of Acquired Immunity*. London: Cambridge Univ. Press.
BURNET, F. M. (1963). *Brit. med. Bull.*, **19**, 245.
GELL, P. G. H., and COOMBS, R. R. A. (1963). *Clinical Aspects of Immunology*. Oxford: Blackwell Scientific Publications.
HOLBOROW, E. J. (1963). *Clinical Aspects of Immunology*, Chapt. 29, Edited by P. G. H. Gell and R. R. A. Coombs. Oxford: Blackwell Scientific Publications.
MILLER, J. F. A. P. (1963). *Brit. med. Bull.*, **19**, 214.
SCHLESINGER, B. E., FORSYTH, C. C., WHITE, R. H. R., SMELLIE, J. M., and STROUD, C. E. (1961). *Arch. Dis. Childh.*, **36**, 65.

CHAPTER XXVII

DISORDERS OF BEHAVIOUR
AND THE EMOTIONS

The contents of this chapter are different in many ways from those which have preceded it. The disturbances to be discussed are not based upon "organic" disease; that is to say, they are not causally related to demonstrable pathological changes in the body tissues or to demonstrable chemical changes in the body fluids. This means that there are no reasonably accurate units of measurement, neither of the normal nor the abnormal. It is possible to define the size of a normal or diseased heart or liver; it is not possible to define a psychogenic pain, a degree of depression or the size of a normal appetite in units of any sort. The treatment of most diseases of organic origin is relatively standardized and mostly based upon measurable and reproducible laboratory or clinical tests. In disturbances of the mind the treatment often varies from one case to another presenting with similar symptoms; furthermore, the treatment of the same case might be very different in the hands of different physicians or psychiatrists. Finally, in organic disease there is usually a primary cause such as an infective agent, a mutant gene, or the immaturity of an enzyme system; whereas, in psychological disturbances the interplay between the patient and his parents, or sibs or school-teachers, the conflicts between him and his cultural surroundings, and the relative importance of his heredity *v.* his environment all go to make up a complex situation, and one which the physician is frequently unable to alter in any radical measure.

It is not proposed in a book of this kind to enter into a discussion of the normal child's mental and emotional development, or to engage in analysis of the psychopathology of the behaviour problems which are so common in the children of the so-called advanced countries. The interested reader is referred to the textbooks by Apley and MacKeith (1962), Cameron (1946), Kanner (1955) and Soddy (1960). These problems appear to be less pressing in more primitive and simple communities. In our Western civilization the more serious ones require the skill of the specially trained child psychiatrist. None the less, most are relatively simple. They can and should be dealt with by the interested family doctor or the paediatrician. Many indeed are almost physiological and demand only that over-anxious and often humourless parents are reassured. Some so-called behaviour problems, in fact, exist only in the minds of parents who would mistakenly "mould" their child into what they would have liked to be themselves, and who have in fact forgotten what it was to be young; indeed it would almost seem as though some of them never had been.

A consultation over a psychologically disturbed child should pursue the usual pattern of history-taking followed by full clinical examination. The history is of even more importance than in organic illness because its object is not only to ascertain the facts, but also to have some therapeutic effect. If the latter objective is to be achieved the physician must be a good listener, appear sympathetic, emotionally detached, and never an inquisitor or judge. An intimate knowledge of the child's home environment will place the good family doctor in an advantageous position. The child psychiatrist must use the trained psychiatric social worker to obtain the same information.

NEGATIVISM

Between the age of 2 and 4 years some degree of negativism is a normal process of the development of the child's individual personality. He resists domination. He stands up for himself. With most children a little tact and a sense of humour will overcome the difficulties but if the parents react with excessive anxiety towards the situation, or with undue restriction or compulsion, a problem can arise which soon is outwith their ability to control. The most common situation is probably negativistic anorexia. The author has become only too familiar through the years with the child who refuses to eat in spite of bribery, coaxing and bullying by his anxious and near-obsessional parents. This type of anorexia may result in some loss of weight but never to any dangerous degree. In some children negativism, the refusal to be too restrictively dominated, takes the form of refusal to sleep. He may demand that his mother goes to bed with him or that some fantastic ritual be completed. The more the parents try bullying, leaving him to cry it out, or staying with him the worse he gets. Another common negativistic reaction is a temper-tantrum and he may resort to kicking, biting, stamping and so on.

The management of these cases is never easy. The parents come for advice on how to make the child eat, or sleep or co-operate. The problem is that he has already suffered from too much pressure to do these very things. The physician can sometimes bring the parents to a realization of their unwisdom, *not* by direct explanation but by guiding the discussion along lines that lead towards a self-realization. They should never be blamed. They require help, never judgment. Some positive advice can be given, e.g. *not* to force him to eat; to stop making mealtimes a battle of wills; to assure them confidently that the child is in no danger of doing himself harm. In the end, spontaneous recovery is certain.

HABIT SPASMS (SIMPLE TICS)

Tics are exceedingly common in childhood. It is probable that the mildest ones of short duration are never seen by the physician. They tend to occur in rather tense, easily worried "highly strung" children who may be suffering from too much pushing by ambitious or perfectionist parents. Only a few have arisen after a physical source of irritation such as conjunctivitis, minor trauma or an attack of chorea. The child with a tic often shows other manifestations of psychological upset, e.g. nail-biting, temper-tantrums, sleep disturbances and nightmares.

Tics may take very many forms. Common are eye-blinking, frowning, head-shaking, shrugging one shoulder, clearing the throat repeatedly, a "nervous" purposeless cough, sighing, or jerking an arm. In any one child the tic is always repetitive, unlike the completely bizarre movements of chorea. The movements of a tic involve a group of muscles which normally act together for a purpose, although in a tic the original purpose of the movements has long been forgotten. Muscle tone is normal in contrast to the hypotonia of chorea in which the outstretched hands show flexion at the wrists and some hyperextension at the metacarpophalangeal joints; this characteristic posture is never seen in tics.

The most important therapeutic requirement is correct diagnosis. Too often the child is put to bed on sedation under suspicion of having chorea. The differentiation is almost always easy and has been discussed above. It is generally agreed that the tic itself should not be directly "forbidden" or attacked. This can only aggravate any anxiety and tension. Indeed, the tic should never be alluded to by anyone in the child's presence. Unfortunately, other children can readily imitate a tic and may cause great distress to some sensitive sufferers. The physician can often relieve the tension in the home by simply letting the parents talk of their anxieties about the child. He must then reassure the parents of the benign character of tics and that most spontaneously disappear. They are only likely to accept this from the physician who has first taken a detailed unhurried history followed by a careful clinical examination in the parents' presence. There is no indication for drugs. Psychiatric advice is only necessary in severe tics which are associated with other marked disturbances of behaviour.

MASTURBATION

This is a common habit in both sexes. Indeed, it is almost physiological at some stage in childhood or adolescence. It is obviously done for pleasure and the child seen indulging in the habit looks flushed and excited. Unfortunately, this habit tends to arouse feelings of shame, horror, disgust or guilt in the minds of lay persons and they may transmit these to the child who becomes more secretive and guilt-ridden than ever. There are many ways by which these children stimulate the genitalia. In girls there may be resultant redness of the vaginal introitus, sometimes a discharge; in boys damage to the urethra may occasionally result from the introduction of a foreign body.

The treatment merely consists in assuring the parents that the habit is entirely benign, that their fears of madness or loss of health are totally without foundation. Perhaps the most effective weapon is the physician's obvious unconcern about their story, the fact that he is not in the least "shocked". The explanation that masturbation is almost universal and usually a transient phase gives parents great comfort. It is only if there are more severe accompanying disturbances that psychotherapy is required and these are not very common.

THUMB SUCKING

In the infant, sucking the thumb or fingers is normal. Some have regarded this as seeking a breast substitute. Freud stressed that it was a form of oral eroticism. As the child gets older he tends to suck his thumb less frequently, but it is a common pre-sleep ritual. Other children at this stage substitute some inanimate object. For example, a child may refuse to settle down to sleep without clutching or sucking a favourite shawl or a toy. Some children persist in the habit for much longer than is usual (e.g. 5–6 years) and it may then become socially embarrassing for the parents. It must be stressed, however, that thumb sucking is really quite unimportant. The only danger attendant upon it lies in the possibility that the parents may introduce a greater or lesser degree of tension and anxiety into the situation by their persistent attempts to stop the habit. They are motivated in this direction by their vague understanding that it may have sexual significance, or by the dentist's warnings that malocclusion can result, or by the thought that it must be unhygienic and introduce germs. None of these dangers has any real substance and parents should be assured to this effect.

NAIL BITING

This too is an extremely common habit in children reflecting often a degree of anxiety and insecurity. It may start on first going to school. The child may even copy other children who have the habit. It is by no means unknown in adults. In most children direct attempts to stop the habit fail and only aggravate the tension. Occasionally appeals to the child's pride, especially in girls, is remarkably successful. In the majority of children the habit ceases spontaneously. This is less likely in children who have other signs of nervous disturbance such as masturbation to excess, nightmares, and restless behaviour. Some such children also bite their toenails. As a general rule the best approach is the negative one of leaving the child alone to adapt to his environment spontaneously.

The exception is when the environment is disadvantageous and capable of alteration, e.g. when a child is afraid of a severe school teacher, or when the parental demands on his performance in school are excessive.

NIGHTMARES AND NIGHT TERRORS

In the *nightmare* the child awakens terrified and able to describe his fearful dream. The episode lasts only a few minutes and he is usually susceptible of reassurance and comfort after which he may soon go off to sleep. In the *night terror* the child is obviously living through a horrific experience but he remains asleep and cannot recall the events of his dream afterwards. The episode can last 15–20 minutes. There is often profuse sweating during the attack and the eyes are wide open with dilated pupils and a terrified expression on the face. Nightmares and night terrors rarely persist into adolescence save in those who have been subjected to severe psychological trauma. Closely related to night terrors is the habit of sleep walking.

There is no specific treatment or physical cause for these manifestations. Apart from shielding the child from injury during sleep walking, and correcting any obvious psychological stresses, the only measure required is reassurance of the parents about their child's physical and mental well-being.

PICA

Common, surely?

Pica or dirt eating is an uncommon but potentially dangerous habit seen in toddlers. Some are from squalid homes in which malnutrition, marital disharmony and drunkenness are common. Some are physically ill, e.g. with coeliac disease. The principal danger is of lead poisoning from eating bits of wood painted with lead-containing paint. A few very disturbed children pluck out their hair and eat it; this occasionally leads to the formation of a hair-ball or trichobezoar in the stomach which causes vomiting and a hard palpable mass in the epigastrium. Pica is to be regarded as an indication that the child's nutritional *to the* requirements are not being met. Its treatment frequently involves *true?* admission of the child to hospital for correction of malnutrition or anaemia, followed by a period of convalescence in healthy open-air surroundings. Meantime an attempt should be made with the help of the almoner or social worker to improve the home situation. Unfortunately, this is often impossible on a long-term basis, and sometimes legal proceedings are necessary to place the child in a foster home.

RHYTHMIC HEAD MOVEMENTS

There is a variety of head movements frequently seen in infants and children in the first three years of life. In *head banging* the infant, apparently voluntarily, intermittently has spells of banging his head against the cot-sides. In other cases there is such continuous *head rolling* on the pillow that an area of baldness is produced over the occiput. Another variant is *head nodding* in which the head movements are vertical rather than lateral or rotatory. In *spasmus nutans* head rolling or nodding is associated with bilateral (occasionally unilateral) nystagmus which can be horizontal, vertical or rotary. These habits are more common in poorly cared-for undernourished children, some of whom are mentally backward. They are, however, also seen in otherwise normal children. Other contributory factors of doubtful validity are neurosis, being kept in dark rooms, visual defects and rickets. The condition ceases spontaneously and does not require direct treatment, although attention should be directed towards any possible improvements in environment, nutrition etc.

PSYCHONEUROSIS

A large variety of behaviour disturbances occur in psychologically unbalanced children. It is often impossible to fit a case into a nice "tidy" diagnosis, although the psychogenic origin of the child's symptoms is usually obvious. It may also be a matter of detailed enquiry and prolonged observation, in the home as well as at the clinic, before the aetiological factors can be clearly understood. A host of inter-related influences exist in many cases, e.g. heredity, parental influences, school experiences, religious influences, economic status, home environment, sexual experiences etc. On the other hand, the majority of psychological problems in childhood can be resolved by the interested and sympathetic physician lacking specialized training in child psychiatry. Indeed, it is probable that most children who suffer a psychological upset never see a physician at all; either they recover spontaneously, or they find help from some understanding layman such as a parent, school teacher, youth leader or older child. In the more severe and persistent illnesses, however, the child psychiatrist supported by his psychiatric social workers, psychologists and play therapists can bring much needed relief from unhappiness and social incompetence.

In many cases the child's symptoms are related to a pathological degree of *anxiety*. This may result in somatic symptoms, e.g. palpitations, left inframammary pain and moist cold hands; abdominal pain, anorexia and nausea; trembling and shaking; or dizzy spells. In other instances there may be a deterioration in school work, or a reaction of agitated depression. A true melancholia is less uncommon in childhood than used to be thought, and suicidal attempts are not uncommon although they frequently go undetected by the unsuspecting physician. The obviously unhappy child, often solitary and disinclined to mix much with other children, is urgently in need of investigation and help; this is the duty of any responsible adult whether or not he be a trained physician.

In other psychologically disturbed children severe *obsessional tendencies* may make life well nigh intolerable, and interfere with both learning and social intercourse. The obsessions (or compulsions) take an infinite variety of forms. There may be obsessive recurrent thoughts which interfere with the child's normal logical thought processes; or a compulsion to touch every lamp post or to avoid every crack on the pavement; or obsessive doubting as to whether the light has been put out or the door closed; or the compulsion to think or perform acts in combinations of certain numbers. It is, of course, quite usual to find anxiety states and obsessional states in the same child. The compulsive child is frequently by nature an excessively orderly "perfectionist". He may become morbidly anxious when he thinks he is failing to reach his own personally set standards.

A third group of children manifest their disturbance in the form of *hysteria*. They are often by nature the "showmen", the seekers after more than their fair share of attention. Characteristically, the hysterical child shows a remarkable indifference towards his somatic manifestations; he may even appear to enjoy them. They may take many forms, e.g. "glove-and-stocking" anaesthesia, paralysis of a limb, aphonia (although singing or laughing may be loud), visual disturbances such as micropsia, polyopia or photophobia and various contractures or deformities. *Astasia-abasia* is the inability to stand or walk while the lower limbs are fully capable of other motor functions. Occasionally the hysterical child can develop anorexia to such a degree that health is impaired. This is associated with a total indifference to their plight and towards their parents' anxiety which is not seen in simple negativistic anorexia. True anorexia nervosa of the type seen in adults probably does not occur before puberty.

The treatment of psychoneurosis in the child is often simple, requiring no more of the physician than the willingness to listen patiently to the parents' story and then to the child. This alone can apparently achieve the most dramatic relief from tension, anxiety and somatic symptoms. The author has experienced this measure of success many times and never failed to be amazed by the excellent results of his own inactivity. Where there are physical symptoms the physician's reassurance that they do not indicate organic disease is often remarkably effective in relieving anxiety *but it will have the desired effect only when it has been preceded by a thorough physical examination of the child.* The child tormented by obsessions can be greatly relieved by simply being encouraged to talk. The fact that the physician is apparently not horrified or surprised by his odd thoughts or actions is in itself therapeutic. The physician should be prepared to see this type of child on several occasions during which he is mostly the sympathetic listener. The parents may also be helped the better to understand their child's difficulties, and in some instances to resolve their own. In conversion hysteria it is often a good plan to admit the child to hospital for a period. Frequently the somatic phenomenon suddenly disappears spontaneously, especially if nobody has paid the slightest attention to it, because it has then lost its effectiveness. It is obvious that the treatment of behaviour problems in most children is not too difficult, but it demands a lot of time. Some physicians are unwilling to spend this time on a case; others are temperamentally incapable of the necessary patient listening and relative inactivity. It is much better that they accept the situation and refer this type of patient to another colleague than that they prescribe a sedative or tranquilliser and send child and parents off with a totally un-justified reassurance. The child with a severe psychoneurotic illness which seems likely to be deep-rooted, and particularly where there is evidence of parental disharmony, gross lack of understanding, or mental breakdown, should be referred to the child psychiatrist. A long period of psychotherapy is likely to be required.

SCHOOL PHOBIA

This must be distinguished from the normal child's disinclination to put attendance at school before outdoor pursuits such as fishing or foot-ball. In its milder forms the child shows a fear of going to school for a variety of reasons, e.g. dislike of a particular teacher, because he finds learning difficult in a class of children more intelligent than himself, because his parents push him too hard in relation to his capabilities, because he is being bullied by an older or bigger boy. In these circum-stances the physician can usually discover the cause and advise parents or teachers or both how it may be removed. In its more severe form school phobia constitutes a psychiatric emergency. Here the child has an intense fear of going to school. His parents may deliver him inside the school gates but yet he will escape and later return home. This is really a serious problem of disharmony between the child and his parents rather than between the child and his school (Apley, 1965). There is often an uninterested father, and a dominant, over-protective and essentially inadequate mother. Severe school phobia requires expert psychiatric handling. It may be best initiated after admission to hospital. It is important to realize that the longer a child is permitted to stay away from school the harder the final solution is going to prove.

SPEECH DIFFICULTIES

As speech and the ability to communicate in a complex fashion mark man apart from all other mammals, and are largely responsible for his successes over the forces of nature, it is not surprising that speech disorders are exceedingly complicated and often constitute a grave disability. Indeed, learning becomes impossible without a properly functioning speech mechanism and we are still handicapped by an imperfect knowledge of this mechanism. It depends on the integrity of the brain, the auditory apparatus and the organs of articulation and phonation. The following is a list taken from Kanner (1955) of speech disorders:

Absence of speech—mutism.
Delayed onset of speech.
Disorders of articulation, e.g. lisping and burring.
Disorders of phonation.
Disorders of rhythm, e.g. stuttering.
Disorders of comprehension, e.g. word deafness (auditory aphasia) and word blindness (developmental dyslexia).
Disorders of symbolization, e.g. motor aphasia.

Their study is a highly specialized business best undertaken by the specialist. When the physician is consulted about such a problem he must take a careful history including enquiries into possible noxious influences during pregnancy (e.g. rubella, drug or irradiation), the presence of neonatal anoxia or jaundice, illnesses such as meningitis and encephalitis, and the presence of otorrhoea. He should look for evidence of mental retardation, deafness, or cerebral palsy, because in these conditions speech problems are common. Defects in the tongue, lips or palate are readily observed. Appropriate treatment should then be arranged.

However, when such marked abnormalities are lacking, more subtle signs of neurological deficit should be sought by detailed examination. Thus, manual dexterity may be less than that expected at a particular age, and when associated with instability of posture or small involuntary movements (dyskinesia) may be a sign of minimal cerebral damage. The laterality of hand, eye and foot should be tested because many children with developmental dyslexia show weak lateralization of hand and foot, and a considerable proportion are left eyed. Most children with dyslexia have also shown slow speech development which is also frequently associated with a poor auditory memory, and this, of course, leads to slowness in learning (Ingram and Mason, 1965). The most difficult type of case to understand and treat is that of developmental aphasia in which delay in the acquisition of speech is not associated with any other obvious neurological deficit. There may, however, be secondary psychological disturbances such as aggressive behaviour and destructiveness. Cases of developmental aphasia may show a deficiency of "expression" more than "reception" in that they fail to develop a vocabulary and their speech remains unintelligible, or the opposite may be the predominant problem in that there is no apparent understanding of speech. These disorders are, in fact, poorly understood by doctors and educationalists, and facilities for their treatment are as yet meagre in both quantity and quality (Court and Harris, 1965).

Faced with the child whose speech is defective the doctor must, by taking a careful history and making a detailed physical examination, exclude mental retardation, cerebral palsy, deafness and local defects in the speech apparatus. The full assessment of disordered speech in the absence of the above causes demands the skills of a variety of specialists including speech therapists, audiologists, neurologists, child psychiatrists, medical social workers and paediatricians. The paediatrician is usually the first specialist upon whom to call because he can most readily provide the contact with other members of the team. It should be stressed that operations for "tongue-tie" and for removal of the tonsils or adenoids, so often advised, are of no value whatsoever in alleviating speech disturbances.

THE PERIODIC SYNDROME

This condition may take various forms, the factors common to all being the periodicity of the attacks, the absence of signs of physical disease between attacks, and the frequency with which a family history is obtainable of "bilious attacks" during childhood or of migraine in adult life. The syndrome has sometimes been called "acidosis", and on the hypothesis that the child has some defect in fat metabolism it used to be fashionable to prescribe a high-carbohydrate low-fat diet. In fact, acidosis is not a feature of the great majority of affected children so that the word is quite inappropriate, and there is not the slightest scientific evidence of a disordered fat metabolism. The precise aetiology is not understood. The majority of affected children are of good intelligence, they tend to be tense "nervous" children, they are usually thin, and the author has been impressed by the regularity with which the parents have been anxious, humourless "perfectionists". Frequently the patient is an only child.

The best known form of the syndrome is *cyclical vomiting* in which there are recurrent attacks of severe vomiting which last from 12–72 hours. The mother will often claim that she knows when an attack is coming on because the child develops "dark rings under his eyes", loses his appetite and may become irritable. Attacks seem sometimes to be precipitated by upper respiratory infections or emotional upsets of a minor nature. After a day or so he starts to vomit, at first food, then bile, and ultimately even sips of water are returned. In severe cases he becomes "hollow-eyed" and dehydrated with a dry tongue and scaphoid somewhat tender abdomen. The breath has the sweet smell of acetone and there is gross acetonuria. In only a few cases, however, is there a true metabolic acidosis with the deep pauseless type of "acidotic" breathing. There may be fever up to 103° F. when the child's cheeks are likely to be flushed. In some children headache is a constant feature in the attacks of vomiting. Recovery always occurs spontaneously and after the attack the child may seem to be exceptionally well and vigorous.

In many children the periodic syndrome assumes a less severe and dramatic form. Attacks of para-umbilical abdominal pain ("button pain") are frequently associated with headache while vomiting is slight or absent. In only an occasional child does the headache take the form of classical migraine with unilateral distribution and visual disturbances. On the other hand, although cyclical vomiting or attacks of periodic abdominal pain usually disappear at puberty a considerable proportion of these patients develop migraine during adolescence or early adult life. Some physicians have included asthmatic attacks among the varieties of the periodic syndrome; they are certainly "periodic" and often psychologically triggered.

The treatment of the periodic syndrome can only be symptomatic. An appropriate start is to explain the nature of the condition to the parents who, like their child, are usually intelligent. They should be assured that the attacks will not harm the child's future health. In cyclical vomiting sips of glucose drinks should be given frequently. Vomiting can often be stopped with intramuscular promazine hydrochloride, 25 mg. eight-hourly, to be followed by oral administration for a day or two after the vomiting has stopped and solid food is being reintroduced. Anti-emetic drugs must not be given, however, until the physician has satisfied himself that there is no organic basis to the vomiting such as appendicitis, high intestinal obstruction or pyelonephritis. When dehydration is marked, or if there is air-hunger due to acidosis, a continuous intravenous infusion of 5 per cent dextrose in physiological saline should be set up. There is no indication for a special diet of any sort between attacks. Undue excitement should be avoided as far as possible and the child should not be permitted to become overwrought on special occasions. It is important, however, that he is not overprotected and surrounded by a host of irksome restrictions or he will rebel against them in other and even more tiresome directions. The periodic nature of the attacks and the finding of electroencephalographic abnormalities in some patients has led some physicians to suggest that the periodic syndrome is a variety of epilepsy. While few paediatricians would feel disposed towards accepting this hypothesis the administration of phenobarbitone, ½ gr. (30 mg.) twice or thrice daily, on a long-term basis is often remarkably successful in diminishing the frequency and severity of the attacks.

ENURESIS

The fact that this problem has been left until the last few pages of this book could well reflect the author's lack of satisfaction with his own attempts to deal with it in practice. A good many paediatricians would probably admit to similar reactions; although from the point of view of treatment they would be unwise to make their admissions to the parents of these unfortunate children. Many theories have been advanced to explain enuresis, by which is meant nocturnal and sometimes also diurnal urinary incontinence having no demonstrable organic basis. Most affected children have always been bed-wetters, but a few have developed control only to lose it subsequently. Sometimes there is a history of one parent, usually the father, having been similarly affected. Some have suggested a delayed maturation of the neurogenic control of the bladder. Others a bladder of unduly small capacity. Excessively zealous "potting" in infancy may sometimes have had a part to play. In some cases lack of reasonable toilet facilities in squalid surroundings may have made the child reluctant to get out of bed. In other children the enuresis has been associated with an unreasonably strict father, or rejection by the mother. It is certain that local irritations from balanitis or acid urine, or reflex irritation from infected tonsils and adenoids have no part to play in causation. The epileptic may wet his bed if he has a seizure during sleep, but this is not enuresis.

Very many forms of treatment by mechanical means, drugs and psychotherapy have been advocated at different times. Indeed, the enthusiast who really believes in his method will always achieve better results with it than other less credulous physicians. *It cannot be over emphasized that organic disease as a cause of bed wetting must be excluded by a thorough clinical examination, including urine analysis, before a child is treated for functional enuresis.* It is not at all uncommon to obtain a history of wet pants or wet beds in pyelonephritis, diabetes mellitus, chronic renal failure and diabetes insipidus. The physician has an obvious duty to exclude these diseases *before* he embarks on the treatment of enuresis. The first essential thereafter is to give the parents some explanation of the nature of enuresis, and to put an immediate stop to any punitive measures which may have been previously employed. Some of these unhappy children have been subjected to the most demoralizing indignities and physical punishments. The only reasonable attitude is one of encouragement with praise for a dry night and understanding sympathy after a wet one. It is logical even if often unsuccessful to advise fluid restriction after 5 p.m., and that the child be fully wakened to empty his bladder at the parents' bed-time. Success can sometimes be attained by training the child in a systematic fashion to go longer and longer during the day between visits to the toilet, the purpose being to increase the intravesical pressure necessary to initiate the micturition reflexes. There can be no doubt that the more thoroughly the measures described above are put into effect, and the more understanding and willing to help by giving of his time the physician seems to be, the better are the results. Formal psychotherapy is only necessary in the few enuretic children who show severe anxiety-depression symptoms or other disturbances; its effect upon the enuresis is sometimes less impressive than upon the purely psychological difficulties.

The place of drugs is difficult to assess but the wide variety which has been tried at one time or another reflects their relative inadequacy. When the child is a deep sleeper amphetamine sulphate 5–20 mg. at bed-time, or ephedrine hydrochloride ½–1 gr. (30–60 mg.) may help. The attempt to reduce the urinary volume during the night by means of pituitary snuff (Disipidin or Pitocin) 10–30 mg. at bed-time seems occasionally to help. An anticholinergic drug which the author has tended to favour is propantheline bromide, 15 mg. thrice daily, and 30 mg. at the parents' bed-time when the child is wakened to empty the bladder. In recent years a form of treatment which involves the induction of a conditioned reflex has given some good results. It is contra-indicated in the severely disturbed child, especially if the parental attitudes are seriously wrong. The apparatus consists of a wired pad which is placed under the child's buttocks. The first drops of urine complete an electrical circuit which rings a loud bell in the room; the child is awakened and gets up to empty his bladder. In successful cases the child will begin to awaken spontaneously without the bell and he will empty his bladder without having wet the bed. The increased self-confidence which results completes the "cure". This apparatus can be constructed for a few pounds sterling and the gross exploitation which some commercial firms have engaged in is much to be deplored.

At the end of the day most children recover from their affliction, but the experience of the Army Medical Services during the second World War showed that a surprising number of young adult males still carry their distressing disability with them.

REFERENCES

APLEY, J. (1965). *Brit. med. J.*, **2**, 157, 213, 281.
APLEY, J., and MACKEITH, R. (1962). *The Child and his Symptoms*. Oxford: Blackwell Scientific Publications.
CAMERON, H. C. (1946). *The Nervous Child*, 5th edit. London: Oxford Univ. Press.
COURT, D., and HARRIS, M. (1965). *Brit. med. J.*, **2**, 345, 409.
INGRAM, T. T. S., and Mason, A. W. (1965). *Brit. med. J.*, **2**, 463.
KANNER, L. (1955). *Child Psychiatry*, 2nd edit. Springfield, Ill.: Chas. C. Thomas.
SODDY, K. (1960). *Clinical Child Psychiatry*. London: Baillière, Tindall and Cox.

CHAPTER XXVIII

ACCIDENTAL POISONING IN CHILDHOOD

The peak incidence of poisoning in paediatric practice is between the ages of 1 and 4 years. Certain children with strong oral tendencies can be identified as especially likely to poison themselves by ingesting tablets or liquids, particularly if these have a pleasing colour or are held in an attractively labelled bottle or container (Craig, 1955). The most dangerous cases involve drugs, particularly salicylates and iron. Poisoning by barbiturates, tranquillizers and antihistamines is not uncommon but, in contrast to experience with adults, is not often severe or fatal. Other common but rarely fatal sources of poisoning are household substances, especially those containing kerosene, and plants such as laburnum, deadly nightshade and foxglove. All cases of possible poisoning should be taken seriously, and it is usually wise to admit the child to hospital as the effects are sometimes delayed for several hours. It is much to be preferred that a symptomless child be kept overnight in hospital than that a deeply unconscious child should be admitted moribund because of failure to take prompt action earlier in the day. It has been the experience of all paediatric departments in the United Kingdom that serious poisoning by drugs has become much more common in recent years as new potent remedies have found their way into so many households. New household cleaners and disinfectants also abound. In a somewhat different category is lead poisoning which usually involves ingestion over a fairly prolonged period and which is probably more common in its milder forms than has always been appreciated. In this chapter it is proposed to describe the general therapeutic measures applicable to acute poisoning, and then to consider some of the more common individual poisonings. The possibility of poisoning should always be entertained in an acute illness of sudden onset if no cause is immediately discoverable, particularly if it is associated with vomiting and diarrhoea, or if there are marked disturbances of consciousness or behaviour.

In the United Kingdom the physician, confronted by a patient suffering from a form of poisoning about which he lacks information, can obtain assistance, day or night, by telephoning one of the following Poisons Centres:

BELFAST: Royal Victoria Infirmary: Tel. Belfast 30503.
CARDIFF: Royal Infirmary: Tel. Cardiff 33101.

EDINBURGH: Royal Infirmary: Tel. FOUntainbridge 2477.
LEEDS: General Infirmary: Tel. 3–2799.
LONDON: Guy's Hospital: Tel. HOP 7600.
NEWCASTLE: Royal Victoria Infirmary: Tel. Newcastle 25131.

GENERAL THERAPEUTIC MEASURES

Unless the child has swallowed kerosene, corrosive, acid or strong alkali he should immediately be made to vomit by inserting a finger deep down his throat. Emetics are less rapid and often not available. In the hospital gastric lavage should be carried out with half-strength physiological saline, or with 1 per cent sodium bicarbonate in the case of iron poisoning. If the child is unconscious his airway must be assured with an oropharyngeal or intratracheal tube, and he should be nursed on his side or semi-prone. Oxygen should be administered if there is respiratory depression, cyanosis or shock. It is only rarely in children that tracheostomy or mechanical ventilation are required when the services of a skilled anaesthetist are invaluable. Severe shock and hypotension are also uncommon in children and may be combated with intravenous plasma or with metaraminol (Aramine) given intravenously or intramuscularly in doses of 1 to 5 mg. according to age and blood pressure response. In severe poisonings intravenous fluids, such as 5 per cent dextrose in quarter-strength physiological saline, will usually be necessary and it is important that periodic measurements be made of the serum electrolytes and of the acid-base status. Intramuscular benzylpenicillin should be administered to all unconscious patients to decrease the risk of aspiration pneumonia, and also in cases of kerosene poisoning. In corrosive poisonings, which are not very common in children, milk is the best oral fluid because the poison is likely to react with the protein. In poisoning with the alkaloids or glycosides of plants the poison can be adsorbed with activated medicinal charcoal (known commercially as Active Carbon). This can be placed in the stomach, 8 to 12 gm. in 300 ml., after the gastric lavage has been completed. When convulsions occur, as in poisoning by strychnine, picrotoxin or nicotine, intramuscular paraldehyde, 0·15 ml./Kg. (1 ml. per stone), may be sufficient but intravenous thiopentone (Pentothal) is sometimes required. The restlessness and excitement of amphetamine poisoning is best treated with chlorpromazine (Largactil) or promazine (Sparine) in intramuscular doses of 25 to 50 mg.; they antagonize both the central and peripheral effects of the poison. One of the few groups of true antidotes comprises the competitive antagonists of the narcotic analgesics such as morphine, pethidine and related substances. Poisoning by these drugs is uncommon in paediatric practice and should be antagonized promptly with intravenous nalorphine,

0·1 mg./Kg., or levallorphan, 0·02 mg./Kg. These antidotes act immediately, and the dose can be repeated if necessary.

SALICYLATE POISONING

This is the most commonly fatal poisoning of childhood (Craig *et al.*, 1966). The salicylate is usually ingested in the form of aspirin. This is often accidental but sometimes it has been given with therapeutic intent by the parents, and even by the doctor. On occasion the source of the salicylate has been swallowed oil of wintergreen (methyl salicylate), one teaspoonful of which contains the equivalent of 60 grains (4 gm.) aspirin.

The prognosis in the individual case is determined much more by the interval of time which has elapsed between the ingestion of the poison and the start of treatment than by the level of the serum salicylate. Indeed, the toddler can show signs of severe poisoning with a salicylate level as low as 40 mg. per 100 ml. "Therapeutic" cases tend to be of longer duration and more often fatal because the deterioration in the child's condition is at first attributed to the disease for which the aspirin was initially prescribed. In the series reported by Craig *et al.* (1966) only 2 of 12 cases of "therapeutic" aspirin poisoning were referred to hospital with the correct diagnosis. "Accidental" cases are promptly recognized by the parents who seek treatment and usually give a clear history that aspirin has been taken so that a fatal outcome is much less likely. Aspirin has become such a familiar household remedy that its dangers in children have often been overlooked. *The author is of the opinion that, with the exceptions of rheumatic fever and rheumatoid arthritis, aspirin should not be prescribed for infants or children.* A raised body temperature can be more effectively lowered by tepid sponging. Paracetamol is an equally effective and safer analgesic.

Clinical Features

The sign of real diagnostic value in salicylate poisoning is the presence of rapid, deep, pauseless and acyanotic breathing, or *air hunger*. Cases are too frequently referred to hospital with the diagnosis of "pneumonia" but the hyperpnoea of salicylate poisoning is quite different from the short, grunting respirations of pneumonia. This sign has been stressed so strongly because of its diagnostic importance. The other early manifestations of salicylate poisoning in infants and toddlers, such as nausea and vomiting, are difficult to evaluate, and they cannot often describe tinnitus.

The hyperpnoea has a double aetiology. It is due initially to the direct excitatory action of salicylate on the respiratory centre in the brain. The resultant overbreathing washes out CO_2 from the lungs and a respiratory alkalosis results. This is reflected in a raised blood pH ($> 7·42$) and a lowered Pco_2 (<35 mm. Hg). This alkalotic phase is commonly seen in adults with salicylate poisoning, but in young children an accelerated fatty-acid catabolism with excess production of ketones results in the early establishment of a metabolic acidosis. By the time the poisoned toddler reaches hospital the blood pH is usually reduced (<7·35), and the metabolic acidosis is reflected in a lowered plasma CO_2 content (Van Slyke method) or plasma standard bicarbonate (Astrup method). The hyperventilation of metabolic acidosis is thus added to the stimulant effect of salicylate on the respiratory centre so that the overbreathing of the poisoned child is often extreme.

As doctors we have all been taught that aspirin is an antipyretic and this probably explains the frequent failure to recognize that a common effect of salicylate overdosage is fever. The author has seen the dose of aspirin actually increased to relieve the fever of aspirin poisoning, with dire effects upon the patient. There is also a disturbance of carbohydrate metabolism and the blood sugar may rise above 200 mg. per 100 ml., although not above 300 mg. per 100 ml. Hypoglycaemia has also been recorded but it must be uncommon.

The child with salicylate poisoning shows peripheral dilatation until he is near to death. There is then a very significant change to peripheral circulatory collapse with restlessness and greyish cyanosis. Finally, death is preceded by twitching, rigidity or coma.

Diagnosis

Doctors, both in and outside the hospitals, must become more aware that aspirin is widely used by mothers for the real or imaginary ills of their offspring, and that its dangers are poorly appreciated by parents. Indeed, they may not even think it relevant to mention the fact of aspirin ingestion to the doctor. The physician who first sees the child in hospital should test the urine, *after boiling*, with ferric chloride solution or Phenistix; a negative result excludes salicylate poisoning, whereas a purple colour reaction demands the immediate estimation of the serum salicylate level. It may, of course, only signify that the child has been given a small non-poisonous dose of aspirin but a positive Phenistix test in a child who is overbreathing is extremely likely to indicate salicylate poisoning. Diabetic pre-coma is associated with hyperpnoea and a positive Phenistix test on *unboiled* urine, but the test will be negative on boiled urine and the blood sugar is always above 300 mg. per 100 ml. unless the child has been given insulin.

Treatment

The immediate treatment in the child's home is to induce vomiting. On arrival at hospital gastric lavage should be performed, and blood taken for estimation of the serum salicylate level and acid-base state. If there is marked air-hunger and dehydration an intravenous infusion of 5 per cent dextrose in quarter strength physiological saline should be set up to deliver 90 ml./lb. (200 ml./Kg.) in 24 hours. Metabolic acidosis, which is usually severe in the toddler, can be safely corrected with 5 mEq. sodium bicarbonate per Kg. of body weight given intravenously every four hours until the urine is alkaline. When the Astrup micro-apparatus is available the acid-base state can be checked at hourly intervals and more rapid correction achieved. The dose of 8·4 per cent sodium bicarbonate (1 ml. = 1 mEq.) can be determined from the base excess value (always negative in acidosis) thus:

Mls. 8·4 per cent sodium bicarbonate required
= body weight in Kg. × base excess in mEq./litre × 0·35.

This calculation assumes that the extracellular fluid volume is 35 per cent of the body weight. Doses of sodium bicarbonate are given at hourly intervals to maintain the base excess value near zero. We have found this to be a safe and effective line of treatment in the toddler but it requires frequent biochemical estimations.

In older children and adults the initial respiratory alkalosis is frequently more marked than metabolic acidosis, and alkalinizing salts must be used more cautiously. None the less, sodium bicarbonate also hastens the excretion of salicylate by the kidney and Dukes *et al.* (1963) have reported good results in adults with forced alkaline diuresis. These workers give, in rotation, 500 ml. each of 0·9 per cent sodium chloride, 5 per cent dextrose, and 2 per cent sodium bicarbonate at an initial rate of 2 litres per hour. The alkali is omitted when a urinary pH of 8·0 is attained.

Whatever intravenous regime is employed it is desirable to measure the serum electrolytes at intervals. It is important to avoid hypernatraemia. If hypokalaemia develops potassium chloride, 10–20 mEq/litre, should be added to the infusion fluid. Haemorrhagic manifestations are uncommon and should be treated with 10 mg. of intramuscular vitamin K_1 (phytomenadione).

In cases of severe oliguria or anuria good results have been obtained with peritoneal dialysis or haemodialysis. This is likely to be available only in special units, and treatment as described above must never be delayed while the special apparatus or personnel are being assembled. Exchange transfusion is another effective method of treatment for the worst cases but it is not free from risk and should not be lightly undertaken.

Iron Poisoning

The most common source of iron poisoning are tablets of ferrous sulphate which the young child mistakes for sweets. Other ferrous salts such as gluconate or succinate are less dangerous. Iron poisoning ranks second only to salicylate in the frequency with which it causes death in the United Kingdom. A child of 2 years can be fatally poisoned by 30 gr. (2 gm.) of ferrous sulphate.

Clinical Features

Four phases can be distinguished in iron poisoning (Henderson *et al.*, 1963). The first begins $\frac{1}{2}$ to 1 hour after ingestion of the tablets with severe vomiting, diarrhoea, haematemesis, melaena, pallor, metabolic acidosis and, in fatal cases, pre-terminal coma. In the child who survives, the second phase is associated with a misleading abatement of symptoms which may persist for a period of 8 to 16 hours. The highly dangerous third phase is then likely to ensue. Iron encephalopathy may cause convulsions and unconsciousness; liver parenchyma damage can result in jaundice and other metabolic derangements; progressive circulatory collapse may end in death. Finally, for the survivors the fourth phase of recovery follows. Even later, severe fibrosis and cicatricial scarring of the pyloric end of the stomach may develop and so interfere with nutrition that surgical intervention is required (Shepherd, 1955). The author has seen this late sequela lead to profound emaciation in one child before its existence was suspected.

Treatment

Vomiting should be induced as soon as possible after ingestion of the tablets. On arrival in hospital gastric lavage should be performed with 1 per cent solution of sodium bicarbonate. Blood should be taken for estimation of the serum iron (sometimes over 2,500 μg. per 100 ml.). The iron-chelating agent desferrioxamine has proved of great value in recent years. Immediately after completion of the gastric lavage 5,000 mg. desferrioxamine should be left in the stomach in 50 to 100 ml of water. At this time 2,000 mg. of the drug should be given intramuscularly. If the child is severely ill and vomiting persistently, an intravenous infusion of 5 per cent dextrose in quarter strength physiological saline should be set up and desferrioxamine should be added to the solution to give not more than 15 mg./Kg. per hour to a maximum of 80 mg./Kg. in 24 hours. The intramuscular dose of desferrioxamine, 2,000 mg., should be repeated every 12 hours until the serum iron level falls to normal. While we have seen a serum level above 3,000 μg. per 100 ml. fall to below 300 μg. per 100 ml. in a few hours on this regime, there is evidence that it must be started before the third phase is well established to prove effective. It is probable that desferrioxamine is preferable to calcium disodium versenate (EDTA) in the treatment of iron poisoning with chelating agents.

BARBITURATE POISONING

While poisoning by long-acting or intermediate-acting barbiturates is now the commonest form of poisoning seen in adult hospital practice, this is not true of children's hospitals. In adults overdosage with barbiturates is usually due to their self-administration, whereas accidental overdosage is the common cause of barbiturate poisoning in young children. The bitter taste of the derivatives of barbituric acid partly explains the relative infrequency of this form of poisoning in toddlers, and also its usually mild degree. The physician should not forget, however, that self-administration of dangerous quantities of barbiturate is occasionally encountered in the unhappy older child. It is important that this situation be recognized and that, after the acute situation has been overcome, expert psychiatric advice be obtained.

Clinical Features

In most cases the child is only extremely drowsy but he can be roused and can answer simple questions. Infrequently he is flushed, excited and restless. Vomiting is common and helps to explain the rarity of severe degrees of poisoning. In severe cases the child is comatose, unresponsive to stimuli, and may show respiratory depression with cyanosis, absence of the deep reflexes, and circulatory failure with hypotension.

Treatment

On admission to hospital gastric lavage should be performed (unless the child is in deep coma), and blood should be withdrawn for estimation of the blood barbiturate level. *In most children no further measures are required.* In severe cases where response to painful stimuli is minimal or absent, a patent airway must be assured by thorough pharyngeal suction followed by the insertion of an oro-pharyngeal airway to prevent the tongue falling backwards. In the worst cases, which are extremely rare in childhood, a cuffed endotracheal tube must be inserted and the co-operation of an anaesthetist is necessary for this. Cyanosis would be an indication for oxygen administration in a suitable tent. In the comatose child showing signs of respiratory depression prophylactic benzylpenicillin is commonly advised by the intramuscular route. While this is the author's practice, Mackintosh and Matthew (1965) do not consider it to be of benefit, at least in the poisoned adult.

Intravenous therapy is required only in comatose children, but the volumes of fluid recommended for forced diuresis in the adult (Linton *et al.*, 1964), or the use of diuretics, would be dangerous in all but the largest children. A satisfactory urinary output can usually be obtained with 5 per cent dextrose in quarter-strength physiological saline, 90 ml./lb./day (200 ml./Kg./day). In such severe cases the serum electrolytes and acid-base status should be assessed periodically. Metabolic acidosis can be corrected with intravenous sodium bicarbonate, and hypokalaemia with potassium chloride. Severe hypotension is rarely a problem in children. It can be alleviated by intravenous plasma.

Alternatively, metaraminol may be given intravenously or intramuscularly in doses of 1 to 5 mg. according to the response. The foot of the bed should also be raised in such cases.

Alternative methods of promoting the removal of barbiturate from the body are haemodialysis and peritoneal dialysis. The indications for such measures have varied in different centres and their need in children is exceedingly infrequent. Linton et al. (1964) have given as their criteria: (i) initial blood barbiturate levels above 15 mg. per 100 ml. (long-acting) or 4 mg. per 100 ml. (intermediate-acting), (ii) a rising blood barbiturate level despite forced diuresis, (iii) a deteriorating clinical state in spite of intravenous therapy.

It is now generally accepted that the so-called respiratory stimulants such as bemigride or amiphenazole should not be used. Indeed, it is again stressed that even in a centre treating more severely poisoned adults 95 per cent of cases can be treated successfully with gastric lavage, care of the respiratory passages and general supportive measures alone (Matthew and Lawson, 1966). Measures to enhance the removal of the poison are only required in children who are comatose.

POISONING BY PHENOTHIAZINE DERIVATIVES AND ANTIHISTAMINES

The much more common prescribing of "tranquillizers" of many kinds has, unfortunately, increased the opportunity of young children to ingest them accidentally. There is sometimes a fairly long period between ingestion and the appearance of symptoms. These include anorexia, progressive drowsiness, stupor and extrapyramidal signs such as inco-ordinated movements, rigidity or tremor. This form of poisoning is, however, rarely fatal in children.

Treatment

This should be along the lines already recommended for barbiturate poisoning, in particular gastric lavage and the maintenance of the airway.

ATROPINE POISONING

This type of poisoning may arise from ingestion of the plant deadly nightshade. It may also occur when drugs such as tincture of belladonna, atropine or hyoscine are taken accidentally, or prescribed in excessive doses. We have seen severe poisoning develop in a child who drank about 4 ml. (40 mg.) of his own 1 per cent atropine eye drops.

Clinical Features

The onset of symptoms is soon after ingestion with thirst, dryness of the mouth, blurring of vision, and photophobia. The child is markedly flushed with widely dilated pupils. Tachycardia is severe and there may be high fever. Extreme restlessness, confusion, delirium and incoordination are characteristic. Indeed, the picture may be mistaken for an acute psychosis. In babies there may be gross gaseous abdominal distension. In fatal cases circulatory collapse and respiratory failure precede death.

Treatment

This can only be symptomatic and supportive. Gastric lavage is essential. It can be followed by the instillation of activated charcoal as described on page 533. Fever should be reduced by tepid sponging. Severe restlessness is best treated with intramuscular paraldehyde, 0·15 ml./Kg. (1 ml./stone).

AMPHETAMINE POISONING

Acute poisoning can arise from accidental ingestion or inhalation. Symptoms include nausea and vomiting, excitement and delirium, blurred vision, fever and convulsions. Death is preceded by coma and respiratory depression.

Treatment

This is along the lines advised for atropine poisoning, but the sedation required is best obtained with intramuscular chlorpromazine or promazine, 25 to 50 mg.

LEAD POISONING

Lead is usually ingested in small quantities over long periods and the manifestations of poisoning develop insidiously. There are various possible sources of lead such as lead-containing paint which may be used by fathers to apply to the child's cot, flakes of paint from plaster-work or woodwork in old Victorian houses, burnt old lead batteries, or swallowed pieces of yellow crayon. Pica is common in children suffering from lead poisoning and is a valuable clue to the diagnosis. It is more common in children from the poorest homes. An early diagnosis is extremely important in lead poisoning because if it is left untreated lead encephalopathy may result in death or permanent brain damage (Smith, 1964). Doctors must become more aware of the condition, which is more common than has usually been realized.

Clinical Features

The earliest symptoms such as lethargy, anorexia, vomiting and abdominal pain are too common to arouse suspicion in themselves, but their persistence without other discoverable cause should do so. The pallor of anaemia is a frequent and characteristic sign. Insomnia and headache frequently precede the onset of lead encephalopathy with convulsions, papilloedema and a cracked-pot sound on percussion of the skull. Radiographs of the skull may then reveal separation of the sutures. Peripheral neuropathy is uncommon in the young child but may develop with paralysis of the dorsiflexors of the wrist or feet. Radiographs of the bones may show characteristic bands of increased density at the metaphyses (Fig. 93) but this is a relatively late sign and,

(lead lines)

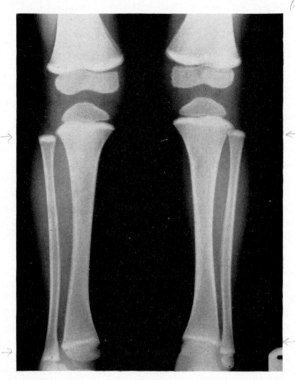

FIG. 93.—Radiograph of legs in chronic lead poisoning. Note bands of increased density ("lead lines") at metaphyseal ends of the long bones.

therefore, of limited diagnostic value. Excess amino-aciduria is a common manifestation of renal tubular damage, and glycosuria may also occur. Renal hypertension has also been reported.

The most dangerous development, both in regard to life and future mental health, is lead encephalopathy. Depending upon the amount of lead ingested this dread complication may develop quite quickly, or only following a long period of relatively mild ill-health.

Diagnosis

The diagnosis of lead poisoning can be justified in the presence of two or more of the following findings (Byers, 1959):

× (i) microcytic hypochromic anaemia with punctate basophilia,
× (ii) radio-opaque foreign bodies in the bowel lumen and lines of increased density at the growing ends of the long bones,
× (iii) coproporphinuria,
(iv) renal glycosuria and amino-aciduria,
(v) raised pressure and protein in the cerebrospinal fluid.

However, the most sensitive test in the author's experience is a marked increase in the urinary excretion of lead after an oral dose of D-penicillamine, 20 mg./Kg./day. On the other hand, an abnormal excretion of delta-aminolaevulic acid is less constantly found in the child than in the adult with chronic lead poisoning.

Interpretation of the blood lead levels is, unfortunately, much more difficult. While levels below 40 μg. per 100 ml. exclude lead poisoning, and high levels would confirm it, levels in the region of 60 μg. per 100 ml. are not uncommon and of uncertain significance. Thus Moncrieff *et al.* (1964) found such levels in 45 per cent of a series of mentally defective children, although a level over 40 μg. per 100 ml. was rarely found in normal children. While it is possible that lead was the cause of the brain damage in the retarded children, it is equally probable that because of their already existing mental abnormality they were more prone than normal children to eat foreign lead-containing materials.

Treatment

It is obviously essential that the child be immediately removed from all sources of lead. Deposition of lead in the bones should be encouraged by giving a diet rich in calcium, phosphorus and vitamin D thereby lowering the level of lead in the blood. The most important measure is to increase the excretion of lead in the urine. In chronic lead poisoning the chelating agent of choice is probably D-penicillamine. It has the advantage of being extremely effective when given orally (Goldberg *et al.*, 1963). A suitable dosage is 20 mg./Kg./day for seven days. Further courses may be required if the blood lead level rises again or if symptoms recur.

The most acute situation arises in lead encephalopathy. Here combination of the metal with sulphhydryl groups leads to inhibition of the intracellular enzyme systems. The resultant cellular injury is followed by oedema which adds further injury to the brain. It seems that the most effective and rapid method of removing lead from the brain is a combination of calcium sodium versenate (CaEDTA) and British antilewisite (BAL). This therapy must be combined with measures designed to diminish cerebral oedema (Coffin *et al.*, 1966). As soon as the diagnosis has been made CaEDTA (75 mg./Kg./day) is given intravenously or intramuscularly in four divided doses per 24 hours for 5 to 7 days. BAL is started simultaneously, or within 24 hours after,

CaEDTA. It is given in a dosage of 3 to 4 mg./Kg./dose every four hours intramuscularly for 3 days. A second course of CaEDTA alone should be given some 3 to 10 days after the end of the first course. Subsequent courses may be required if the blood lead level remains elevated, or at this stage oral D-penicillamine might be employed as described above.

The dangers of cerebral oedema are sufficiently great to demand palliative measures while CaEDTA and BAL are being used. Various measures, including surgical decompression, have been tried in this emergency. Possibly mannitol is the safest and most effective diuretic agent. It can be given in a dosage of 2·5 gm. per Kg. by intravenous infusion of a 20 per cent solution. Dexamethasone has also been advised by the intravenous route in doses of 1 mg./Kg./day given in four equal six-hourly injections for 48 hours. Intravenous urea has also been used to decrease cerebral oedema, but as its use can be followed by a rebound of cerebrospinal fluid pressure to the pre-treatment level or higher it should probably be reserved for cases in which surgical decompression is planned to follow immediately. Once lead encephalopathy has been allowed to develop, the risks to life and subsequent mental development are very great and can only be obviated by intense therapeutic measures.

REFERENCES

BYERS, R. K. (1959). *Pediatrics*, **23**, 585.
COFFIN, R., PHILLIPS, J. L., STAPLES, W. I., and SPECTOR, S. (1966). *J. Pediat.*, **69**, 198.
CRAIG, J. O. (1955). *Arch. Dis. Childh.*, **30**, 419.
CRAIG, J. O., FERGUSON, I. C., and SYME, J. (1966). *Brit. med. J.*, **1**, 757.
DUKES, D. C., BLAINEY, J. D., CUMMING, G., and WIDDOWSON, G. (1963). *Lancet* **2**, 329.
GOLDBERG, A., SMITH, J. A., and LOCHHEAD, A. C. (1963). *Brit. med. J.*, **1**, 1270.
HENDERSON, F., VIETTI, T. J., and BROWN, E. B. (1963). *J. Amer. med. Ass.*, **186**, 1139.
LINTON, A. L., LUKE, R. G., SPEIRS, I., and KENNEDY, A. C. (1964). *Lancet*, **1**, 1008.
MACKINTOSH, T. F., and MATTHEW, H. (1965). *Lancet*, **1**, 1252.
MATTHEW, H., and LAWSON, A. A. H. (1966). *Quart. J. Med.*, **35**, 539.
MONCRIEFF, A. A., KOUMIDES, O. P., CLAYTON, B. E., PATRICK, A. D., RENWICK, A. G. C., and ROBERTS, G. E. (1964). *Arch. Dis. Childh.*, 39, 1.
SHEPHERD, J. A. (1955). *Brit. med. J.*, **2**, 418.
SMITH, H. D. (1964). *Arch. environm. Hlth.*, **8**, 256.

INDEX

Abdomen, tuberculosis of, 143, 144
Abnormalities, congenital
  alimentary, **259**
  of the central nervous system, **431**
  of the heart, **238–258**
  of the renal tract, **321**
  respiratory, **193**
ABO incompatibility (*see*
  Haemolytic disease of
  newborn).
Abscess
  appendix, 282
  brain, 412
  breast, in newborn, 77
  Brodie's, 474
  kidney, 315
  liver, 79
  peritonsillar (*see* also Quinsy), **200**
  pulmonary, 204, 205, 294
  retropharyngeal, **200**
Absorption collapse, of lungs (*see*
  Atelectasis)
Accidental poisoning, **532–543**
Acholuric jaundice (*see also* Congenital
  spherocytosis), **53, 387**
Achondroplasia, 336, 498
Acidosis
  diabetic, 373
  hyperchloraemic, **326**
  in gastroenteritis, 73, 277
  in glycogen storage disease, 115
  in haemolytic disease of newborn,
    51
  in periodic syndrome, 528
  in renal failure, 325
  respiratory, in pulmonary syndrome
    of newborn, 21
Acrodynia, infantile (*see also* Pink
  disease), **435**
Acromegaly, 339
Addison's disease, **364**
Adenitis, non-specific mesenteric, 283
Adenoma of bronchus, 195
  parathyroid gland, 356
  basophil, 339, 363
  chromophobe, 339, 363
  eosinophil, 339
Adenoma sebaceum, in tuberous
  sclerosis, 427
Adenovirus, 196
Adrenals
  apoplexy, 415
  disorders of, **357**
  function of, 358
  haemorrhage, 39, 415
    in newborn, 39

Adrenals—*cont.*
  in Waterhouse-Friderichsen
    syndrome, **415**
  hyperplasia, congenital, **357**
  hypoplasia, congenital, 365
Adynamia episodica hereditaria, 488
Afibrinogenaemia, congenital, **409**
Agammaglobulinaemia (*see*
  Hypogammaglobulinaemia)
Agenesis
  pulmonary, **194**
  renal, **322**
Agranulocytosis, 409
Albers-Schönberg disease (*see also*
  Osteopetrosis), **398**
Albinism, total, 108
Albuminuria
  in nephritis, 308
  in nephrosis, 312
Alimentary diseases, **259–304**
Alkalosis
  in duodenal obstruction, 265
  in intestinal obstruction, 268
  in pyloric stenosis, 273
Alkaptonuria, 108
Alymphoplasia, thymic 123
Amaurotic family idiocy (*see also*
  Tay-Sachs disease), **189**
Amentia (*see also* Mental deficiency),
  455
Amniocentesis, in haemolytic disease,
  49
Amphetamine poisoning, **540**
Amyloid disease, 212, 511
Amylopectinosis, 117
Amyoplasia congenita (*see also*
  Arthrogryposis multiplex), **489**
Amyotonia congenita, 425
Anaphylactoid purpura (*see also*
  Henoch Schönlein purpura), **400**
Anaemia
  Addisonian, 386
  Cooley's, **388**
  early, of prematurity, **25**
  haemolytic, **386**
    acquired, **392**
    congenital spherocytosis, **53, 387**
    due to G-6-P dehydrogenase
      deficiency, **52**
    in sickle cell disease, **390**
    in other haemoglobinopathies, **391**
    in thalassaemia, **388**
    of the newborn, 48
  haemolytic-uraemic syndrome of
    infancy, **394**
  hypoplastic, **394**